T0140073

Cancer Drug Discovery and Development

Series editor:

Beverly A. Teicher
Bethesda, MD, USA

The Cancer Drug Discovery and Development series (Beverly A Teicher, series editor) is the definitive book series in cancer research and oncology, providing comprehensive coverage of specific topics and the field. Volumes cover the process of drug discovery, preclinical models in cancer research, specific drug target groups and experimental and approved therapeutic agents. The volumes are current and timely, anticipating areas where experimental agents are reaching FDA approval. Each volume is edited by an expert in the field covered and chapters are authored by renowned scientists and physicians in their fields of interest.

More information about this series at http://www.springer.com/series/7625

Atsushi Kaneda • Yu-ichi Tsukada
Editors

DNA and Histone Methylation as Cancer Targets

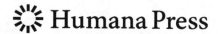 Humana Press

Editors
Atsushi Kaneda
Graduate School of Medicine
Chiba University
Chiba, Chiba, Japan

Yu-ichi Tsukada
Advanced Biological Information Research
  Division, INAMORI Frontier Research
  Center
Kyushu University
Fukuoka, Fukuoka, Japan

ISSN 2196-9906   ISSN 2196-9914   (electronic)
Cancer Drug Discovery and Development
ISBN 978-3-319-86700-7   ISBN 978-3-319-59786-7   (eBook)
DOI 10.1007/978-3-319-59786-7

Printed on acid-free paper

This Humana Press imprint is published by Springer Nature
The registered company is Springer International Publishing AG
The registered company address is: Gewerbestrasse 11, 6330 Cham, Switzerland

Foreword

Epigenetics is a novel dogma that regulates gene expression profiles in the cells and is known to be involved in cancer. Among numerous epigenetic factors, DNA and histone methylation has a unique feature that this covalent modification is stable compared to other covalent modifications, thereby its reversibility had been unknown until recently. The significant advance of epigenetics has also occurred in methylation. Histone methylation was revealed to be reversible by the discoveries of histone demethylases, and DNA demethylation pathway was elucidated by the discovery of DNA oxidases.

This book focuses on DNA and histone methylation in epigenetics and describes how it is involved in the molecular mechanisms responsible for the development of cancer. Each chapter summarizes the current knowledge of the molecular basis of DNA and histone methylation to explain its involvement in cancer, and describes the features of DNA and histone methylation associated with a particular type of cancer, the current diagnostic/therapeutic applications, and future directions of study on DNA and histone methylation as cancer targets.

Yu-ichi Tsukada

Contents

DNA and Histone Methylation in Epigenetics

Hengbin Wang, Jinrong Min, and Trygve Tollefsbol

Abstract Epigenetics, the mechanism that defines gene expression patterns without changing the DNA sequence, has far-reaching consequences on normal and pathological development including but not limited to cell fate determination, maintenance of tissue differentiation, and cancer occurrence. Methylation of DNA and histones, the two components of chromatin, constitutes important epigenetic mechanisms that govern chromatin-based nuclear processes. In this chapter, we briefly summarize the key enzymes involved, mechanisms, and function of these two modifications. We envision that DNA and histone methylation will increasingly become important targets for cancer treatment.

Keywords Epigenetics • DNA methylation • Histone methylation

1 Introduction

Epigenetics refers to mechanisms that control gene expression patterns across cell generations but do not involve changes in the DNA sequence [1]. Since virtually all somatic cells contain the same DNA sequence, epigenetic mechanisms must lie outside of the DNA sequence. Specific to eukaryotes, the genomic DNA is associated with a set of highly conserved histone proteins that form the structure of chromatin. Compared to the linearly organized genetic information in the DNA sequence, which is identical in virtually all somatic cells, chromatin adapts distinct local

H. Wang (✉)
Department of Biochemistry and Molecular Genetics, University of Alabama at Birmingham,
Kaul Human Genetics Building 402A, 720 20th Street South, Birmingham, AL 35294, USA
e-mail: hbwang@uab.edu

J. Min
Structural Genomics Consortium and Department of Physiology, University of Toronto,
101 College Street, MaRS South Tower, Toronto, ON M5G 1L7, Canada

T. Tollefsbol
Department of Biology, University of Alabama at Birmingham,
Campbell Hall 175, 1300 University Boulevard, Birmingham, AL 35294, USA

© Springer International Publishing AG 2017
A. Kaneda, Y.-i. Tsukada (eds.), *DNA and Histone Methylation as Cancer Targets*,
Cancer Drug Discovery and Development, DOI 10.1007/978-3-319-59786-7_1

conformation, permissive or repressive to protein factor binding, allowing gene expression at programs specific to each cell type. Therefore, the organized information in chromatin constitutes an additional layer of mechanisms that control the use of genetic information (Fig. 1). This organized information is unique to each cell type and also specific to any given cellular functional status. As the physical carrier of epigenetic regulation, chromatin integrates signals from endogenous development and the exogenous environment to define the functional output of the underlying DNA sequences. It is due to the epigenetic mechanism that eukaryotes can have many different cell types, which corresponds to distinct gene expression programs (the so-called epigenomes), from a single genome. This fundamental function endows essential roles of epigenetics in normal development as well as disease progression.

Studies in the past decades have revealed multiple mechanisms that modulate chromatin structure and affect the functional output of chromatin. These mechanisms include, but are not limited to, DNA methylation, ATP-dependent chromatin remodeling, posttranslational histone modifications, and non-coding RNAs [1]. Of these mechanisms, both DNA and histone methylation involve the addition of a methyl group, a single carbon metabolite, to the essential components of chromatin. Both DNA and histone methylation may profoundly affect the chromatin conformation and functional output of the underlying DNA sequence. While the mechanism that mediates the transmission of DNA methylation from mother cells to daughter cells has been revealed, the mechanism that mediates the transmission of histone methylation remains largely obscure. Although the formation of C-C bond in DNA methylation and N-C bound in histone methylation render these modifications relatively stable, recent studies reveal the reversibility of both modifications. The stability as well as the plasticity of both modifications entitles important regulatory functions of both modifications in chromatin conformation during cell proliferation and differentiation. Both DNA and histone methylation are tightly regulated to ensure proper cellular function during normal development. Deregulation of either modification system, including mutations in the enzymes catalyzing DNA and histone methylations, dysregulation of proteins binding to and mediating the function of DNA and histone methylation, and even histone protein itself are frequently

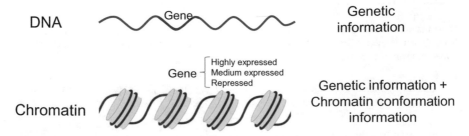

Fig. 1 Genetics vs epigenetics. Genetic information is stored in the DNA sequence while chromatin contains organized structural information in addition to the genetic information. This epigenetic mechanism allows genes to be expressed at different levels according to requirement

observed in many human diseases including cancers. Therefore, both DNA and histone methylation are appealing targets for cancer treatment.

2 DNA Methylation

2.1 DNA Methylation in Mammals

Of the four nucleotides that make up the DNA, adenosine, thymine, cytosine, and guanine, both adenine and cytosine can be methylated; however, methylated cytosine is mainly detected in mammals [15]. The methyl group is added to the 5 position of the pyridmidine ring to form the 5-methylcytosine (5mC). The methyl group is positioned in the major groove of the DNA and this methylation does not interfere with the Watson-Crick pairing of cytosine and guanine. Therefore, cytosine methylation by itself does not affect the stability of DNA double helix. In mammals, DNA methylation occurs predominantly in a CpG dinucleotide context, where cytosine is positioned 5' to a guanine nucleotide. 60–90% of CpGs are methylated and methylation is generally evenly distributed in mammals. In contrast, CpG methylation is often grouped into clusters in invertebrates.

In mammals, unmethylated CpGs are often clustered together and form the so-called CpG islands [5]. CpG islands are often located upstream of transcription initiation sites of protein coding genes and modulate the expression of downstream genes. These DNA sequences destabilize nucleosomes and recruit proteins that help establish a transcriptionally permissive chromatin status. When these CpGs are methylated, methylated DNA binding proteins (MBDs) are often recruited. These MBDs may complex with histone deacetylases and chromatin remodeling factors and create a chromatin status that is repressive to gene transcription. In many human diseases including cancer, CpGs are aberrantly methylated at many gene promoters. CpG methylation may result in the repression of many important genes that regulate cell cycle, apoptosis, DNA repair, etc. The silencing of these genes causes the damaged DNA unrepaired in daughter cells and may preposition these cells for cancer progression. Alterations in DNA methylation patterns have been recognized as an important feature of cancer development. On the other hand, a decrease of DNA methylation (so called hypomethylation) is linked to chromosome instability, due to essential roles of DNA methylation in repressing repetitive DNA sequences at pericentromeric regions. Genome instability also constitutes an important component of cancer development. Therefore, both DNA hyper- and hypo-methylation may contribute to the development of cancers.

DNA methylation undergoes dynamic changes during development [6]. Genomic DNA methylation is greatly reduced as the zygote develops into the gastrulation stages of embryos. During this process, DNA methylation in the female genome is passively removed by dilution as cells undergo division, whereas it is erased in the male genome by a faster, active DNA demethylation process. As a result, embryos at gastrulation stages have low levels of DNA methylation. DNA methylation is re-established via *de novo* DNA methylation during successive cell divisions as the gastrulation stage of embryos initiates differentiation and further develops into the next stages. DNA methylation is usually heritable through mitotic cell division and some methylation is also heritable through the specialized meiotic cell division that creates egg and sperm cells, resulting in genomic imprinting.

DNA methylation can be offset by the activity of ten-eleven translocation (TET) methylcytosine dioxygenase family of proteins [11]. Instead of direct removal of methyl groups, TET family of proteins hydroxylates the methyl group to form the 5-hydromethylcytisine (5hmC). The 5hmC can be further oxidized and finally removed from DNA sequence by the demethylation DNA repair system. This allows for the removal of the DNA methylation. Both DNA methylation and demethylation are tightly regulated. Misregulation of either process can result in dysregulation of gene expression that leads to increased susceptibility to human diseases such as cancer.

2.2 DNA Methyltransferase

The enzyme that catalyzes DNA methylation is DNA methyltransferase (DNMT) [17]. DNMT uses S-adenosyl methionine (SAM) as the methyl group donor to methylate cytosine at the 5 position of the pyrimidine ring. In mammals, there are four members of DNMTs that share the same catalytic domains: DNMT1, DNMT2, DNMT3a, and DNMT3b (Fig. 2). One additional protein, DNMT3L, although containing the ATRX domain that is also present in DNMT3A and DNMT3B, does not contain an active catalytic domain. Based on the function of these DNMTs in DNA methylation, DNMTs can be divided into two subgroups: maintenance DNMT and *de novo* DNMT.

DNMT1 is the maintenance DNA methyltransferase (Fig. 2A). Through multiple regions, DNMT1 interacts with the replication fork, and uses the methylated cytosine from the parental strand as hemimethylated templates to methylate cytosine in the newly synthesized daughter strand during DNA replication. Therefore, this enzyme is required for preserving the DNA methylation pattern during successive cell division. Without the function of this enzyme, the replication machinery would produce daughter strands that are unmethylated, leading to passive DNA demethylation as cells undergo division. Deletion of DNMT1 results in genome-wide loss of DNA methylation. However, DNMT1 can only methylate DNA when one strand is methylated and cannot initiate DNA methylation when there is no methylated cytosine in either strand. DNMT3A and DNMT3B are the enzymes that initiate DNA methylation without the dependence on preexisting methylated cytosine (Fig. 2B). These two proteins are responsible for setting up the DNA methylation patterns during early embryonic development. After fertilization, the male genome is actively demethylated and the female genome is passively demethyated as the embryos develop to the blastocyst stages. At this stage, the majority of genome DNA methylation is removed except for the imprinting

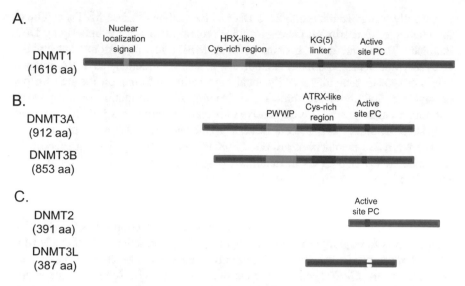

Fig. 2 Mammalian DNA methyltransferases. (**a**) Maintenance DNA methyltransferase DNMT1. (**b**) De novo DNA methyltransferases DNMT3A and DNMT3B. (**c**) Proteins sharing sequence homologues with DNA methyltransferase. Functional domains are denoted

regions. As embryos further develop and progress into the next stage, the DNA methylation pattern is re-established and DNMT3A and DNMT3B are responsible for the establishment of the DNA methylation pattern during this development stage. These two proteins may be partially redundant, as only deletion of both DNMT3A and DNMT3B in mouse leads to a failure to initiate *de novo* methylation after implantation.

DNMT2 also contains the catalytic domain for DNA methylation (Fig. 2C); however, the substrate for DNMT2 is not DNA but is the cytosine 38 in the anticodon loop of aspartic acid transfer RNA (tRNA-Asp) [8]. Methylation of tRNA-Asp increases its affinity for aspartyl-tRNA synthetase and therefore controls the synthesis of a group of proteins containing poly-Asp sequences. Although DNM3L itself does not have DNA methylation activity (Fig. 2C), this protein can interact with the *de novo* DNMT 3A and 3B and contribute to the establishment of DNA methylation patterns. Interaction with DNMT3L increases the binding affinity of these two DNMTs to DNA and stimulates the methyltransferase activity.

2.3 Methylated DNA Binding Protein

DNA methylation may affect the conformation and function of chromatin through several ways [9]. First, the methyl group on cytosine itself may physically impede the binding of transcription factors or other proteins to the underlying DNA template. Second, a group of proteins, named methylated DNA binding proteins (MBDs), can specifically recognize the methylated DNA. The binding of these MBDs can block the binding of transcription factors or other protein factors to the underlying DNA template. Third and more generally, these MBDs recruit histone deacetylases (HDACs) and other chromatin remodeling proteins to methylated DNA regions. These enzymatic activities modify local chromatin conformation through histone deactylation and chromatin remodeling, leading to the formation of a repressive chromatin environment. This repressive chromatin environment inhibits transcription and other processes that require access to the underlying DNA template.

There are five members of proteins, MeCP2 and MBD1-4 that can specifically recognize methylated CpGs in mammals (Fig. 3) [9]. These proteins bind to the methylated CpGs through a methyl-CpG-binding domain (MBD). The MBD domain contains 75 amino acids and adapt to a structural fold of four beta strands, three loops and one alpha helix, forming the interfacial surface with methylated DNA. The interaction occurs in the major groove of the double DNA helix. The interaction is through hydrophilic and hydrophobic interactions. Of these MBDs, MeCP2 appears to be specifically important for the normal function of nerve cells. Mutations of the *MeCP2* gene are the cause of most cases of Rett syndrome, a progressive neurologic developmental disorder and one of the most common causes of mental retardation in females. In addition to the MBD domain, the MBD1 protein contains two to three cysteine-rich (CXXC) type zinc finger domains, and an additional transcriptional repression domain (TRD). MBD1 not only represses transcription from methylated promoters but also repress unmethylated promoter activity through the variation of the CXXC domain. MBD2 has been reported to interact with HDAC1/2, MBD3, and Sin3, and mediates the repressive function of DNA methylation, by histone deacetylation. MBD3 is a subunit of the NuRD, a multisubunit complex containing nucleosome remodeling and histone deacetylase activities. MBD3 has been reported to interact with MTA2, HDAC1/2, and MBD2, and mediates the repressive function of DNA methylation. In addition to the MBD domain, MBD4 also contains a DNA glycosylase domain at its C-terminus. MBD4 can also bind to the deamination derivatives of CpG G:U and G:T base pairs, and function in the initial step of base excision repair. MBD4 can specifically remove T and U paired with guanine (G) within the CpG sites, and contributes to the stability

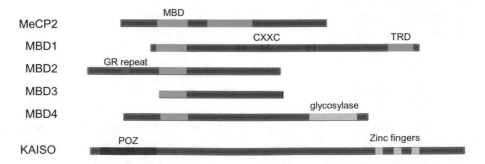

Fig. 3 Methyl DNA binding proteins. Functional domains are denoted

of CpG at promoters. In addition to these MBD proteins, mammals also contain a KAISO protein. This protein exhibits bimodal DNA-binding specificity. KAISO binds to methylated DNA and also to the non-methylated DNA within the TCCTGCNA sequence. KAISO can recruit the N-CoR repressor complex, which contains the histone deacetylation activity and helps form the repressive chromatin structures in target gene promoters.

2.4 Function of DNA Methylation

Although methylated cytosine can be further hydroxylated to form 5hmC, DNA methylation is often stable and therefore the effects of DNA methylation on gene expression are normally permanent and unidirectional. The stable nature of DNA methylation helps the maintenance of the gene expression program specific to each cell type and prevents cells from reverting to stem cells or trans-converting into different cell types. The function of DNA methylation in mammals includes transcription silencing, X chromosome inactivation, genome stability, as well as in many other biological processes [6, 13].

DNA methylation has been generally associated with transcription repression. Through the recruitment of HDACs and chromatin remodeling complexes, methylation of DNA often results in a compact chromatin conformation and transcription silencing. One special case of DNA methylation-mediated gene silencing is gene imprinting. Gene imprinting refers to a phenomenon where the expression of a given gene depends on which allele the gene is located on, i.e., only one allele from either the paternal (sperm derived) or maternal (egg-derived) genome is expressed. DNA methylation on imprinted genes escapes the global DNA demethylation after fertilization. One of the best characterized examples of gene imprinting is the insulin-like growth factor *Igf2/H19* genes. These two genes are located 70 kb away in human chromosome 11. The *Ifg2* gene is preferentially expressed from the paternal allele while the *H19* gene is preferentially expressed from the maternal allele. This allele-specific expression is controlled by a region located upstream of the *H19* gene. This region is methylated in the paternal allele, which recruits MBDs to form a closed chromatin conformation, and represses the expression of *H19* gene. In this case, the tissue-specific enhancer interacts with the promoter of the *Igf2* gene and allows the expression of this gene from the paternal allele. In contrast, this region is not methylated in maternal allele, which recruits CTCF to form an open chromatin conformation, allowing the expression of *H19* gene only from maternal allele. The engagement of tissue-specific enhancer with the *H19* gene prevents the expression of *Igf2* gene from the maternal allele. Gene imprinting prevents the reproduction of organisms from unfertilized eggs and contributes to the stability and variability of species. The gene imprinting system is often disrupted in congenital malformation syndromes, tumors, or cloned animals.

Another important function of DNA methylation is X inactivation. In female mammals, one of the two X chromosomes is silenced to achieve equal gene doses between male and female individuals. The silencing is achieved by packaging the entire X chromosome into a highly compact inactive structure called heterochromatin. This chromosome-wide phenomenon has long been considered a paradigm for the study of the effect of heterochromatin formation and DNA methylation on gene expression in mammals. The inactivated X chromosome contains high levels of DNA methylation, which may contribute to the packaging of the X chromosome into the highly compacted inactive status. The inactivation process consists of three components—initiation, spreading and maintenance. DNA methylation may play a role in all three of these processes; however, the exact mechanism remains unclear.

DNA methylation is also required for the establishment of heterochromatic regions such as the centromere and telomere regions. These heterochromatic regions play important roles in genome stability. The centromere is required for proper segregation of mitotic chromosomes to daughter cells. Malfunction of the centromeric region is often accompanied by inappropriate partition of genetic materials into two daughter cells. DNA methylation may also be responsible for maintaining telomere integrity through indirect regulation. DNMT knockout mice exhibit increased telomeric recombination and variations in telomere length. One particular example of DNA methylation in affecting genome stability is the ICF (immunodeficiency, centromere instability, facial anomalies) syndrome. The majority of ICF patients carry mutations in the *de novo* DNA methyltransferase DNMT3B. Of these patients, hypomethylation is observed in centromeric heterochromatic regions, which may account for the genomic instability in ICF syndrome patients. Genome instability arising from aberrant DNA methylation particularly contributes to cancer initiation and development. DNA methylation has appeared as an appealing target for cancer treatment. Currently, small inhibitors for DNA methylation have undergone clinical trials for certain cancer treatment and have been approved by the FDA.

3   Histone Methylation

3.1   *Methylation Sites*

As the building block of chromatin, nucleosomes are subject to a variety of modifications that modulate the dynamics and metabolism of chromatin. Once thought merely as a static structural component for DNA packaging, histones are now recognized as important regulators for nucleosome function. Histones, particularly the N-terminal tails, are modified by a variety of posttranslational modifications. These modifications include, but are not limited to, methylation, acetylation, phosphorylation, and ubiquitination [16]. These modifications regulate the interaction between DNA and histones within the nucleosome, the interaction between adjacent nucleosomes, and even the interaction between nucleosomes from different chromosomes. Among these modifications, histone methylation is a prevalent modification and can modulate gene expression in either a positive or negative manner.

Of the four histones, histones H3 and H4 are predominately methylated (Fig. 4). Both histone lysine (K) and arginine (R) residues, which contain the free amino groups on their side chains, can be modified by methylation. The prominent methylation sites on histone H3 include R2, K4, K9, R17, R26, K27, K36, and K79 (Fig. 4). The prominent sites on histone H4 include R3 and K20 (Fig. 4). Furthermore, lysine residues can be methylated to mono-, di-, and tri-methylation status. Meanwhile, the arginine residue can be mono- and di- methylated, and based on the location of the methyl groups, arginine methylation can occur in symmetrical or asymmetrical manners. While methylation of arginine is generally linked to gene activation, lysine methylation can lead to both gene activation and repression, depending on the specific amino acids being modified and the methylation status. It should be pointed out that the advance of the mass spectrometry technology and the development of the specific software allow more methylation sites being identified.

The formation of N-C bond in histone methylation renders the stable nature of this modification. Once thought to be a unidirectional modification, histone methylation has now been recognized as a reversible modification [10]. Two families of proteins targeting lysine methylation have been identified, and both employ an oxidation mechanism. The lysine-specific demethylase 1 (LSD1) is a flavin-dependent monoamino oxidase, which coverts mono- and di- methylated H3K4 or H3K9 to unmethylated lysine residues. The JmjC domain-containing protein family catalyzes lysine demethylation with Fe(II) and α-ketoglutarate as cofactors. In contrast to LSD1, JmjC domain-containing demethylase can remove all three lysine methylation states and constitutes the larger family of histone demethylases. As compared to lysine demethylation, arginine methylation is reversed in a different way. While the enzymes for demethylation of arginine residues remains to be identified, a dimi-

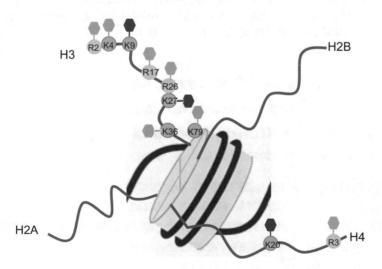

Fig. 4 Histone methylation sites. Repressive histone methylations are marked with *red* while active histone methylation sites are marked with *green*. Both lysine and arginine methylation are indicated

nase PADI4 can convert the methylated arginine to citrulline residue and thus antagonize the effects of arginine methylation. However, PADI4 can also convert non-methylated arginine residues to citrulline residue, rendering the specificity of this enzyme in antagonizing the function of arginine methylation in question.

3.2   Histone Methyltransferases

The enzymes that catalyze histone methylation are histone methyltransferases (HMTs). Based on specific residues targeted by these enzymes, HMTs can be further divided into different subgroups [14]. HMTs that specifically target the arginine residues are protein arginine methyltransferases (PRMTs) [7]. All PRMTs contain the conserved catalytic core, with signature motif I, post-I, II, III, and the THW loop (Fig. 5). The catalytic core adapts a doughnut-like head-to-tail homodimer. Each monomer contains an active site that binds the methyl group donor SAM and the targeted peptide or protein substrate. A pair of highly conserved glutamate residues in the active core uses its negative charge to coordinate the positively charged guanidino group of the arginine residue into the correct orientation for methylation.

HMTs that specifically catalyze the methylation of lysine resides can be further divided into two subgroups [14]. One subgroup contains a conserved SET (stands for Su(var)3-9, Enhancer of Zeste, Trithorax) domain, a pre-SET domain, and a post-SET domain (Fig. 6). The structures involved in the methyltransferase activity are the SET domain, which is composed of approximately 130 amino acids, the pre-SET, and the post-SET domains. The pre-SET domain often contains cysteine residues and forms zinc clusters to bind zinc ions. The SET domain is enriched in β-strands, which together with the β-sheets in pre-SET domain, forms the catalytic core. For methylation, the catalytic core binds to both the SAM and the substrate

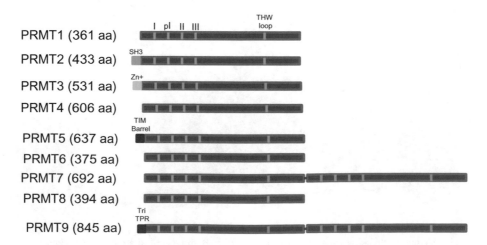

Fig. 5 Protein arginine methyltransferases. Functional domains are denoted

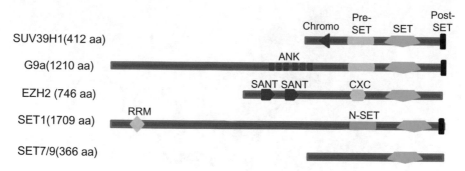

Fig. 6 Selected Histone lysine methyltransferases. Functional domains are denoted

histone tail and orients them in a proper position. A tyrosine residue in the catalytic core then deprotonates the ε-amino group of the lysine residue allowing the lysine chain to make a nucleophilic attack on the methyl group on the sulfur atom of the SAM molecule and thereby transferring the methyl group to the lysine side chain. This family of HMTs constitutes the largest family of histone methyltransferases. The variations of the SET domain structure allow these SET domain methyltransferases to target many different residues and perform different degrees of methylation. Interestingly, some of the HMTs targeting lysine methylation do not contain the SET domain. The only enzyme in this family of HMTs is Dot1 or Dot1L in humans. Dot1 or Dot1L methylates histone H3 at K79 that is at its globular region. The active site of Dot1 is at its N-terminal. The methyl group donor SAM binds to a loop linking the N-terminal catalytic domain and the C-terminal domain. The C-terminal is important for the substrate specificity and Dot1 binding to DNA. The structural constraints define that Dot1 can only methylate histone H3.

3.3 Methylated Histone Binding Protein

Although methylation does not change the overall charge of the residue, each replacement of the proton from the ε-amino decreases the possibility of hydrogen bound formation and increases hydrophobicity. Therefore, methylation of histones by itself could affect the interactions of protein factors with the chromatin template. More generally, methylation of histones provides a binding platform for other downstream proteins [12]. The diverse function of histone methylation in chromatin regulation is largely attributed to the various binding proteins for lysine residues modified at different sites and different states (Fig. 7).

Domains that specifically recognize methylated lysine residues include the plant homeodomain (PHD), the Royal family domains, CW domain and some WD40 domains, such as those of WDR5 and EED. The Royal family includes the Tudor, plant agent, chromo, PWWP, and malignant brain tumor (MBT) domains. The PHD finger constitutes a large family of proteins that specifically bind to methylated

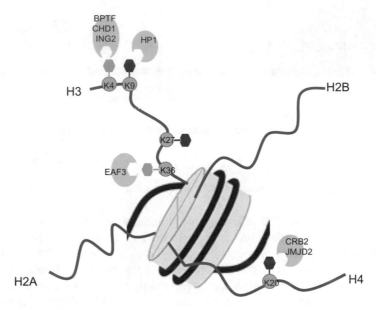

Fig. 7 Proteins bound to methylated lysine residues in histones

H3K4. The PHD fingers of ING family proteins bind to H3K4me3 through aromatic side chains of Y215 and W238 residues. The binding of H3K4me3 stabilizes the association of mSin3a-HDAC1 complex, where ING2 is a core subunit, to chromatin. The association results in histone deacetylation and formation of repressive chromatin conformation in response to DNA damage. On the other hand, the PHD finger in the BPTF protein recognizes H3K4me3 through the anti-parallel β-sheet and the H3K4me3 is inserted into the deep packets on the BPTF surface. Since BPTF is a component of the ATP-dependent chromatin remodeling complex, the binding may contribute to chromatin remodeling during transcription activation. The PHD finger in RAG2 proteins can influence V(D)J recombination through recognition of H3K4me3. Another big family of proteins that recognize methylated lysine residues is the "Royal family" domain. The chromodomains in HP1 and PC recognize methylated H3K9 and H3K27, respectively. The binding may help trigger the formation of heterochromatin and/or recruitment of downstream of repressive complexes. The Tudor domain has high degrees of structural and functional diversity. Similar to the chromodomain, the Tudor domain recognizes methylated lysine through an hydrophobic packet formed by 2–4 aromatic amino acids. The tandem Tudor domain in 53BP1 and JMJD2A has been implicated in the binding of methylated histones. In this case, the tandem Tudor domain of 53BP1 has been implicated in binding of H4K20me2. The two Tudor domains in JMJD2A are interdigitated and form the binding surface of H3K4me3 and H4K20mes. Many MBT domain proteins belong to the Polycomb protein family. This domain shows structural similarity to the "Royal family" of histone binding domains. However, MBT domain may bind to methylated lysine with low methylation level (e.g. mono- and di-).

A subgroup of Tudor domains, such as those in the SMN, SPF30 and TDRDs, can specifically recognize arginine methylation [2, 3]. Yet, it is difficult to predict which Tudor domain recognizes methylated lysine or arginine just based on the protein sequences. Tudor domain proteins that bind to methylarginine are often linked to RNA metabolism. For example, both SMN and SPF30 are involved in regulation of pre-mRNA splicing, and many members of the TDRD family of proteins regulate small interference RNA (siRNA) silencing pathway through recognition of methylated arginine residues. Interestingly, the expression of most TDRD proteins is particularly high in the germ cells, which might implicate their involvement in the piRNA pathway during gametogenesis. TDRD3 is the only known Tudor protein that was shown to recognize arginine-methylated histones. TDRD3 preferentially recognizes H3R17me2a and H4R3me2a mark and promotes transcription.

3.4 Function of Histone Methylation

Although histone methylation does not alter chromatin function directly, methylation can affect the binding of protein factors, in turn repressing or activating transcription (Fig. 4, repressive marks are colored red and permissive marks are colored green) [14]. Furthermore, different degrees of histone methylation can have different functional outputs. For example, methylation of H3K4 at di- or tri-methylated status usually locates on the promoter regions of active genes. Methylation of H3K4 at mono- methylated status often locates at enhancer regions. These methylation events are believed to activate transcription, directly or indirectly. Indeed, the enzymes that catalyze H3K4 methylation are associated with actively transcribed RNA polymerases and add these histone marks as transcription occurs. These methylation events may help establish chromatin status for the next round of transcription. In contrast, methylated H3K36 is localized in gene coding regions. This mark is deposited on chromatin by association of the enzymes with elongating form of RNA polymerases. This mark may help contribute to the stability of nucleosomes after transcription and may also modulate the pre-mRNA splicing processes. Methylation of H3K79 is also located in gene coding regions. Both H3K4 and H3K79 methylation are controlled by H2B ubiquitination and ongoing transcription. In addition to these lysine modifications, H3R2, H3R16, and R26 are also correlated with gene activation. Methylation of these three arginine residues is carried out by the co-activator CARM1. Arginine methylation may enhance the histone acetylation and contribute to gene activation. Similarly, H4R3 can also be methylated, and this methylation facilitates downstream histone acetylation and positively contributes to gene activation.

Histone methylation sites that are linked to gene repression include H3K9, H3K27, and H4K20 methylation (Fig. 4). These modifications may contribute to the closed chromatin conformation and transcription repression, directly or indirectly. Methylations of H3K9 di- and tri- status are involved in heterochromatin formation and thus gene repression. These modifications are mediated by SUV39H1 and are particularly enriched at percentermatic regions. These modifications recruit the HP1 proteins and serve as seeding sites for heterochromatin spreading. This modification is important in the formation of constitutive heterochromatic structure and thus genomic stability. In contrast, H3K9 di- and tri- methylation in eurochromatic regions is mediated by G9a. This modification facilitates the formation of faculta-tive heterochromatin and transcription repression. Methylation of H3K27 is cata-lyzed by Polycomb repressive complex 2 and therefore this modification is believed to create a binding site for downstream PRC1. Therefore, H3K27 methylation is specifically linked to polycomb group protein-mediated gene silencing. Methylation of H4K20 is also associated with a closed chromatin status and may function in DNA damage repair. In this case, H4K20 methylation is recognized by 53BP1 pro-tein and helps localize 53BP1 to damaged DNA foci, in conjunction with H2AK15 ubiquitination. Although histone demethylases have been identified, histone modifications are generally stable and can be passed down to progeny with the mechanism remains to be elucidated.

4   Perspective

Methylation of DNA and histones are important components of the epigenetic machinery. These two modifications, together with other epigenetic regulatory mechanisms, contribute to the stable expression of gene expression program spe-cific to a given cell type. The epigenetic mechanism is particularly important as cells undergo normal programming during development and undertake reprogram-ing to acquire a cancerous phenotype. Compared to gene mutation and deletion, epigenetic mechanisms are reversible and can be targeted by small molecule inhibi-tors, and thus epigenetics has appeared as an appealing target for cancer treatment.

   As important components of epigenetics, both DNA and histone methylation depends on the availability of methyl group donor SAM. In humans, there are three major resources of methyl group donor: methionine (~ 10 mmol of methyl/day), one carbon metabolism via methylfolate (~5–10 mmol of methyl/day), and choline (~30 mmoles methyl/day). The three methyl group donors can compensate each other; however, when severely depleted from diet, methylation of DNA and histones can be affected. Since proper methylation of DNA and histones may be important for normal cell functions, scientists recommend adequate methyl donors in the diet such as green tea, red wine, spinach, walnuts, and pomegranate [4]. This diet may be of benefit in repressing the expression of harmful genes.

   Since the epigenetic system plays a key role in the cell gene expression program, this system has to undergo profound reprograming as cells revert to acquire uncon-trolled proliferative features. As important components of epigenetics, there has been a wealth of literature that both DNA and histone methylation undergo signifi-cant changes during the carcinogenesis processes. Consequently, DNA methylation inhibitors have been used in certain cancer treatments, in conjunction with other treatments. The specific effects on cancer cells are enhanced by the relatively rapid division of these cells *vs* normal somatic cells. Along this line, a number of novel inhibitors for HMTs are under way for clinical trial. One side effect for these inhibitors and possibly all inhibitors targeting epigenetic revenue is that epigenetics are also essential for normal cell function. How to specifically target these inhibitors to cancer cells may be a long way for future studies. However, strong basic science and mechanism-based clinical trials will overcome the issue.

References

1. Allis CD, Caparros M-L, Jenuwein T, Reinberg D, Lachlan M (2015) Epigenetics, 2nd edn. Cold Spring Harbor Laboratory Press, Cold Spring Harbor, New York
2. Beaver JE, Waters ML (2016) Molecular recognition of Lys and Arg methylation. ACS Chem Biol 11:643–653
3. Chen C, Nott TJ, Jin J, Pawson T (2011) Deciphering arginine methylation: Tudor tells the tale. Nat Rev Mol Cell Biol 12:629–642
4. Choi SW, Friso S (2010) Epigenetics: a new bridge between nutrition and health. Adv Nutr (Bethesda, Md) 1:8–16
5. Deaton AM, Bird A (2011) CpG islands and the regulation of transcription. Genes Dev 25:1010–1022
6. Hackett JA, Surani MA (2013) DNA methylation dynamics during the mammalian life cycle. Philos Trans R Soc Lond Ser B Biol Sci 368:20110328
7. Jahan S, Davie JR (2015) Protein arginine methyltransferases (PRMTs): role in chromatin organization. Adv Biol Regul 57:173–184
8. Jeltsch A, Ehrenhofer-Murray A, Jurkowski TP, Lyko F, Reuter G, Ankri S, Nellen W, Schaefer M, Helm M (2016) Mechanism and biological role of Dnmt2 in nucleic acid methylation. RNA Biol:1–16
9. Klose RJ, Bird AP (2006) Genomic DNA methylation: the mark and its mediators. Trends Biochem Sci 31:89–97
10. Klose RJ, Zhang Y (2007) Regulation of histone methylation by demethylimination and demethylation. Nat Rev Mol Cell Biol 8:307–318
11. Kohli RM, Zhang Y (2013) TET enzymes, TDG and the dynamics of DNA demethylation. Nature 502:472–479
12. Patel DJ, Wang Z (2013) Readout of epigenetic modifications. Annu Rev Biochem 82:81–118
13. Rottach A, Leonhardt H, Spada F (2009) DNA methylation-mediated epigenetic control. J Cell Biochem 108:43–51
14. Shilatifard A (2006) Chromatin modifications by methylation and ubiquitination: implications in the regulation of gene expression. Annu Rev Biochem 75:243–269
15. Smith ZD, Meissner A (2013) DNA methylation: roles in mammalian development. Nat Rev Genet 14:204–220
16. Tessarz P, Kouzarides T (2014) Histone core modifications regulating nucleosome structure and dynamics. Nat Rev Mol Cell Biol 15:703–708
17. Turek-Plewa J, Jagodzinski PP (2005) The role of mammalian DNA methyltransferases in the regulation of gene expression. Cell Mol Biol Lett 10:631–647

Part I
DNA Methylation and Cancer

The Molecular Basis of DNA Methylation

Isao Suetake, Mikio Watanebe, Kohei Takeshita, Saori Takahashi, and Peter Carlton

Abstract In mammals, cytosine in CpG sequences in genomic DNA is often methylated at the 5th position. DNA methylation acts as a regulator of gene expression, and is crucial for development, especially in higher eukaryotes. Three DNA (cytosine-5)-methyltransferases, Dnmt1, Dnmt3a, and Dnmt3b, have been identified. Dnmt3a and Dnmt3b are mainly responsible for establishing DNA methylation patterns in the genome. Factors interacting with Dnmt3a or Dnmt3b, histone modifications, and their timing of expression act as determinants for sites to be methylated. Once DNA methylation patterns are established, the patterns are maintained by Dnmt1, which favors methylation of hemi-methylated DNA (where only one DNA strand is methylated) after DNA replication and repair. For maintenance DNA methylation, interacting factors and histone modifications are also necessary in vivo. In this chapter, the function of DNA methylation and the molecular mechanisms to establish and maintain DNA methylation are described.

Keywords DNA methylation • DNA methyltransferase • Dnmt1 • Dnmt3a • Dnmt3b • Histone modifications

I. Suetake (✉)
College of Nutrition, Koshien University, 10-1 Momijigaoka, Takaradura 665-0006, Japan

Center for Twin Research, Graduate School of Medicine, Osaka University,
1-7 Yamadaoka, Suita, Osaka 565-0871, Japan
e-mail: suetake@koshien.ac.jp

M. Watanebe
Center for Twin Research, Graduate School of Medicine, Osaka University,
1-7 Yamadaoka, Suita, Osaka 565-0871, Japan

K. Takeshita
Laboratory of Supermolecular Crystallography, Institute for Protein Research, Osaka University, 3-2 Yamadaoka, Suita, Osaka 565-0871, Japan

S. Takahashi
Laboratory for Developmental Epigenetics, RIKEN CDB, 2-2-3 Minatojima, Kobe 650-0047, Japan

P. Carlton
Laboratory of Chromosome Function and Inheritance, Graduate School of Biostudies, Kyoto University, Yoshida-konoe-cho, Sakyo-ku, Kyoto 606-8501, Japan

© Springer International Publishing AG 2017
A. Kaneda, Y.-i. Tsukada (eds.), *DNA and Histone Methylation as Cancer Targets*, Cancer Drug Discovery and Development, DOI 10.1007/978-3-319-59786-7_2

1   Introduction

DNA methylation is a covalent functional modification of genomic DNA, providing a layer of information in addition to the nucleotide sequence [15]. In mammals, DNA methylation mainly occurs at the C-5 position of cytosine, mostly within CpG sequences [15], though recently N^6-methyladenine has also been reported [197]. In the human and mouse genomes, about 4% of cytosine residues are methylated in differentiated tissues. 5-methylcytosine (5mC) is widespread throughout the mammalian genome and observed on about 80% of CpG dinucleotides. 5mC is thought to contribute to the formation of heterochromatin at pericentromeric regions, transcriptional repression of the inactive X chromosome in females, and expression regulation at imprinting control regions in a parent-of-origin specific manner [162]. CpG-rich regions of approximately 1 kb, known as CpG islands, are found in more than half of genes, and are often observed in or near promoter regions [52]. 5mC in CpG islands is negatively correlated with gene expression, and this correlation contributes to cell type-specific gene expression patterns [77]. In contrast, DNA methylation in gene bodies is generally associated with high expression levels [174, 70]. Levels of DNA methylation are higher in exons than introns in diverse organisms [56]. While DNA methylation has only a minor influence on the regulation of splicing of constitutive exons, it has a major effect on alternative exon splicing [97].

In mammals, global DNA methylation is reduced during the early stages of germ cell development, and re-established in gonocytes in males and growing oocytes in females [149]. The expression of roughly 100 autosomal genes, referred to as imprinted genes, is differentially regulated between the two parental genomes. Imprinted genes are characterized by distinct DNA methylation regions in the male and female genomes, termed differentially methylated regions (DMRs). The DMR methylation states are established in germ cells at the same time as global DNA methylation [81, 160].

After cell differentiation, DNA methylation is thought to be a stable epigenetic signal; however, DNA methylation patterns are changed during biological and pathological processes [142, 11]. Several relationships between DNA methylation and disease have been reported. Hypermethylation of tumour suppressor genes is often associated with transcriptional silencing [41]. Changes of DNA methylation are associated with other diseases such as rheumatoid arthritis [110] and neuronal disorders [34, 114, 130]. Moreover, DNA methylation can be periodically changed in a strand-specific manner during transcriptional cycling of the p52/TFF1 gene promoter upon activation by oestrogens on a time scale as short as 1 h [116, 83].

DNA methylation drifts in an age-specific manner, in which global hypomethylation and local hypermethylation are observed [78]. Dynamic changes in DNA methylation are also critical in the consolidation of contextual fear-conditioned memories [117]. In summary, DNA methylation contributes to many biological phenomena mainly by regulating gene expression.

2 DNA Methylation and Gene Silencing

Generally, DNA methylation on promoter regions represses gene expression. Genes that are tissue-specifically expressed are generally heavily methylated and in a condensed chromatin state in tissues that are not expressing the genes. It has also been reported that methylation contributes to the silencing of transposons, which occupy a significant proportion of mammalian genomes. The level of DNA methylation increases in proportion to the size of the genome. This could be due to the fact that the numbers of transcriptional factors does not increase in proportion to genome size in higher eukaryotes. Except for a small number of transcription factors such as SP1 [67], many transcription factors such as CTCF [10, 66], E-box-binding transcription factor c-Myc [134], and Ets transcription proteins [183], are inhibited in their binding to target DNA sequences due to target sequence methylation. Repression of binding of transcriptional factors by DNA methylation could contribute to the efficient utilization of a limited number of transcription factors to manage the increased genome size.

In addition to this direct effect of DNA methylation on the recognition of transcription factors, methylated DNA is recognized by several methylated DNA-binding proteins, which form complexes or associate with co-repressor complexes such as NuRD, Sin3A, or NCoR, by coupling histone modifications and chromatin states [33].

3 DNA Methyltransferases in Mammals

DNA methylation is established and maintained by the coordinated activity of DNA methyltransferases [13] (Fig. 1). DNA methylation patterns are established by the de novo methyltransferases Dnmt3a and Dnmt3b. One member of the Dnmt3 family, Dnmt3L, does not possess DNA methylation activity, but the protein is indispensable

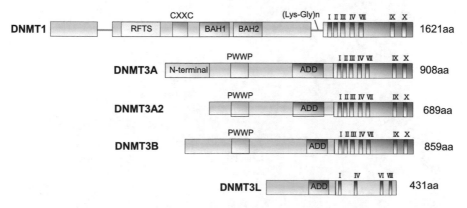

Fig. 1 Schematic illustration of mouse Dnmts. RFTS, CXXC, BAH, PWWP, ADD, and catalytic domain are indicated by *yellow*, *purple*, *gray*, *light green*, *red*, and *pink*, respectively. Conserved motif I, IV, VI, VIII, IX, and X in catalytic domain is shown by *blue*. In Dnmt1, lysine-glycine repeats are followed by catalytic domain

for DNA methylation for global genomic regions in germ cells [69]. As Dnmt1 preferentially methylates hemimethylated DNA in which only one of the two strands is methylated, Dnmt1 maintains the established DNA methylation patterns through the cell cycle. Dnmt2 was found to be another DNA methyltransferase [203]; however, the enzyme has turned out to catalyze tRNA methylation [57].

3.1 Proposed Mechanism of Methylation Reaction

The reaction of DNA methylation is a two-substrate reaction involving S-adenosyl-L-methionine (SAM) as a methyl-group donor and cytosine bases in DNA as a methyl-group acceptor (Fig. 2). The SH group of cysteine at the catalytic center of DNA methyltransferase nucleophilically attacks the 6th carbon in the pyrimidine ring of cytosine, and forms a covalent bond to cytosine. This activates the 5th carbon and promotes the transfer of a methyl-group from SAM. Finally, the enzyme is released from the DNA [92].

The sequence responsible for the catalytic reaction comprises ten motifs that are conserved in prokaryotes and eukaryotes. Among these motifs, six, i.e. I, IV, VI, VIII, IX, and X, are conserved in all cytosine methyltransferases. Motif I is responsible for the binding of SAM, and the Cys of the Pro-Cys sequence in motif IV covalently binds to the carbon at the 6th position to become the intermediate of the methylation reaction, as described above. The sequence between motifs VIII and IX, which exhibits no homology among the enzymes, is called the "target recognition domain (TRD)", and specifies the catalysis target sequence for methylation [92]. In fact, the TRDs of Dnmt1 and bacterial methyltransferase show clear differences in their structures derived from x-ray crystallography (Fig. 3).

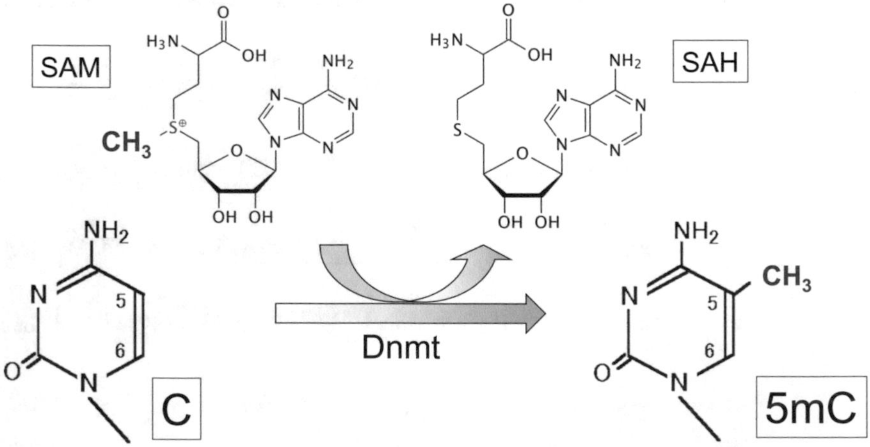

Fig. 2 Cytosine methylation. By transferring methyl group from s-adenosyl methyonine (SAM) to 5th position of cytosine (C), with DNA methyltransferase (Dnmt), cytosine is converted to 5-methyl cytosine (5mC). After the transfer, S-adenosyl-homocysteine (SAH) is produced

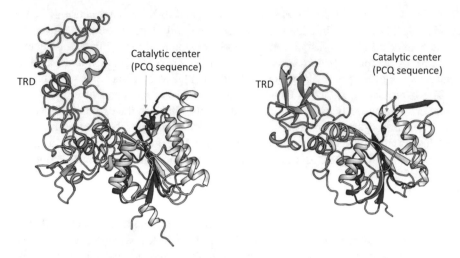

Fig. 3 Disposition of motifs within catalytic domain of Dnmt1. The comparison of the catalytic domain of mouse Dnmt1 (*left panel*; PDB ID: 3AV4) and bacterial methyltransferase, M.HhaI, (*right panel*; ID: 1MHT). Motif I, IV, VI, VIII, IX and X in catalytic domain in both Dnmt1 and Hha I are indicated by *red, blue, purple, yellow, pink*, and *cyan*, respectively. TRD region is indicated by *green*. These catalytic center (PCQ sequence) are showed by stick model, respectively. TRD region Dnmt1 and M. HhaI is 1398–1547 and 189–271 amino acids, respectively

3.2   Establishment of DNA Methylation Patterns

3.2.1   Properties of the de novo Methyltransferases Dnmt3a and 3b

In mammals, two of the three cytosine DNA-methyltransferases, Dnmt3a and Dnmt3b, are responsible for establishing methylation patterns with their de novo-type DNA methylation activity [123, 2]. Both Dnmt3a and Dnmt3b knockout mice show severe defects in establishment of DNA methylation patterns at early stages of embryogenesis, and consequently do not develop normally [123], indicating that Dnmt3a and Dnmt3b play crucial roles in creating DNA methylation patterns. Double knockout mice, in which Dnmt3a and Dnmt3b genes are simultaneously removed, show a more severe phenotype during development compared to single knockout of either gene. Thus, Dnmt3a and Dnmt3b are partially redundant for the establishment of DNA methylation.

Several phenotypes of Dnmt3 mutants have been reported. Centromeric heterochromatin regions are prominent, specific methylation sites of Dnmt3b [123]. Knockout or mutation of the *Dnmt3b* gene induces hypomethylation in the centromeric hetrochromatin region, which is a cause of the autosomal recessive disorder, immunodeficiency-centromeric instability-facial anomalies (ICF) syndrome [123, 65, 199]. Induced hypomethylation in a pericentric region can induce genome instability.

Recently, a mutation in the *Dnmt3a* gene was found to be a major cause of acute myeloid leukemia [99]. In addition, both Dnmt3a and Dnmt3b are upregulated in cornu ammonis 1 (CA1) of hippocampus, and blocking their methyltransferase activity prevents neuronal memory consolidation [117]. Together, Dnmt3a and Dnmt3b play essential roles in normal development and regulation of the nervous system.

The expression patterns of Dnmt3a and Dnmt3b are independently regulated. Dnmt3a is ubiquitously expressed in somatic cells, although the expression level is low. Exceptionally, an isoform named Dnmt3a2 (de novo type DNA methyltransferase) that is missing roughly 200 amino acid residues found at Dnmt3a's aminoterminus is highly expressed during germ cell development and in early embryos (Fig. 1) [22, 194, 150, 151]. In contrast to Dnmt3a, the expression of Dnmt3b is strictly regulated. Dnmt3b is highly expressed in pluripotent stem cells and progenitor cells at the stage of pre- and post-implantation [192].

Recently, the genome-wide localization of both Dnmt3 genes has been analyzed in ES cells [9]. Dnmt3a and Dnmt3b localize to methylated, CpG-dense regions in mouse stem cells, but are excluded from active promoters and enhancers. Dnmt3b selectively binds to the bodies of transcribed genes, which leads to their preferential methylation, and its targeting to transcribed sequences requires SETD2-mediated methylation of lysine 36 on histone H3 [9].

Many alternative splicing isoforms have been reported for Dnmt3b [143, 126]. Most of the Dnmt3b isoforms have a deletion in the C-terminal catalytic region and thus exhibit no DNA methylation activity. Among the translation products, only Dnmt3b1 and Dnmt3b2 possess DNA methylation activity [2]. Recently, a new splicing isoform that skips exon 6 has been reported to be highly expressed in in vitro fertilized embryos and shows relatively low DNA methylation activity, leading to low DNA methylation in these embryos [71]. A major isoform, Dnmt3b3, which lacks the exon of the middle part of the catalytic domain, exhibits no DNA methylation activity [2]. Dnmt3b3 has also been reported to play a role in modulating DNA methylation [195, 186].

3.2.2   Structural Properties of Dnmt3

Both Dnmt3a and Dnmt3b have similar domain arrangements: a Pro-Trp-Trp-Pro (PWWP) domain, Atrx-Dnmt3-Dnmt3L (ADD) domain (also known as the plant homeodomain (PHD)), and C-terminal catalytic methyltransferase domain (Fig. 1). An amino-terminal region, which is located ahead of the PWWP domain, is unique to the long isoform of Dnmt3a and exhibits DNA-binding capability [171, 135], and is reported to bind to the silenced Oct4 promoter region in mouse embryonic stem cells [87]. The PWWP domain is reported to bind DNA in vitro [135, 137]. The targeting of Dnmt3b to transcribed sequences requires a functional PWWP domain of Dnmt3b [9]. The ADD domain interacts with various proteins, such as HDAC1 (histone deacetylase) and Ezh2 (histone H3K27 methyltransferase) [48, 189]. Ezh2 binds to the amino-terminal region of Dnmt3a, in addition to its ADD domain [189].

   A dimer of the Dnmt3a catalytic domain with Dnmt3L (described in detail in following section) shows a "butterfly" structure (Fig. 4a) [75]. The distance of catalytic pockets in the dimer is 40 Å, which corresponding to single turn of DNA helix [75]. Similar periodic DNA methylation patterns are observed for the frequency of CpG sites in the DMRs of 12 maternally imprinted mouse genes [75]. Thus, periodic methylation in the genome is proposed to be created by Dnmt3a [75]. ADD domain structure of Dnmt3a is similar to that of the ADD domains of DNMT3L and ATRX [4, 125], and is composed of two C4-type zinc fingers [127]. Recently, the co-crystal of truncated DNMT3a (ADD and catalytic region) and histone H3 amino-terminal peptide has been solved [63] (Fig. 4b). DNMT3A exists in an autoinhibitory form, as the ADD domain inhibits DNA binding activity of the catalytic domain. ADD domain of Dnmt3a specifically binds to unmodified histone H3 [127], and its binding is clearly visible in the crystal structure [63]. In addition, the histone H3

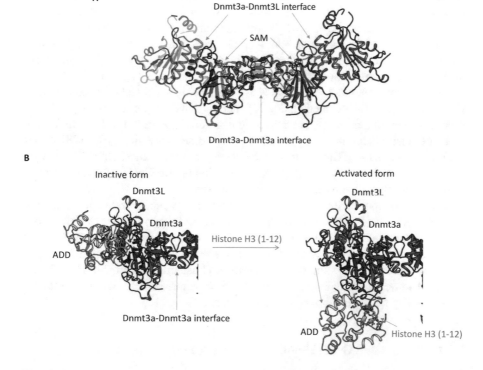

Fig. 4 Structure of Dnmt3a and Dnmt3L. (**a**) Co-Crystal of Dnmt3a catalytic domain and Dnmt3L. Dnmt3a catalytic domain and Dnmt3L are shown as *red* and *blue*, respectively. SAM is shown by stick model (*yellow*). (**b**) The activation mechanism of Dnmt3a by the orientational change of Dnmt3a ADD domain. Catalytic domain and ADD of Dnmt3a, and Dnmt3L are shown by *red*, *green*, and *blue*, respectively. The H3 peptide was drown by stick model (*light-blue*)

N-terminal tail stimulates its activity in a Dnmt3L-independent manner, when the H3 tail interacts with the ADD domain, causing a positional change (Fig. 4b) [63]. Thus, recent extensive studies have opened a window on the relationship between function and domain structure of Dnmt3.

3.2.3   Sequence Specificity of de novo Methyltransferases

Using whole-genome bisulfite sequencing methylome analyses, non-CpG methylation was observed in human and mouse ES cells, human induced pluripotent stem cells and mouse brain [107, 93, 141], and mouse oocyte [159], but is not present in most somatic cells,. The major methylation target sequence of Dnmt3a and Dnmt3b is CpG sequence, however, Dnmt3a and Dnmt3b cause non-CpG methylation of CpA, and CpC and CpT, respectively, in vitro [2, 167].

Knockout of the maintenance methyltransferase Dnmt1 induces little effect on non-CpG methylation in mouse ES cells [3]. Dnmt3a deficiency and knockout reduced non-CpG methylation in ES cells [3, 114], oocytes [159] and neurons [62]. In addition, deletion of the *DNMT3b* gene results in a dramatic reduction of non-CpG methylation in human ES cells [3, 103], and knockdown of Dnmt3b following DNMT3a shows a further reduction of non-CpG methylation in human ES cells [210]. Non-CpG methylation is therefore dependent on both Dnmt3a and Dnmt3b, and each is able to partially compensate for loss of the other's methylation activity. Most non-CpG methylation is observed at CpApG sequences in human ES cells [93, 107].

In particular, 25% of total methylated cytosines are in a non-CpG context in human ES cells [107]. Non-CpG methylation is generally lower in promoters [93, 107] and more abundant in gene bodies, compared to intergenic regions [108, 198]. Intragenic non-CpG methylation is closely correlated with gene expression [108, 198]. Lister et al. reported that non-CpGs are not methylated on both strands, but rather only on the antisense strand [108]. Although the localization of non-CpG methylation is clear in some cells, its function in mammals is still elusive.

It was also reported that Dnmt3a and Dnmt3b likely recognize adjacent nucleotides of CpG sites: Dnmt3a prefers CpG sites flanked by pyrimidines (Y) over those flanked by purines (R) [104]. Furthermore, Dnmt3a and Dnmt3b prefer RCGY, and disfavor YCGR [64]. However, such sequence specificity is not sufficient for targeting of methylation to specific genomic regions. Thus, either Dnmt3a or Dnmt3b are recruited to target methylation regions by other factors, or the state of chromatin structure may determine the methylation regions.

3.2.4   Factors that Guide Dnmt3 to Target Sites for Methylation

Sequence-specific DNA-binding proteins are involved for the targeting of Dnmts. Dnmt3a binds the co-repressor complex of PR48/HDAC1 or proto-oncogene c-Myc through the ADD domain [48, 19]. Both Dnmt3a and Dnmt3b cooperate with EVI1 (oncogene product) to bind and methylate the expression-controlling region of miRNA 124-3 [155]. Recently, noncoding RNA is reported to be involved in targeting of Dnmt3b to de novo methylation sites. pRNA, which binds the promoter of rRNA coding genes and forms a DNA:RNA triplex, recruits Dnmt3b for DNA methylation [153]. On the contrary, Ross et al. have reported that the DNA:RNA heteroduplex inhibits the de novo methylation activities of both Dnmt3a and Dnmt3b in vitro [145].

In addition, guiding by factors that bind to sequence-specific DNA-binding proteins has been reported. ZFP57, which is one of the KRAB zinc-finger proteins, plays crucial roles in the establishment and maintenance of imprinted gene methylation specifically through interaction with Trim28 (KAP1 or TIF1β) [138, 139], to which Dnmt3a and Dnmt1 bind [211]. The KRAB zinc-finger protein family, which comprises more than 300 genes, determines target regions [111]. Trim28 contributes as a scaffold for guiding Dnmts to a variety of target sequences using sequence-specific KRAB zinc-finger proteins. In a similar category, NEDD8, which is an ubiquitin-like small protein modifier, acts as a tag in guiding Dnmt3b to NEDDylated proteins [156]. The main target of NEDDylation is Cullin protein, which plays a role in heterochromatin formation. Dnmt3b is reported to be tethered to centromeric and pericentromeric heterochromatin regions through interaction with CENP-C [58].

Contrarily, the recruitment of Dnmt3a is not coupled with introduction of methylation. Dnmt3a can be recruited to target sequences by Ezh2, a component of polycomb repressive complex 2 (PRC2) [148], MBD3, an intrinsic component of the co-repressor complex NuRD, Brg1, an ATPase subunit of Swi/Snf chromatin remodeling factor [31], or p53 [190]; however, the recruitment does not affect the DNA methylation state. Thus, while proteins that interact with Dnmt3s, either directly or indirectly, have been identified, the regulation of de novo methylation still remains elusive.

3.2.5 Function of Dnmt3L in Establishing DNA Methylation Patterns

Dnmt3a and Dnmt3b also strongly interact with Dnmt3L, whose sequence is similar to that of Dnmt3a or Dnmt3b, but has no catalytic activity [72]. The expression of Dnmt3L is not observed in differentiated somatic cells, and its expression is restricted to germ cells and very early stage embryos. The expression of Dnmt3L in germ cells is necessary for global DNA methylation as well as the DMRs of imprinted genes [69]. The C-terminal half of Dnmt3L directly interacts with Dnmt3a or Dnmt3b and thereby enhances their DNA methylation activity [168, 25]. In male germ cells in gonocytes at 14–18 day postcoitum (dpc) when global methylation occurs, Dnmt3L and Dnmt3a2 show high expression levels [150]. Loss of Dnmt3L also causes overexpression of retrotransposons and defects in synaptonemal complex formation required for mature meiotic spermatocytes, leading to meiotic catastrophe and spermatogenic arrest [18, 193].

Biochemical analysis showed that the activity of Dnmt3a2 is more sensitive to salt conditions compared with Dnmt3a, in vitro, and thus cannot exhibit DNA methylation activity under physiological salt conditions; however, it is resistant to salt in the presence of Dnmt3L [169]. Dnmt3L interacts with the polycomb complex

PRC2 in competition with Dnmt3a and Dnmt3b to maintain low methylation levels in chromatin regions enriched with lysine 27 tri-methylated histone H3 (H3K27me3). It has been proposed that, in ES cells, Dnmt3L counteracts the activity of de novo DNA methylation to maintain hypomethylation at promoters of H3K27-methylated genes [120].

3.2.6   Chromatin Structure and Establishment of DNA Methylation

Biochemical studies showed that the DNA in nucleosome core regions is a poor substrate for Dnmt3a or Dnmt3b [144, 178, 179]. Dnmt3b, however, weakly but significantly methylates DNA in the nucleosome core region [178]. Dnmt3b is the major DNA methyltransferase that contributes to global DNA methylation at an early stage of embryogenesis [123, 191]. Thus, the ability of Dnmt3b to methylate the nucleosome core region may contribute to this global methylation. In addition to nucleosome structure, the effect of the linker histone (histone H1) on Dnmt3 has been investigated. Dnmt3a and Dnmt3b preferentially methylate a naked linker portion, which is inhibited by the binding of linker histone H1 (H1) [178, 179]. Interestingly, however, in vivo, H1 is necessary for the maintenance of methylation in *Arabidopsis* with the aid of a chromatin remodeling factor [205]. Since it has been reported that the half-life of H1 at the same position is less than 10 min [20], the replacement of H1 may provide a naked linker to Dnmt3a for de novo methylation. DNA methylation occurs mainly in the linker region not only in ES cells [182] but also in HeLa cells [46], while it is also reported that nucleosome position-dependent DNA methylation distribution is not detected by methylome mapping [140]. Histone H1 promotes epigenetic silencing at the H19 and Gtl2 imprinting loci in mouse ES cells, by either direct interaction between H1 and DNMT3B as well as DNMT1, leading to their recruitment to DNA, or by interfering with binding of the SET7/9 methyltransferase to chromatin, leading to inhibition of methylation of H3K4 in nucleosomes [201]. However, direct interaction between H1 and DNMT3a has not been observed, and interaction of H1 with DNMT1 or DNMT3b differs between H1 isoforms [201]. Furthermore, the effect of nucleosome remodeling on the activity of Dnmt3 has been studied. The Swi/Snf-type chromatin remodeling factor *Lsh* associates with Dnmt3a or Dnmt3b in embryonic cells [209]. Knockout of *Lsh* induces hypomethylation in the genome [209]. Similar to this, DDM1, which is an *Arabidopsis* Lsh ortholog, also contributes to global DNA methylation [205]. Dnmt3a and Dnmt3b are reported to be in complexes with the remodeling factor Brg1 [31]. Considering these observations, it is reasonable that the regulation of exposure of naked DNA is an important step for de novo DNA methylation.

The PWWP domain of Dnmt3a and Dnmt3b is reported to be a motif for DNA binding [137, 135], and to bring Dnmt3a or Dnmt3b to heterochromatin [24, 55]. Thus, the PWWP in the amino-terminal half of Dnmt3a or Dnmt3b is one of the determinants for targeting of methylation sites. It is not known yet, however, how the PWWP of Dnmt3a or Dnmt3b selectively recognizes heterochromatin. Such recruitment of Dnmt3a or Dnmt3b to specific regions is strongly correlated with the chromatin state.

Lysine 44 (K44) of the amino-terminal domain of Dnmt3a is dimethylated by G9a, a histone H3K9 methyltransferase, and is important for interactions with G9a and/or EHMT1 (also called GLP) [21]. The interaction between Dnmt3a and G9a is necessary for the DNA methylation of some loci, such as the OCT3 promoter, which is involved in embryonic stem cell pluripotency. Many reports have shown that Dnmt3a recognizes both modified and unmodified histone tails. Trim28, which is reported to interact directly with Dnmt3a [211], also interacts with Setdb1, a histone H3K9 methyltransferase, and HP1, which recognizes di- and tri-methylated K9 of histone H3 (H3K9me2,3). The PWWP domain of Dnmt3a recognizes tri-methylated lysine 36 of histone H3 (H3K36me3) to enhance DNA methylation activity [36], and the ADD domain binds unmethylated lysine 4 of histone H3 (H3K4) [127, 101] and enhances DNA methylation activity [101]. Tri-methylation at Lys 4 of histone H3 (H3K4me3) inhibits DNA methylation by Dnmt3a, and the inhibition is more effective compared with H3K9me3 [206, 101]. Dnmt3L, which lacks methylation activity, also contains an ADD domain and recognizes an unmethylated state of H3K4 [125]. As H3K4me3 is the hallmark of open, transcriptionally-active chromatin, it is reasonable that an un-methylated form of H3K4 recruits a de novo methyltransferase complex including Dnmt3a and Dnmt3L. In addition, symmetric di-methylation of arginine 3 of histone H4 (H4R3me2S) is a target of Dnmt3a *via* the ADD domain for DNA methylation [208]. From screening with a peptide array, H3K36me2,3 was shown to be directly recognized by Dnmt3a, and its activity is repressed by histone modification [36]. Genome-wide analysis also indicates that SERD2-mediated H3K36me3 can guide DNMT3 binding and de novo methylation at transcribed gene bodies in mouse ES cells [9]. The amino-terminal portion of Dnmt3b, which includes its PWWP domain, specifically interacts with Hela mononucleosomes containing histone K36me3 [9].

Recently, a study using oocytes in which DNA methylation patterns are established has elucidated relationships between histone modifications and DNA methylation. Reduction of DNMT3a2 and HDAC2 levels in *sin3a^-/-* oocytes leads to decreased DNA methylation of imprinting control regions of specific genes, and DNMT3a2 co-immunoprecipitated with HDAC2 in mouse ES cells. The authors proposed that DNMT3a2-HDAC2 complex is essential for establishment of genomic imprinting [113]. Methylome profiling of mouse oocytes deficient for H3K4 demethylase shows that H3K4 methylation is crucial for proper DNA methylation establishment at CGI [165]. Thus, histone tail modifications recruit de novo-type Dnmt3a or Dnmt3b to the site of DNA methylation, leading proper mouse development.

In plants, a DNA methyltransferase CMT (chromomethylase) of *Arabidopsis*, which methylates the CpHpG and/or CpHpH sequence, also recognizes methylated histone H3 (H3K9me) with its chromodomain [166]. Similar to CMT, DNA methyltransferase Dim2 of *Neurospora crassa* also contains a chromodomain and is guided to H3K9me [181]. Therefore, CMT and Dim2 show H3K9me-dependent methylation of DNA. Although mammalian Dnmts do not directly recognize H3K9me, the Dnmts are reported to interact with heterochromatin protein 1 (HP1) [49, 161, 40], which specifically recognizes H3K9me2,3. Because of this, H3K9 methylation is proposed to be a cause and/or result of DNA methylation.

3.3   Maintenance DNA Methylation

Once genome methylation patterns are established in an early stage of embryogenesis, the patterns are faithfully propagated to the next generation *via* replication in a cell lineage-dependent manner. By virtue of the fact that CpG dinucleotides are symmetrically methylated, the modification plays roles to maintain parental DNA methylation patterns on the daughter strand during semiconsevative DNA replication. Dnmt1 is the first identified DNA methyltransferase [13], and preferentially methylates hemi-methylated DNA in vitro [188]. Due to this preference, it was expected that Dnmt1 is responsible for maintenance DNA methylation during replication, at which stage hemi-methylated DNA is present on both daughter strands. Dnmt1$^{-/-}$ mice show global DNA demethylation during development, and do not survive past mid-gestation, demonstrating that Dnmt1 is responsible for the maintenance DNA methylation [100].

3.3.1   Structure and Properties of Dnmt1

Dnmt1 is a large protein with many subdomains. Mouse Dnmt1 contains 1620 amino acid residues (Fig. 1). The replication foci targeting sequence (RFTS) domain, the CXXC motif that contains two Zn-finger-like motifs, two bromo-adjacent homology (BAH) domains, and the C-terminal catalytic domain, follows the amino-terminal independently-folded domain. These motifs are folded independently, and the RFTS, CXXC, and two BAH domains surround and interact with the catalytic domain [180] (Fig. 5a).

The amino-terminal domain (1–243) is also folded independently [170], and binds many factors such as DMAP1, which is a factor that represses transcription in concert with histone deacetylase HDAC2 and binds Dnmt1 at replication foci to help maintain the heterochromatin state [147], and proliferating cell nuclear antigen (PCNA), which binds DNA polymerase δ, is a prerequisite factor for replication, and helps Dnmt1 in maintaining the methylation profile of the daughter DNA [29]. Dnmt1 interacts with the de novo DNA methyltransferases Dnmt3a and Dnmt3b [84], H3K9me2,3 binding protein HP1β [49], H3K9 methyltransferase, G9a [161], cyclin-dependent kinase-like 5 (CDKL5) [80], and casein kinase [172]. Dnmt1 can also bind directly to DNA itself [170].

The amino-terminal region of Dnmt1 (119–197 amino acids) binds to DNA, and preferentially binds to the minor groove of AT-rich sequences. We hypothesized that this DNA-binding activity of the domain contributes to the localization of Dnmt1 to AT-rich genome regions such as LINE1, satellite, and the promoters of tissue-specific silent genes, to maintain the fully methylated state of repaired regions that are non-replicatively hemi-methylated [170]. As the DNA binding domain of Dnmt1 overlaps with the PCNA-binding motif, the entire amino-terminal independent domain may act as a platform for factors that regulate Dnmt1.

The kinase CDKL5, which specifically phosphorylates the amino-terminal domain of Dnmt1, is reported to be a causative kinase for Rett syndrome. Rett syndrome is known to be caused by a mutation in the *MeCP2* gene, whose product specifically binds to methylated DNA and is a component of the co-repressor complex. We expect that the interaction between Dnmt1 and CDKL5 may contribute to the pathogenic process of Rett syndrome [80]. We have also identified another kinase, casein kinase 1, that interacts with the amino-terminal domain of Dnmt1. Phosphorylation by casein kinase 1 inhibits the DNA-binding activity of the amino-terminal domain [172]. Thus, the ability of the amino-terminal domain to act as a platform for regulatory factors of Dnmt1 seems to be regulated by different types of kinases [43, 94].

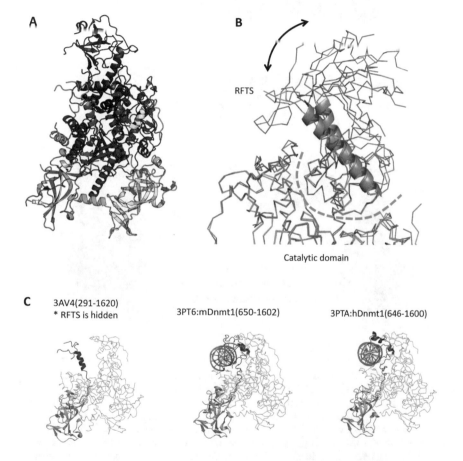

Fig. 5 Structural properties of Dnmt1. (**a**) The crystal structure of mouse Dnmt1 (291-1620). The domains in mouse Dnmt1 structure, which are RFTS, BAH1, BAH2, and catalytic domain are indicated by *purple, green, yellow*, and *red*, respectively. The connective helix between BAH1 and BAH2 showed by *light-green*. (**b**) Structural Change of RFTS. The comparison of RFTS orientation depending on the structural property of α-helix which connects the two halves of the RFTS domain. The α-helix in hDnmt1 (495–519 residues, *green*) is a straight conformation. On the other hand, the α-helix in mDnmt1 (502–524 residues, *orange*) is kinked. The *dotted-line* showed the interface between RFTS and catalytic domain. (**c**) Superimposition of CXXC-BAH1 regions.

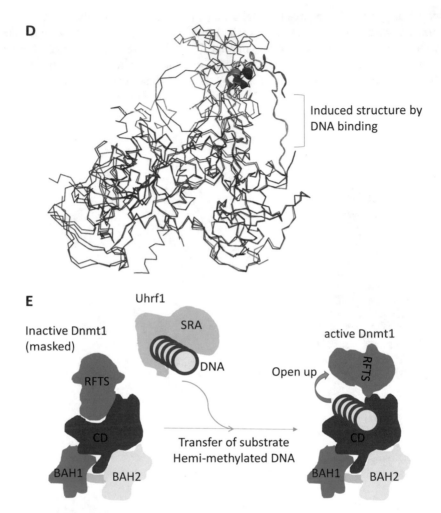

Fig. 5 (continued) The structural comparisons between three reported states of Dnmt1. The region of CXXC, CXXC-BAH1 loop, and BAH1 are shown in *magenta, blue*, and *green* color, respectively. The structure of CXXC-BAH1 loop in the auto-inhibition state (3PT6, 3PTA) is disordered, and surrounded along DNA, which is indicated with *orange*. The structure in non-substrate structure (3AV4) is shown in *left panel*. (**d**) Conformational change of BAH2 loop by DNA binding. The structure of mDnmt1 without DNA (*blue*; 3av4), and that of hDNMT1 with DNA (*brown*; 3 pt6 (active form), or *purple*; 3PTA (autoinhibited form)) is superimposed. (**e**) The release of RFTS from DNA binding pocket in exchange for DNA binding. The speculative conformational change of Dnmt1 is expected to be induced by substrate DNA. RFTS is competitively released form the catalytic domain (CD), in conjunction with a substrate DNA binding

The RFTS domain is responsible for tethering Dnmt1 to replication foci [96]. In mouse ES cells, the truncation of DNMT1's RFTS region leads to aberrant DNA methylation, corresponding to depletion of DNMT1 activity at replication foci [53]. The RFTS domain occupies the DNA binding pocket of the enzyme in the absence of DNA [175, 180]. Thus, the RFTS domain strongly inhibits DNA binding and methylation [175] and increases the methyltransferase reaction's activation energy [180]. This could be due to the evidence that the RFTS domain binds to the catalytic domain via several hydrogen bonds in mDnmt1 (291-1620) (E531, D532, D554, and L593 in RFTS and K1597, K1576, S1495, T1505 in the catalytic domain) [180]. In addition to mDnmt1, a similar hydrogen bond network is also found in hDNMT1 [207]. In hDNMT1, a unique hydrogen bond between D583 and K1535 is observed, which cannot exist in mDNMT1 because the residue corresponding to hDNMT1's D583 is substituted with alanine. Two additional associations between the RFTS domain and the catalytic domain are water-mediated hydrogen bonds (between D547's side chain and both the amide nitrogen of M1533 and the side chain hydroxyl group of Y1514) are identified in hDNMT1 [207]. In mouse, E553 interacts with M1535 and Y1615. Other structural differences in the RFTS domain between human and mouse Dnmt1 have also been reported. The main conformational difference between mDnmt1 (291–1620) and hDNMT1 (351-1600) is the amino-terminal half of the RFTS domain, despite possessing conserved folds [180, 207]. The α-helix (residues 495–519 in hDNMT1) that connects the two halves of the RFTS domain is a straight conformation, but is kinked within residues 502–524 in mDnmt1 (291-1620) (Fig. 5b). Consequently, the orientation of the first half of the RFTS domain relative to the rest of the protein deviates by 19° between the mouse and human structures [207]. It is interesting that, for mDnmt1 dimerization, both bipartite interfaces in the RTFS domain (310–409 and 476–502) are located on the amino-terminal subdomain of RFTS [47].

The CXXC domain specifically binds unmethylated CpG sites [132]. The function of the CXXC domain's DNA binding activity is controversial. Binding of unmethylated CpG sites to the CXXC domain prevents their methylation, because truncated Dnmt1 containing an intact CXXC domain shows a higher preference for methylation of hemimethylated over unmethylated substrates (17 fold) than shorter Dnmt1 not containing the CXXC domain that shows only a 2.2-fold preference [163]. In contrast, full-length Dnmt1 carrying mutations in the CXXC domain, which leads complete loss of DNA binding activity in the recombinant CXXC region, does not affect DNA substrate specify [8].

The CXXC motif sequence (694–705 amino acids in mDnmt1) forms an α-helix in crystal structure without DNA [180]. On the other hand, the structure reported by Song et al., in which RFTS deleted, is complexed with non-methylated DNA interestingly showed a unfolded loop structure (Fig.5c) [164]. Between the CXXC and BAH1 domains, a highly acidic sequence (D703-D711 in hDNMT1) is reported to negatively regulate de novo methylation [164]. The helical linker between CXXC and BAH1 in mDnmt1 binds to RFTS via hydrogen bonding. Two BAH domains, which are connected by an alpha helix and form a dumbbell-like configuration in all determined Dnmt1 structures (Fig. 5a) [163, 164, 180, 207], are linked to the catalytic domain via a (Lys-Gly)$_n$ linker (Fig. 1). A conformational change in the BAH2 loop is induced by binding to DNA, in which the loop moves towards DNA along with the target recognition domain (TRD) (Fig. 5d) [164]. The region is disordered in both DNA-free mDnmt1 (291-1620) and in the autoinhibited mDnmt1-DNA complex [163, 180]; thus, the interaction between the phosphate backbone of DNA and the amino acids in the loop (K985, Y983 and S981 in hDNMT1) support the conformation.

In contrast to other methyltransferases, Dnmt1 possesses a unique substrate specificity that favors methylation of hemi-methylated CpG-containing DNA. This unique catalytic property can be achieved by two BAH and catalytic domains, because bacterial methyltransferases do not contain BAH domains [163, 164]. The BAH2 domain loop (V956-E993 in mDnmt1) is anchored to the TRD of the methyltransferase domain, as well as hDNMT1 [180]. The main catalytic domain contains two subdomains, the TRD and the catalytic core, which are separated by a large cleft in the protein, which in turn is occupied with DNA. A co-crystal structure of the catalytic domain of Dnmt1 (721-1602) and short hemi-methylated fluorocytosine-containing DNA, in which the 5th position of the target methylation site is fluorinated, revealed that the TRD inserts into the major groove [164]. The catalytic site cysteine in the PCQ loop of mouse Dnmt1 undergoes a conformational change in response to AdoMet binding [180], while human DNMT1 (351-1600) does not [207]. Following the PCQ loop, a straight helix from residues 1243 to 1261 is observed in a productive Dnmt1 (721-1602) complex with DNA [164], while the helix is kinked in both Dnmt1 (291-1620) alone and the autoinhibited Dnmt1 complex with DNA [163, 180], indicating that the catalytic domain structure could be changed during catalysis. In mDnmt1 (291-1620), F1238, Y1243, and F1246 in the helix that follows the PCQ-loop form hydrophobic interactions with F631, F634, and F635 in the linker region between the RFTS domain and CXXC motif, and the interactions contribute to narrowing the entrance of the DNA-binding pocket and to anchoring the RFTS domain to the DNA-binding pocket, and consequently the catalytic center is completely masked (Fig. 5e) [180]. In the bacterial DNA methyltransferase M. HhaI-DNA complex, the target cytosine is no longer buried within the double helix, but rotates on its flanking sugar-phosphate bonds and leads to base flipping and projection into the catalytic pocket [26, 85]. In contrast to bacterial methyltransferase, not only the target cytosine but also a base on the opposite strand located at the neighboring CpG site are flipped out in hDNMT1(731-1602) [164]. Further investigations and integrating with the reported properties could elucidate the molecular mechanism of maintenance methylation and species-specific differences in reaction mechanism.

3.3.2 Factors Necessary for Maintenance DNA Methylation

In the process of DNA replication, Dnmt1 methylates hemi-methylated CpG sites that are generated at the replication fork. Dnmt1 methylates hemi-methylated DNA in a processive manner even in the absence of the amino-terminal domain containing the PCNA-binding sequence [188]. However, the fidelity as to maintenance of full-methylation patterns seems to be surprisingly low, being about 95% in vitro [188]. Since the fidelity in vivo is reported to be more than 99% [184], other factor(s) may help to maintain DNA methylation patterns. Dnmt1 binds to PCNA, which forms a ring shaped trimer, and PCNA clamp-bound DNA is methylated more efficiently by Dnmt1 than free DNA [73]; thus, PCNA promotes DNA methylation processivity in vivo.

Uhrf1 (Ubiquitin-like, containing PHD and RING finger domains, 1), also known as Np95 in mouse and ICBP (Inverted CCAAT box Binding Protein) in human, is required for the propagation of methylation patterns to the next generation (maintenance methylation) in vivo [157, 17]. Uhrf1 knockout mice show similar phenotypes to Dnmt1 null mice including genomic DNA hypomethylation and developmental arrest at embryonic day 9.5 [157, 100]. Uhrf1 contains a domain called SET and Ring finger Associated (SRA), which specifically binds hemi-methylated DNA and flips the methylated cytosine out of double-stranded DNA [5, 7, 68]. Since the RFTS domain of Dnmt1 is reported to be necessary for Dnmt1localization to replication foci [96], it is reasonable to expect that the RFTS and SRA domains functionally interact during maintenance methylation. The direct interaction of the RFTS domain of Dnmt1 with the SRA domain of Uhrf1 is necessary for faithful propagation of methylation patterns to the next generation in vivo. In addition, Uhrf1 increases Dnmt1's activity and specificity in vitro [12, 8]. As hemimethylated DNA is not simultaneously recognized by SRA and the catalytic domain of Dnmt1, the DNA substrate is expected to be transferred from SRA to Dnmt1 (Fig. 5e); the corresponding molecular mechanism has yet to be elucidated.

Dnmt1 selectively binds to the di-ubiquitylated Lys23 of histone H3 (H3K23ub2) to perform maintenance methylation [121]. Abrogation of the interaction between RFTS and catalytic domain rather results in non-ubiquitinated H3 binding by using Xenopus lysate [118]. Interestingly, the Ring-finger motif of Uhrf1, which is a prerequisite factor for maintenance methylation, is involved in the ubiquitylation as an E3 ligase. In mouse ES cells, H3K18 instead of H3K23 is identified as the ubiquitination target on H3 by Uhrf1 using mass spectrometry, and the modification is recognized by the ubiquitin interaction motif of Dnmt1's RTFS domain [136]. Qin et al. also reported that RFTS recognizes H2AK119Ub [136]. Further, the tandem tudor domain and the PHD finger of Uhrf1 are readers of H3K9me3 and unmethylated H3R2 [6], and mutations that inhibit recognition of H3K9me3 also partly inhibit maintenance DNA methylation [146]. Recognition of histone H3R2, H3K9me3 and hemimethylated DNA by Uhrf1 is necessary for DNA methylation by Dnmt1 [136]. Thus, Uhrf1 exerts a multifaceted influence on maintenance DNA methylation, in concert with histone modifications.

Nucleosomal structure also regulates Dnmt1 activity [59, 124, 144, 154]. When mononucleosomes that were reconstituted with unmodified histones and DNA containing several hemimethylated sites is used as a substrate, DNMT1 is able to methylate a number of CpG sites even when the DNA major groove is oriented toward the histone surface [124]. However the ability of DNMT1 to methylate nucleosomal sites is highly dependent on the DNA sequence, because nucleosomes containing the *Air* promoter are refractory to methylation irrespective of target cytosine location, whereas ones reconstituted with the H19 imprinting control region are more accessible [124]. Robertson et al. showed that the steady-state activity of Dnmt1 towards mononucleosomes is similar to that towards naked DNA, but K_m values for mononucleosomes are increased [144]. Gowher et al. reported that Dnmt1 can efficiently methylate nucleosomal DNA without dissociation of the histone octamer from the DNA. In addition, Schrander et al. recently reported that nucleosome structure inhibits Dnmt1 activity [154]. The effect of nucleosome structure on Dnmt1 activity is controversial, and remains to be elucidated.

DNMT1 also interacts with the hSNF2H chromatin remodeling enzyme [144]. Addition of hSNF2H increases the binding affinity of DNMT1 for mononucleosomes in in vitro assays; however, the activity of Dnmt1 is not stimulated by hSNF2H [144]. Another recent report shows that Dnmt1 activity towards oligonucleosomes reconstituted with hemimethylated DNA is stimulated by the chromatin remodeling factors Brg1 or ACF [154]. Thus, chromosome structure and histone modifications could regulate site-specific DNA methylation.

3.3.3   Exceptional Expression of Dnmt1 and Its Localization

Expression of Dnmt1 is regulated in a cell cycle-dependent manner. The localization of Dnmt1 in nuclei is changed throughout the cell cycle, reflecting the contributions of both the PCNA binding motif during S phase and RFTS domain-mediated heterochromatin association during late S and G2 phase [39]. Dnmt1 is stable in proliferating cells and during S phase. Its half-life becomes short when cells are terminally differentiated or outside of S-phase [109]. This makes sense in light of Dnmt1's main role in methylating hemi-methylated DNA produced during replication. As exceptions, however, the expression levels of Dnmt1 in oocytes and neurons, which are not proliferating and post-mitotic, respectively, are quite high, and Dnmt1 is localized outside of nuclei [115, 74] in these cell types. In mouse oocytes, an oocyte-specific Dnmt1 isoform missing the amino-terminal 118 amino acid residues is expressed, and Dnmt1 is excluded from nuclei [115, 54]. This localization contributes to the global demethylation observed in early-stage embryos prior to implantation. As DNA methylation in neurons is dynamically regulated, and Dnmt1 mutants lead to neurological disorders such as cerebellar ataxia, deafness, and narcolepsy [196], the localization of Dnmt1 outside of nuclei in a large quantity might function as a pool for occasional writing of DNA methylation patterns for establishing or erasing memory.

Since *Dnmt1* null mice die as early embryos and Dnmt1 is crucial for maintenance of established DNA methylation patterns, it has been hard to reconcile the fact that that milder phenotypes, such as disease, are caused by mutation of Dnmt1. Recently, however, point mutations in Dnmt1 that cause autosomal neuropathy were reported by independent groups [196, 129]. All the mutations that cause neuronal diseases are located in the RFTS and on the interaction surface to the catalytic domain. As the diseases caused by these mutations are of late onset, Dnmt1 is likely to have interesting post-developmental roles.

3.4   Cross-Talk Between de novo- and Maintenance-Type DNA Methyltransferases

Establishment of DNA methylation patterns is mainly performed by the de novo DNA methyltransferases, Dnmt3a and Dnmt3b, while Dnmt1 maintains methylation patterns during replication, as described above. However, for maintaining the methylation of repetitive elements, it was reported that both Dnmt1 and Dnmt3a and/or Dnmt3b are necessary [102]. In *Dnmt3a* and *Dnmt3b* double-knockout ES cells, which are expected not to establish novel DNA methylation patterns, DNA methylation gradually decreases during cell culture [23]. DNA methylation gradually decreases in mouse embryonic fibroblasts due to *Dnmt3b* but not *Dnmt3a* deletion [37]. These reports indicate that not only Dnmt1 but also de novo-type DNA methyltransferases Dnmt3a and/or Dnmt3b contribute to the maintenance of DNA methylation. Consistent with this, there has been a report that Dnmt3a and Dnmt3b interact with Dnmt1 at the amino-terminal region [84]. It is unlikely, however, that Dnmt3a and Dnmt3b co-exist with Dnmt1 at replication foci since Dnmt1 is loaded at an early stage of replication, and Dnmt3a and Dnmt3b at a rather late stage of replication [1].

As for the establishment of DNA methylation patterns, it was expected that Dnmt1 would exhibit de novo methylation activity in vivo [28]. In fact, Dnmt1 exhibits a significant level of de novo-type DNA methylation activity in vitro [45, 100]. Ectopically overexpressed Dnmt1 introduces de novo DNA methylation [176, 187, 14]. In *Dnmt3a* and *Dnmt3b* knockout embryonic stem cells, ectopically introduced DNA [112] as well as endogenous regions [3], received de novo DNA methylation. This could be due to the fact that Dnmt1 apparently favors de novo methylation near pre-existing methylation sites [188, 3].

4 Modifications of Dnmts

It has been reported that Dnmts are post-translationally modified by methylation, phosphorylation, acetylation, sumoylation, and that some of these modifications alter their activity and stability. SET7 is a large family of lysine methyltransferases containing a SET domain [43]. Although the major target of SET7 is histone H3 lysine 4, which promotes a euchromatin state, lysine 142 of Dnmt1 is also methylated by SET7 during S and G2 phase [43]. Methylated Dnmt1 is less stable, because the modification facilitates proteasome-mediated degradation. Mono-methylated lysine 142 on Dnmt1 is recognized by PHF20L1, and its binding blocks proteasomal degradation of Dnmt1 [42]. Methylation on Dnmt1 is removed by lysine specific demethylase (LSD) [133], implying that a balance between SET7 and LSD may finely tune the expression level of Dnmt1.

Adjacent to lysine 142, serine 143 on Dnmt1 is phosphorylated by AKT kinase [43]. Phosphorylation of this residue blocks SET7 methylation of peptides in vitro, and the phosphorylated Dnmt1 displays increased half-life compared with methylated Dnmt1 [43]. Because Dnmt1 contains an AKT1 target sequence, the overexpression of AKT1 leads to increased phosphorylation levels of Dnmt1, and the AKT1 inhibitor causes Dnmt1 degradation and DNA hypomethylation [43]. In addition, S515 located in the RFTS domain is phosphorylated, and exogenously added peptides phosphorylated at S515 inhibit Dnmt1 activity to a greater extent than unmodified peptide, in vitro [60].

Recently, USP7 was shown to bind to KG repeats on DNMT1, and this interaction is required for USP7-mediated stabilization of DNMT1 [27]. Acetylation of KG repeats impairs the DNMT1-USP7 interaction and promotes degradation of DNMT1 [27]. In addition, DNMT1 is destabilized by acetylation by the acetyltransferase,

Tip60, as acetylation-triggered ubiquitination by the E3 ligase UHRF1 targets DNMT1 for proteasomal degradation [38]. In contrast, histone deacetylase 1 (HDAC1) and herpes virus-associated ubiquitin-specific protease (HAUSP) protect DNMT1 from degradation by deacetylation and deubiquitination, respectively [38]. Dnmt1 binds to Ubc9, a member of the E2 family, as well as SUMO-1, and is sumoylated at several lysine residues throughout the protein. The sumoylation significantly enhances DNA methylation activity of Dnmt1 [95].

In addition to Dnmt1, Dnmt3a and Dnmt3b are also posttranslationally modified. Sumoylation on Dnmt3a occurs in its PWWP domain [106, 82]. The sumoylation of Dnmt3a disrupts the interaction between Dnmt3a and HDACs, allowing abolishment of transcriptional repression [106]. The amino-terminal region of Dnmt3b is also sumoylated, but the function is not elucidated [82].

Two amino acid residues (S386 and S389) in the PWWP domain of Dnmt3a are phosphorylated by CK2, and the phosphorylation represses the methylation activity of Dnmt3a [35]. CK2 phosphorylation modulates CpG methylation of several repeats, and is required for localization of Dnmt3a to heterochromatin [35]. ERK2 interacts with L373 and/or L637 in human DNMT3a and this interaction supports the efficient phosphorylation of S255A in mesenchymal cells [91]. The ERK and Dnmt3a interaction and phosphorylation attenuates binding of DNMT3a to SOX9 promoters, which contributes to cell signaling in these cells [91].

5   DNA Methylation and Aging

Global levels of 5mC are reduced in senescent cells, compared with actively dividing cells [30]. Age-associated DNA methylation alterations have been reported in blood, brain, kidney and muscle tissue, and both common and unique methylation alterations between different tissues are identified [32]. Aging-associated DNA methylation alteration is also observed in sperm [122].

Since the function of the hematopoietic system declines and autoimmune and inflammatory disorders with age are increased, it is important to analyze epigenetic modification and gene expression in hematopoietic stem cells in young and older animals. Recently, whole genome bisulfite sequencing in hematopoietic stem cells from 4 and 24 month old mice unearthed a small increment in global DNA methylation in older mice and hypomethylation of specific genes [173]. The hematopoietic stem cell-specific genes, Gata2 and Hinga2, are hypomethylated and upregulated in older mice, while the binding sites for a transcription factor associated with differentiation, Pu.1, are hypermethylated [173]. The change of methylation could misregulate gene expression by regulating the targeting of transcriptional factor(s). To understand the epigenetic changes during aging, detailed epigenetic maps will be required. Further insights into the epigenetics of aging may hold great promise in the treatment of aging and aging-related diseases.

6 Inhibitors of Dnmts

The pharmacological inhibition of DNA methylation represents an attractive strategy for treatment of the cancer patient [44], because DNA methylation, as well as genetic mutations, contributes to tumorigenesis [131]. Among the several potential DNA methyltransferase inhibitors, the nucleotide analogues 5-azacytidine and 5-aza-2'-deoxycytidine (decitbine) are the most well-known. The cytosine analogues in which the carbon atom in position 5 is replaced by a nitrogen atom, and the analogies cause covalent trapping and subsequent depletion of Dnmts, after incorporation into DNA [152, 89]. Substantial cellular and clinical toxicity of azanucleotide has led to the development of a number of substances to inhibit Dnmt1. Following the azanucleotides, other analogues such as 5,6-dihydro-5 azacytidine and 5-fluoro-2'-deoxycytidine have also been synthesized and examined for inhibition activity. In addition to the nucleotide analogues, sinefungin is reported to act as a SAM or SAH analogue to inhibit Dnmt [105]. Future study of drugs to regulate the activity of Dnmt enzymes, and to reduce side effects, will contribute to cancer treatments and for manipulating stem cell aging. Site-specific introduction of DNA methylation activity could also play a role in treatment or delay of disease. Recently, an oxime compound has been identified as binding to the 5mC pocket of Uhrf1 [119]. The compound reduces the interaction between Dnmt1 and Uhrf1 in vivo, and reduces the global DNA methylation level to around half of the level in wild type cells.

7 DNA Demethylation

CpG methylation is physiologically removed through both active and passive mechanisms. Active demethylation is dependent on enzymatic process, while passive demethylation happens as a result of semiconservative DNA replication. In active demethylation, hydroxymethylated cytosine (5hmC) is noted to be an intermediate [88, 158]. The TET (ten-eleven translocation) enzymes successively oxidize 5mC to 5hmC, 5-formyl C (5fC), and 5-carboxyl C (5caC), in an Fe(II) and 2-oxoglutarate-dependent oxidization reaction [88]. 5hmC is the most abundant among the 5mC oxidants, and 0.67% of 5mC is hydroxymethylated in human brain [98]. Specific roles for 5hmC in gene expression control through chromatin regulation have been recently shown [158], leading to 5hmC's designation as the "6th base". The level of 5hmC in cancers of the breast, liver, lung, pancreas, and prostate is dramatically lower than that in surrounding noncancerous tissues, and the reduction of 5hmC is associated with the declining expression of TET proteins [90]. Further oxidized methylcytosine derivatives, 5fC and 5caC are processed by thymine-DNA glycosylase (TDG) followed by base excision repair, completing the active DNA demethylation process [86]. Deamination of 5hmC by AID/APOBEC can also promote the decrease of 5hmC, as the resulting 5-hydroxymethyluracil (hmU) is excised by TDG, SMUG1 or MBD4 glycosylases [61].

On the other hand, 5hmC also contributes to passive demethylation. As 5hmC is not strongly recognized by Dnmt1, and the SRA domain of Uhrf1only weakly binds to hemi-hydroxymethylated DNA [185, 128], 5hmC at hemi-hydroxymethylated CpG sites leads to the addition of unmodified cytosines on the daughter strand during DNA replication and repair. Recently, 5hmC has been shown to accumulate locally at damaged DNA when mammalian culture cells or primary neurons are treated with DNA-damaging compounds, laser microirradiation, UV, or γ-rays [76, 79]. Deficiency of Tet enzymes was further shown to elicit chromosome segregation defects in mouse embryonic stem cells treated with aphidicolin [79], and telomere fusions were shown to result [202] from misregulated subtelomeric methylation due to combined deficiency for Tet1 and Tet2. Therefore, 5hmC likely functions in aspects of chromosome biology, including DNA repair, in addition to its roles in DNA methylation and gene expression. With the recent advance of techniques to analyze 5hmC in genomic DNA at single-base resolution [204, 16, 177, 50, 51], the contribution of 5hmC to DNA demethylation and other process will be unraveled in the near future.

8 Perspective

By genome-wide analysis, the patterns of DNA methylation and histone modification(s) have been collected, and the correlation and functional interaction(s) is proposed. Dnmts directly and indirectly recognize histone tail peptides carrying specific modifications. The molecular mechanism(s) underlying establishment of DNA methylation pattern has elucidated. In spite of recent advances, how Dnmts recognize the modifications on nucleosome structure is not clear. A full understanding of the molecular mechanisms regulating DNA methylation awaits future biochemical, structural, and functional studies. These molecular-level analyses will help us to figure out the detailed function and/or regulatory mechanism(s) of DNA methylation in vivo.

References

1. Alabert C, Bukowski-Wills J-C, Lee S-B, Kustatscher G, Nakamura K, de Lima Alves F, Menard P, Mejlvang J, Rappsilber J, Groth A (2014) Nascent chromatin capture proteomics determines chromatin dynamics during DNA replication and identifies unknown fork components. Nat Cell Biol 16:281–293
2. Aoki A, Suetake I, Miyagawa J, Fujio T, Chijiwa T, Sasaki H, Tajima S (2001) Enzymatic properties of de novo-type mouse DNA (cytosine-5) methyltransferases. Nucleic Acids Res 29:3506–3512
3. Arand J, Spieler D, Karius T, Branco MR, Meilinger D, Meissner A, Jenuwein T, Xu G, Leonhardt H, Wolf V et al (2012) In vivo control of CpG and non-CpG DNA methylation by DNA methyltransferases. PLoS Genet 8:1–11
4. Argentaro A, Yang J-C, Chapman L, Kowalczyk MS, Gibbons RJ, Higgs DR, Neuhaus D, Rhodes D (2007) Structural consequences of disease-causing mutations in the ATRX-DNMT3-DNMT3L (ADD) domain of the chromatin-associated protein ATRX. Proc Natl Acad Sci U S A 104:11939–11944

5. Arita K, Ariyoshi M, Tochio H, Nakamura Y, Shirakawa M (2008) Recognition of hemi-methylated DNA by the SRA protein UHRF1 by a base-flipping mechanism. Nature 455:818–821

6. Arita K, Isogai S, Oda T, Unoki M, Sugita K, Sekiyama N, Kuwata K, Hamamoto R, Tochio H, Sato M et al (2012) Recognition of modification status on a histone H3 tail by linked histone reader modules of the epigenetic regulator UHRF1. Proc Natl Acad Sci U S A 109:12950–12955

7. Avvakumov GV, Walker JR, Xue S, Li Y, Duan S, Bronner C, Arrowsmith CH, Dhe-Paganon S (2008) Structural basis for recognition of hemi-methylated DNA by the SRA domain of human UHRF1. Nature 455:822–825

8. Bashtrykov P, Jankevicius G, Smarandache A, Jurkowska RZ, Ragozin S, Jeltsch A (2012) Specificity of dnmt1 for methylation of hemimethylated CpG sites resides in its catalytic domain. Chem Biol 19:572–578

9. Baubec T, Colombo DF, Wirbelauer C, Schmidt J, Burger L, Krebs AR, Akalin A, Schübeler D (2015) Genomic profiling of DNA methyltransferases reveals a role for DNMT3B in genic methylation. Nature 520:243–247

10. Bell AC, Felsenfeld G (2000) Methylation of a CTCF-dependent boundary controls imprinted expression of the Igf2 gene. Nature 405:482–485

11. Bergman Y, Cedar H (2013) DNA methylation dynamics in health and disease. Nat Struct Mol Biol 20:274–281

12. Berkyurek AC, Suetake I, Arita K, Takeshita K, Nakagawa A, Shirakawa M, Tajima S (2014) The DNA methyltransferase Dnmt1 directly interacts with the SET and RING finger-associated (SRA) domain of the multifunctional protein Uhrf1 to facilitate accession of the catalytic center to hemi-methylated DNA. J Biol Chem 289:379–386

13. Bestor T, Laudano A, Mattaliano R, Ingram V (1988) Cloning and sequencing of a cDNA encoding DNA methyltransferase of mouse cells. J Mol Biol 203:971–983

14. Biniszkiewicz D, Gribnau J, Ramsahoye B, Gaudet F, Eggan K, Humpherys D, Mastrangelo M, Jun Z, Walter J, Jaenisch R (2002) Dnmt1 Overexpression Causes Genomic Hypermethylation , Loss of Imprinting , and Embryonic Lethality. Mol Cell Biol 22:2124–2135

15. Bird A (2002) DNA methylation patterns and epigenetic memory DNA methylation patterns and epigenetic memory. Genes Dev 16:6–21

16. Booth MJ, Branco MR, Ficz G, Oxley D, Krueger F, Reik W, Balasubramanian S (2012) Quantitative sequencing of 5-Methylcytosine and 5-Hydroxymethylcytosine at Single-Base resolution. Science 336:934–937

17. Bostick M, Kim JK, Estève P-O, Clark A, Pradhan S, Jacobsen SE (2007) UHRF1 plays a role in maintaining DNA methylation in mammalian cells. Science 317:1760–1764

18. Bourc'his D, Bestor TH (2004) Meiotic catastrophe and retrotransposon reactivation in male germ cells lacking Dnmt3L. Nature 431:96–99

19. Brenner C, Deplus R, Line Didelot C, Loriot A, Viré E, De Smet C, Gutierrez A, Danovi D, Bernard D, Boon T et al (2005) Myc represses transcription through recruitment of DNA methyltransferase corepressor. EMBO J 24:336–346

20. Catez F, Ueda T, Bustin M (2006) Determinants of histone H1 mobility and chromatin binding in living cells. Nat Struct Mol Biol 13:305–310

21. Chang Y, Sun L, Kokura K, Horton JR, Fukuda M, Espejo A, Izumi V, Koomen JM, Bedford MT, Zhang X et al (2011) MPP8 mediates the interactions between DNA methyltransferase Dnmt3a and H3K9 methyltransferase GLP/G9a. Nat Commun 2:533

22. Chen T, Ueda Y, Xie S, Li E (2002) A novel Dnmt3a isoform produced from an alternative promoter localizes to euchromatin and its expression correlates with active de novo methylation. J Biol Chem 277:38746–38754

23. Chen T, Ueda Y, Dodge JE, Wang Z, Li E (2003) Establishment and maintenance of genomic methylation patterns in mouse embryonic stem cells by Dnmt3a and Dnmt3b. Mol Cell Biol 23:5594–5605

24. Chen T, Tsujimoto N, Li E (2004) The PWWP domain of Dnmt3a and Dnmt3b is required for directing DNA methylation to the major satellite repeats at pericentric heterochromatin. Mol Cell Biol 24:9048–9058

25. Chen ZX, Mann JR, Hsieh CL, Riggs AD, Chédin F (2005) Physical and functional interactions between the human DNMT3L protein and members of the de novo methyltransferase family. J Cell Biochem 95:902–917

26. Cheng X, Roberts RJ (2001) AdoMet-dependent methylation, DNA methyltransferases and base flipping. Nucleic Acids Res 29:3784–3795

27. Cheng J, Yang H, Fang J, Ma L, Gong R, Wang P, Li Z, Xu Y (2015) Molecular mechanism for USP7-mediated DNMT1 stabilization by acetylation. Nat Commun 6:7023

28. Christman JK, Sheikhnejad G, Marasco CJ, Sufrin JR (1995) 5-methyl-2′-deoxycytidine in single-stranded DNA can act in cis to signal de novo DNA methylation. Proc Natl Acad Sci U S A 92:7347–7351

29. Chuang LSH, Ian HI, Koh TW, Ng HH, Xu GL, Li BFL (1997) Human DNA (cytosine-5) methyltransferase PCNA complex as a target for p21 (WAF1). Science 277:1996–2000

30. Cruickshanks HA, McBryan T, Nelson DM, Vanderkraats ND, Shah PP, van Tuyn J, Singh Rai T, Brock C, Donahue G, Dunican DS et al (2013) Senescent cells harbour features of the cancer epigenome. Nat Cell Biol 15:1495–1506

31. Datta J, Majumder S, Bai S, Ghoshal K, Kutay H, Smith DS, Crabb JW, Jacob ST (2005) Physical and functional interaction of DNA methyltransferase 3A with Mbd3 and Brg1 in mouse lymphosarcoma cells. Cancer Res 65:10891–10900

32. Day K, Waite LL, Thalacker-Mercer A, West A, Bamman MM, Brooks JD, Myers RM, Absher D (2013) Differential DNA methylation with age displays both common and dynamic features across human tissues that are influenced by CpG landscape. Genome Biol 14:R102

33. Defossez PA, Stancheva I (2011) Biological functions of methyl-CpG-binding proteins. 1st ed. Elsevier Inc.. Prog Mol Biol Transl Sci 101:377–98. doi: 10.1016/B978-0-12-387685-0.00012-3

34. Dempster EL, Pidsley R, Schalkwyk LC, Owens S, Georgiades A, Kane F, Kalidindi S, Picchioni M, Kravariti E, Toulopoulou T et al (2011) Disease-associated epigenetic changes in monozygotic twins discordant for schizophrenia and bipolar disorder. Hum Mol Genet 20:4786–4796

35. Deplus R, Blanchon L, Rajavelu A, Boukaba A, Defrance M, Luciani J, Rothe F, Dedeurwaerder S, Denis H, Brinkman AB et al (2014) Regulation of DNA methylation patterns by CK2-mediated phosphorylation of Dnmt3a. Cell Rep 8:743–753

36. Dhayalan A, Rajavelu A, Rathert P, Tamas R, Jurkowska RZ, Ragozin S, Jeltsch A (2010) The Dnmt3a PWWP domain reads histone 3 lysine 36 trimethylation and guides DNA methylation. J Biol Chem 285:26114–26120

37. Dodget JE, Okano M, Dick F, Tsujimoto N, Chen T, Wang S, Ueda Y, Dyson N, Li E (2005) Inactivation of Dnmt3b in mouse embryonic fibroblasts results in DNA hypomethylation, chromosomal instability, and spontaneous immortalization. J Biol Chem 280:17986–17991

38. Du Z, Song J, Wang Y, Zhao Y, Guda K, Yang S, Kao H-Y, Xu Y, Willis J, Markowitz SD et al (2010) DNMT1 stability is regulated by proteins coordinating Deubiquitination and acetylation-driven Ubiquitination. Sci. Signal. 3:ra80

39. Easwaran HP, Schermelleh L, Leonhardt H, Cardoso MC (2004) Replication-independent chromatin loading of Dnmt1 during G2 and M phases. EMBO Rep 5:1181–1186

40. El Gazzar M, Yoza BK, Chen X, Hu J, Hawkins GA, McCall CE (2008) G9a and HP1 couple histone and DNA methylation to TNFα transcription silencing during endotoxin tolerance. J Biol Chem 283:32198–32208

41. Esteller M (2007) Cancer epigenomics: DNA methylomes and histone-modification maps. Nat Rev Genet 8:286–298

42. Esteve PO, Terragni J, Deepti K, Chin HG, Dai N, Espejo A, Corrêa IR, Bedford MT, Pradhan S (2014) Methyllysine reader plant homeodomain (PHD) finger protein 20-like 1 (PHF20L1) antagonizes DNA (cytosine-5) methyltransferase 1 (DNMT1) proteasomal degradation. J Biol Chem 289:8277–8287

43. Estève P-O, Chang Y, Samaranayake M, Upadhyay AK, Horton JR, Feehery GR, Cheng X, Pradhan S (2011) A methylation and phosphorylation switch between an adjacent lysine and serine determines human DNMT1 stability. Nat Struct Mol Biol 18:42–48

44. Fahy J, Jeltsch A, Arimondo PB (2012) DNA methyltransferase inhibitors in cancer: a chemical and therapeutic patent overview and selected clinical studies. Expert Opin Ther Pat 22:1–16

45. Fatemi M, Hermann A, Pradhan S, Jeltsch A (2001) The activity of the murine DNA methyltransferase Dnmt1 is controlled by interaction of the catalytic domain with the N-terminal part of the enzyme leading to an allosteric activation of the enzyme after binding to methylated DNA. J Mol Biol 309:1189–1199

46. Felle M, Hoffmeister H, Rothammer J, Fuchs A, Exler JH, Längst G (2011) Nucleosomes protect DNA from DNA methylation in vivo and in vitro. Nucleic Acids Res 39:6956–6969

47. Fellinger K, Rothbauer U, Felle M, Längst G, Leonhardt H (2009) Dimerization of DNA methyltransferase 1 is mediated by its regulatory domain. J Cell Biochem 106:521–528

48. Fuks F, Burgers WA, Godin N, Kasai M, Kouzarides T (2001) Dnmt3a binds deacetylases and is recruited by a sequence-specific repressor to silence transcription. EMBO J 20:2536–2544

49. Fuks F, Hurd PJ, Deplus R, Kouzarides T (2003) The DNA methyltransferases associate with HP1 and the SUV39H1 histone methyltransferase. Nucleic Acids Res 31:2305–2312

50. Fukuzawa S, Tachibana K, Tajima S, Suetake I (2015) Selective oxidation of 5-hydroxymethylcytosine with micelle incarcerated oxidants to determine it at single base resolution. Bioorganic Med Chem Lett 25:5667–5671

51. Fukuzawa S, Takahashi S, Tachibana K, Tajima S, Suetake I (2016) Simple and accurate single base resolution analysis of 5-hydroxymethylcytosine by catalytic oxidative bisulfite sequencing using micelle incarcerated oxidants. Bioorg Med Chem 24:4254–4262

52. Gardiner-Garden M, Frommer M (1987) CpG Islands in Vertebrate Genomes. JMolBiol 196:261–282

53. Garvilles RG, Hasegawa T, Kimura H, Sharif J, Muto M, Koseki H, Takahashi S, Suetake I, Tajima S (2015) Dual functions of the RFTS domain of dnmt1 in replication-coupled DNA methylation and in protection of the genome from aberrant methylation. PLoS One 10:1–19

54. Gaudet F, Talbot D, Leonhardt H, Jaenisch R (1998) A short DNA methyltransferase isoform restores methylation in vivo. J Biol Chem 273:32725–32729

55. Ge YZ, Pu MT, Gowher H, Wu HP, Ding JP, Jeltsch A, Xu GL (2004) Chromatin targeting of de novo DNA methyltransferases by the PWWP domain. J Biol Chem 279:25447–25454

56. Gelfman S, Cohen N, Yearim A, Ast G (2013) DNA-methylation effect on cotranscriptional splicing is dependent on GC architecture of the exon – intron structure DNA-methylation effect on cotranscriptional splicing is dependent on GC architecture of the exon – intron structure. Genome Res 23:789–799

57. Goll MG, Kirpekar F, Maggert KA, Yoder JA, Hsieh C-L, Zhang X, Golic KG, Jacobsen SE, Bestor TH (2006) Methylation of tRNAAsp by the DNA methyltransferase homolog Dnmt2. Science 311:395–398

58. Gopalakrishnan S, Sullivan BA, Trazzi S, Della Valle G, Robertson KD (2009) DNMT3B interacts with constitutive centromere protein CENP-C to modulate DNA methylation and the histone code at centromeric regions. Hum Mol Genet 18:3178–3193

59. Gowher H, Stockdale CJ, Goyal R, Ferreira H, Owen-Hughes T, Jeltsch A (2005) De novo methylation of nucleosomal DNA by the mammalian Dnmt1 and Dnmt3A DNA methyltransferases. Biochemistry 44:9899–9904

60. Goyal R, Rathert P, Laser H, Gowher H, Jeltsch A (2007) Phosphorylation of serine-515 activates the mammalian maintenance methyltransferase Dnmt1. Epigenetics 2:155–160

61. Guo JU, Su Y, Zhong C, Ming GL, Song H (2011) Hydroxylation of 5-methylcytosine by TET1 promotes active DNA demethylation in the adult brain. Cell 145:423–434

62. Guo JU, Su Y, Shin JH, Shin J, Li H, Xie B, Zhong C, Hu S, Le T, Fan G et al (2014) Distribution, recognition and regulation of non-CpG methylation in the adult mammalian brain. Nat Neurosci 17:215–222

63. Guo X, Wang L, Li J, Ding Z, Xiao J, Yin X, He S, Shi P, Dong L, Li G et al (2015) Structural insight into autoinhibition and histone H3-induced activation of DNMT3A. Nature 517:640–644

64. Handa V, Jeltsch A (2005) Profound flanking sequence preference of Dnmt3a and Dnmt3b mammalian DNA methyltransferases shape the human epigenome. J Mol Biol 348:1103–1112
65. Hansen RS, Wijmenga C, Luo P, Stanek AM, Canfield TK, Weemaes CM, Gartler SM (1999) The DNMT3B DNA methyltransferase gene is mutated in the ICF immunodeficiency syndrome. Proc Natl Acad Sci U S A 96:14412–14417
66. Hark AT, Schoenherr CJ, Katz DJ, Ingram RS, Levorse JM, Tilghman SM (2000) CTCF mediates methylation-sensitive enhancer-blocking activity at the H19/Igf2 locus. Nature 405:486–489
67. Harrington MA, Jones PA, Imagawa M, Karin M (1988) Cytosine methylation does not affect binding of transcription factor Sp1. Proc Natl Acad Sci 85:2066–2070
68. Hashimoto H, Horton JR, Zhang X, Bostick M, Jacobsen SE, Cheng X (2008) The SRA domain of UHRF1 flips 5-methylcytosine out of the DNA helix. Nature 455:826–829
69. Hata K, Okano M, Lei H, Li E (2002) Dnmt3L cooperates with the Dnmt3 family of de novo DNA methyltransferases to establish maternal imprints in mice. Development 129:1983–1993
70. Hellman A (2007) Gene body – specific methylation. Science 315:1141–1143
71. Horii T, Suetake I, Yanagisawa E, Morita S, Kimura M, Nagao Y, Imai H, Tajima S, Hatada I (2011) The Dnmt3b splice variant is specifically expressed in in vitro-manipulated blastocysts and their derivative ES cells. J Reprod Dev 57:579–585
72. Hu YG, Hirasawa R, Hu JL, Hata K, Li CL, Jin Y, Chen T, Li E, Rigolet M, Viegas-Pequignot E et al (2008) Regulation of DNA methylation activity through Dnmt3L promoter methylation by Dnmt3 enzymes in embryonic development. Hum Mol Genet 17:2654–2664
73. Iida T, Suetake I, Tajima S, Morioka H, Ohta S, Obuse C, Tsurimoto T (2002) PCNA clamp facilitates action of DNA cytosine methyltransferase 1 on hemimethylated DNA. Genes Cells 7:997–1007
74. Inano K, Suetake I, Ueda T, Miyake Y, Nakamura M, Okada M, Tajima S (2000) Maintenance-type DNA Methyltransferase is highly expressed in post-mitotic neurons and localized in the cytoplasmic compartment. J Biochem 128:315–321
75. Jia D, Jurkowska RZ, Zhang X, Jeltsch A, Cheng X (2007) Structure of Dnmt3a bound to Dnmt3L suggests a model for de novo DNA methylation. Nature 449:248–251
76. Jiang D, Zhang Y, Hart RP, Chen J, Herrup K, Li J (2015) Alteration in 5-hydroxymethylcytosine-mediated epigenetic regulation leads to Purkinje cell vulnerability in ATM deficiency. Brain 138:3520–3536
77. Jones P, Baylin SB (2002) The fundamental role of epigenetic events in cancer. Nat Rev Genet 3:415–428
78. Jung M, Pfeifer GP (2015) Aging and DNA methylation. BMC Biol 13:7
79. Kafer GR, Li X, Horii T, Suetake I, Tajima S, Hatada I, Carlton PM, Kafer GR, Li X, Horii T et al (2016) 5-Hydroxymethylcytosine marks sites of DNA damage and promotes genome stability 5-Hydroxymethylcytosine marks sites of DNA damage and promotes genome stability. Cell Rep 14:1283–1292
80. Kameshita I, Sekiguchi M, Hamasaki D, Sugiyama Y, Hatano N, Suetake I, Tajima S, Sueyoshi N (2008) Cyclin-dependent kinase-like 5 binds and phosphorylates DNA methyltransferase 1. Biochem Biophys Res Commun 377:1162–1167
81. Kaneda M, Okano M, Hata K, Sado T, Tsujimoto N, Li E, Sasaki H (2004) Essential role for de novo DNA methyltransferase Dnmt3a in paternal and maternal imprinting. Nature 429:900–903
82. Kang ES, Chang W, Jae H (2001) Dnmt3b, de novo DNA Methyltransferase, interacts with SUMO-1 and Ubc9 through its N-terminal region and is subject to modification by SUMO-1. Biochem Biophys Res Commun 289:862–868
83. Kangaspeska S, Stride B, Métivier R, Polycarpou-Schwarz M, Ibberson D, Carmouche RP, Benes V, Gannon F, Reid G (2008) Transient cyclical methylation of promoter DNA. Nature 452:112–115
84. Kim GD, Ni J, Kelesoglu N, Roberts RJ, Pradhan S (2002) Co-operation and communication between the human maintenance and de novo DNA (cytosine-5) methyltransferases. EMBO J 21:4183–4195

85. Klimasauskas S, Kumar S, Roberts RJ, Cheng X (1994) HhaI methyltransferase flips its target base out of the DNA helix. Cell 76:357–369
86. Kohli RM, Zhang Y (2013) TET enzymes, TDG and the dynamics of DNA demethylation. Nature 502:472–479
87. Kotini AG, Mpakali A, Agalioti T (2011) Dnmt3a1 upregulates transcription of distinct genes and targets chromosomal gene clusters for epigenetic silencing in mouse embryonic stem cells. Mol Cell Biol 31:1577–1592
88. Kriukienė E, Liutkevičiūtė Z, Klimašauskas S (2012) 5-Hydroxymethylcytosine--the elusive epigenetic mark in mammalian DNA. Chem Soc Rev 41:6916–6930
89. Kuck D, Singh N, Lyko F, Medina-Franco JL (2010) Novel and selective DNA methyltransferase inhibitors: docking-based virtual screening and experimental evaluation. Bioorganic Med Chem 18:822–829
90. Kudo Y, Tateishi K, Yamamoto K, Yamamoto S, Asaoka Y, Ijichi H, Nagae G, Yoshida H, Aburatani H, Koike K (2012) Loss of 5-hydroxymethylcytosine is accompanied with malignant cellular transformation. Cancer Sci 103:670–676
91. Kumar D, Lassar AB (2014) Fibroblast growth factor maintains Chondrogenic potential of limb bud Mesenchymal cells by modulating DNMT3A recruitment. Cell Rep 8:1419–1431
92. Kumar S, Cheng X, Klimasauskas S, Mi S, Posfai J, Roberts RJ, Wilson GG (1994) The DNA (cytosine-5) methyltransferases. Nucleic Acids Res 22:1–10
93. Laurent L, Wong E, Li G, Laurent L, Wong E, Li G, Huynh T, Tsirigos A, Ong CT, Low HM et al (2010) Dynamic changes in the human methylome during differentiation dynamic changes in the human methylome during differentiation. Genome Res 20:320–331
94. Lavoie G, St-Pierre Y (2011) Phosphorylation of human DNMT1: implication of cyclin-dependent kinases. Biochem Biophys Res Commun 409:187–192
95. Lee B, Muller MT (2009) SUMOylation enhances DNA methylation activity. Biochem J 421:449–461
96. Leonhardt H, Page AW, Weier HU, Bestor TH (1992) A targeting sequence directs DNA methyltransferase to sites of DNA replication in mammalian nuclei. Cell 71:865–873
97. Lev Maor G, Yearim A, Ast G (2015) The alternative role of DNA methylation in splicing regulation. Trends Genet 31:274–280
98. Li W, Liu M (2011) Distribution of 5-Hydroxymethylcytosine in Different human tissues. Journal of Nucleic Acids 2011:1–5
99. Li Y, Zhu B (2014) Acute myeloid leukemia with DNMT3A mutations. Leuk Lymphoma 55:2002–2012
100. Li E, Bestor TH, Jaenisch R (1992) Targeted mutation of the DNA methyltransferase gene results in embryonic lethality. Cell 69:915–926
101. Li B-Z, Huang Z, Cui Q-Y, Song X-H, Du L, Jeltsch A, Chen P, Li G, Li E, Xu G-L (2011) Histone tails regulate DNA methylation by allosterically activating de novo methyltransferase. Cell Res 21:1172–1181
102. Liang G, Chan MF, Tomigahara Y, Tsai YC, Gonzales FA, Li E, Laird PW, Jones PA (2002) Cooperativity between DNA methyltransferases in the maintenance methylation of repetitive elements. Mol Cell Biol 22:480–491
103. Liao J, Karnik R, Gu H, Ziller MJ, Clement K, Tsankov AM, Akopian V, Gifford C a, Donaghey J, Galonska C et al (2015) Targeted disruption of DNMT1, DNMT3A and DNMT3B in human embryonic stem cells. Nat Genet 47:469–478
104. Lin IG, Han L, Taghva A, O'Brien LE, Hsieh C-L (2002) Murine de novo methyltransferase Dnmt3a demonstrates strand asymmetry and site preference in the methylation of DNA in vitro. Mol Cell Biol 22:704–723
105. Lin Y, Fan H, Frederiksen M, Zhao K, Jiang L, Wang Z, Zhou S, Guo W, Gao J, Li S et al (2012) Detecting S-adenosyl-l-methionine-induced conformational change of a histone methyltransferase using a homogeneous time-resolved fluorescence-based binding assay. Anal Biochem 423:171–177

106. Ling Y, Sankpal UT, Robertson AK, McNally JG, Karpova T, Robertson KD (2004) Modification of de novo DNA methyltransferase 3a (Dnmt3a) by SUMO-1 modulates its interaction with histone deacetylases (HDACs) and its capacity to repress transcription. Nucleic Acids Res 32:598–610

107. Lister R, Pelizzola M, Dowen RH, Hawkins RD, Hon G, Tonti-Filippini J, Nery JR, Lee L, Ye Z, Ngo Q-M et al (2009) Human DNA methylomes at base resolution show widespread epigenomic differences. Nature 462:315–322

108. Lister R, Pelizzola M, Kida YS, Hawkins RD, Nery JR, Hon G, Antosiewicz-Bourget J, O'Malley R, Castanon R, Klugman S et al (2011) Hotspots of aberrant epigenomic reprogramming in human induced pluripotent stem cells. Nature 471:68–73

109. Liu Y, Sun L, Jost JP (1996) In differentiating mouse myoblasts DNA methyltransferase is posttranscriptionally and posttranslationally regulated. Nucleic Acids Res 24:2718–2722

110. Liu Y, Aryee MJ, Padyukov L, Fallin MD, Hesselberg E, Runarsson A, Reinius L, Acevedo N, Taub M, Ronninger M et al (2013) Epigenome-wide association data implicate DNA methylation as an intermediary of genetic risk in rheumatoid arthritis. Nat Biotechnol 31:142–147

111. Liu Y, Zhang X, Blumenthal RM, Cheng X (2013) A common mode of recognition for methylated CpG. Trends Biochem Sci 38:177–183

112. Lorincz MC, Schübeler D, Hutchinson SR, Dickerson DR, Groudine M (2002) DNA methylation density influences the stability of an epigenetic imprint and Dnmt3a/b-independent de novo methylation. Mol Cell Biol 22:7572–7580

113. Ma P, de Waal E, Weaver JR, Bartolomei MS, Schultz RM (2015) A DNMT3A2-HDAC2 complex is essential for genomic imprinting and genome integrity in mouse oocytes. Cell Rep 13:1552–1560

114. Meissner A, Gnirke A, Bell GW, Ramsahoye B, Lander ES, Jaenisch R (2005) Reduced representation bisulfite sequencing for comparative high-resolution DNA methylation analysis. Nucleic Acids Res 33:5868–5877

115. Mertineit C, Yoder JA, Taketo T, Laird DW, Trasler JM, Bestor TH (1998) Sex-specific exons control DNA methyltransferase in mammalian germ cells. Development 125:889–897

116. Métivier R, Gallais R, Tiffoche C, Le Péron C, Jurkowska RZ, Carmouche RP, Ibberson D, Barath P, Demay F, Reid G et al (2008) Cyclical DNA methylation of a transcriptionally active promoter. Nature 452:45–50

117. Miller CA, Sweatt JD (2007) Covalent modification of DNA regulates memory formation. Neuron 53:857–869

118. Misaki T, Yamaguchi L, Sun J, Orii M, Nishiyama A, Nakanishi M (2016) The replication foci targeting sequence (RFTS) of DNMT1 functions as a potent histone H3 binding domain regulated by autoinhibition. Biochem Biophys Res Commun 470:741–747

119. Myrianthopoulos V, Cartron PF, Liutkevičiūtė Z, Klimašauskas S, Matulis D, Bronner C, Martinet N, Mikros E (2016) Tandem virtual screening targeting the SRA domain of UHRF1 identifies a novel chemical tool modulating DNA methylation. Eur J Med Chem 114:390–396

120. Neri F, Krepelova A, Incarnato D, Maldotti M, Parlato C, Galvagni F, Matarese F, Stunnenberg HG, Oliviero S (2013) XDnmt3L antagonizes DNA methylation at bivalent promoters and favors DNA methylation at gene bodies in ESCs. Cell 155:121–134

121. Nishiyama A, Yamaguchi L, Sharif J, Johmura Y, Kawamura T, Nakanishi K, Shimamura S, Arita K, Kodama T, Ishikawa F et al (2013) Uhrf1-dependent H3K23 ubiquitylation couples maintenance DNA methylation and replication. Nature 502:249–253

122. Oakes CC, Smiraglia DJ, Plass C, Trasler JM, Robaire B (2003) Aging results in hypermethylation of ribosomal DNA in sperm and liver of male rats. Proc Natl Acad Sci U S A 100:1775–1780

123. Okano M, Bell DW, Haber DA (1999) DNA methyltransferases Dnmt3a and Dnmt3b are essential for de novo methylation and mammalian development. Cell 99:247–257

124. Okuwaki M, Verreault A (2004) Maintenance DNA methylation of nucleosome Core particles. J Biol Chem 279:2904–2912

125. Ooi SKT, Qiu C, Bernstein E, Li K, Jia D, Yang Z, Erdjument-Bromage H, Tempst P, Lin S-P, Allis CD et al (2007) DNMT3L connects unmethylated lysine 4 of histone H3 to de novo methylation of DNA. Nature 448:714–717

126. Ostler KR, Davis EM, Payne SL, Gosalia BB, Expósito-Céspedes J, Le Beau MM, Godley LA (2007) Cancer cells express aberrant DNMT3B transcripts encoding truncated proteins. Oncogene 26:5553–5563

127. Otani J, Nankumo T, Arita K, Inamoto S, Ariyoshi M, Shirakawa M (2009) Structural basis for recognition of H3K4 methylation status by the DNA methyltransferase 3A ATRX-DNMT3-DNMT3L domain. EMBO Rep 10:1235–1241

128. Otani J, Kimura H, Sharif J, Endo TA, Mishima Y, Kawakami T, Koseki H, Shirakawa M, Suetake I, Tajima S (2013) Cell cycle-dependent turnover of 5-hydroxymethyl cytosine in mouse embryonic stem cells. PLoS One 8:1–11

129. Pedroso JL, Povoas Barsottini OG, Lin L, Melberg A, Oliveira ASB, Mignot E (2013) A novel de novo exon 21 DNMT1 mutation causes cerebellar ataxia, deafness, and narcolepsy in a Brazilian patient. Sleep 36(1257–9):1259A

130. Pidsley R, Viana J, Hannon E, Spiers H, Troakes C, Al-Saraj S, Mechawar N, Turecki G, Schalkwyk LC, Bray NJ et al (2014) Methylomic profiling of human brain tissue supports a neurodevelopmental origin for schizophrenia. Genome Biol 15.483

131. Portela A, Esteller M (2010) Epigenetic modifications and human disease. Nat Biotechnol 28:1057–1068

132. Pradhan M, Estève PO, Hang GC, Samaranayke M, Kim GD, Pradhan S (2008) CXXC domain of human DNMT1 is essential for enzymatic activity. Biochemistry 47:10000–10009

133. Pradhan S, Chin HG, Estève PO, Jacobsen SE (2009) SET7/9 mediated methylation of non-histone proteins in mammalian cells. Epigenetics 4:383–387

134. Prendergast GC, Ziff EB (1991) Methylation-sensitive sequence-specific DNA binding by the c-Myc basic region. Science 251:186–189

135. Purdy MM, Holz-Schietinger C, Reich NO (2010) Identification of a second DNA binding site in human DNA methyltransferase 3A by substrate inhibition and domain deletion. Arch Biochem Biophys 498:13–22

136. Qin W, Wolf P, Liu N, Link S, Smets M, Mastra FL, Forné I, Pichler G, Hörl D, Fellinger K et al (2015) DNA methylation requires a DNMT1 ubiquitin interacting motif (UIM) and histone ubiquitination. Cell Res 25:911–929

137. Qiu C, Sawada K, Zhang X, Cheng X (2002) The PWWP domain of mammalian DNA methyltransferase Dnmt3b defines a new family of DNA-binding folds. Nat Struct Biol 9:217–224

138. Quenneville S, Verde G, Corsinotti A, Kapopoulou A, Jakobsson J, Offner S, Baglivo I, Pedone PV, Grimaldi G, Riccio A et al (2011) In embryonic stem cells, ZFP57/KAP1 recognize a methylated hexanucleotide to affect chromatin and DNA methylation of imprinting control regions. Mol Cell 44:361–372

139. Quenneville S, Turelli P, Bojkowska K, Raclot C, Offner S, Kapopoulou A, Trono D (2012) The KRAB-ZFP/KAP1 system contributes to the early embryonic establishment of site-specific DNA methylation patterns maintained during development. Cell Rep 2:766–773

140. Radman-Livaja M, Rando OJ (2010) Nucleosome positioning: how is it established, and why does it matter? Dev Biol 339:258–266

141. Ramsahoye BH, Biniszkiewicz D, Lyko F, Clark V, Bird AP, Jaenisch R (2000) Non-CpG methylation is prevalent in embryonic stem cells and may be mediated by DNA methyltransferase 3a. Proc Natl Acad Sci U S A 97:5237–5242

142. Robertson KD (2005) DNA methylation and human disease. Nat Rev Genet 6:597–610

143. Robertson KD, Uzvolgyi E, Liang G, Talmadge C, Sumegi J, Gonzales FA, Jones PA (1999) The human DNA methyltransferases (DNMTs) 1, 3a and 3b: coordinate mRNA expression in normal tissues and overexpression in tumors. Nucleic Acids Res 27:2291–2298

144. Robertson AK, Geiman TM, Sankpal UT, Hager GL, Robertson KD (2004) Effects of chromatin structure on the enzymatic and DNA binding functions of DNA methyltransferases DNMT1 and Dnmt3a in vitro. Biochem Biophys Res Commun 322:110–118

145. Ross JP, Suetake I, Tajima S, Molloy PL (2010) Recombinant mammalian DNA methyltransferase activity on model transcriptional gene silencing short RNA-DNA heteroduplex substrates. Biochem J 432:323–332

146. Rothbart SB, Dickson BM, Ong MS, Krajewski K, Houliston S, Kireev DB, Arrowsmith CH, Strahl BD (2013) Multivalent histone engagement by the linked tandem tudor and PHD domains of UHRF1 is required for the epigenetic inheritance of DNA methylation. Genes Dev 27:1288–1298

147. Rountree MR, Bachman KE, Baylin SB (2000) DNMT1 binds HDAC2 and a new co-repressor, DMAP1, to form a complex at replication foci. Nat Genet 25:269–277

148. Rush M, Appanah R, Lee S, Lam LL, Goyal P, Lorincz MC (2009) Targeting of EZII2 to a defined genomic site is sufficient for recruitment of Dnmt3a but not de novo DNA methylation. Epigenetics 4:404–414

149. Saitou M, Kagiwada S, Kurimoto K (2012) Epigenetic reprogramming in mouse pre-implantation development and primordial germ cells. Development 139:15–31

150. Sakai Y, Suetake I, Shinozaki F, Yamashina S, Tajima S (2004) Co-expression of de novo DNA methyltransferases Dnmt3a2 and Dnmt3L in gonocytes of mouse embryos. Gene Expr Patterns 5:231–237

151. Sato N, Kondo M, Arai K (2006) The orphan nuclear receptor GCNF recruits DNA methyltransferase for Oct-3/4 silencing. Biochem Biophys Res Commun 344:845–851

152. Schermelleh L, Spada F, Easwaran HP, Zolghadr K, Margot JB, Cardoso MC, Leonhardt H (2005) Trapped in action: direct visualization of DNA methyltransferase activity in living cells. Nat Methods 2:751–756

153. Schmitz KM, Mayer C, Postepska A, Grummt I (2010) Interaction of noncoding RNA with the rDNA promoter mediates recruitment of DNMT3b and silencing of rRNA genes. Genes Dev 24:2264–2269

154. Schrader A, Gross T, Thalhammer V, Langst G (2015) Characterization of Dnmt1 binding and DNA methylation on nucleosomes and nucleosomal arrays. PLoS One 10:e0140076

155. Senyuk V, Premanand K, Xu P, Qian Z, Nucifora G (2011) The oncoprotein EVI1 and the DNA methyltransferase Dnmt3 co-operate in binding and de novo methylation of target DNA. PLoS One 6:e0020793

156. Shamay M, Greenway M, Liao G, Ambinder RF, Hayward SD (2010) De novo DNA methyltransferase DNMT3b interacts with NEDD8-modified proteins. J Biol Chem 285:36377–36386

157. Sharif J, Muto M, Takebayashi S, Suetake I, Iwamatsu A, Endo T a, Shinga J, Mizutani-Koseki Y, Toyoda T, Okamura K et al (2007) The SRA protein Np95 mediates epigenetic inheritance by recruiting Dnmt1 to methylated DNA. Nature 450:908–912

158. Shen L, Zhang Y (2013) 5-Hydroxymethylcytosine: generation, fate, and genomic distribution. Curr Opin Cell Biol 25:289–296

159. Shirane K, Toh H, Kobayashi H, Miura F, Chiba H, Ito T, Kono T, Sasaki H (2013) Mouse oocyte Methylomes at base resolution reveal genome-wide accumulation of non-CpG methylation and role of DNA Methyltransferases. PLoS Genet 9:e1003439

160. Smallwood SA, Kelsey G (2012) De novo DNA methylation: a germ cell perspective. Trends Genet 28:33–42

161. Smallwood A, Estève PO, Pradhan S, Carey M (2007) Functional cooperation between HP1 and DNMT1 mediates gene silencing. Genes Dev 21:1169–1178

162. Smith ZD, Meissner A (2013) DNA methylation: roles in mammalian development. Nat Rev Genet 14:204–220

163. Song J, Rechkoblit O, Bestor TH, Patel DJ (2011) Structure of DNMT1-DNA complex reveals a role for autoinhibition in maintenance DNA methylation. Science 331:1036–1040

164. Song J, Teplova M, Ishibe-Murakami S, Patel DJ (2012) Structure-based mechanistic insights into DNMT1-mediated maintenance DNA methylation. Science 335:709–712

165. Stewart KR, Veselovska L, Kim J, Huang J, Saadeh H, Tomizawa S, Smallwood SA, Chen T, Kelsey G (2015) Dynamic changes in histone modifications precede de novo DNA methylation in oocytes. Genes Dev 29:2449–2462

166. Stroud H, Do T, Du J, Zhong X, Feng S, Johnson L, Patel DJ, Jacobsen SE (2014) Non-CG methylation patterns shape the epigenetic landscape in Arabidopsis. Nat Struct Mol Biol 21:64–72

167. Suetake I, Miyazaki J, Murakami C, Takeshima H, Tajima S (2003) Distinct enzymatic properties of recombinant mouse DNA methyltransferases Dnmt3a and Dnmt3b. J Biochem 133:737–744

168. Suetake I, Shinozaki F, Miyagawa J, Takeshima H, Tajima S (2004) DNMT3L stimulates the DNA methylation activity of Dnmt3a and Dnmt3b through a direct interaction. J Biol Chem 279:27816–27823
169. Suetake I, Morimoto Y, Fuchikami T, Abe K, Tajima S (2006) Stimulation effect of Dnmt3L on the DNA methylation activity of Dnmt3a2. J Biochem 140:553–559
170. Suetake I, Hayata D, Tajima S (2006) The amino-terminus of mouse DNA methyltransferase 1 forms an independent domain and binds to DNA with the sequence involving PCNA binding motif. J Biochem 140:763–776
171. Suetake I, Mishima Y, Kimura H, Lee Y-H, Goto Y, Takeshima H, Ikegami T, Tajima S (2011) Characterization of DNA-binding activity in the N-terminal domain of the DNA methyltransferase Dnmt3a. Biochem J 437:141–148
172. Sugiyama Y, Hatano N, Sueyoshi N, Suetake I, Tajima S, Kinoshita E, Kinoshita-Kikuta E, Koike T, Kameshita I (2010) The DNA-binding activity of mouse DNA methyltransferase 1 is regulated by phosphorylation with casein kinase 1delta/epsilon. Biochem J 427:489–497
173. Sun D, Luo M, Jeong M, Rodriguez B, Xia Z, Hannah R, Wang H, Le T, Faull KF, Chen R et al (2014) Epigenomic profiling of young and aged HSCs reveals concerted changes during aging that reinforce self-renewal. Cell Stem Cell 14:673–688
174. Suzuki MM, Bird A (2008) DNA methylation landscapes: provocative insights from epigenomics. Nat Rev Genet 9:465–476
175. Syeda F, Fagan RL, Wean M, Avvakumov GV, Walker JR, Xue S, Dhe-Paganon S, Brenner C (2011) The replication focus targeting sequence (RFTS) domain is a DNA-competitive inhibitor of Dnmt1. J Biol Chem 286:15344–15351
176. Takagi H, Tajima S, Asano A (1995) Overexpression of DNA methyltransferase in myoblast cells accelerates myotube formation. Eur J Biochem 231:282–291
177. Takahashi S, Suetake I, Engelhardt J, Tajima S (2015) A novel method to analyze 5-hydroxymethylcytosine in CpG sequences using maintenance DNA methyltransferase, DNMT1. FEBS Open Bio 5:741–747
178. Takeshima H, Suetake I, Shimahara H, Ura K, Tate SI, Tajima S (2006) Distinct DNA methylation activity of Dnmt3a and Dnmt3b towards naked and nucleosomal DNA. J Biochem 139:503–515
179. Takeshima H, Suetake I, Tajima S (2008) Mouse Dnmt3a preferentially Methylates linker DNA and is inhibited by histone H1. J Mol Biol 383:810–821
180. Takeshita K, Suetake I, Yamashita E, Suga M, Narita H, Nakagawa A, Tajima S (2011) Structural insight into maintenance methylation by mouse DNA methyltransferase 1 (Dnmt1). Proc Natl Acad Sci U S A 108:9055–9059
181. Tamaru H, Selker EU (2001) A histone H3 methyltransferase controls DNA methylation in Neurospora crassa. Nature 414:277–283
182. Teif VB, Beshnova DA, Vainshtein Y, Marth C, Mallm JP, Rippe TH (2014) Nucleosome repositioning links DNA (de)methylation and differential CTCF binding during stem cell development. Genome Res 24:1285–1295
183. Umezawa A, Yamamoto H, Rhodes K, Klemsz MJ, Maki R a, Oshima RG (1997) Methylation of an ETS site in the intron enhancer of the keratin 18 gene participates in tissue-specific repression. Mol Cell Biol 17:4885–4894
184. Ushijima T, Watanabe N, Okochi E, Kaneda A, Sugimura T, Miyamoto K (2003) Fidelity of the methylation pattern and its variation in the genome. Genome Res 13:868–874
185. Valinluck V, Sowers LC (2007) Endogenous cytosine damage products alter the site selectivity of human DNA maintenance methyltransferase DNMT1. Cancer Res 67:946–950
186. Van Emburgh BO, Robertson KD (2011) Modulation of Dnmt3b function in vitro by interactions with Dnmt3L, Dnmt3a and Dnmt3b splice variants. Nucleic Acids Res 39:4984–5002
187. Vertino PM, Yen RW, Gao J, Baylin SB (1996) De novo methylation of CpG island sequences in human fibroblasts overexpressing DNA (cytosine-5-)-methyltransferase. Mol Cell Biol 16:4555–4565
188. Vilkaitis G, Suetake I, Klimasauskas S, Tajima S (2005) Processive methylation of hemi-methylated CpG sites by mouse Dnmt1 DNA methyltransferase. J Biol Chem 280:64–72

189. Viré E, Brenner C, Deplus R, Blanchon L, Fraga M, Didelot C, Morey L, Van Eynde A, Bernard D, Vanderwinden J-M et al (2005) The Polycomb group protein EZH2 directly controls DNA methylation. Nature 439:871–874

190. Wang YA, Kamarova Y, Shen KC, Jiang Z, Hahn MJ, Wang Y, Brooks SC (2005) DNA methyltransferase-3a interacts with p53 and represses p53-mediated gene expression. Cancer Biol Ther 4:1138–1143

191. Watanabe D, Suetake I, Tada T, Tajima S (2002) Stage- and cell-specific expression of Dnmt3a and Dnmt3b during embryogenesis. Mech Dev 118:187–190

192. Watanabe D, Suetake I, Tajima S, Hanaoka K (2004) Expression of Dnmt3b in mouse hematopoietic progenitor cells and spermatogonia at specific stages. Gene Expr Patterns 5:43–49

193. Webster KE, O'Bryan MK, Fletcher S, Crewther PE, Aapola U, Craig J, Harrison DK, Aung H, Phutikanit N, Lyle R et al (2005) Meiotic and epigenetic defects in Dnmt3L-knockout mouse spermatogenesis. Proc Natl Acad Sci U S A 102:4068–4073

194. Weisenberger DJ, Velicescu M, Preciado-Lopez MA, Gonzales FA, Tsai YC, Liang G, Jones PA (2002) Identification and characterization of alternatively spliced variants of DNA methyltransferase 3a in mammalian cells. Gene 298:91–99

195. Weisenberger DJ, Velicescu M, Cheng JC, Gonzales F a, Liang G, Jones P a (2004) Role of the DNA methyltransferase variant DNMT3b3 in DNA methylation. Mol Cancer Res 2:62–72

196. Winkelmann J, Lin L, Schormair B, Kornum BR, Faraco J, Plazzi G, Melberg A, Cornelio F, Urban AE, Pizza F et al (2012) Mutations in DNMT1 cause autosomal dominant cerebellar ataxia, deafness and narcolepsy. Hum Mol Genet 21:2205–2210

197. Wu TP, Wang T, Seetin MG, Lai Y, Zhu S, Lin K, Liu Y, Byrum SD, Mackintosh SG, Zhong M, Tackett A, Wang G, Hon LS, Fang G, Swenberg JA, Xiao AZ (2016) DNA methylation on N6-adenine in mammalian embryonic stem cells. Nature 532:329–333

198. Xie W, Barr CL, Kim A, Yue F, Lee AY, Eubanks J, Dempster EL, Ren B (2012) Base-resolution analyses of sequence and parent-of-origin dependent DNA methylation in the mouse genome. Cell 148:816–831

199. Xu GL, Bestor TH, Bourc'his D, Hsieh CL, Tommerup N, Bugge M, Hulten M, Qu X, Russo JJ, Viegas-Péquignot E (1999) Chromosome instability and immunodeficiency syndrome caused by mutations in a DNA methyltransferase gene. Nature 402:187–191

200. Yang H, Liu Y, Bai F, Zhang JY, Ma SH, Liu J, Xu ZD, Zhu HG, Ling ZQ, Ye D, Guan KL, Xiong Y (2013) Tumor development is associated with decrease of TET gene expression and 5-methylcytosine hydroxylation. Oncogene 32:663–669

201. Yang S-M, Kim BJ, Norwood Toro L, Skoultchi AI (2013) H1 linker histone promotes epigenetic silencing by regulating both DNA methylation and histone H3 methylation. Proc Natl Acad Sci 110:1708–1713

202. Yang J, Guo R, Wang H, Ye X, Zhou Z, Dan J, Wang H, Gong P, Deng W, Yin Y, Mao S, Wang L, Ding J, Li J, Keefe DL, Dawlaty MM, Wang J, Xu G, Liu L (2016) Tet enzymes regulate telomere maintenance and chromosomal stability of mouse ESCs. Cell Rep 15:1809–1821

203. Yoder JA, Bestor TH (1998) A candidate mammalian DNA methyltransferase related to pmt1p of fission yeast. Hum Mol Genet 7:279–284

204. Yu M, Hon GC, Szulwach KE, Song C, Zhang L, Kim A, Li X, Dai Q, Shen Y, Park B et al (2012) Resource Base-resolution analysis of 5-Hydroxymethylcytosine in the mammalian genome. Cell 149:1368–1380

205. Zemach A, Kim MY, Hsieh PH, Coleman-Derr D, Eshed-Williams L, Thao K, Harmer SL, Zilberman D (2013) The arabidopsis nucleosome remodeler DDM1 allows DNA methyltransferases to access H1-containing heterochromatin. Cell 153:193–205

206. Zhang Y, Jurkowska R, Soeroes S, Rajavelu A, Dhayalan A, Bock I, Rathert P, Brandt O, Reinhardt R, Fischle W et al (2010) Chromatin methylation activity of Dnmt3a and Dnmt3a/3L is guided by interaction of the ADD domain with the histone H3 tail. Nucleic Acids Res 38:4246–4253

207. Zhang Z-M, Liu S, Lin K, Luo Y, Perry JJ, Wang Y, Song J (2015) Crystal structure of human DNA Methyltransferase 1. J Mol Biol 427:2520–2531

208. Zhao Q, Rank G, Tan YT, Li H, Moritz RL, Simpson RJ, Cerruti L, Curtis DJ, Patel DJ, Allis CD et al (2009) PRMT5-mediated methylation of histone H4R3 recruits DNMT3A, coupling histone and DNA methylation in gene silencing. Nat Struct Mol Biol 16:304–311

209. Zhu H, Geiman TM, Xi S, Jiang Q, Schmidtmann A, Chen T, Li E, Muegge K (2006) Lsh is involved in de novo methylation of DNA. EMBO J 25:335–345

210. Ziller MJ, Gu H, Müller F, Donaghey J, Tsai LT-Y, Kohlbacher O, De Jager PL, Rosen ED, Bennett DA, Bernstein BE et al (2013) Charting a dynamic DNA methylation landscape of the human genome. Nature 500:477–481

211. Zuo X, Sheng J, Lau HT, McDonald CM, Andrade M, Cullen DE, Bell FT, Iacovino M, Kyba M, Xu G et al (2012) Zinc finger protein ZFP57 requires its co-factor to recruit DNA methyltransferases and maintains DNA methylation imprint in embryonic stem cells via its transcriptional repression domain. J Biol Chem 287:2107–2118

The Molecular Basis of DNA Demethylation

Miao Shi and Li Shen

Abstract DNA methylation is a key epigenetic modification in mammalian genomes and is dynamically regulated in development and diseases. While enzymes catalyzing DNA methylation have been well characterized, those involved in demethylation have remained elusive until recently. Mounting evidence now suggests that the TET proteins, a family of AlkB-like Fe(II)/α-ketoglutarate-dependent dioxygenases, initiate active DNA demethylation by oxidizing 5-methylcytosine (5mC) to generate 5-hydroxymethylcytosine (5hmC), 5-formylcytosine (5fC), and 5-carboxylcytosine (5caC). In this chapter, we discuss the molecular basis of DNA demethylation in mammalian genomes, focusing on TET proteins and TET-mediated oxidative DNA demethylation. Other potential DNA demethylation pathways are also summarized.

Keywords DNA methylation • DNA demethylation • TET proteins • Dioxygenase • 5-methylcytosine • 5-hydroxymethylcytosine • 5-formylcytosine • 5-carboxylcytosine • TDG

1 Introduction

The chromatin of a multicellular organism stores a vast quantity of information that defines the complex gene expression patterns in diverse cell types, and is indispensable for growth and development. This information is stored both genetically in DNA sequences and epigenetically through DNA and histone modifications [1–4]. However, nearly all cells in an organism (except gametes and some immune cells) contain the same genomic sequences as the zygotic genome and therefore, it is the epigenetic information residing in chromatin that determines a cell's identity and its corresponding gene expression profiles [5]. Generally, epigenetic information is faithfully propagated to each progeny cell upon division to maintain cell identity, but epigenetic states can also undergo dynamic changes during lineage specification

M. Shi • L. Shen (✉)
Life Sciences Institute, Zhejiang University, Hangzhou 310058, China
e-mail: li_shen@zju.edu.cn

© Springer International Publishing AG 2017
A. Kaneda, Y.-i. Tsukada (eds.), *DNA and Histone Methylation as Cancer Targets*,
Cancer Drug Discovery and Development, DOI 10.1007/978-3-319-59786-7_3

or upon certain environmental stimuli [6]. Aberrant alterations of epigenetic information, such as DNA and histone modifications, are frequently associated with the onset of various human diseases, including cancers [7].

DNA methylation, in particular, is the most common covalent modification of DNA. The best-studied form of DNA methylation is 5-methylcytosine (5mC), which is generated by S-adenosyl-L-methionine (SAM)-dependent DNA methyltransferases (DNMTs), and does not interfere with Watson-Crick base pairing [8, 9]. In mammals, this enzymatically introduced DNA methylation exists predominantly in the CpG dinucleotide context (a cytosine followed by a guanine) and carries epigenetic information typically required for long-term gene silencing. Notably, over 70% of CpGs in somatic mammalian cells are methylated, therefore 5mC has long been the focus of compelling biochemical and genomics studies. In addition to 5mC, other forms of DNA methylation also exist. However, it is important to note that not all DNA methylation is the carrier of epigenetic information. For example, methylation can be introduced by endogenous or exogenous methylation agents-mediated DNA damage [9]. These methylated bases, such as N1-methyladenosine (m1A) and N3-methylcytosine (m3C), are considered cytotoxic or mutagenic as they tend to block or alter Watson-Crick base pairing. In the following sections, we will focus on the demethylation of 5mC, and will use the term DNA methylation to refer to 5mC only.

2   DNA Methylation Machinery

In mammals, three enzymatically active DNMTs, namely DNMT1, DNMT3A and DNMT3B, catalyze the transfer of a methyl group from SAM to the carbon-5 position of cytosine residues in DNA, generating 5mC [8]. DNMT1 preferentially methylates hemimethylated DNA [10], and in the presence of its cofactor UHRF1 (also known as NP95) [11, 12], DNMT1 is mainly responsible for copying DNA methylation patterns to the daughter strands during DNA replication (maintenance methylation). In contrast, DNMT3A and DNMT3B are the main enzymes to establish initial DNA methylation patterns during early embryonic development (de novo methylation), and do not show any preference for hemimethylated DNA [13]. Nevertheless, both maintenance and de novo methylation activities are required for normal development as depletion of DNMT1 or DNMT3B in mice results in embryonic lethality, and Dnmt3a-knockout mice die 4–8 weeks after birth [13, 14].

Structurally, the methyl group of 5mC is located in the major groove of DNA double helix, and is involved in either attracting or repelling many DNA binding proteins [15]. For example, three of the methyl-CpG binding domain (MBD) containing proteins, MeCP2, MBD1, MBD2, and a transcriptional regulator KAISO, have been shown to preferentially bind to methylated DNA and recruit repressor complexes to methylated promoters, leading to subsequent chromatin condensation and gene silencing [16]. On the contrary, DNA methylation can also prevent binding of some transcription factors (TFs), such as YY1 and CTCF [17, 18], to their specific recognition sites. DNA methylation has been demonstrated to play critical roles in various of cellular processes such as genomic imprinting, X-chromosome inactivation, retrotransposon silencing as well as maintenance of cell identity, supporting its general transcription repression function and heritable nature [15].

3   Passive and Active DNA Demethylation

While most histone modifications are readily reversible [19], DNA methylation has been generally viewed as a relatively stable epigenetic mark. Indeed, there is a dedicated maintenance enzyme, DNMT1, to faithfully copy DNA methylation patterns to daughter strands during DNA replication; in addition, the methyl group on 5mC is connected to the base through a C-C bond which exhibits high chemical stability under physiological conditions; furthermore, no DNA demethylase could be identified by 2009 when a large number of histone demethylases had been discovered. Nevertheless, studies in the past decade have indicated that DNA methylation is not as static as once thought. Loss of DNA methylation, or DNA demethylation, has been reported in various biological contexts and can be achieved through either passive or active mechanisms.

As illustrated in Fig. 1, passive DNA demethylation, or replication-dependent dilution of 5mC, refers to loss of 5mC instead of semi conservatively replicating methylation patterns during DNA replication. In the absence of functional maintenance methylation machinery, i.e., DNMT1 and UHRF1, successive cycles of DNA replication can result in gradual dilution of 5mC to achieve global DNA demethylation. Passive DNA demethylation has been demonstrated to play a major role in maternal-genome demethylation of zygotes [20–22], and in the whole-genome demethylation of primordial germ cells (PGCs) [23–25].

By contrast, active DNA demethylation refers to direct removal of the methyl group from 5mC, or an enzymatic process that removes or modifies 5mC with regeneration of unmodified cytosine. Processes that are initiated with active modification (AM) of 5mC can be further divided into two forms by whether the modified 5mC is converted to unmodified cytosine through passive dilution (PD) or active restoration (AR). Similar to passive DNA demethylation, the AM-PD pathway may be well suited for large-scale DNA demethylation events observed in PGCs and zygotes, which we will discuss in Sect. 4.4. However, the AM-AR pathway and direct removal of the methyl group or the 5mC base may take place rapidly, and are implicated in locus-specific demethylation which requires rapid response towards environmental stimuli. For example, rapid active DNA demethylation was observed at the interleukin-2 (IL-2) promoter-enhancer region in activated T lymphocytes within 20 minutes upon stimulation [26], at the promoter of brain-derived neurotrophic factor (BDNF) in KCl-stimulated postmitotic neurons without DNA replication [27], at several other specific genomic loci in response to nuclear hormone and growth factors [28–30]. Thus, these studies suggest that active DNA demethylation could function in the dynamic regulation of genes that require rapid responses to specific environmental stimuli.

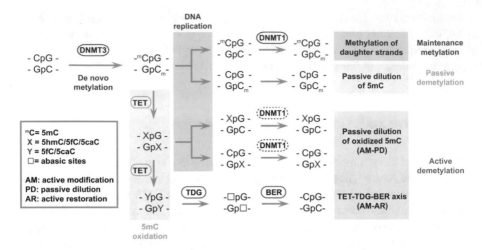

Fig. 1 Major mechanisms of passive and active DNA demethylation in the mammalian genome. DNA methylation patterns are established by DNMT3 proteins and maintained by DNMT1 during DNA replication, and passive DNA demethylation occurs when DNMT1 is inhibited. TET proteins can oxidize 5-methylcytosine (5mC) to generate 5-hydroxymethylcytosine (5hmC), 5-formylcytosine (5fC), and 5-carboxylcytosine (5caC), which are inefficient substrates for DNMT1 and are passively diluted during DNA replication. This form of active DNA demethylation is termed as active modification followed by passive dilution (AM-PD). Among the three 5mC oxidation derivatives, 5fC and 5caC can be excised by TDG to form abasic sites, which are further repaired by base excision repair (BER) pathway to complete DNA demethylation. This form of active DNA demethylation is termed as active modification followed by active restoration (AM-AR)

4   TET-Mediated Oxidative DNA Demethylation

4.1   TET Family Dioxygenases

While passive DNA demethylation has long been understood and accepted, the mechanism of active DNA demethylation was not understood until recently, following the discovery that TET (ten-eleven translocation) proteins can convert 5mC to its oxidized forms, namely 5-hydroxymethylcytosine (5hmC), 5-formylcytosine (5fC), and 5-carboxylcytosine (5caC). Interestingly, the names of TET genes trace back to the involvement of the human *TET1* gene in the ten-eleven translocation [t(10;11)(q22;q23)] in rare cases of acute myeloid leukemia (AML), which fuses the *TET1* gene on chromosome 10 with the mixed-lineage leukemia gene (*MLL*; also known as *KMT2A*) on chromosome 11 [31, 32]. Along with *TET1*, two additional genes in this protein family, *TET2* and *TET3* are also identified based on their sequence homology. Sequence comparison and structural studies have shown that TET proteins are a distinct family of the Fe(II)/α-ketoglutarate (αKG)-dependent dioxygenase superfamily [33, 34], members of which also include JmjC domain containing histone demethylases and AlkB family DNA/RNA repair proteins.

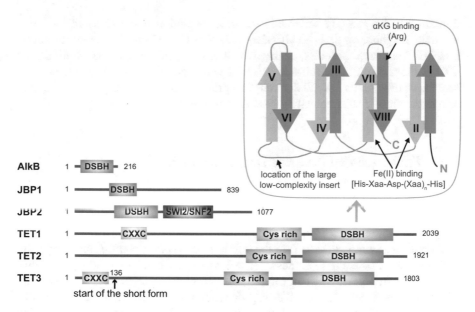

Fig. 2 Schematic diagrams of the TET proteins. Three conserved domains are indicated in mouse TET proteins, including CXXC zinc finger, cysteine-rich region (Cys-rich), and the double-stranded β-helix (DSBH) fold of the Fe(II)/α-ketoglutarate (αKG)-dependent dioxygenases. Locations of Fe(II) and the αKG-binding sites in the conserved DSBH fold are shown in the topology diagram. Also presented are the domain structures of three other enzymes in the super family: *Trypanosoma brucei* JBP1, JBP2, and *Escherichia coli* AlkB. Note that TET3 has a shorter form, which starts at amino acid 136, that does not contain the CXXC domain

Similar to most Fe(II)/αKG-dependent dioxygenase superfamily members, TET proteins share a conserved DSBH fold (or jelly-roll fold) in their catalytic domains, consisting of eight antiparallel β-strands (I–VIII) and an iron-binding motif (Fig. 2). Unique characteristics are also present in the catalytic domain of TET proteins, such as a cysteine-rich domain adjacent to the N terminus of the DSBH fold, and a large non-conserved low-complexity region between conserved β-strands IV and V [33, 35, 36]. Although the low-complexity region's function is not clear, the cysteine-rich domain has been shown to stabilize substrate DNA by wrapping around the DSBH core, and is essential for the enzymatic activity [37]. Outside of the catalytic domain, a CXXC (Cysteine-X-X-cysteine) domain is present at the N terminus of both TET1 and TET3. Indeed, TET1 is also known as CXXC6 (CXXC zinc finger 6) and LCX (leukemia-associated CXXC protein). Both in vitro DNA binding assay and structural analyses have revealed that TET proteins' CXXC domain strongly binds to unmethylated DNA [38]. However, the catalytic domains of TET proteins alone can also bind to DNA and oxidize 5mC without the help of a CXXC domain [39]. Therefore, the catalytic domains of TET proteins may possess a non-sequence-specific DNA-binding capacity whereas the CXXC domain may increase the sequence selectivity to facilitate and regulate binding of TET proteins to their genomic targets [38, 40, 41]. Surprisingly, TET2 does not possess a CXXC domain, which was suggested to be lost during evolution, and is now encoded by a separate, neighboring gene IDAX (also known as CXXC4)[41]. It is worth noting that TET3 has three isoforms, among which only the full-length form contains the CXXC domain [42]. The full-length TET3 was reported to bind to 5caC at CCG sequences through its CXXC domain, and promote DNA demethylation by acting as a regulator of 5caC removal by base excision repair [42].

4.2   TET-Mediated Iterative Oxidation of 5mC

The finding that TET proteins can convert 5mC of DNA to 5hmC by oxidation was a great advance in understanding the mechanisms of DNA demethylation [34]. This finding was initially inspired by the biosynthesis of glucosylated 5-hydroxymethyluracil (base J) in the genome of *Trypanosoma brucei*, a parasite causing African sleeping sickness. Base J synthesis involves oxidation of thymine to 5-hydroxymethyluracil (5hmU) by J-binding proteins 1 and 2 (JBP1 and JBP2), two enzymes of the Fe(II)/αKG-dependent dioxygenase superfamily [43]. Because of the structural similarity between 5mC and thymine, mammalian homologs of JBP proteins were thought to possess 5mC oxidation activity, and TET family proteins were identified as the mammalian homologs of JBP proteins [33, 34]. Interestingly, the presence of TET genes in animals seems to coincide with the presence of 5mC in the genome [33, 36]. It was then convincingly demonstrated by in vitro biochemical experiments that TET proteins can oxidize 5mC to 5hmC [34]. Moreover, 5hmC is relatively abundant in mouse embryonic stem cells (ESCs) where both TET1 and TET2 are highly expressed, and its presence is TET dependent [34, 39], providing in vivo evidence that 5hmC is generated by TET-mediated oxidation of 5mC.

Fe(II)/αKG-dependent dioxygenase-mediated oxidation reactions typically consist of two stages: dioxygen activation and substrate oxidation (Fig. 3). The dioxygen activation stage is a four-electron process, where Fe(II) and αKG may each contribute two electrons to activate a dioxygen molecule first into bridged peroxo and then into the Fe(IV)-oxo intermediate. In the following substrate oxidation stage, the inert C-H bond of the substrate can be oxidized by the highly active Fe(IV)-oxo species, and finally Fe(IV) is reduced back into Fe(II) to complete the catalytic cycle [44]. During the whole process, four electrons, two from αKG and another two from the substrate C-H bond, are consumed to fully reduce a dioxygen molecule. The two oxygen atoms of the dioxygen molecule are incorporated into the succinate (the oxidized and decarboxylated product of αKG) and the oxidized product (Fig. 3).

Interestingly, some Fe(II)/αKG-dependent dioxygenase are capable to iteratively oxidize the substrate methyl group to carboxyl group. For instance, the thymine-7-hydroxylase, a Fe(II)/αKG-dependent dioxygenase in the thymidine salvage pathway, is known to catalyze a three-step oxidation of thymine to generate 5-carboxyluracil (isoorotate), where the methyl group of thymine is sequentially oxidized to hydroxymethyl group, formyl group, and finally to the carboxyl group,

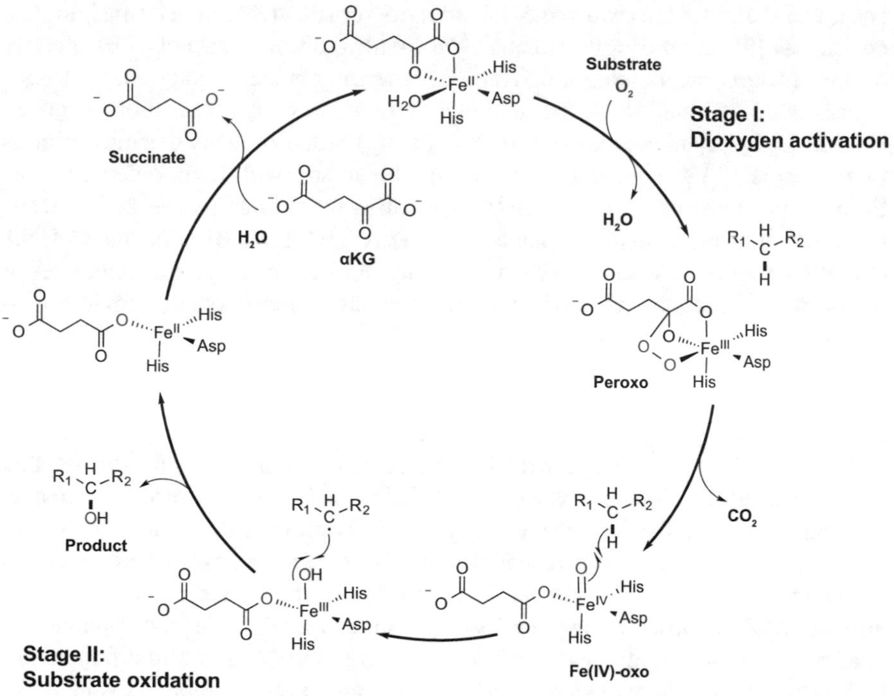

Fig. 3 The chemical mechanism underlying TET–mediated 5mC oxidation. In the dioxygen activation stage, Fe(II) and αKG activate dioxygen to form a highly active Fe(IV)-oxo species; and in the substrate oxidation stage, Fe(IV)-oxo inserts the oxygen atom into the C–H bond of the substrate, and Fe(IV) is reduced back to Fe(II) to complete the catalytic cycle

which is subsequently removed by an isoorotate decarboxylase (IDase) to generate uracil [45]. Enlightened by this example, it was proposed that TET proteins might oxidize 5mC not only to 5hmC, but also to 5fC and 5caC [46]. This hypothesis was soon experimentally proved both in vitro and in vivo [47, 48], and was further supported by a structural study that TET2's active cavity could recognize CpG dinucleotide regardless of its methylation/oxidation status [37].

4.3   TDG-Mediated Excision of 5fC/5caC

Because 5mC can be converted to 5hmC, 5fC and 5caC, these modified bases are naturally considered to be involved in DNA demethylation. However, unlike the N-methyl group in m1A, m3C and methylated histones, which is unstable on the C-N bond and go through spontaneous hydrolytic deformylation upon enzymatic oxidation (i.e., direct removal of the oxidized methyl group) [19], the methyl group of 5mC is connected through a highly stable C-C bond to the rest of the base, and therefore the oxidized 5-substituents remain stable under physiological conditions [9]. Interestingly, although the 5-substituents seem not to be directly removed from 5mC oxidation derivatives, emerging evidence suggests that once converted to 5fC and 5caC, the modified cytosine base can be entirely removed from DNA by thymine-DNA glycosylase (TDG) [48, 49]. DNA demethylation is then completed by replacing the resulting abasic site with unmodified cytosine through the base excision repair (BER) pathway, similar to the active DNA demethylation mechanism in plants [50]. This TET-TDG-BER-mediated DNA demethylation process may take place rapidly, and seems a perfect candidate for locus-specific demethylation which requires rapid response towards environmental stimuli.

TDG belongs to the uracil-DNA glycosylase (UDG) superfamily. It has been well established that TDG can excise pyrimidine moiety from G/U and G/T mispairs in dsDNA by a base-flipping mechanism [51]. Interestingly, TDG also excises properly base-paired cytosine bases with 5-position substituents that destabilize the base-sugar bond (N-glycosidic bond), such as 5-fluorocytosine, indicating that the stability of the N-glycosidic bond contributes to TDG's substrate specificity [52]. More recent studies further demonstrated that TDG can recognize and remove 5fC and 5caC, but not 5mC, 5hmC, and unmodified cytosine, from DNA duplex when paired with guanine [48, 49]. Indeed, computational analyses suggest that 5fC and 5caC form a more labile N-glycosidic bond compared to unmodified cytosine, 5mC, 5hmC, and even 5-fluorocytosine [53]. Consistently, TDG has a slightly higher binding affinity towards G/5fC and G/5caC pairs than to G/U and G/T mismatches [49]. When co-overexpressed in HEK293 cells [48, 54], TDG efficiently depletes TET-generated 5fC and 5caC; and in contrast, TDG knockdown in mouse ESCs results in a 5–10-fold increase of endogenous 5fC and 5caC [55, 56], providing in vivo evidence that TDG is responsible for 5fC/5caC removal.

Intriguingly, among the four enzymes with UDG activity in mammals (i.e., TDG, UNG, MBD4, and SMUG1), only TDG is required during mouse embryonic development [57–60], where global DNA methylation reprogramming takes place, implicating that the DNA glycosylase activity of TDG is essential for DNA demethylation. Compared with the other UDGs, the active site of TDG is indeed uniquely configured to accommodate 5fC/5caC and facilitate its cleavage, as revealed by the crystal structure of human TDG in complex with 5caC-containing dsDNA [61]. Consistently, both *Tdg*-null-mutant and *Tdg*-catalytic-mutant mice exhibit abnormal DNA methylation and die around embryonic day (E)12.5 [57, 58], confirming a crucial role of the TET-TDG-BER axis in DNA demethylation during embryonic development.

4.4 Replication-Dependent Dilution of 5mC Oxidation Derivatives

TET mediated 5mC oxidation not only initiates the TET-TDG-BER demethylation pathway, but also generates DNA demethylation intermediates (i.e., 5hmC, 5fC, and 5caC) that can be passively diluted in a replication-dependent manner. Mechanistically, hemi-modified CpGs carrying 5hmC, 5fC or 5caC (XG:GC, where X = 5hmC/5fC/5caC) have been demonstrated to be significantly less efficient in being methylated by DNMT1 compared with hemimethylated CpGs (i.e., 5mCG:GC) [62–64], therefore, TET-mediated 5mC oxidation can block the maintenance methylation machinery, facilitating replication-dependent DNA demethylation. Because this DNA demethylation process starts with active modification of 5mC, it has been suggested to be regarded as active DNA demethylation (Fig. 1) [65]. The replication-dependent active DNA demethylation has been observed in the paternal genome (to a less extent in the maternal genome) of zygotes and in developing PGCs [21, 22, 66, 67]. However, it is worth noting that global DNA demethylation in zygotes could be largely achieved without 5mC oxidation due to the inhibition of DNMT1 at this stage. Therefore, 5mC oxidation probably only facilitates, but is not indispensable for, replication-dependent whole genome DNA demethylation. The extent to which 5mC oxidation is required for demethylation may depend on the genomic context of the DNA sequence.

4.5 Other Potential TET-Initiated Active DNA Demethylation Pathways

In addition to the two major TET-mediated DNA demethylation pathways discussed above (i.e., the TET-TDG-BER axis and the replication-dependent dilution of 5mC oxidation derivatives) which have been extensively supported by recent biochemical and genetic studies [65], evidence for the existence of other TET-initiated DNA demethylation pathways, in which 5mC oxidation derivatives act as demethylation intermediates, have also been reported.

Firstly, the 5-carboxyl group on 5caC might be removed by a putative decarboxylase to complete DNA demethylation. This mechanism was proposed under the inspiration of the thymidine salvage pathway that we discussed above [46], where the thymine-7-hydroxylase oxidizes the methyl group of thymine to a carboxyl group that is subsequently removed by an isoorotate decarboxylase to convert thymine to uracil [45]. Although the idea of decarboxylation is more energy-efficient compared with the TET-TDG-BER pathway, only one study reported weak 5caC decarboxylase activity in mouse ESC extracts [68]. In addition, the pronounced increase of endogenous 5caC upon TDG depletion has already indicated that TDG is the major enzyme for 5caC removal [55, 56]. Therefore, whether a 5caC decarboxylase exists remains to be explored.

Secondly, the 5-position substituents may be directly removed by DNMTs. It has been reported that both bacteria and mammalian DNMTs could remove the 5-hydroxymethyl group of 5hmC and the 5-carboxyl group of 5caC in vitro to generate unmodified cytosine in the absence of SAM, the methyl donor in a DNMT-mediated DNA methylation reaction [69–71]. However, given that SAM is present in all cell types as a general methyl donor of many other essential biochemical reactions, whether DNMT-mediated 5-position substituent removal of 5hmC/5caC can take place in vivo remains questionable.

Thirdly, 5hmC deamination followed by BER has also been implicated in active DNA demethylation. AID (activation-induced deaminase)/APOBEC (apolipoprotein B mRNA editing enzyme, catalytic polypeptide) family of cytidine deaminases typically target unmodified cytosine in single-strand DNA or RNA to generate mutations, which are required for the generation of antibody diversity in B cells, RNA editing, and retroviral defense [72]. Interestingly, one study showed that AID/APOBEC deaminases might deaminate 5hmC to produce 5hmU in HEK293 cells and in the mouse brain [73], indicating a TET-AID/APOBEC-BER axis for active DNA demethylation. But this potential pathway has been questioned due to the following reasons: 1) AID only acts robustly on single-strand DNA but not on double-strand DNA [74]; 2) AID/APOBEC deaminases exhibit no detectable in vitro deamination activity on 5hmC [54, 75]. Therefore, further evidence is required to support this potential active DNA demethylation mechanism.

5 Potential TET-Independent Active DNA Demethylation Mechanisms

While TET proteins have been widely accepted as major players for active DNA demethylation, many other proteins were also historically proposed to play direct roles in demethylating DNA [46, 76]. Here we list some of the putative mechanisms that are independent of TET proteins, however, due to lack of direct evidence or conflicting observations, these demethylation mechanisms must be reexamined to confirm their biological relevance.

Firstly, despite the difficult nature of breaking a C-C bond, enzymatic removal of the 5-methyl group from 5mC is the simplest way to achieve DNA demethylation. The first protein reported to possess this activity is the methylated DNA binding protein MBD2. It was shown that MBD2-mediated 5-methyl group excision could take place in vitro without any cofactors [77]. However, this observation could not be reproduced by other laboratories and MBD-null mice were viable with normal DNA methylation patterns [78], raising the certain whether MBD2 could serve as a functional DNA demethylase in vivo. In addition to MBD2, elongator complex protein3 (ELP3) was also proposed to achieve DNA demethylation by breaking the C-C bond through a radical SAM mechanism [46]. While ELP3 bears a Fe-S radical SAM domain, and was reported to play a role in the paternal genome demethylation in mouse zygotes [79], direct biochemical evidence demonstrating its enzymatic activity is still lacking. Interestingly, an in vitro study has showed that, in the absence of SAM, the mammalian DNMTs (i.e., DNMT3A, DNMT3B, and DNMT1) themselves could also remove the 5-methyl group from 5mC [80], but the physiological relevance of this observation remains unclear due to the widespread presence of SAM in all cell types as discussed above.

Secondly, the entire 5mC base can be erased by a DNA glycosylase to form an abasic site, followed by BER DNA repair pathway to complete active DNA demethylation. In plants, compelling biochemical and genetic evidence has validated this mechanism with the discovery of a family of specialized DNA glycosylases responsible for 5mC excision, namely Demeter (Dme) family proteins [81]. While no obvious mammalian orthologues of Dme family proteins have been identified, two mammalian DNA glycosylases, TDG and MBD4, were reported to have incision activity against 5mC [82, 83]. However, 5mC incision activity of the two enzymes is about 30 times lower compared with that against G/T mismatches. In addition, *Mbd4*-null mice were viable and exhibit normal DNA methylation patterns [59]. Although *Tdg*-deficient mice exhibit abnormal DNA methylation and die around E12.5 [57, 58], the phenotype is more likely to be attributed to the loss of 5fC/5caC incision activity of TDG required in the TET/TDG-mediated DNA demethylation as discussed in Sect. 4.3. Thus, whether BER of 5mC by a DNA glycosylase can contribute to DNA demethylation in mammals has yet to be determined.

Thirdly, active DNA demethylation may also be achieved through deamination of 5mC to generate thymine, followed by BER to replace this mismatched thymine to unmodified cytosine. As discussed earlier, AID/APOBEC family proteins show no detectable in vitro deamination activity on 5hmC, however, these deaminases do deaminate 5mC in the context of single-strand DNA in vitro, despite at a 10-fold slower rate compared with that towards their canonical substrate cytosine [54, 75, 84]. Indeed, several lines of evidence has suggested that AID/APOBEC family deaminases play a role in active DNA demethylation, including studies in zebrafish embryos [85], in mouse PGCs [86], in promoting pluripotency in somatic nuclei after fusion with ESCs [87], and in reprogramming of somatic cells to induced pluripotent stem cells (iPSCs) [88]. Nevertheless, due to conflicting observations and the fact that these deaminases only act robustly on single-strand DNA, further mechanistic studies are required to clarify the function of AID/APOBEC proteins in active DNA demethylation. Interestingly, DNMTs, in addition to AID/APOBEC proteins, have also been shown to deaminate 5mC in the absence of SAM in vitro [29]. But again, the physiological relevance of DNMTs' in vitro deamination activity is uncertain as depletion of SAM is unlikely in living cells.

Fourthly, nucleotide excision repair (NER), which typically repairs bulky DNA lesions generated by exposure to chemicals and radiation, has also been implicated in active DNA demethylation. Multiple lines of evidence have shown that GADD45 (growth arrest and DNA-damage-inducible 45) family proteins could stimulate active DNA demethylation via NER in frog, zebrafish, and mammals [85, 89–91]. However, evidence to the contrary also exists [92, 93]. More importantly, the exact underlying mechanism is still unclear. Therefore, the role of GADD45 family proteins and NER in DNA demethylation remains to be elucidated.

6 Regulation of TET-Mediated DNA Demethylation

Precise control of DNA methylation is critical to the maintenance of genome stability as well as cell-type- and developmental-stage-specific gene expression. Therefore, proper regulation of both DNA methylation and demethylation is required in many biological processes, such as development and the onset of diseases. Compared with the regulation of DNA methylation, which has been extensively studied [8, 15], the regulation of DNA demethylation has just begun to be understood. Because TET-mediated 5mC oxidation has become the most accepted mechanism of active DNA demethylation [9, 94], we only discuss factors involved in the regulation of TET-mediated DNA demethylation in the following sections.

6.1 Regulation of TET Expression

Regulation of enzyme abundance is a common way to control its activity in cells. In mouse E10.5 PGCs, transient conversion of 5mC to 5hmC can be readily detected together with a dramatic TET1 upregulation [67, 95, 96], indicating that regulation of TET expression is an important way to regulate DNA demethylation. Indeed, the three TET genes exhibit different expression patterns in a cell-type- and developmental-stage-specific manner: TET1 shows a high-level of expression specifically in mouse E10.5–12.5 PGCs, the inner cell mass (ICM) of blastocysts, as well as ESCs [39, 95]; TET2 is highly expressed in ESCs, and is broadly expressed in various mouse adult tissues [39]; TET3 is the only TET family member that is highly expressed in mouse oocytes and zygotes [97, 98], although it also shows a broad expression pattern in mouse adult tissues.

The regulation of TET expression has been reported at different levels. At the transcriptional level, cell-type-specific transcription factors (TFs) may play a major role. For example, a large cluster of binding sites for core pluripotency TFs are present in the upstream promoter of mouse *Tet1* gene [99], in line with the rapid reduction of TET1 expression upon ESC differentiation [47, 100]. At the posttranscriptional level, it has been shown that an oncogenic microRNA miR-22 could negatively regulate TET family proteins in breast cancer development and in hematopoietic stem cell transformation [101, 102]. In addition, one study reported that the CXXC domain-containing protein IDAX could directly interact with the catalytic domain of TET2 to downregulate TET2 protein through caspase-mediated degradation [41]. Moreover, all three TET proteins are direct substrates of calpains, a family of calcium-dependent proteases. Specifically, calpain1 mediates TET1 and TET2 turnover in mouse ESCs, and calpain2 regulates TET3 level during differentiation [103]. Such multiple layers of regulation on TET expression provides a robust control of TET activity in cells.

6.2 Regulation of TET Activity by Metabolites and Nutrients

Given the importance of precise regulation of DNA methylation in various biological processes, it is not surprising that TET activity can be regulated in multiple ways, including the metabolic states and the milieu of cells (e.g., nutritional and developmental signals, stress, and chemical exposure). For example, both adenosine-5'-triphosphate (ATP) and hydroquinone were reported to stimulate TET-mediated 5mC oxidation [48, 104]. More importantly, the five-carbon dicarboxylic acid αKG, which is part of the tricarboxylic acid (TCA) cycle, is an essential co-factor for TET-mediated 5mC oxidation (as discussed in Sect. 4.2,). Therefore, metabolic states of cells, which affect intracellular αKG levels, may influence TET activity. Indeed, it has been reported that global 5hmC levels were rapidly increased together with αKG levels in mouse livers within 30 min after glucose, glutamine or glutamate injection [105].

In contrast, another five-carbon dicarboxylic acid, 2-hydroxyglutarate (2HG), which is chemically analogous to αKG, has been shown to inhibit TET activity by competing with αKG [106, 107]. Cellular accumulation of 2HG is often caused by tumor-associated mutations in the $NADP^+$-dependent isocitrate dehydrogenase genes (*IDH1/IDH2*), which encode enzymes that normally produce αKG in the cell. These tumor-associated *IDH1/IDH2* mutations (R132 of IDH1 and R140/R172 of IDH2) impair αKG production, and obtain an enzymatic activity to convert αKG to 2HG [108, 109], which inhibits TET activity. Consistently, co-expression of mutant IDH enzymes and TET proteins inhibits TET-mediated 5mC to 5hmC conversion [106, 107]. It was hypothesized that the substitution of the keto group on αKG to a hydroxyl group on 2HG might interfere with Fe(II) binding and stabilize the reaction intermediate. In line with this hypothesis, another two metabolites, fumarate and succinate, which also share structural similarity with αKG, both function as competitive inhibitors of Fe(II)/αKG-dependent dioxygenases, including TET proteins. Similar to 2HG, these metabolites are accumulated in a subset of human cancers with inactivation mutations of fumarate hydratase (FH) and succinate dehydrogenase (SDH), respectively [110]. Thus, multiple intracellular metabolites may regulate TET-mediated oxidative DNA demethylation, at least under certain pathological conditions.

Ascorbate (also known as vitamin C), an essential nutrient for humans and certain other animal species, has also been demonstrated to positively regulate TET activity [111–113]. In wild-type, but not *Tet1/Tet2* deficient mouse ESCs, ascorbate significantly increases the levels of all 5mC oxidation products, particularly 5fC and 5caC by more than an order of magnitude, leading to a global loss of 5mC (~40%) [111, 113]. Ascorbate uniquely interacts with the catalytic domain of TET enzymes, enhancing their catalytic activities likely by promoting their folding and/or recycling of Fe(II) [111]. Intriguingly, ascorbate-induced demethylation has stronger effect on the DNA sequences that gain methylation in cultured ES cells compared to blastocysts, which are typically methylated only after implantation in vivo [113]. These studies suggest that ascorbate is a positive modulator of TET activity and may play a critical role in regulating DNA methylation during development. Further studies are needed to elucidate the sequence specificity of ascorbate-mediated stimulation of TET activity.

6.3 Regulation by TET-Interacting Proteins and DNA-Binding Proteins

In addition to the overall TET activity in cells, the specific targeting of TET proteins, and the regulation of their processivity (i.e., why TET-mediated 5mC oxidation tends to stall at 5hmC, and only proceed to 5fC and 5caC at specific loci) provide another important layer of demethylation control. Emerging evidence indicates that the genomic targeting, activity, and processivity of TET enzymes can be modulated by their interacting proteins and some DNA-binding proteins. The O-linked N-acetylglucosamine (O-GlcNAc) transferase OGT, has been reported to directly interact with, and also GlcNAcylate TET proteins [114–118]. Although OGT binding and GlcNAcylation appear not to regulate the enzymatic activity of TET proteins [115], OGT regulates the subcellular location of TET3 by promoting its nuclear export in high-glucose conditions [118]. Moreover, depletion of OGT in mouse ESCs decreases the association of TET1 with chromatin and alters 5hmC enrichment at certain loci [116, 117], suggesting that OGT plays a specific role in targeting and stabilizing TET proteins to the chromatin. In addition to OGT, the CXXC domain protein IDAX was shown to interact with TET2 and was suggested to recruit TET2 to promoters and CpG islands [41]. Recently, a sequence specific transcription factor WT1 (Wilms tumor protein 1) has also been shown to physically interacts with and recruits TET2 to its target genes to activate their expression [119]. Furthermore, PGC7 (also known as STELLA or DPPA3), a maternal factor essential for early development, was demonstrated in one-cell zygotes to protect maternal genome and the imprinting control regions (ICRs) in paternal genome by inhibiting TET activity through direct interaction [97, 120, 121]. These findings suggest an important role of TET interacting partners in targeting and restricting TET activity in the cell.

In addition to TET interacting proteins, some DNA binding proteins can also regulate DNA demethylation. For example, one study showed that knockdown of methyl-CpG binding domain protein 3 (MBD3), which also binds to 5hmC, caused a strong reduction in global 5hmC level in mouse ESCs [122]. In another study, UHRF2 was identified as a 5hmC-specific binding protein in neuronal progenitor cells, and was shown to be capable of stimulating the processivity of TET1 when co-overexpressed with the catalytic domain of TET1 in HEK293T cells [123]. These observations demonstrate that proteins bound to the substrate DNA of TET enzymes may regulate the enzymes' activity and processivity, therefore implying a role of DNA binding proteins in controlling DNA demethylation.

7 Concluding Remarks

Ever since the discovery of 5mC oxidation by TET family proteins, there has been tremendous progress in understanding the molecular basis of DNA demethylation. Accumulating biochemical and genetic studies have demonstrated that TET family proteins play a critical role in active DNA demethylation during dynamic regulation of DNA methylation patterns in development and diseases. While the TET-TDG-BER pathway and replication-dependent dilution of 5hmC/5fC/5caC have been generally accepted as the major forces of active DNA demethylation, other potential active DNA demethylation mechanisms have also been reported. It is worth noting that most of those observations were made before knowing the existence of 5hmC/5fC/5caC, and by immunostaining of 5mC or bisulfite sequencing that do not distinguish 5mC from 5hmC or unmodified cytosine from 5fC and 5caC [9]. Therefore, with many new technologies recently developed to map various new modifications in the genome, historically reported active DNA demethylation pathways should be revisited to further advance this exciting field by revealing a more comprehensive understanding on how DNA methylation is dynamically regulated.

References

1. Bird A (2002) DNA methylation patterns and epigenetic memory. Genes Dev 16(1):6–21
2. Jenuwein T, Allis CD (2001) Translating the histone code. Science 293(5532):1074–1080
3. Holliday R, Pugh JE (1975) DNA modification mechanisms and gene activity during development. Science 187(4173):226–232
4. Riggs AD (1975) X inactivation, differentiation, and DNA methylation. Cytogenet Cell Genet 14(1):9–25
5. Henikoff S, Greally JM (2016) Epigenetics, cellular memory and gene regulation. Curr Biol 26(14):R644–R648
6. Bonasio R, Tu S, Reinberg D (2010) Molecular signals of epigenetic states. Science 330(6004):612–616
7. Easwaran H, Tsai HC, Baylin SB (2014) Cancer epigenetics: tumor heterogeneity, plasticity of stem-like states, and drug resistance. Mol Cell 54(5):716–727
8. Goll MG, Bestor TH (2005) Eukaryotic cytosine methyltransferases. Annu Rev Biochem 74:481–514
9. Shen L, Song CX, He C, Zhang Y (2014) Mechanism and function of oxidative reversal of DNA and RNA methylation. Annu Rev Biochem 83:585–614
10. Hermann A, Goyal R, Jeltsch A (2004) The Dnmt1 DNA-(cytosine-C5)-methyltransferase methylates DNA processively with high preference for hemimethylated target sites. J Biol Chem 279(46):48350–48359
11. Sharif J, Muto M, Takebayashi S, Suetake I, Iwamatsu A, Endo TA, Shinga J, Mizutani-Koseki Y, Toyoda T, Okamura K, Tajima S, Mitsuya K, Okano M, Koseki H (2007) The SRA protein Np95 mediates epigenetic inheritance by recruiting Dnmt1 to methylated DNA. Nature 450(7171):908–912
12. Bostick M, Kim JK, Esteve PO, Clark A, Pradhan S, Jacobsen SE (2007) UHRF1 plays a role in maintaining DNA methylation in mammalian cells. Science 317(5845):1760–1764
13. Okano M, Bell DW, Haber DA, Li E (1999) DNA methyltransferases Dnmt3a and Dnmt3b are essential for de novo methylation and mammalian development. Cell 99(3):247–257

14. Li E, Bestor TH, Jaenisch R (1992) Targeted mutation of the DNA methyltransferase gene results in embryonic lethality. Cell 69(6):915–926
15. Li E, Zhang Y (2014) DNA methylation in mammals. Cold Spring Harb Perspect Biol 6(5):a019133
16. Liu Y, Zhang X, Blumenthal RM, Cheng X (2013) A common mode of recognition for methylated CpG. Trends Biochem Sci 38(4):177–183
17. Bell AC, Felsenfeld G (2000) Methylation of a CTCF-dependent boundary controls imprinted expression of the Igf2 gene. Nature 405(6785):482–485
18. Kim J, Kollhoff A, Bergmann A, Stubbs L (2003) Methylation-sensitive binding of transcription factor YY1 to an insulator sequence within the paternally expressed imprinted gene, Peg3. Hum Mol Genet 12(3):233–245
19. Mosammaparast N, Shi Y (2010) Reversal of histone methylation: biochemical and molecular mechanisms of histone demethylases. Annu Rev Biochem 79:155–179
20. Rougier N, Bourc'his D, Gomes DM, Niveleau A, Plachot M, Paldi A, Viegas-Pequignot E (1998) Chromosome methylation patterns during mammalian preimplantation development. Genes Dev 12(14):2108–2113
21. Shen L, Inoue A, He J, Liu Y, Lu F, Zhang Y (2014) Tet3 and DNA replication mediate demethylation of both the maternal and paternal genomes in mouse zygotes. Cell Stem Cell 15(4):459–470
22. Guo F, Li X, Liang D, Li T, Zhu P, Guo H, Wu X, Wen L, Gu TP, Hu B, Walsh CP, Li J, Tang F, Xu GL (2014) Active and passive demethylation of male and female pronuclear DNA in the mammalian zygote. Cell Stem Cell 15(4):447–458
23. Seisenberger S, Andrews S, Krueger F, Arand J, Walter J, Santos F, Popp C, Thienpont B, Dean W, Reik W (2012) The dynamics of genome-wide DNA methylation reprogramming in mouse primordial germ cells. Mol Cell 48(6):849–862
24. Kagiwada S, Kurimoto K, Hirota T, Yamaji M, Saitou M (2013) Replication-coupled passive DNA demethylation for the erasure of genome imprints in mice. EMBO J 32(3):340–353
25. Vincent JJ, Huang Y, Chen PY, Feng S, Calvopina JH, Nee K, Lee SA, Le T, Yoon AJ, Faull K, Fan G, Rao A, Jacobsen SE, Pellegrini M, Clark AT (2013) Stage-specific roles for tet1 and tet2 in DNA demethylation in primordial germ cells. Cell Stem Cell 12(4):470–478
26. Bruniquel D, Schwartz RH (2003) Selective, stable demethylation of the interleukin-2 gene enhances transcription by an active process. Nat Immunol 4(3):235–240
27. Martinowich K, Hattori D, Wu H, Fouse S, He F, Hu Y, Fan G, Sun YE (2003) DNA methylation-related chromatin remodeling in activity-dependent BDNF gene regulation. Science 302(5646):890–893
28. Kangaspeska S, Stride B, Metivier R, Polycarpou-Schwarz M, Ibberson D, Carmouche RP, Benes V, Gannon F, Reid G (2008) Transient cyclical methylation of promoter DNA. Nature 452(7183):112–115
29. Metivier R, Gallais R, Tiffoche C, Le Peron C, Jurkowska RZ, Carmouche RP, Ibberson D, Barath P, Demay F, Reid G, Benes V, Jeltsch A, Gannon F, Salbert G (2008) Cyclical DNA methylation of a transcriptionally active promoter. Nature 452(7183):45–50
30. Thillainadesan G, Chitilian JM, Isovic M, Ablack JN, Mymryk JS, Tini M, Torchia J (2012) TGF-beta-dependent active demethylation and expression of the p15ink4b tumor suppressor are impaired by the ZNF217/CoREST complex. Mol Cell 46(5):636–649
31. Ono R, Taki T, Taketani T, Taniwaki M, Kobayashi H, Hayashi Y (2002) LCX, leukemia-associated protein with a CXXC domain, is fused to MLL in acute myeloid leukemia with trilineage dysplasia having t(10;11)(q22;q23). Cancer Res 62(14):4075–4080
32. Lorsbach RB, Moore J, Mathew S, Raimondi SC, Mukatira ST, Downing JR (2003) TET1, a member of a novel protein family, is fused to MLL in acute myeloid leukemia containing the t(10;11)(q22;q23). Leuk Off J Leuk Soc Am Leuk Res Fund UK 17(3):637–641
33. Iyer LM, Tahiliani M, Rao A, Aravind L (2009) Prediction of novel families of enzymes involved in oxidative and other complex modifications of bases in nucleic acids. Cell Cycle 8(11):1698–1710

34. Tahiliani M, Koh KP, Shen Y, Pastor WA, Bandukwala H, Brudno Y, Agarwal S, Iyer LM, Liu DR, Aravind L, Rao A (2009) Conversion of 5-methylcytosine to 5-hydroxymethylcytosine in mammalian DNA by MLL partner TET1. Science 324(5929):930–935

35. McDonough MA, Loenarz C, Chowdhury R, Clifton IJ, Schofield CJ (2010) Structural studies on human 2-oxoglutarate dependent oxygenases. Curr Opin Struct Biol 20(6):659–672

36. Iyer LM, Abhiman S, Aravind L (2011) Natural history of eukaryotic DNA methylation systems. Prog Mol Biol Transl Sci 101:25–104

37. Hu L, Li Z, Cheng J, Rao Q, Gong W, Liu M, Shi YG, Zhu J, Wang P, Xu Y (2013) Crystal structure of TET2-DNA complex: insight into TET-mediated 5mC oxidation. Cell 155(7):1545–1555

38. Xu Y, Xu C, Kato A, Tempel W, Abreu JG, Bian C, Hu Y, Hu D, Zhao B, Cerovina T, Diao J, Wu F, He HH, Cui Q, Clark E, Ma C, Barbara A, Veenstra GJ, Xu G, Kaiser UB, Liu XS, Sugrue SP, He X, Min J, Kato Y, Shi YG (2012) Tet3 CXXC domain and dioxygenase activity cooperatively regulate key genes for Xenopus eye and neural development. Cell 151(6):1200–1213

39. Ito S, D'Alessio AC, Taranova OV, Hong K, Sowers LC, Zhang Y (2010) Role of Tet proteins in 5mC to 5hmC conversion, ES-cell self-renewal and inner cell mass specification. Nature 466(7310):1129–1133

40. Liu N, Wang M, Deng W, Schmidt CS, Qin W, Leonhardt H, Spada F (2013) Intrinsic and extrinsic connections of Tet3 Dioxygenase with CXXC zinc finger modules. PLoS One 8(5):e62755

41. Ko M, An J, Bandukwala H, Chavez L (2013) Modulation of TET2 expression and 5-methylcytosine oxidation by the CXXC domain protein IDAX. Nature 497:122–126

42. Jin SG, Zhang ZM, Dunwell TL, Harter MR, Wu X, Johnson J, Li Z, Liu J, Szabo PE, Lu Q, Xu GL, Song J, Pfeifer GP (2016) Tet3 reads 5-Carboxylcytosine through its CXXC domain and is a potential Guardian against Neurodegeneration. Cell Rep 14(3):493–505

43. Borst P, Sabatini R (2008) Base J: discovery, biosynthesis, and possible functions. Annu Rev Microbiol 62:235–251

44. Krebs C, Galonic Fujimori D, Walsh CT, Bollinger JM Jr (2007) Non-heme Fe(IV)-oxo intermediates. Acc Chem Res 40(7):484–492

45. Smiley JA, Kundracik M, Landfried DA, Barnes VR Sr, Axhemi AA (2005) Genes of the thymidine salvage pathway: thymine-7-hydroxylase from a *Rhodotorula glutinis* cDNA library and iso-orotate decarboxylase from Neurospora crassa. Biochim Biophys Acta 1723(1–3):256–264

46. Wu SC, Zhang Y (2010) Active DNA demethylation: many roads lead to Rome. Nat Rev Mol Cell Biol 11(9):607–620

47. Ito S, Shen L, Dai Q, Wu SC, Collins LB, Swenberg JA, He C, Zhang Y (2011) Tet proteins can convert 5-methylcytosine to 5-formylcytosine and 5-carboxylcytosine. Science 333(6047):1300–1303

48. He YF, Li BZ, Li Z, Liu P, Wang Y, Tang Q, Ding J, Jia Y, Chen Z, Li L, Sun Y, Li X, Dai Q, Song CX, Zhang K, He C, Xu GL (2011) Tet-mediated formation of 5-carboxylcytosine and its excision by TDG in mammalian DNA. Science 333(6047):1303–1307

49. Maiti A, Drohat AC (2011) Thymine DNA glycosylase can rapidly excise 5-formylcytosine and 5-carboxylcytosine: potential implications for active demethylation of CpG sites. J Biol Chem 286(41):35334–35338

50. Zhang H, Zhu JK (2012) Active DNA demethylation in plants and animals. Cold Spring Harb Symp Quant Biol 77:161–173

51. Stivers JT, Jiang YL (2003) A mechanistic perspective on the chemistry of DNA repair glycosylases. Chem Rev 103(7):2729–2759

52. Bennett MT, Rodgers MT, Hebert AS, Ruslander LE, Eisele L, Drohat AC (2006) Specificity of human thymine DNA glycosylase depends on N-glycosidic bond stability. J Am Chem Soc 128(38):12510–12519

53. Williams RT, Wang Y (2012) A density functional theory study on the kinetics and thermo-dynamics of N-glycosidic bond cleavage in 5-substituted 2′-deoxycytidines. Biochemistry 51(32):6458–6462
54. Nabel CS, Jia H, Ye Y, Shen L, Goldschmidt HL, Stivers JT, Zhang Y, Kohli RM (2012) AID/APOBEC deaminases disfavor modified cytosines implicated in DNA demethylation. Nat Chem Biol 8(9):751–758
55. Shen L, Wu H, Diep D, Yamaguchi S, D'Alessio AC, Fung HL, Zhang K, Zhang Y (2013) Genome-wide analysis reveals TET and TDG-dependent 5-methylcytosine oxidation dynamics. Cell 153(3):692–706
56. Song C-X, Szulwach KE, Dai Q, Fu Y, Mao S-Q, Lin L, Street C, Li Y, Poidevin M, Wu H, Gao J, Liu P, Li L, Xu G-L, Jin P, He C (2013) Genome-wide profiling of 5-Formylcytosine reveals its roles in epigenetic priming. Cell 153:678–691
57. Cortellino S, Xu J, Sannai M, Moore R, Caretti E, Cigliano A, Le Coz M, Devarajan K, Wessels A, Soprano D, Abramowitz LK, Bartolomei MS, Rambow F, Bassi MR, Bruno T, Fanciulli M, Renner C, Klein-Szanto AJ, Matsumoto Y, Kobi D, Davidson I, Alberti C, Larue L, Bellacosa A (2011) Thymine DNA glycosylase is essential for active DNA demethylation by linked deamination-base excision repair. Cell 146(1):67–79
58. Cortazar D, Kunz C, Selfridge J, Lettieri T, Saito Y, MacDougall E, Wirz A, Schuermann D, Jacobs AL, Siegrist F, Steinacher R, Jiricny J, Bird A, Schar P (2011) Embryonic lethal pheno-type reveals a function of TDG in maintaining epigenetic stability. Nature 470(7334):419–423
59. Millar CB, Guy J, Sansom OJ, Selfridge J, MacDougall E, Hendrich B, Keightley PD, Bishop SM, Clarke AR, Bird A (2002) Enhanced CpG mutability and tumorigenesis in MBD4-deficient mice. Science 297(5580):403–405
60. Kemmerich K, Dingler FA, Rada C, Neuberger MS (2012) Germline ablation of SMUG1 DNA glycosylase causes loss of 5-hydroxymethyluracil- and UNG-backup uracil-excision activities and increases cancer predisposition of Ung−/−Msh2−/− mice. Nucleic Acids Res 40(13):6016–6025
61. Zhang L, Lu X, Lu J, Liang H, Dai Q, Xu GL, Luo C, Jiang H, He C (2012) Thymine DNA glycosylase specifically recognizes 5-carboxylcytosine-modified DNA. Nat Chem Biol 8(4):328–330
62. Hashimoto H, Liu Y, Upadhyay AK, Chang Y, Howerton SB, Vertino PM, Zhang X, Cheng X (2012) Recognition and potential mechanisms for replication and erasure of cytosine hydroxymethylation. Nucleic Acids Res 40(11):4841–4849
63. Valinluck V, Sowers LC (2007) Endogenous cytosine damage products alter the site selectiv-ity of human DNA maintenance methyltransferase DNMT1. Cancer Res 67(3):946–950
64. Ji D, Lin K, Song J, Wang Y (2014) Effects of Tet-induced oxidation products of 5-methylcytosine on Dnmt1- and DNMT3a-mediated cytosine methylation. Mol BioSyst 10(7):1749–1752
65. Kohli RM, Zhang Y (2013) TET enzymes, TDG and the dynamics of DNA demethylation. Nature 502(7472):472–479
66. Inoue A, Zhang Y (2011) Replication-dependent loss of 5-hydroxymethylcytosine in mouse preimplantation embryos. Science 334(6053):194
67. Hackett JA, Sengupta R, Zylicz JJ, Murakami K, Lee C, Down TA, Surani MA (2013) Germline DNA demethylation dynamics and imprint erasure through 5-hydroxymethylcytosine. Science 339(6118):448–452
68. Schiesser S, Hackner B, Pfaffeneder T, Muller M, Hagemeier C, Truss M, Carell T (2012) Mechanism and stem-cell activity of 5-carboxycytosine decarboxylation determined by iso-tope tracing. Angew Chem Int Ed 51(26):6516–6520
69. Chen CC, Wang KY, Shen CK (2012) The mammalian de novo DNA methyltransferases DNMT3A and DNMT3B are also DNA 5-hydroxymethylcytosine dehydroxymethylases. J Biol Chem 287(40):33116–33121
70. Liutkeviciute Z, Lukinavicius G, Masevicius V, Daujotyte D, Klimasauskas S (2009) Cytosine-5-methyltransferases add aldehydes to DNA. Nat Chem Biol 5(6):400–402

71. Liutkeviciute Z, Kriukiene E, Licyte J, Rudyte M, Urbanaviciute G, Klimasauskas S (2014) Direct decarboxylation of 5-carboxylcytosine by DNA C5-methyltransferases. J Am Chem Soc 136(16):5884–5887
72. Conticello SG (2008) The AID/APOBEC family of nucleic acid mutators. Genome Biol 9(6):229
73. Guo JU, Su Y, Zhong C, Ming GL, Song H (2011) Hydroxylation of 5-methylcytosine by TET1 promotes active DNA demethylation in the adult brain. Cell 145(3):423–434
74. Bransteitter R, Pham P, Scharff MD, Goodman MF (2003) Activation-induced cytidine deaminase deaminates deoxycytidine on single-stranded DNA but requires the action of RNase. Proc Natl Acad Sci U S A 100(7):4102–4107
75. Rangam G, Schmitz KM, Cobb AJ, Petersen-Mahrt SK (2012) AID enzymatic activity is inversely proportional to the size of cytosine C5 orbital cloud. PLoS One 7(8):e43279
76. Ooi SK, Bestor TH (2008) The colorful history of active DNA demethylation. Cell 133(7):1145–1148
77. Bhattacharya SK, Ramchandani S, Cervoni N, Szyf M (1999) A mammalian protein with specific demethylase activity for mCpG DNA. Nature 397(6720):579–583
78. Santos F, Hendrich B, Reik W, Dean W (2002) Dynamic reprogramming of DNA methylation in the early mouse embryo. Dev Biol 241(1):172–182
79. Okada Y, Yamagata K, Hong K, Wakayama T, Zhang Y (2010) A role for the elongator complex in zygotic paternal genome demethylation. Nature 463(7280):554–558
80. Chen CC, Wang KY, Shen CK (2013) DNA 5-methylcytosine demethylation activities of the mammalian DNA methyltransferases. J Biol Chem 288(13):9084–9091
81. Zhu JK (2009) Active DNA demethylation mediated by DNA glycosylases. Annu Rev Genet 43:143–166
82. Zhu B, Zheng Y, Hess D, Angliker H, Schwarz S, Siegmann M, Thiry S, Jost JP (2000) 5-methylcytosine-DNA glycosylase activity is present in a cloned G/T mismatch DNA glycosylase associated with the chicken embryo DNA demethylation complex. Proc Natl Acad Sci U S A 97(10):5135–5139
83. Zhu B, Zheng Y, Angliker H, Schwarz S, Thiry S, Siegmann M, Jost JP (2000) 5-methylcytosine DNA glycosylase activity is also present in the human MBD4 (G/T mismatch glycosylase) and in a related avian sequence. Nucleic Acids Res 28(21):4157–4165
84. Morgan HD, Dean W, Coker HA, Reik W, Petersen-Mahrt SK (2004) Activation-induced cytidine deaminase deaminates 5-methylcytosine in DNA and is expressed in pluripotent tissues: implications for epigenetic reprogramming. J Biol Chem 279(50):52353–52360
85. Rai K, Huggins IJ, James SR, Karpf AR, Jones DA, Cairns BR (2008) DNA demethylation in zebrafish involves the coupling of a deaminase, a glycosylase, and gadd45. Cell 135(7):1201–1212
86. Popp C, Dean W, Feng S, Cokus SJ, Andrews S, Pellegrini M, Jacobsen SE, Reik W (2010) Genome-wide erasure of DNA methylation in mouse primordial germ cells is affected by AID deficiency. Nature 463(7284):1101–1105
87. Bhutani N, Brady JJ, Damian M, Sacco A, Corbel SY, Blau HM (2010) Reprogramming towards pluripotency requires AID-dependent DNA demethylation. Nature 463(7284):1042–1047
88. Kumar R, DiMenna L, Schrode N, Liu TC, Franck P, Munoz-Descalzo S, Hadjantonakis AK, Zarrin AA, Chaudhuri J, Elemento O, Evans T (2013) AID stabilizes stem-cell phenotype by removing epigenetic memory of pluripotency genes. Nature 500(7460):89–92
89. Barreto G, Schafer A, Marhold J, Stach D, Swaminathan SK, Handa V, Doderlein G, Maltry N, Wu W, Lyko F, Niehrs C (2007) Gadd45a promotes epigenetic gene activation by repair-mediated DNA demethylation. Nature 445(7128):671–675
90. Ma DK, Jang MH, Guo JU, Kitabatake Y, Chang ML, Pow-Anpongkul N, Flavell RA, Lu B, Ming GL, Song H (2009) Neuronal activity-induced Gadd45b promotes epigenetic DNA demethylation and adult neurogenesis. Science 323(5917):1074–1077

91. Schmitz KM, Schmitt N, Hoffmann-Rohrer U, Schafer A, Grummt I, Mayer C (2009) TAF12 recruits Gadd45a and the nucleotide excision repair complex to the promoter of rRNA genes leading to active DNA demethylation. Mol Cell 33(3):344–353

92. Engel N, Tront JS, Erinle T, Nguyen N, Latham KE, Sapienza C, Hoffman B, Liebermann DA (2009) Conserved DNA methylation in Gadd45a(−/−) mice. Epigenetics 4(2):98–99

93. Jin SG, Guo C, Pfeifer GP (2008) GADD45A does not promote DNA demethylation. PLoS Genet 4(3):e1000013

94. Wu H, Zhang Y (2014) Reversing DNA methylation: mechanisms, genomics, and biological functions. Cell 156(1–2):45–68

95. Yamaguchi S, Hong K, Liu R, Shen L, Inoue A, Diep D, Zhang K, Zhang Y (2012) Tet1 controls meiosis by regulating meiotic gene expression. Nature 492(7429):443–447

96. Yamaguchi S, Hong K, Liu R, Inoue A, Shen L, Zhang K, Zhang Y (2013) Dynamics of 5-methylcytosine and 5-hydroxymethylcytosine during germ cell reprogramming. Cell Res 23(3):329–339

97. Wossidlo M, Nakamura T, Lepikhov K, Marques CJ, Zakhartchenko V, Boiani M, Arand J, Nakano T, Reik W, Walter J (2011) 5-hydroxymethylcytosine in the mammalian zygote is linked with epigenetic reprogramming. Nat Commun 2:241

98. Iqbal K, Jin SG, Pfeifer GP, Szabo PE (2011) Reprogramming of the paternal genome upon fertilization involves genome-wide oxidation of 5-methylcytosine. Proc Natl Acad Sci U S A 108(9):3642–3647

99. Ficz G, Branco MR, Seisenberger S, Santos F, Krueger F, Hore TA, Marques CJ, Andrews S, Reik W (2011) Dynamic regulation of 5-hydroxymethylcytosine in mouse ES cells and during differentiation. Nature 473(7347):398–402

100. Koh KP, Yabuuchi A, Rao S, Huang Y, Cunniff K, Nardone J, Laiho A, Tahiliani M, Sommer CA, Mostoslavsky G, Lahesmaa R, Orkin SH, Rodig SJ, Daley GQ, Rao A (2011) Tet1 and Tet2 regulate 5-hydroxymethylcytosine production and cell lineage specification in mouse embryonic stem cells. Cell Stem Cell 8(2):200–213

101. Song SJ, Poliseno L, Song MS, Ala U, Webster K, Ng C, Beringer G, Brikbak NJ, Yuan X, Cantley LC, Richardson AL, Pandolfi PP (2013) MicroRNA-antagonism regulates breast cancer Stemness and metastasis via TET-family-dependent chromatin remodeling. Cell 154(2):311–324

102. Song Su J, Ito K, Ala U, Kats L, Webster K, Sun Su M, Jongen-Lavrencic M, Manova-Todorova K, Teruya-Feldstein J, Avigan David E, Delwel R, Pandolfi Pier P (2013) The oncogenic microRNA miR-22 targets the TET2 tumor suppressor to promote hematopoietic stem cell self-renewal and transformation. Cell Stem Cell 13:87–101

103. Wang Y, Zhang Y (2014) Regulation of TET protein stability by Calpains. Cell Rep 6(2):278–284

104. Coulter JB, O'Driscoll CM, Bressler JP (2013) Hydroquinone increases 5-hydroxymethylcytosine formation through ten eleven translocation 1 (Tet1) 5-methylcytosine dioxygenase. J Biol Chem 288(40):28792–28800

105. Yang H, Lin H, Xu H, Zhang L, Cheng L, Wen B, Shou J, Guan K, Xiong Y, Ye D (2014) TET-catalyzed 5-methylcytosine hydroxylation is dynamically regulated by metabolites. Cell Res 24(8):1017–1020

106. Figueroa ME, Abdel-Wahab O, Lu C, Ward PS, Patel J, Shih A, Li Y, Bhagwat N, Vasanthakumar A, Fernandez HF, Tallman MS, Sun Z, Wolniak K, Peeters JK, Liu W, Choe SE, Fantin VR, Paietta E, Lowenberg B, Licht JD, Godley LA, Delwel R, Valk PJ, Thompson CB, Levine RL, Melnick A (2010) Leukemic IDH1 and IDH2 mutations result in a hypermethylation phenotype, disrupt TET2 function, and impair hematopoietic differentiation. Cancer Cell 18(6):553–567

107. Xu W, Yang H, Liu Y, Yang Y, Wang P, Kim SH, Ito S, Yang C, Xiao MT, Liu LX, Jiang WQ, Liu J, Zhang JY, Wang B, Frye S, Zhang Y, Xu YH, Lei QY, Guan KL, Zhao SM, Xiong Y (2011) Oncometabolite 2-hydroxyglutarate is a competitive inhibitor of alpha-ketoglutarate-dependent dioxygenases. Cancer Cell 19(1):17–30

108. Ward PS, Patel J, Wise DR, Abdel-Wahab O, Bennett BD, Coller HA, Cross JR, Fantin VR, Hedvat CV, Perl AE, Rabinowitz JD, Carroll M, Su SM, Sharp KA, Levine RL, Thompson CB (2010) The common feature of leukemia-associated IDH1 and IDH2 mutations is a neomorphic enzyme activity converting alpha-ketoglutarate to 2-hydroxyglutarate. Cancer Cell 17(3):225–234

109. Dang L, White DW, Gross S, Bennett BD, Bittinger MA, Driggers EM, Fantin VR, Jang HG, Jin S, Keenan MC, Marks KM, Prins RM, Ward PS, Yen KE, Liau LM, Rabinowitz JD, Cantley LC, Thompson CB, Vander Heiden MG, Su SM (2009) Cancer-associated IDH1 mutations produce 2-hydroxyglutarate. Nature 462(7274):739–744

110. Xiao M, Yang H, Xu W, Ma S, Lin H, Zhu H, Liu L, Liu Y, Yang C, Xu Y, Zhao S, Ye D, Xiong Y, Guan KL (2012) Inhibition of alpha-KG-dependent histone and DNA demethylases by fumarate and succinate that are accumulated in mutations of FH and SDH tumor suppressors. Genes Dev 26(12):1326–1338

111. Yin R, Mao S-Q, Zhao B, Chong Z, Yang Y, Zhao C, Zhang D, Huang H, Gao J, Li Z, Jiao Y, Li C, Liu S, Wu D, Gu W, Yang Y-G, Xu G-L, Wang H (2013) Ascorbic acid enhances TET-mediated 5-methylcytosine oxidation and promotes DNA demethylation in mammals. J Am Chem Soc 135(28):10396–10403

112. Minor EA, Court BL, Young JI, Wang G (2013) Ascorbate induces ten-eleven translocation (Tet) methylcytosine dioxygenase-mediated generation of 5-hydroxymethylcytosine. J Biol Chem 288(19):13669–13674

113. Blaschke K, Ebata KT, Karimi MM, Zepeda-Martínez JA, Goyal P, Mahapatra S, Tam A, Laird DJ, Hirst M, Rao A, Lorincz MC, Ramalho-Santos M (2013) Vitamin C induces Tet-dependent DNA demethylation and a blastocyst-like state in ES cells. Nature 500(7461):222–226

114. Deplus R, Delatte B, Schwinn MK, Defrance M, Méndez J, Murphy N, Ma D, Volkmar M, Putmans P, Calonne E, Shih AH, Levine RL, Bernard O, Mercher T, Solary E, Urh M, Daniels DL, Fuks F (2013) TET2 and TET3 regulate GlcNAcylation and H3K4 methylation through OGT and SET1/COMPASS. EMBO J 32:645–655

115. Chen Q, Chen Y, Bian C, Fujiki R, Yu X (2013) TET2 promotes histone O-GlcNAcylation during gene transcription. Nature 493:561–564

116. Vella P, Scelfo A, Jammula S, Chiacchiera F, Williams K, Cuomo A, Roberto A, Christensen J, Bonaldi T, Helin K, Pasini D (2013) Tet proteins connect the O-linked N-acetylglucosamine transferase Ogt to chromatin in embryonic stem cells. Mol Cell 49:645–656

117. Shi FT, Kim H, Lu W, He Q, Liu D, Goodell MA, Wan M, Songyang Z (2013) Ten-eleven translocation 1 (tet1) is regulated by o-linked N-acetylglucosamine transferase (ogt) for target gene repression in mouse embryonic stem cells. J Biol Chem 288(29):20776–20784

118. Zhang Q, Liu X, Gao W, Li P, Hou J, Li J, Wong J (2014) Differential regulation of the ten-eleven translocation (TET) family of dioxygenases by O-linked beta-N-acetylglucosamine transferase (OGT). J Biol Chem 289(9):5986–5996

119. Wang Y, Xiao M, Chen X, Chen L, Xu Y, Lv L, Wang P, Yang H, Ma S, Lin H, Jiao B, Ren R, Ye D, Guan KL, Xiong Y (2015) WT1 recruits TET2 to regulate its target gene expression and suppress leukemia cell proliferation. Mol Cell 57(4):662–673

120. Nakamura T, Liu YJ, Nakashima H, Umehara H, Inoue K, Matoba S, Tachibana M, Ogura A, Shinkai Y, Nakano T (2012) PGC7 binds histone H3K9me2 to protect against conversion of 5mC to 5hmC in early embryos. Nature 486(7403):415–419

121. Bian C, Yu X (2014) PGC7 suppresses TET3 for protecting DNA methylation. Nucleic Acids Res 42(5):2893–2905

122. Yildirim O, Li R, Hung JH, Chen PB, Dong X, Ee LS, Weng Z, Rando OJ, Fazzio TG (2011) Mbd3/NURD complex regulates expression of 5-hydroxymethylcytosine marked genes in embryonic stem cells. Cell 147(7):1498–1510

123. Spruijt CG, Gnerlich F, Smits AH, Pfaffeneder T, Jansen PWTC, Bauer C, Münzel M, Wagner M, Müller M, Khan F, Eberl HC, Mensinga A, Brinkman AB, Lephikov K, Müller U, Walter J, Boelens R, van Ingen H, Leonhardt H, Carell T, Vermeulen M (2013) Dynamic readers for 5-(hydroxy)methylcytosine and its oxidized derivatives. Cell 152:1146–1159

DNA Methylation Changes in Cancer

John P. Thomson and Richard R. Meehan

Abstract Although cancer is a genetic disease, broad changes in epigenomic profiles are a key observation in many distinct cancer types that can be diagnostic, reflect altered signalling/gene regulatory networks and may directly contribute to the disease state. In this short review we will focus on how DNA modification changes have contributed to our understanding of cancer progression and the hypothesis that cancer cells have an epigenome reflecting altered dependencies compared to the tissue of origin.

Keywords DNA methylation reprogramming • 5-hydroxymethylcytosine landscapes • Cancer diagnostics • Tet-1/2/3 enzymes

1 Introduction

The concept of 'epigenetics' was originated by Conrad Waddington to resolve a potential paradox of cellular differentiation; how can embryological cells with similar genetic material differentiate into multiple and distinct cell types [1, 2]. Importantly, whatever the epigenetic mechanism is, it had to incorporate the idea of inheritance of altered gene expression states during subsequent divisions of committed cells, even after the signals that initiated epigenetic changes may have long ceased [2–5]. This concept runs in parallel with the idea that signalling pathways and gene regulatory networks organise the development of an organism from a fertilized egg through embryogenesis and adulthood, a fundamentally genetic basis of development and disease [6–8]. Waddington's illustrative 'epigenetic landscapes' are bedded on the action of genes, which influence the epigenetic states adopted by differentiating cells [1, 9]. In Waddington's landscape, as the cell progresses down the valleys, its genetic information becomes modified (but not lost) which restricts its developmental potential. Subsequent molecular analysis identified chromatin-centred mechanisms which can promote the selective gene silencing and activation

J.P. Thomson • R.R. Meehan (✉)
MRC Human Genetics Unit, Institute of Genetics and Molecular Medicine,
University of Edinburgh, Crewe Road, Edinburgh EH4 2XU, UK
e-mail: John.Thomson@igmm.ed.ac.uk; richard.meehan@igmm.ed.ac.uk

© Springer International Publishing AG 2017   75
A. Kaneda, Y.-i. Tsukada (eds.), *DNA and Histone Methylation as Cancer Targets*,
Cancer Drug Discovery and Development, DOI 10.1007/978-3-319-59786-7_4

profiles that are characteristic of cell types [10]. However, the ability to transdifferentiate cells with core transcription factors offers strong evidence for gene regulatory networks (GRN) as the dominant mode of development specification and it is within this context that epigenetic mechanisms operate [11]. One question that then arises, can embryo development or cancer transformation occur without active epigenetic pathways? Understanding the potential roles of epigenetic processes in cancer is predicated on comprehending their role in development, how and why they are altered during cellular transformation and what are the functional consequences of these alterations [12, 13]. It is becoming increasingly clear that disruption of the "epigenome" as a result of alterations in epigenetic regulators is a fundamental mechanism in cancer, which has implications for both molecular diagnostics and small molecule cancer therapies.

2   DNA Methylation Machinery

A core feature of 'epigenetics' is that developmental potential is linked with changes in gene activity independently of genetic alterations. This concept has driven the identification of DNA and chromatin modifying activities which participate in regulating gene expression profiles in development and disease states [9, 10]. However, the targeting of many of these activities depends on a classical transcriptional mechanism, where DNA-binding proteins recruit chromatin/DNA-modifying activities in concert with the transcriptional machinery [7].

In mammals, DNA methylation is the best studied epigenetic mark in development and disease contexts, especially in cancer studies [14]. This is partly due the relatively simple models that correlate changes in chromatin function with altered DNA methylation profiles, efficient data generation and sophisticated bioinformatics analysis [15–20]. It is well established that CpG Island (CGI) methylation can provide strong and heritable repression of transcription, and that ectopic de novo methylation of CGI's associated with tumour suppressor genes can potentially contribute to establishing the cancer state [21–23]. However, there is still strong debate as to whether observed promoter methylation alterations are a cause or consequence of gene inactivation in cancer, as much of the analysis relies on correlative evidence [21, 22]?

The maintenance methyltransferase Dnmt1 and its cofactors have been classically considered responsible for the perpetuation of DNA methylation during cell divisions, whereas de novo DNA methylation is initially established in development by a combination of Dnmt3A and Dnmt3B acting in concert with the cofactor Dnmt3L [24–27]. Dnmt3L itself is essential during germ cell development to ensure that endogenous retrotransposons are inactivated [28]. Somatic patterns of DNA methylation participate at multiple levels (locus specific, genome stability and indirectly) in most epigenetic mechanisms, including X-chromosome inactivation, ensuring genomic imprinting, retrotransposon silencing and gene repression [16, 29–32]. 5-methyl cytosine (5mC) is enzymatically generated on mammalian DNA by the addition of a methyl group to the carbon-5 position of the pyrimidine ring of cytosine, mostly in the context of the dinucleotide CpG [33]. Both DNA strands are symmetrically methylated at CpGs and during replication hemi-methylated DNA is potent substrate for the maintenance DNA methyltransferase, Dnmt1; perpetuating the parental pattern [33]. Genome-wide profiling demonstrate that methylated CpG (MeCpGs) are pervasive throughout mammalian genomes, with the exception of discrete non-methylated CGI which feature as regulatory landmarks, as they are mostly associated with gene promoters [34–38]. Changes in DNA methylation profiles and content are indicative of an altered cellular state, as first exemplified in early cancer studies [39–42]. This has been replicated many times culminating in nucleotide resolution modification maps of cancer cell lines and tumours, for example colon cancer, which exhibit characteristic alterations [19, 43]. DNA methylation data from many cancer genome consortia are being continuously incorporated with comprehensive resources of somatic mutations in human cancer to improve definitions of disease types at presentation, remission and reoccurrence [44]. DNA methylation profiling has also been used extensively in reprogramming and disease studies to chart changes in cell state, which can also be linked to physiological processes, such as ageing and metabolism [45–51].

The attraction of DNA methylation as an epigenetic mark was the observation that symmetrically methylated DNA is relatively stable in the originating cell and the patterns can be propagated through cell division by the DNA methylation machinery, which integrates with DNA replication pathways [23, 52]. In general, the occurrence of DNA methylation at regulatory regions such as enhancers or active CGI promoters is associated with induced transcriptional repression, which may be mediated by direct inhibition of Transcription Factor (TF) binding or by attracting chromatin silencing activities [13, 16]. Differentially methylated promoters associated with gene inactivation in different tissues types have been identified, but these may correspond to a remarkably small number of genes that are normally expressed in the germline [29, 30]. Most silent non-methylated CGI genes are associated with a histone repressive modification profile that is dependent on Polycomb Repressive Complex's 1 and 2, which are responsible for adding a ubiquityl moiety to histone H2A at Lys119 (H2AK119ub1; PRC1)) and the addition of one to three methyl groups to histone H3 at Lys27, leading to H3K27me1, H3K27me2 and H3K27me3 (PRC2) respectively [53, 54]. It is the H3K27me3 mark that is resolutely associated with gene repression.

DNA methylation undergoes extensive reprogramming during early embryo development and in primordial germ cell (PGC) progression (PGCs), which have been linked with signal induced pathways that shift DNA methylation profiles in mouse ES cells [32, 50, 55–58]. Similar developmental changes have been observed in other somatic cell contexts [59, 60]. Until recently it was unclear what the molecular mechanisms were that underpinned 'DNA demethylation' pathways, whose disruption could account for the altered patterns of hyper- and hypo-DNA methylation observed in many cancers [61–63].

3 DNA De-methylation

Two basic mechanisms leading to DNA demethylation can be considered; (A) a passive mechanism in which re-methylation of hemi-methylated substrates during DNA replication is prevented, thus leading to progressive loss of 5mC in concert with cellular proliferation and (B) active processes that remove the modification or modified bases from DNA [64–69]. 5mC marks can be converted back to an unmodified state via methylcytosine dioxygenase enzymes known as the Ten-Eleven-Translocases (TETs 1, 2 & 3) that can generate intermediates in a potential DNA demethylation pathway; 5-hydroxymethylcytosine (5hmC), 5-formylcytosine (5fC) and 5-carboxylcytosine (5caC) [70–72] (Fig. 1). 5hmC has gathered much interest in recent years as its stable relative abundance predicts that it may have biological functions in addition to its role as a DNA demethylation intermediate [72–75]. The presence of oxidation derivatives may also lead to passive demethylation because

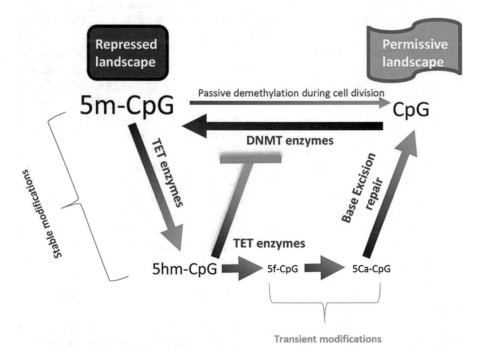

Fig. 1 Overview of the DNA methylation cycle. DNA modification occurs largely at CpG (cytosine-phosphodiester-guanine) dinucleotides in the mammalian genome. The bulk of CpGs are modified by methylation (5m–CpG). Recent reports reveal that these methylated cytosines can be converted to 5-hydroxymethylcytosine (5hm-CpG) through the actions of the TET enzymes. 5hmC is relatively stable but can be further converted into 5-formylcytosine (5f–CpG) and 5-carboxylcytosine (5Ca–CpG) which are rapidly removed by base excision repair, resulting in an unmodified CpG dinucleotide. Relative amounts of each modification are suggested through the font size of the CpG text. The presence of 5hmC in the genome can dampen the activity of DNA methyltransferases (DNMTs) leading to passive hypomethylation via DNA replication

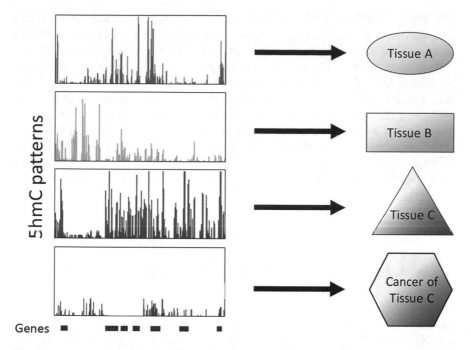

Fig. 2 DNA modification patterns act as identifiers of cell state. Both 5mC and 5hmC patterns are unique to given cell types and are strongly altered in cancer. Understanding how these epigenetic changes relate to transcriptional outcomes for a given cell is important for understanding their significance in cancer

they are not properly recognized by the methylation maintenance machinery, for example DNMT1 is not active on hemi-hydroxymethylated DNA [76]. Another possibility is that 5hmC, 5caC, or 5fC trigger erasure by DNA glycosylases such as thymine DNA glycosylase (TDG), followed by base excision repair [77–79]. However oocyte-specific *Tdg* conditional knockout gives rise to normal offspring which do not exhibit altered levels of zygotic 5hmC [80]. This result may indicate the existence of as-yet-unknown demethylation mechanisms downstream of 5mC oxidation [81].

TET enzyme conversion of 5-methyl modified cytosine bases to 5-hydroxymethyl marked bases by oxidation occurs in an iron and α-ketoglutarate (αKG) dependent manner [70, 71]. Changes in TET activity is linked with altered 5mC patterns in many cancers [82–87]. Although less abundant in absolute terms than 5mC (between 0.1% and 0.7% of all cytosines) the levels of 5-hydroxy-marked cytosines are far greater than the downstream DNA demethylation modifications; 5fC and 5caC; the more abundant 5hmC may also have a functional role throughout the genome [69, 74].

The patterns of the modifications vary greatly between tissue and cell types – to the extent that 5hmC profiling can be used as an exquisite identifier of cell state or tissue type [49, 59, 88, 89] (Fig. 2). A consensus view is such that 5hmC modified

CpGs are generally depleted over the majority of promoter elements but are enriched over the bodies of transcriptionally active genes and enhancer elements as well as a small number of transcriptional starts sites associated with silenced genes [90, 91]. This contrasts with 5mC profiles which are present genome wide and enriched at satellite and repeat DNA sequences [90]. Proximal enrichment of 5hmC at enhancers upstream of annotated transcriptional start sites (TSS) suggests a role for these regions in the regulation of gene expression [92]. Histone modification profiles around genes strongly overlaps with peaks of 5hmC in normal tissues, for example active enhancer marks, H3K4me1/H3K27ac, are associated with 5hmC at regions flanking transcription start sites (TSS) [59, 93]. The fact that 5hmC profiles are related to the transcriptional landscape means that it is a far more dynamic modification than 5mC – which is typically thought of as a stable lock on inactive chromatin states.

4   DNA Modification Perturbations in Cancer

Disruption of epigenetic landscapes, including 5hmC and 5mC patterns, is a hallmark of cancer [93–97] (Fig. 3). Although the underlying mechanisms of cancer-specific methylation changes are still largely unclear, it is apparent that they can occur early in both cancer initiation and progression [98]. Focal hypermethylation of specific regions of the genome was first reported in 1986 and inactivation of the RB1 gene in retinoblastoma cells by de novo methylation of its CGI was reported in 1989 [99, 100]. Subsequently causation, mechanism, scope, and the potential for experimental artefacts were addressed in multiple studies investigating the relationship between alterations in genomic methylation patterns and carcinogenesis [12, 14, 101]. Accumulative evidence suggests that DNA methylation patterns are often drastically different in cancer compared to those found in the normal healthy tissue, which can create altered epigenetic dependencies [23]. Three major epigenetic alterations are frequently observed: (A) global DNA hypo-methylation in cancer across large domains and affecting repetitive DNA sequences, (B) global hypo-hydroxymethylation across the majority of the genome including over promoters and gene bodies, and (C) discrete gene-specific hypermethylation of CGIs, CGI shores and enhancer elements affecting hundreds of loci [82, 101–104]. Given the dynamic interplay that 5mC and 5hmC exhibit, the observed changes in each modification throughout cancer are dynamically linked [87, 105, 106].

5   Discrete Hyper-Methylation Events in Cancer

Recent evidence suggests that disruption of the normal DNA methylation/demethylation cycle during carcinogenesis may be one mechanism that is responsible for aberrant CGI hyper-methylation events [87, 93, 97, 99, 102, 103] (Figs. 1 and 2).

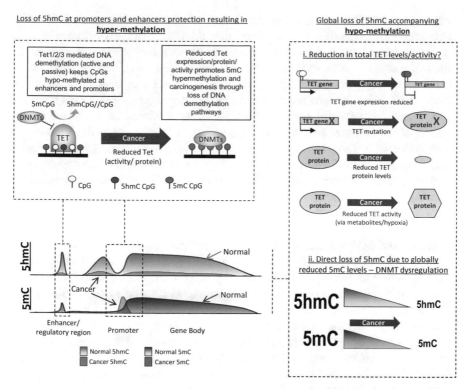

Fig. 3 Schematic for 5hmC and 5mC patterns across the genome in normal and cancer cells. Coloured plots show typical 5hmC and 5mC patterns across the genome. Typically 5hmC is found enriched over enhancers, promoter proximal and genic regions, whilst 5mC is found at enhancer, genic and repetitive elements (not shown). In cancer 5hmC is lost from promoter and enhancer regions contributing to aberrant hypermethylation events. In contrast, genic 5hmC loss accompanies loss of 5mC. *Dashed boxes* indicate possible mechanisms for these two observations

Mutations in the *TET1* gene are associated with hematopoietic malignancy where loss of 5hmC and/or gain of 5mC on promoters in *tet1*$^{-/-}$ cells may result in down-regulation of expression and derailment of the differentiation process [107]. Of interest is the observation that oncogenic KRAS can inhibit TET1 expression via the ERK-signalling pathway; restoration of TET1 expression by ERK pathway inhibition or ectopic TET1 reintroduction in KRAS-transformed cells reactivates a select number of target genes [85]. This indicates a dichotomy between signalling induced regulation of methylation of a discrete number of CGI target genes and generalised tissue determined CGI methylator profiles that are variable within tumour types [3, 97]. In the latter case, *de novo* methylation occurs predominantly at already silenced genes (passenger genes) and therefore does not affect their expression status while in the former silencing by DNA methylation of select target genes is dependent on an active signalling pathway and therefore is not strictly epigenetic in character [85, 96]. Oncogenic RAS or BRAF is required for both initiation of the pathway and maintenance of repression via the activation of pathway intermediates which can direct methylation at select target CGI genes [108–110]. This consideration leads to two questions; how do tumour suppressor genes become methylated and how is DNA methylation of tumour suppressor genes inherited through multiple generations [3]? One idea would be that DNA methylation at TSGs is not epigenetically inherited, but is maintained by an instructive transcriptional mechanism that can potentially repress multiple genes [3]. In contrast, we have recently shown that the aberrant CGI hyper-methylation in several mouse models of liver cancer occurs at sites marked by a unique chromatin state in the healthy liver [87]. The promoter proximal sites destined to become hyper-methylated in liver cancer were found to be rich in 5hmC and associated with "bivalently" marked histone tail modifications (H3K27me3 and H3K4me3), which are typically associated with a transcriptionally poised but not active expression states. We observe loss of 5hmC occurs at these sites prior to accumulation of 5mC and this is related to a reduction in the levels of the TET1 enzyme, which has previously been shown to bind preferentially to CGIs. Loss or reduced binding of TET1 from these CGIs would ultimately result in a loss of active, 'protective' DNA demethylation and acquisition of 5mC (Fig. 3). The activity of TET enzymes can also be reduced by tumour hypoxia in human and mouse cells, which occurs independently of hypoxia-associated alterations in TET expression and depends directly on oxygen shortage [86]. This can result in increased hypermethylation at gene promoters in vitro, patients exhibit markedly more methylated at selected promoters in hypoxic tumour tissue, independently of proliferation, stromal cell infiltration and tumour characteristics. Increased hypoxia in mouse breast tumours also increases hyper-methylation, while restoration of tumour oxygenation abrogates this effect.

Hyper-methylation at CGIs is often invoked as a mechanism of transcriptional inactivation of tumour suppressor genes that directly drives the carcinogenic process, however many of the genes associated with hyperethylated CGIs in cancer are already silent in the host tissue to begin with [12, 87, 96, 97, 111–113]. Recent data suggests that changes in 5mC profiles over enhancer elements may instead be related to the phenotypic and transcriptomic changes observed during cancer progression [93]. Enhancers are consistently the most differentially methylated regions during the progression from normal tissue to primary tumours and subsequently to metastases, compared to other genomic features. Changes in the 5mC levels at these loci have been linked to cancer type as well as the overall patient outcome [93, 103].

The anti-cancer effects of DNA methyltransferase inhibitors has been linked with upregulation of immune signalling in cancer through the viral defence pathway, independently of CpG island methylator profiles [114, 115]. In these examples, upregulation of intergenic hypomethylated endogenous retrovirus (ERV) genes accompanies, and may drive, the response. This anti-viral response may underlie some of the anti-tumour activity of these drugs, e.g. 5-Azacytidine (AZA), as transfection of dsRNA derived from AZA-treated cells, but not control cells, induced an antiviral response in recipient cells. Interferon pathway genes were also upregulated by AZA, and this was correlated with increased expression of endogenous retroviral transcripts rather than de-repression of interferon pathway transcription factors [114, 115] (Fig. 4).

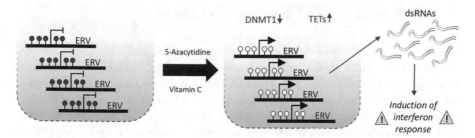

Fig. 4 Schematic of the molecular mechanisms of combined 5-Azacytidine and Vitamin C treatment in generating an anti-tumour response. Loss of 5mC at multiple endogenous retrovirus (ERV) genes occurs through inhibition of DNMT1 by 5-Azacytidine and stimulation of active DNA demethylation through elevated TET enzyme activity following vitamin C treatment. This results in the induction of double stranded RNAs (dsRNAs) which are recognised by the cell and stimulate an interferon response, enhanced immune signalling resulting in reduced cell proliferation and ultimately apoptosis of tumour cells

6 Changes to the 5hmC Landscape in Cancer

Studies using immunohistochemistry, immuno-dot blot and mass spectroscopy, consistently report a strong global loss of 5hmC in cancer cell lines and tumours [87, 88, 104, 116–120] (Fig. 3). In concert with these reduced global levels of 5hmC, genome-wide patterns of 5hmC are also markedly altered between tumour samples and normal surrounding tissue [87, 93, 104, 120, 121]. In melanoma, there is both loss and gain of genic 5hmC at a large number of gene bodies: although the changes in 5mC are far more subtle than for 5hmC. These genes tended to be associated with melanoma related pathways, Wnt signalling components and not surprisingly, general cancer progression. In lung and liver cancers the specific relationships between 5hmC and sets of chromatin marks present in normal tissue is largely absent in tumours, which may drive or reflect altered regulation of gene expression [93]. In both mouse liver cancer and in human cancer cell lines, 5hmC is lost from a series of promoter regions, resulting in aberrant hyper-methylation event at such sites and reinforcing the reciprocity between these two marks in the regulation of DNA modification landscapes [86, 87, 122]. As well as genic and promoter regions, 5hmC is typically strongly enriched over promoter–proximal enhancer elements. In mouse ES cells, loss of TET enzymes results in hypermethylation at such enhancer elements and delays nearby gene induction during differentiation [123]. Similar results have also been observed in acute myeloid leukemia (AML) where loss of the TET2 enzyme was linked to hypermethylation of ~25% of active enhancer elements [124]. These results indicate that the TET enzymes are fundamentally required to maintain normal epigenetic and transcriptomic landscapes in a given cell at least in part through the protection of key regulatory loci such as enhancers and promoter elements. This dysregulation can, in turn, provide the cell with a growth advantage through increases stem cell-like proliferation and silencing of tumour suppressor genes (Fig. 3). Studies comparing 5hmC changes between tumour types and subtypes are essential to shed light on the molecular events associated with cancer progression, and to the identification of biomarkers for clinical use.

7   The Role of the TET Enzymes in Cancer

The TET methyl cystosine dioxygenase enzymes (TET1, 2 and 3) – as well as several of their cofactors, are often mutated, transcriptionally downregulated or reduced at the protein level [86, 87, 125]. There is substantial amount of overlap in 5hmC deposition by the three members as Tet-1, -2 or -3 null mice are viable and that loss of 5hmC is not absolute in *Tet1* null mouse livers [87, 126]. Short hairpin RNA (shRNA) reduction of each of the TET enzymes in human embryonic carcinoma cells has shown that loss of TET1 resulted in the greatest elevation of 5mC at promoter elements as well as widespread reduction of 5hmC, while depletion of TET2 and TET3 reduces 5hmC at a subset of TET1 targets suggesting functional co-dependence [122]. All TET mediated 5hmC can prevent hypermethylation throughout the genome, particularly at CGI shores where loss of all three TETs was related to hypermethylation events [93, 104, 121]. Loss of 5hmC at enhancers in Tet2$^{-/-}$ mouse ES cells resulted in their hypermethylation and impacted on gene expression during early stages of ES cell differentiation [123].

Analysis of large numbers of human cancer studies (such as those recorded in the Catalogue of Somatic Mutations in Cancer – "COSMIC" – database) reveals a differing number of mutations across the three TET enzymes. TET2 is the most frequently mutated of the three however such mutations are more or less exclusively found in haematopoietic and lymphoid cancers (14.18% COSMIC datasets). TET1 and TET3 are by comparison only found mutated in a rare number of cases (both typically <0.5% of human cancers; TET3 mutated ~5% of skin cancers and 3% of colorectal cancers) [44]. Although specific mutations within the TET1 gene have not been directly associated with cancer progression, reduced transcriptional and/or protein levels of TET1 has been reported in colon, gastric, lung and liver cancers whilst TET2 transcription/protein levels are more typically reduced in leukaemia and melanoma [83, 105, 116, 120, 127–129]. TET1 downregulation has also been shown to promote malignancy in breast cancer and to act as a tumour suppressor that can inhibit colon cancer growth by de-repressing inhibitors of the WNT pathway [83]. In addition, reduced levels of TET1 has also been shown to result in elevated rates of metastasis in gastric cancer through the miss-regulation of downstream pathways required for tumour migration [128]. Interestingly TET1 is itself found both methylated and transcriptionally repressed in a series of cell lines and primary tumours of multiple carcinomas and lymphoma although, whether or not the methylation is itself causative or reflective of TET transcriptional inactivation is still to be fully elucidated [85, 127].

The activity of TET enzymes can be inhibited or stimulated by several cofactors, metabolites, and post-translational modifications. This is most evident in cancers harbouring gain-of-function mutations in the genes *IDH1* and *IDH2* – the Krebs cycle enzymes isocitrate dehydrogenase 1 and 2 – which results in the aberrant conversion of αKG into 2-hydroxyglutarate (2HG), a potent inhibitor of TET activity [105]. Mutations in two other Krebs cycle proteins; Fumarate hydratase (FH) and succinate dehydrogenase (SDH) are relatively common in a subset of human cancers including Gastrointestinal stromal tumours (3–8% of SDH cases), Renal cell carcinomas (1–4% of SDH and 71–93% of FH cases) and Paraganglioma (12–15% of SDH cases) [130–132]. Mutations in FH and SDH lead to an accumulation of fumarate and succinate which can inhibit multiple αKG-dependent dioxygenases, including the TET family of enzymes. Loss of TET activity in tumour hypoxia was found to result in a loss of 5hmC and gain of 5mC over gene promoters and enhancer elements, once again reinforcing the "protective" role that these enzymes play at these loci in the normal cell [86].

In contrast, it has been shown that increasing the levels of ascorbic acid (vitamin C) stimulates TET protein enzymatic activity in both cultured cells as well as mouse tissues [49, 133]. The addition of vitamin C to low doses with AZA results in a synergistic inhibition of cancer-cell proliferation and increased apoptosis. These effects are associated with enhanced immune signals including increased expression of bidirectionally transcribed ERVs, increased cytosolic dsRNA, and activation of an IFN-inducing cellular response [134]. Many patients with hematological neoplasia are markedly vitamin C deficient, treatment of patients with hematological and other cancers with vitamin C may improve responses to epigenetic therapy with DNA methyltransferase inhibitors [134]. Treatment with DNA methylation inhibitors to activate a growth-inhibiting immune response may also be an effective therapeutic approach for colon cancers [135]. Taken together, these results highlight the complex relationship between 5hmC disruption and cancer progression that is not only reliant directly on the transcriptional state of the TET enzymes but also the overall environment in the cancer cell [136].

8 Indirect Impact of DNA Methylation Reprogramming on Cancer Epigenomes

Two major differences can be observed between normal mammalian DNA methylation landscapes and those found in cancer cell lines and tumours, (i) as discussed above, many CGIs become aberrantly hypermethylated in cancerous cells whereas (ii) hypo-DNA methylation occurs at other genomic regions [137]. Genes that are subject to CGI promoter hypermethylation are frequently marked by PRC2-deposited H3K27me3 in early development [138, 139]. The persistence of H3K27me3 at these regions in normal cells and in development is dependent on the global 5mC content [50, 140–142]. Induced hypomethylation results in loss of H3K27me3 from previously unmethylated CGIs, which in a somatic cell context can lead to gene activation [142]. Importantly, DNA hypomethylation results in the accumulation of the PRC2 complex components and H3K27me3 to genomic locations that were previously DNA methylated, suggesting that dense DNA methylation prevents PRC2 binding to chromatin. In addition, TET1 is required for a significant proportion of PRC targeting in mouse ES cells, connecting this putative demethylation pathway to PRC recruitment [87, 143]. In this context it is formally possible that delocalisation of PRC complexes in tandem with loss of demethylation activities makes CGI genes formerly marked by H3K27me3 susceptible to *de novo* methylation during the epigenomic reprogramming phase of carcinogenesis [18]. This brings the relationship between DNA methylation and the Polycomb system to the forefront of cancer epigenomics, and also has implications for genome regulation [144]. An important inference is that reprogramming of DNA methylation patterns in cancer could trigger mis-regulation of transcriptional programs through subsequent redistribution of the repressive activity of PRCs, that in addition also feeds back on ectopic targeting of de novo methylation to CGIs previously marked by H3K27me3 [18]. These targets include a large number of genes with key functions in cell lineage decisions and the regulation of the cell cycle, which have a major impact on the development and progression of cancer [54]. Mutations resulting in histone variants in cancers that are resistant to modification can impact on diverse aspects of chromatin biology including DNA methylation and gene expression [20]. The functional interplay between DNA methylation and PRC pathways are also likely to be important in other biological systems, especially ageing [46, 145]. In cancer, these mechanisms promote a transcriptome that facilitates cancer formation, plasticity, and progression; analysis of multiple cancer DNA methylomes implies that altered TF binding occurs contributing to altered enhancer activities, which impacts on the transforming processes during carcinogenesis [87, 113, 146]. The checkpoints that enable correct preservation of transcriptional circuits and metabolic programs are often absent in tumorigenic lesions, thus imparting cancer cells with the ability to generate novel transcriptional, metabolic and epigenetic dependencies [147].

9   Future Perspectives

Future studies should concentrate on dissecting the cause-consequence relationships involved in cancer transformation, the role of epigenetic plasticity in driving tumour progression and identity, the epigenetics of cellular heterogeneity and exploring potential points of combinatorial therapeutic intervention. This will involve patient/tumour stratification by genetic, metabolic and epigenetic profiling, which in themselves may provide new markers for early diagnosis (Fig. 5).

The ability to identify DNA based markers for liquid biopsies of circulating tumour cells, may be effective in identifying origin of the tumour, especially during metastasis [148]. Regulation of the inhibitory immune receptor programmed cell death-1 (PD-1) is governed by cis-DNA elements, TFs, and epigenetic modifications [149, 150]. Of note is a report that PD-1 promoter methylation is an independent prognostic biomarker for biochemical recurrence-free survival in prostate cancer patients, which may linked with immune surveillance [151, 152]. Finally the availability of new gene-editing tools may enable exquisite manipulation of cancer epigenetic profiles, including Tet gene function, that promote cell death rather that cell proliferation [13, 153].

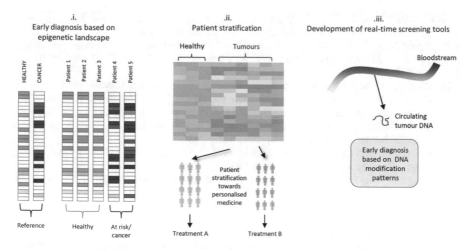

Fig. 5 Utility of DNA modification based assays towards clinical application. Analysis of genome wide DNA modification landscapes holds potential towards the development of novel early stage diagnostic screens (**i**), stratification of tumour subclasses towards more efficient personalised medicine regimes (**ii**) and the development of new real-time screening tools such as epigenetic based liquid biopsy screens (**iii**)

Acknowledgements We would like to thank Colm Nestor (Linköping University) for helpful comments and insight. Part of this work was supported by the Metastasis prize from The Beug Foundation to JT. RM is supported by the Medical Research Council (MRC_MC_PC_U127574433). Work in RM's lab is supported by CEFIC, the BBSRC and the MRC.

References

1. Waddington CH (1957) The strategy of the genes: a discussion of some aspects of theoretical biology. Book – Ruskin House/George Allen and Unwin Ltd, London
2. Waddington CH (2012) The epigenotype. 1942. Int J Epidemiol 41(1):10–13. doi:10.1093/ije/dyr184
3. Struhl K (2014) Is DNA methylation of tumour suppressor genes epigenetic? elife 3:e02475. doi:10.7554/eLife.02475
4. Gilbert SF (2012) Commentary: 'The epigenotype' by C.H. Waddington. Int J Epidemiol 41(1):20–23. doi:10.1093/ije/dyr186
5. Noble D (2015) Conrad Waddington and the origin of epigenetics. J Exp Biol 218(Pt 6):816–818. doi:10.1242/jeb.120071
6. Ptashne M (2013) Epigenetics: core misconcept. Proc Natl Acad Sci U S A 110(18):7101–7103. doi:10.1073/pnas.1305399110
7. Peter IS, Davidson EH (2016) Implications of developmental gene regulatory networks inside and outside developmental biology. Curr Top Dev Biol 117:237–251. doi:10.1016/bs.ctdb.2015.12.014
8. Lander ES (2011) Initial impact of the sequencing of the human genome. Nature 470(7333):187–197. doi:10.1038/nature09792
9. Deichmann U (2016) Epigenetics: the origins and evolution of a fashionable topic. Dev Biol 416(1):249–254. doi:10.1016/j.ydbio.2016.06.005

10. Cantone I, Fisher AG (2013) Epigenetic programming and reprogramming during development. Nat Struct Mol Biol 20(3):282–289. doi:10.1038/nsmb.2489
11. Takahashi K, Yamanaka S (2006) Induction of pluripotent stem cells from mouse embryonic and adult fibroblast cultures by defined factors. Cell 126(4):663–676. doi:10.1016/j.cell.2006.07.024
12. Timp W, Feinberg AP (2013) Cancer as a dysregulated epigenome allowing cellular growth advantage at the expense of the host. Nat Rev Cancer 13(7):497–510. doi:10.1038/nrc3486
13. Amabile A, Migliara A, Capasso P, Riffi M, Cittaro D, Naldini L, Lombardo A (2016) Inheritable silencing of endogenous genes by hit-and-run targeted epigenetic editing. Cell 167(1):219–232. e214. doi:10.1016/j.cell.2016.09.006
14. Razvi E, Oosta G (2016) Epigenetics market landscape: a qualitative and quantitative picture. Genetic Engineering and Biotechnology News
15. Plongthongkum N, Diep DH, Zhang K (2014) Advances in the profiling of DNA modifications: cytosine methylation and beyond. Nat Rev Genet 15(10):647–661
16. Reddington JP, Pennings S, Meehan RR (2013) Non-canonical functions of the DNA methylome in gene regulation. Biochem J 451(1):13–23. doi:10.1042/bj20121585
17. Farlik M, Sheffield NC, Nuzzo A, Datlinger P, Schonegger A, Klughammer J, Bock C (2015) Single-cell DNA methylome sequencing and bioinformatic inference of epigenomic cell-state dynamics. Cell Rep 10(8):1386–1397
18. Hon GC, Hawkins RD, Caballero OL, Lo C, Lister R, Pelizzola M, Valsesia A, Ye Z, Kuan S, Edsall LE, Camargo AA, Stevenson BJ, Ecker JR, Bafna V, Strausberg RL, Simpson AJ, Ren B (2012) Global DNA hypomethylation coupled to repressive chromatin domain formation and gene silencing in breast cancer. Genome Res 22(2):246–258
19. Berman BP, Weisenberger DJ, Aman JF, Hinoue T, Ramjan Z, Liu Y, Noushmehr H, Lange CP, van Dijk CM, Tollenaar RA, Van Den Berg D, Laird PW (2012) Regions of focal DNA hypermethylation and long-range hypomethylation in colorectal cancer coincide with nuclear lamina-associated domains. Nat Genet 44(1):40–46. doi:10.1038/ng.969
20. Plass C, Pfister SM, Lindroth AM, Bogatyrova O, Claus R, Lichter P (2013) Mutations in regulators of the epigenome and their connections to global chromatin patterns in cancer. Nat Rev Genet 14(11):765–780
21. Bestor TH (2003) Unanswered questions about the role of promoter methylation in carcinogenesis. Ann N Y Acad Sci 983:22–27
22. Baylin S, Bestor TH (2002) Altered methylation patterns in cancer cell genomes: cause or consequence? Cancer Cell 1(4):299–305
23. Sharma S, Kelly TK, Jones PA (2010) Epigenetics in cancer. Carcinogenesis 31(1):27–36
24. Hata K, Okano M, Lei H, Li E (2002) Dnmt3L cooperates with the Dnmt3 family of de novo DNA methyltransferases to establish maternal imprints in mice. Development 129(8):1983–1993
25. Li E, Bestor TH, Jaenisch R (1992) Targeted mutation of the DNA methyltransferase gene results in embryonic lethality. Cell 69(6):915–926
26. Okano M, Bell DW, Haber DA, Li E (1999) DNA methyltransferases Dnmt3a and Dnmt3b are essential for de novo methylation and mammalian development. Cell 99(3):247–257
27. Qin W, Leonhardt H, Pichler G (2011) Regulation of DNA methyltransferase 1 by interactions and modifications. Nucleus 2(5):392–402. doi:10.4161/nucl.2.5.17928
28. Bourc'his D, Bestor TH (2004) Meiotic catastrophe and retrotransposon reactivation in male germ cells lacking Dnmt3L. Nature 431(7004):96–99. doi:10.1038/nature02886
29. Crichton JH, Dunican DS, Maclennan M, Meehan RR, Adams IR (2014) Defending the genome from the enemy within: mechanisms of retrotransposon suppression in the mouse germline. Cell Mol Life Sci 71(9):1581–1605. doi:10.1007/s00018-013-1468-0
30. Hackett JA, Reddington JP, Nestor CE, Dunican DS, Branco MR, Reichmann J, Reik W, Surani MA, Adams IR, Meehan RR (2012) Promoter DNA methylation couples genome-defence mechanisms to epigenetic reprogramming in the mouse germline. Development 139(19):3623–3632. doi:10.1242/dev.081661

31. Kelsey G, Feil R (2013) New insights into establishment and maintenance of DNA methylation imprints in mammals. Philos Trans R Soc Lond Ser B Biol Sci 368(1609):20110336. doi:10.1098/rstb.2011.0336

32. Borgel J, Guibert S, Li Y, Chiba H, Schubeler D, Sasaki H, Forne T, Weber M (2010) Targets and dynamics of promoter DNA methylation during early mouse development. Nat Genet 42(12):1093–1100. doi:10.1038/ng.708

33. Jeltsch A, Jurkowska RZ (2016) Allosteric control of mammalian DNA methyltransferases – a new regulatory paradigm. Nucleic Acids Res 44:8556–8575. doi:10.1093/nar/gkw723

34. Lister R, Pelizzola M, Dowen RH, Hawkins RD, Hon G, Tonti-Filippini J, Nery JR, Lee L, Ye Z, Ngo QM, Edsall L, Antosiewicz-Bourget J, Stewart R, Ruotti V, Millar AH, Thomson JA, Ren B, Ecker JR (2009) Human DNA methylomes at base resolution show widespread epigenomic differences. Nature 462(7271):315–322. doi:10.1038/nature08514

35. Meissner A, Mikkelsen TS, Gu H, Wernig M, Hanna J, Sivachenko A, Zhang X, Bernstein BE, Nusbaum C, Jaffe DB, Gnirke A, Jaenisch R, Lander ES (2008) Genome-scale DNA methylation maps of pluripotent and differentiated cells. Nature 454(7205):766–770. doi:10.1038/nature07107

36. Bird A, Taggart M, Frommer M, Miller OJ, Macleod D (1985) A fraction of the mouse genome that is derived from islands of nonmethylated, CpG-rich DNA. Cell 40(1):91–99

37. Bird AP (1986) CpG-rich islands and the function of DNA methylation. Nature 321(6067):209–213. doi:10.1038/321209a0

38. Illingworth RS, Gruenewald-Schneider U, Webb S, Kerr AR, James KD, Turner DJ, Smith C, Harrison DJ, Andrews R, Bird AP (2010) Orphan CpG islands identify numerous conserved promoters in the mammalian genome. PLoS Genet 6(9):e1001134. doi:10.1371/journal.pgen.1001134

39. Feinberg AP, Gehrke CW, Kuo KC, Ehrlich M (1988) Reduced genomic 5-methylcytosine content in human colonic neoplasia. Cancer Res 48(5):1159–1161

40. Feinberg AP, Vogelstein B (1983) Hypomethylation distinguishes genes of some human cancers from their normal counterparts. Nature 301(5895):89–92

41. Gama-Sosa MA, Slagel VA, Trewyn RW, Oxenhandler R, Kuo KC, Gehrke CW, Ehrlich M (1983) The 5-methylcytosine content of DNA from human tumors. Nucleic Acids Res 11(19):6883–6894

42. Goelz SE, Vogelstein B, Hamilton SR, Feinberg AP (1985) Hypomethylation of DNA from benign and malignant human colon neoplasms. Science 228(4696):187–190

43. Comprehensive molecular characterization of human colon and rectal cancer (2012). Nature 487(7407):330–337. doi:10.1038/nature11252

44. Forbes SA, Beare D, Gunasekaran P, Leung K, Bindal N, Boutselakis H, Ding M, Bamford S, Cole C, Ward S, Kok CY, Jia M, De T, Teague JW, Stratton MR, McDermott U, Campbell PJ (2015) COSMIC: exploring the world's knowledge of somatic mutations in human cancer. Nucleic Acids Res 43(Database issue):D805–D811. doi:10.1093/nar/gku1075

45. Cacchiarelli D, Trapnell C, Ziller MJ, Soumillon M, Cesana M, Karnik R, Donaghey J, Smith ZD, Ratanasirintrawoot S, Zhang X, Ho Sui SJ, Wu Z, Akopian V, Gifford CA, Doench J, Rinn JL, Daley GQ, Meissner A, Lander ES, Mikkelsen TS (2015) Integrative analyses of human reprogramming reveal dynamic nature of induced pluripotency. Cell 162(2):412–424. doi:10.1016/j.cell.2015.06.016

46. Cruickshanks HA, McBryan T, Nelson DM, Vanderkraats ND, Shah PP, van Tuyn J, Singh Rai T, Brock C, Donahue G, Dunican DS, Drotar ME, Meehan RR, Edwards JR, Berger SL, Adams PD (2013) Senescent cells harbour features of the cancer epigenome. Nat Cell Biol 15(12):1495–1506. doi:10.1038/ncb2879

47. Horvath S, Gurven M, Levine ME, Trumble BC, Kaplan H, Allayee H, Ritz BR, Chen B, Lu AT, Rickabaugh TM, Jamieson BD, Sun D, Li S, Chen W, Quintana-Murci L, Fagny M, Kobor MS, Tsao PS, Reiner AP, Edlefsen KL, Absher D, Assimes TL (2016) An epigenetic clock analysis of race/ethnicity, sex, and coronary heart disease. Genome Biol 17(1):171. doi:10.1186/s13059-016-1030-0

48. Lee DS, Shin JY, Tonge PD, Puri MC, Lee S, Park H, Lee WC, Hussein SM, Bleazard T, Yun JY, Kim J, Li M, Cloonan N, Wood D, Clancy JL, Mosbergen R, Yi JH, Yang KS, Kim H, Rhee H, Wells CA, Preiss T, Grimmond SM, Rogers IM, Nagy A, Seo JS (2014) An epigenomic roadmap to induced pluripotency reveals DNA methylation as a reprogramming modulator. Nat Commun 5:5619. doi:10.1038/ncomms6619

49. Nestor CE, Ottaviano R, Reinhardt D, Cruickshanks HA, Mjoseng HK, McPherson RC, Lentini A, Thomson JP, Dunican DS, Pennings S, Anderton SM, Benson M, Meehan RR (2015) Rapid reprogramming of epigenetic and transcriptional profiles in mammalian culture systems. Genome Biol 16:11. doi:10.1186/s13059-014-0576-y

50. Marks H, Kalkan T, Menafra R, Denissov S, Jones K, Hofemeister H, Nichols J, Kranz A, Stewart AF, Smith A, Stunnenberg HG (2012) The transcriptional and epigenomic foundations of ground state pluripotency. Cell 149(3):590–604. doi:10.1016/j.cell.2012.03.026

51. Veillard AC, Marks H, Bernardo AS, Jouneau L, Laloe D, Boulanger L, Kaan A, Brochard V, Tosolini M, Pedersen R, Stunnenberg H, Jouneau A (2014) Stable methylation at promoters distinguishes epiblast stem cells from embryonic stem cells and the in vivo epiblasts. Stem Cells Dev 23(17):2014–2029. doi:10.1089/scd.2013.0639

52. Nishiyama A, Yamaguchi L, Sharif J, Johmura Y, Kawamura T, Nakanishi K, Shimamura S, Arita K, Kodama T, Ishikawa F, Koseki H, Nakanishi M (2013) Uhrf1-dependent H3K23 ubiquitylation couples maintenance DNA methylation and replication. Nature 502(7470):249–253. doi:10.1038/nature12488

53. Blackledge NP, Rose NR, Klose RJ (2015) Targeting polycomb systems to regulate gene expression: modifications to a complex story. Nat Rev Mol Cell Biol 16(11):643–649. doi:10.1038/nrm4067

54. Simon JA, Kingston RE (2013) Occupying chromatin: polycomb mechanisms for getting to genomic targets, stopping transcriptional traffic, and staying put. Mol Cell 49(5):808–824

55. Nashun B, Hill PW, Hajkova P (2015) Reprogramming of cell fate: epigenetic memory and the erasure of memories past. EMBO J 34(10):1296–1308

56. Gkountela S, Zhang KX, Shafiq TA, Liao WW, Hargan-Calvopina J, Chen PY, Clark AT (2015) DNA demethylation dynamics in the human prenatal germline. Cell 161(6):1425–1436

57. Smith ZD, Chan MM, Humm KC, Karnik R, Mekhoubad S, Regev A, Eggan K, Meissner A (2014) DNA methylation dynamics of the human preimplantation embryo. Nature 511(7511):611–615

58. Smith ZD, Chan MM, Mikkelsen TS, Gu H, Gnirke A, Regev A, Meissner A (2012) A unique regulatory phase of DNA methylation in the early mammalian embryo. Nature 484(7394):339–344

59. Nestor CE, Lentini A, Hagg Nilsson C, Gawel DR, Gustafsson M, Mattson L, Wang H, Rundquist O, Meehan RR, Klocke B, Seifert M, Hauck SM, Laumen H, Zhang H, Benson M (2016) 5-hydroxymethylcytosine remodeling precedes lineage specification during differentiation of human CD4(+) T cells. Cell Rep 16(2):559–570

60. Hodges E, Molaro A, Dos Santos CO, Thekkat P, Song Q, Uren PJ, Park J, Butler J, Rafii S, McCombie WR, Smith AD, Hannon GJ (2011) Directional DNA methylation changes and complex intermediate states accompany lineage specificity in the adult hematopoietic compartment. Mol Cell 44(1):17–28

61. Bestor TH, Edwards JR, Boulard M (2015) Notes on the role of dynamic DNA methylation in mammalian development. Proc Natl Acad Sci U S A 112(22):6796–6799

62. Ooi SK, Bestor TH (2008) The colorful history of active DNA demethylation. Cell 133(7):1145–1148

63. Huang Y, Rao A (2014) Connections between TET proteins and aberrant DNA modification in cancer. Trends Genet 30(10):464–474

64. Huang Y, Rao A (2014) Connections between TET proteins and aberrant DNA modification in cancer. Trends Genet 30:464–474. doi:S0168-9525(14)00117-6 [pii] 10.1016/j.tig.2014.07.005

65. Inoue A, Shen L, Dai Q, He C, Zhang Y (2011) Generation and replication-dependent dilution of 5fC and 5caC during mouse preimplantation development. Cell Res 21(12):1670–1676. doi:cr2011189 [pii] 10.1038/cr.2011.189

66. Inoue A, Zhang Y (2011) Replication-dependent loss of 5-hydroxymethylcytosine in mouse preimplantation embryos. Science 334(6053):194. doi:10.1126/science.1212483 science.1212483 [pii]

67. Amouroux R, Nashun B, Shirane K, Nakagawa S, Hill PW, D'Souza Z, Nakayama M, Matsuda M, Turp A, Ndjetehe E, Encheva V, Kudo NR, Koseki H, Sasaki H, Hajkova P (2016) De novo DNA methylation drives 5hmC accumulation in mouse zygotes. Nat Cell Biol 18(2):225–233. doi: 10.1038/ncb3296. Epub 2016 Jan 11.

68. Cortellino S, Xu J, Sannai M, Moore R, Caretti E, Cigliano A, Le Coz M, Devarajan K, Wessels A, Soprano D, Abramowitz LK, Bartolomei MS, Rambow F, Bassi MR, Bruno T, Fanciulli M, Renner C, Klein-Szanto AJ, Matsumoto Y, Kobi D, Davidson I, Alberti C, Larue L, Bellacosa A (2011) Thymine DNA glycosylase is essential for active DNA demethylation by linked deamination-base excision repair. Cell 146(1):67–79. doi:S0092-8674(11)00662-3 [pii] 10.1016/j.cell.2011.06.020

69. Shen L, Wu H, Diep D, Yamaguchi S, D'Alessio AC, Fung HL, Zhang K, Zhang Y (2013) Genome-wide analysis reveals TET- and TDG-dependent 5-methylcytosine oxidation dynamics. Cell 153(3):692–706. doi:10.1016/j.cell.2013.04.002 S0092-8674(13)00401-7 [pii]

70. Tahiliani M, Koh KP, Shen Y, Pastor WA, Bandukwala H, Brudno Y, Agarwal S, Iyer LM, Liu DR, Aravind L, Rao A (2009) Conversion of 5-methylcytosine to 5-hydroxymethylcytosine in mammalian DNA by MLL partner TET1. Science 324(5929):930–935. doi:1170116 [pii] 10.1126/science.1170116

71. Kriaucionis S, Heintz N (2009) The nuclear DNA base 5-hydroxymethylcytosine is present in Purkinje neurons and the brain. Science 324(5929):929–930. doi:1169786 [pii] 10.1126/science.1169786

72. Thomson JP, Hunter JM, Meehan RR (2013) Deep C diving: mapping the low-abundance modifications of the DNA demethylation pathway. Genome Biol 14(5):118. doi:gb-2013-14-5-118 [pii] 10.1186/gb-2013-14-5-118

73. Bachman M, Uribe-Lewis S, Yang X, Williams M, Murrell A, Balasubramanian S (2014) 5-hydroxymethylcytosine is a predominantly stable DNA modification. Nat Chem 6(12):1049–1055. doi:10.1038/nchem.2064

74. Laird A, Thomson JP, Harrison DJ, Meehan RR (2013) 5-hydroxymethylcytosine profiling as an indicator of cellular state. Epigenomics 5(6):655–669. doi:10.2217/epi.13.69

75. Matarese F, Carrillo-de Santa Pau E, Stunnenberg HG (2011) 5-hydroxymethylcytosine: a new kid on the epigenetic block? Mol Syst Biol 7:562. doi:10.1038/msb.2011.95 msb201195 [pii]

76. Valinluck V, Sowers LC (2007) Endogenous cytosine damage products alter the site selectivity of human DNA maintenance methyltransferase DNMT1. Cancer Res 67(3):946–950

77. He YF, Li BZ, Li Z, Liu P, Wang Y, Tang Q, Ding J, Jia Y, Chen Z, Li L, Sun Y, Li X, Dai Q, Song CX, Zhang K, He C, Xu GL (2011) Tet-mediated formation of 5-carboxylcytosine and its excision by TDG in mammalian DNA. Science 333(6047):1303–1307

78. Hu X, Zhang L, Mao SQ, Li Z, Chen J, Zhang RR, Wu HP, Gao J, Guo F, Liu W, Xu GF, Dai HQ, Shi YG, Li X, Hu B, Tang F, Pei D, Xu GL (2014) Tet and TDG mediate DNA demethylation essential for mesenchymal-to-epithelial transition in somatic cell reprogramming. Cell Stem Cell 14(4):512–522

79. Xu X, Watt DS, Liu C (2016) Multifaceted roles for thymine DNA glycosylase in embryonic development and human carcinogenesis. Acta Biochim Biophys Sin 48(1):82–89

80. Guo F, Li X, Liang D, Li T, Zhu P, Guo H, Wu X, Wen L, Gu TP, Hu B, Walsh CP, Li J, Tang F, Xu GL (2014) Active and passive demethylation of male and female pronuclear DNA in the mammalian zygote. Cell Stem Cell 15(4):447–458

81. Xu G-L, Wong J (2015) Oxidative DNA demethylation mediated by Tet enzymes. Nat Sci Rev 2:318–328. nwv029

82. Ficz G, Gribben JG (2014) Loss of 5-hydroxymethylcytosine in cancer: cause or consequence? Genomics 104:352–357. doi:S0888-7543(14)00159-1 [pii] 10.1016/j.ygeno.2014.08.017

83. Neri F, Dettori D, Incarnato D, Krepelova A, Rapelli S, Maldotti M, Parlato C, Paliogiannis P, Oliviero S (2014) TET1 is a tumour suppressor that inhibits colon cancer growth by derepressing inhibitors of the WNT pathway. Oncogene 34:4168–4176. doi:10.1038/onc.2014.356 onc2014356 [pii]

84. Ichimura N, Shinjo K, An B, Shimizu Y, Yamao K, Ohka F, Katsushima K, Hatanaka A, Tojo M, Yamamoto E, Suzuki H, Ueda M, Kondo Y (2015) Aberrant TET1 methylation closely associated with CpG island methylator phenotype in colorectal cancer. Cancer Prev Res (Phila) 8(8):702–711. doi:10.1158/1940-6207.capr-14-0306

85. Wu BK, Brenner C (2014) Suppression of TET1-dependent DNA demethylation is essential for KRAS-mediated transformation. Cell Rep 9(5):1827–1840. doi:10.1016/j.celrep.2014.10.063

86. Thienpont B, Steinbacher J, Zhao H, D'Anna F, Kuchnio A, Ploumakis A, Ghesquiere B, Van Dyck L, Boeckx B, Schoonjans L, Hermans E, Amant F, Kristensen VN, Koh KP, Mazzone M, Coleman ML, Carell T, Carmeliet P, Lambrechts D (2016) Tumour hypoxia causes DNA hypermethylation by reducing TET activity. Nature 537(7618):63–68. doi:10.1038/nature19081

87. Thomson JP, Ottaviano R, Unterberger EB, Lempiainen H, Muller A, Terranova R, Illingworth RS, Webb S, Kerr AR, Lyall MJ, Drake AJ, Wolf CR, Moggs JG, Schwarz M, Meehan RR (2016) Loss of Tet1-associated 5-hydroxymethylcytosine is concomitant with aberrant promoter hypermethylation in liver cancer. Cancer Res 76(10):3097–3108. doi:10.1158/0008-5472.CAN-15-1910 0008-5472.CAN-15-1910 [pii]

88. Nestor CE, Ottaviano R, Reddington J, Sproul D, Reinhardt D, Dunican D, Katz E, Dixon JM, Harrison DJ, Meehan RR (2012) Tissue type is a major modifier of the 5-hydroxymethylcytosine content of human genes. Genome Res 22(3):467–477. doi:gr.126417.111 [pii] 10.1101/gr.126417.111

89. Thomson JP, Lempiainen H, Hackett JA, Nestor CE, Muller A, Bolognani F, Oakeley EJ, Schubeler D, Terranova R, Reinhardt D, Moggs JG, Meehan RR (2012) Non-genotoxic carcinogen exposure induces defined changes in the 5-hydroxymethylome. Genome Biol 13(10):R93. doi:gb-2012-13-10-r93 [pii] 10.1186/gb-2012-13-10-r93

90. Song CX, Yi C, He C (2012) Mapping recently identified nucleotide variants in the genome and transcriptome. Nat Biotechnol 30(11):1107–1116. doi:nbt.2398 [pii] 10.1038/nbt.2398

91. Thomson JP, Hunter JM, Nestor CE, Dunican DS, Terranova R, Moggs JG, Meehan RR (2013) Comparative analysis of affinity-based 5-hydroxymethylation enrichment techniques. Nucleic Acids Res 41(22):e206. doi:gkt1080 [pii] 10.1093/nar/gkt1080

92. Bogdanovic O, Smits AH, de la Calle ME, Tena JJ, Ford E, Williams R, Senanayake U, Schultz MD, Hontelez S, van Kruijsbergen I, Rayon T, Gnerlich F, Carell T, Veenstra GJ, Manzanares M, Sauka-Spengler T, Ecker JR, Vermeulen M, Gomez-Skarmeta JL, Lister R (2016) Active DNA demethylation at enhancers during the vertebrate phylotypic period. Nat Genet 48(4):417–426. doi:10.1038/ng.3522

93. Li X, Liu Y, Salz T, Hansen KD, Feinberg AP (2016) Whole genome analysis of the methylome and hydroxymethylome in normal and malignant lung and liver. Genome Res 26:1730–1741. bioRxiv. doi:http://dx.doi.org/10.1101/062588

94. Feinberg AP, Koldobskiy MA, Gondor A (2016) Epigenetic modulators, modifiers and mediators in cancer aetiology and progression. Nat Rev Genet 17(5):284–299. doi:10.1038/nrg.2016.13 nrg.2016.13 [pii]

95. Hanahan D, Weinberg RA (2011) Hallmarks of cancer: the next generation. Cell 144(5):646–674. doi:10.1016/j.cell.2011.02.013

96. Sproul D, Kitchen RR, Nestor CE, Dixon JM, Sims AH, Harrison DJ, Ramsahoye BH, Meehan RR (2012) Tissue of origin determines cancer-associated CpG island promoter hypermethylation patterns. Genome Biol 13(10):R84. doi:gb-2012-13-10-r84 [pii] 10.1186/gb-2012-13-10-r84

97. Sproul D, Meehan RR (2013) Genomic insights into cancer-associated aberrant CpG island hypermethylation. Brief Funct Genomics 12(3):174–190. doi:10.1093/bfgp/els063 els063 [pii]

98. Feinberg AP, Ohlsson R, Henikoff S (2006) The epigenetic progenitor origin of human cancer. Nat Rev Genet 7(1):21–33. doi:nrg1748 [pii] 10.1038/nrg1748

99. Baylin SB, Hoppener JW, de Bustros A, Steenbergh PH, Lips CJ, Nelkin BD (1986) DNA methylation patterns of the calcitonin gene in human lung cancers and lymphomas. Cancer Res 46(6):2917–2922

100. Greger V, Passarge E, Hopping W, Messmer E, Horsthemke B (1989) Epigenetic changes may contribute to the formation and spontaneous regression of retinoblastoma. Hum Genet 83(2):155–158

101. Baylin SB, Jones PA (2011) A decade of exploring the cancer epigenome – biological and translational implications. Nat Rev Cancer 11(10):726–734. doi:10.1038/nrc3130 nrc3130 [pii]

102. Irizarry RA, Ladd-Acosta C, Wen B, Wu Z, Montano C, Onyango P, Cui H, Gabo K, Rongione M, Webster M, Ji H, Potash JB, Sabunciyan S, Feinberg AP (2009) The human colon cancer methylome shows similar hypo- and hypermethylation at conserved tissue-specific CpG island shores. Nat Genet 41(2):178–186. doi:10.1038/ng.298 ng.298 [pii]

103. Bell RE, Golan T, Sheinboim D, Malcov H, Amar D, Salamon A, Liron T, Gelfman S, Gabet Y, Shamir R, Levy C (2016) Enhancer methylation dynamics contribute to cancer plasticity and patient mortality. Genome Res 26(5):601–611. doi:10.1101/gr.197194.115 gr.197194.115 [pii]

104. Gao F, Xia Y, Wang J, Lin Z, Ou Y, Liu X, Liu W, Zhou B, Luo H, Wen B, Zhang X, Huang J (2014) Integrated analyses of DNA methylation and hydroxymethylation reveal tumor suppressive roles of ECM1, ATF5, and EOMES in human hepatocellular carcinoma. Genome Biol 15(12):533. doi:10.1186/s13059-014-0533-9

105. Figueroa ME, Abdel-Wahab O, Lu C, Ward PS, Patel J, Shih A, Li Y, Bhagwat N, Vasanthakumar A, Fernandez HF, Tallman MS, Sun Z, Wolniak K, Peeters JK, Liu W, Choe SE, Fantin VR, Paietta E, Lowenberg B, Licht JD, Godley LA, Delwel R, Valk PJ, Thompson CB, Levine RL, Melnick A (2010) Leukemic IDH1 and IDH2 mutations result in a hypermethylation phenotype, disrupt TET2 function, and impair hematopoietic differentiation. Cancer Cell 18(6):553–567. doi:S1535-6108(10)00483-6 [pii] 10.1016/j.ccr.2010.11.015

106. Rampal R, Alkalin A, Madzo J, Vasanthakumar A, Pronier E, Patel J, Li Y, Ahn J, Abdel-Wahab O, Shih A, Lu C, Ward PS, Tsai JJ, Hricik T, Tosello V, Tallman JE, Zhao X, Daniels D, Dai Q, Ciminio L, Aifantis I, He C, Fuks F, Tallman MS, Ferrando A, Nimer S, Paietta E, Thompson CB, Licht JD, Mason CE, Godley LA, Melnick A, Figueroa ME, Levine RL (2014) DNA hydroxymethylation profiling reveals that WT1 mutations result in loss of TET2 function in acute myeloid leukemia. Cell Rep 9(5):1841–1855. doi:10.1016/j.celrep.2014.11.004

107. Cimmino L, Dawlaty MM, Ndiaye-Lobry D, Yap YS, Bakogianni S, Yu Y, Bhattacharyya S, Shaknovich R, Geng H, Lobry C, Mullenders J, King B, Trimarchi T, Aranda-Orgilles B, Liu C, Shen S, Verma AK, Jaenisch R, Aifantis I (2015) TET1 is a tumor suppressor of hematopoietic malignancy. Nat Immunol 16(6):653–662. doi:10.1038/ni.3148 ni.3148 [pii]

108. Fang M, Ou J, Hutchinson L, Green MR (2014) The BRAF oncoprotein functions through the transcriptional repressor MAFG to mediate the CpG island methylator phenotype. Mol Cell 55(6):904–915. doi:10.1016/j.molcel.2014.08.010

109. Gu J, Stevens M, Xing X, Li D, Zhang B, Payton JE, Oltz EM, Jarvis JN, Jiang K, Cicero T, Costello JF, Wang T (2016) Mapping of variable DNA methylation across multiple cell types defines a dynamic regulatory landscape of the human genome. G3 (Bethesda) 6(4):973–986. doi:10.1534/g3.115.025437

110. Serra RW, Fang M, Park SM, Hutchinson L, Green MR (2014) A KRAS-directed transcriptional silencing pathway that mediates the CpG island methylator phenotype. elife 3:e02313. doi:10.7554/eLife.02313

111. Sproul D, Nestor C, Culley J, Dickson JH, Dixon JM, Harrison DJ, Meehan RR, Sims AH, Ramsahoye BH (2011) Transcriptionally repressed genes become aberrantly methylated and distinguish tumors of different lineages in breast cancer. Proc Natl Acad Sci U S A 108(11):4364–4369. doi:10.1073/pnas.1013224108 1013224108 [pii]

112. Holm K, Staaf J, Lauss M, Aine M, Lindgren D, Bendahl PO, Vallon-Christersson J, Barkardottir RB, Hoglund M, Borg A, Jonsson G, Ringner M (2016) An integrated genomics analysis of epigenetic subtypes in human breast tumors links DNA methylation patterns to chromatin states in normal mammary cells. Breast Cancer Res 18(1):016–0685

113. Teschendorff AE, Zheng SC, Feber A, Yang Z, Beck S, Widschwendter M (2016) The multi-omic landscape of transcription factor inactivation in cancer. Genome Med 8(1):016–0342

114. Chiappinelli KB, Strissel PL, Desrichard A, Li H, Henke C, Akman B, Hein A, Rote NS, Cope LM, Snyder A, Makarov V, Buhu S, Slamon DJ, Wolchok JD, Pardoll DM, Beckmann MW, Zahnow CA, Mergoub T, Chan TA, Baylin SB, Strick R (2015) Inhibiting DNA methylation causes an interferon response in cancer via dsRNA including endogenous retroviruses. Cell 162(5):974–986. doi:10.1016/j.cell.2015.07.011

115. Roulois D, Loo Yau H, Singhania R, Wang Y, Danesh A, Shen SY, Han H, Liang G, Jones PA, Pugh TJ, O'Brien C, De Carvalho DD (2015) DNA-demethylating agents target colorectal cancer cells by inducing viral mimicry by endogenous transcripts. Cell 162(5):961–973. doi:10.1016/j.cell.2015.07.056

116. Liu C, Liu L, Chen X, Shen J, Shan J, Xu Y, Yang Z, Wu L, Xia F, Bie P, Cui Y, Bian XW, Qian C (2013) Decrease of 5-hydroxymethylcytosine is associated with progression of hepatocellular carcinoma through downregulation of TET1. PLoS One 8(5):e62828. doi:10.1371/journal.pone.0062828 PONE-D-13-05782 [pii]

117. Park JL, Kim HJ, Seo EH, Kwon OH, Lim B, Kim M, Kim SY, Song KS, Kang GH, Choi BY, Kim YS (2015) Decrease of 5hmC in gastric cancers is associated with TET1 silencing due to with DNA methylation and bivalent histone marks at TET1 CpG island 3′-shore. Oncotarget 6(35):37647–37662. doi:10.18632/oncotarget.6069 6069 [pii]

118. Chen K, Zhang J, Guo Z, Ma Q, Xu Z, Zhou Y, Li Z, Liu Y, Ye X, Li X, Yuan B, Ke Y, He C, Zhou L, Liu J, Ci W (2015) Loss of 5-hydroxymethylcytosine is linked to gene body hypermethylation in kidney cancer. Cell Res 26(1):103–118. doi:10.1038/cr.2015.150 cr2015150 [pii]

119. Kroeze LI, Aslanyan MG, van Rooij A, Koorenhof-Scheele TN, Massop M, Carell T, Boezeman JB, Marie JP, Halkes CJ, de Witte T, Huls G, Suciu S, Wevers RA, van der Reijden BA, Jansen JH (2014) Characterization of acute myeloid leukemia based on levels of global hydroxymethylation. Blood 124(7):1110–1118. doi:10.1182/blood-2013-08-518514 blood-2013-08-518514 [pii]

120. Lian CG, Xu Y, Ceol C, Wu F, Larson A, Dresser K, Xu W, Tan L, Hu Y, Zhan Q, Lee CW, Hu D, Lian BQ, Kleffel S, Yang Y, Neiswender J, Khorasani AJ, Fang R, Lezcano C, Duncan LM, Scolyer RA, Thompson JF, Kakavand H, Houvras Y, Zon LI, Mihm MC, Jr., Kaiser UB, Schatton T, Woda BA, Murphy GF, Shi YG (2012) Loss of 5-hydroxymethylcytosine is an epigenetic hallmark of melanoma. Cell 150(6):1135–1146. doi:S0092-8674(12)01012-4 [pii] 10.1016/j.cell.2012.07.033

121. Ye C, Tao R, Cao Q, Zhu D, Wang Y, Wang J, Lu J, Chen E, Li L (2016) Whole-genome DNA methylation and hydroxymethylation profiling for HBV-related hepatocellular carcinoma. Int J Oncol 49(2):589–602. doi:10.3892/ijo.2016.3535

122. Putiri EL, Tiedemann RL, Thompson JJ, Liu C, Ho T, Choi JH, Robertson KD (2014) Distinct and overlapping control of 5-methylcytosine and 5-hydroxymethylcytosine by the TET proteins in human cancer cells. Genome Biol 15(6):R81. doi:10.1186/gb-2014-15-6-r81 gb-2014-15-6-r81 [pii]

123. Hon GC, Song CX, Du T, Jin F, Selvaraj S, Lee AY, Yen CA, Ye Z, Mao SQ, Wang BA, Kuan S, Edsall LE, Zhao BS, Xu GL, He C, Ren B (2014) 5mC oxidation by Tet2 modulates enhancer activity and timing of transcriptome reprogramming during differentiation. Mol Cell 56(2):286–297. doi:10.1016/j.molcel.2014.08.026

124. Rasmussen KD, Jia G, Johansen JV, Pedersen MT, Rapin N, Bagger FO, Porse BT, Bernard OA, Christensen J, Helin K (2015) Loss of TET2 in hematopoietic cells leads to DNA hypermethylation of active enhancers and induction of leukemogenesis. Genes Dev 29(9):910–922. doi:10.1101/gad.260174.115 gad.260174.115 [pii]
125. Rasmussen KD, Helin K (2016) Role of TET enzymes in DNA methylation, development, and cancer. Genes Dev 30(7):733–750. doi:10.1101/gad.276568.115 30/7/733 [pii]
126. Dawlaty MM, Ganz K, Powell BE, Hu YC, Markoulaki S, Cheng AW, Gao Q, Kim J, Choi SW, Page DC, Jaenisch R (2011) Tet1 is dispensable for maintaining pluripotency and its loss is compatible with embryonic and postnatal development. Cell Stem Cell 9(2):166–175. doi:10.1016/j.stem.2011.07.010 S1934-5909(11)00340-7 [pii]
127. Li L, Li C, Mao H, Du Z, Chan WY, Murray P, Luo B, Chan AT, Mok TS, Chan FK, Ambinder RF, Tao Q (2016) Epigenetic inactivation of the CpG demethylase TET1 as a DNA methylation feedback loop in human cancers. Sci Rep 6:26591. doi:10.1038/srep26591 srep26591 [pii]
128. Pei YF, Tao R, Li JF, Su LP, Yu BQ, Wu XY, Yan M, Gu QL, Zhu ZG, Liu BY (2016) TET1 inhibits gastric cancer growth and metastasis by PTEN demethylation and re-expression. Oncotarget 7(21):31322–31335. doi:10.18632/oncotarget.8900 8900 [pii]
129. Kroeze LI, van der Reijden BA, Jansen JH (2015) 5-hydroxymethylcytosine: an epigenetic mark frequently deregulated in cancer. Biochim Biophys Acta 1855(2):144–154. doi:10.1016/j.bbcan.2015.01.001
130. Letouze E, Martinelli C, Loriot C, Burnichon N, Abermil N, Ottolenghi C, Janin M, Menara M, Nguyen AT, Benit P, Buffet A, Marcaillou C, Bertherat J, Amar L, Rustin P, De Reynies A, Gimenez-Roqueplo AP, Favier J (2013) SDH mutations establish a hypermethylator phenotype in paraganglioma. Cancer Cell 23(6):739–752. doi:10.1016/j.ccr.2013.04.018 S1535-6108(13)00183-9 [pii]
131. Oermann EK, Wu J, Guan KL, Xiong Y (2012) Alterations of metabolic genes and metabolites in cancer. Semin Cell Dev Biol 23(4):370–380. doi:10.1016/j.semcdb.2012.01.013 S1084-9521(12)00023-7 [pii]
132. Toro JR, Nickerson ML, Wei MH, Warren MB, Glenn GM, Turner ML, Stewart L, Duray P, Tourre O, Sharma N, Choyke P, Stratton P, Merino M, Walther MM, Linehan WM, Schmidt LS, Zbar B (2003) Mutations in the fumarate hydratase gene cause hereditary leiomyomatosis and renal cell cancer in families in North America. Am J Hum Genet 73(1):95–106. doi:S0002-9297(07)63898-1 [pii] 10.1086/376435
133. Yin R, Mao SQ, Zhao B, Chong Z, Yang Y, Zhao C, Zhang D, Huang H, Gao J, Li Z, Jiao Y, Li C, Liu S, Wu D, Gu W, Yang YG, Xu GL, Wang H (2013) Ascorbic acid enhances Tet-mediated 5-methylcytosine oxidation and promotes DNA demethylation in mammals. J Am Chem Soc 135(28):10396–10403. doi:10.1021/ja4028346
134. Liu M, Ohtani H, Zhou W, Orskov AD, Charlet J, Zhang YW, Shen H, Baylin SB, Liang G, Gronbaek K, Jones PA (2016) Vitamin C increases viral mimicry induced by 5-aza-2'-deoxycytidine. Proc Natl Acad Sci U S A 113(37):10238–10244
135. Saito Y, Nakaoka T, Sakai K, Muramatsu T, Toshimitsu K, Kimura M, Kanai T, Sato T, Saito H (2016) Inhibition of DNA methylation suppresses intestinal tumor organoids by inducing an anti-viral response. Sci Rep 6:25311
136. Laukka T, Mariani CJ, Ihantola T, Cao JZ, Hokkanen J, Kaelin WG Jr, Godley LA, Koivunen P (2016) Fumarate and succinate regulate expression of hypoxia-inducible genes via TET enzymes. J Biol Chem 291(8):4256–4265
137. Feinberg AP, Tycko B (2004) The history of cancer epigenetics. Nat Rev Cancer 4(2):143–153
138. Ohm JE, McGarvey KM, Yu X, Cheng L, Schuebel KE, Cope L, Mohammad HP, Chen W, Daniel VC, Yu W, Berman DM, Jenuwein T, Pruitt K, Sharkis SJ, Watkins DN, Herman JG, Baylin SB (2007) A stem cell-like chromatin pattern may predispose tumor suppressor genes to DNA hypermethylation and heritable silencing. Nat Genet 39(2):237–242
139. Schlesinger Y, Straussman R, Keshet I, Farkash S, Hecht M, Zimmerman J, Eden E, Yakhini Z, Ben-Shushan E, Reubinoff BE, Bergman Y, Simon I, Cedar H (2007) Polycomb-mediated

methylation on Lys27 of histone H3 pre-marks genes for de novo methylation in cancer. Nat Genet 39(2):232–236

140. Brinkman AB, Gu H, Bartels SJ, Zhang Y, Matarese F, Simmer F, Marks H, Bock C, Gnirke A, Meissner A, Stunnenberg HG (2012) Sequential ChIP-bisulfite sequencing enables direct genome-scale investigation of chromatin and DNA methylation cross-talk. Genome Res 22(6):1128–1138

141. Hagarman JA, Motley MP, Kristjansdottir K, Soloway PD (2013) Coordinate regulation of DNA methylation and H3K27me3 in mouse embryonic stem cells. PLoS One 8(1):11

142. Reddington JP, Perricone SM, Nestor CE, Reichmann J, Youngson NA, Suzuki M, Reinhardt D, Dunican DS, Prendergast JG, Mjoseng H, Ramsahoye BH, Whitelaw E, Greally JM, Adams IR, Bickmore WA, Meehan RR (2013) Redistribution of H3K27me3 upon DNA hypomethylation results in de-repression of polycomb target genes. Genome Biol 14(3):2013–2014

143. Williams K, Christensen J, Pedersen MT, Johansen JV, Cloos PA, Rappsilber J, Helin K (2011) TET1 and hydroxymethylcytosine in transcription and DNA methylation fidelity. Nature 473(7347):343–348

144. Reddington JP, Sproul D, Meehan RR (2014) DNA methylation reprogramming in cancer: does it act by re-configuring the binding landscape of polycomb repressive complexes? BioEssays 36(2):134–140

145. Shah PP, Donahue G, Otte GL, Capell BC, Nelson DM, Cao K, Aggarwala V, Cruickshanks HA, Rai TS, McBryan T, Gregory BD, Adams PD, Berger SL (2013) Lamin B1 depletion in senescent cells triggers large-scale changes in gene expression and the chromatin landscape. Genes Dev 27(16):1787–1799

146. Heyn H, Vidal E, Ferreira HJ, Vizoso M, Sayols S, Gomez A, Moran S, Boque-Sastre R, Guil S, Martinez-Cardus A, Lin CY, Royo R, Sanchez-Mut JV, Martinez R, Gut M, Torrents D, Orozco M, Gut I, Young RA, Esteller M (2016) Epigenomic analysis detects aberrant super-enhancer DNA methylation in human cancer. Genome Biol 17:11. doi:10.1186/s13059-016-0879-2

147. Cantor JR, Sabatini DM (2012) Cancer cell metabolism: one hallmark, many faces. Cancer Discov 2(10):881–898

148. Wen L, Li J, Guo H, Liu X, Zheng S, Zhang D, Zhu W, Qu J, Guo L, Du D, Jin X, Zhang Y, Gao Y, Shen J, Ge H, Tang F, Huang Y, Peng J (2015) Genome-scale detection of hypermethylated CpG islands in circulating cell-free DNA of hepatocellular carcinoma patients. Cell Res 25(11):1250–1264

149. McPherson RC, Konkel JE, Prendergast CT, Thomson JP, Ottaviano R, Leech MD, Kay O, Zandee SE, Sweenie CH, Wraith DC, Meehan RR, Drake AJ, Anderton SM (2014) Epigenetic modification of the PD-1 (Pdcd1) promoter in effector CD4(+) T cells tolerized by peptide immunotherapy. elife 29(3):03416

150. Youngblood B, Oestreich KJ, Ha SJ, Duraiswamy J, Akondy RS, West EE, Wei Z, Lu P, Austin JW, Riley JL, Boss JM, Ahmed R (2011) Chronic virus infection enforces demethylation of the locus that encodes PD-1 in antigen-specific CD8(+) T cells. Immunity 35(3):400–412

151. Goltz D, Gevensleben H, Dietrich J, Ellinger J, Landsberg J, Kristiansen G, Dietrich D (2016) Promoter methylation of the immune checkpoint receptor PD-1 (PDCD1) is an independent prognostic biomarker for biochemical recurrence-free survival in prostate cancer patients following radical prostatectomy. Oncoimmunology 5:e1221555. doi:10.1080/2162402x.2016.1221555

152. Bally AP, Austin JW, Boss JM (2016) Genetic and epigenetic regulation of PD-1 expression. J Immunol 196(6):2431–2437

153. Mizuguchi Y, Saiki Y, Horii A, Fukushige S (2016) Targeted TET oxidase activity through methyl-CpG-binding domain extensively suppresses cancer cell proliferation. Cancer Med 5(9):2522–2533

Misregulation of DNA Methylation Regulators in Cancer

Joyce J. Thompson and Keith D. Robertson

Abstract Epigenetic modifications at the DNA level play a central role in establishing the chromatin state and thereby influencing biological function. Several disorders arise from aberrant epigenetic patterns on DNA, cancer being widely explored as an epigenetic disorder. In fact several cancers are associated with a hypermethylator phenotype, which essentially functions as a 'driver' of tumorigenesis. Aberrant DNA methylation patterns arise from disrupting the 'writers' or 'erasers' of the DNA methylation pathway, coordinately functioning to regulate DNA epigenetic marks. Cancer associated deregulatory mechanisms targeting functional disruption of the molecular components of the DNA methylation pathway, and their contribution to cancer initiation and progression are being increasingly appreciated. Understanding these mechanisms of deregulation is central to identifying new targets for therapeutic intervention, in both cancer prevention and treatment.

Keywords DNA methylation pathway • Hypermethylator phenotype • DNMT • TET • Epimutation • Oncogenic • Tumorigenesis

Abbreviations

AML	Acute Myeloid Leukemia
CGI	CpG island
CIMP	CpG hypermethylator phenotype
DNMT	DNA methyltransferase
EBF1	Early B-Cell Factor 1
EMT	Epithelial to mesenchymal transition
FH	Fumarate hydratase (fumarase)
G-CIMP	Glioma specific CIMP

J.J. Thompson • K.D. Robertson (✉)
Department of Molecular Pharmacology and Experimental Therapeutics, Mayo Clinic,
Rochester, MN 55905, USA
e-mail: Robertson.Keith@mayo.edu

© Springer International Publishing AG 2017   97
A. Kaneda, Y.-i. Tsukada (eds.), *DNA and Histone Methylation as Cancer Targets*,
Cancer Drug Discovery and Development, DOI 10.1007/978-3-319-59786-7_5

GSC   Glioblastoma Stem Cells
HIF   Hypoxia inducible factor
HPC   Hematopoietic presursor cells
HRE   Hypoxia response element
HSC   Hematopoietic stem cells
IDAX   Inhibition of the Dvl and Axin Complex
IDH   Isocitrate dehydrogenase
MBD   Methyl binding domain
mCG   CpG methylation
mCH   Non-CpG methylation
MDS   Myelodysplastic Syndromes
MLL   Mixed-lineage leukemia
MPN   Myeloproliferative Neoplasm
MTase   Methyltransferase
PCNA   Proliferating cell nuclear antigen
SDH   Succinate dehydrogenase
TDG   Thymine-DNA glycosylase
TET   Ten-eleven translocation
UHRF   Ubiquitin-Like with PHD and Ring Finger Domains
α-KG   Alpha-ketoglutarate

1 Introduction

Cancer is a complex diseased state arising from impaired cellular homeostasis. Cellular homeostasis is essentially defined by the underlying dynamic transcriptome, coding for the functional proteome, which is temporally modulated by intrinsic and extrinsic cues. However, the transcriptome is only an effector of the epigenetic changes occurring at the different components of chromatin – DNA, histones, and nucleosomes, which essentially control the progression of central biological processes. At the DNA level, epigenetic information is carried in the form of cyclic modifications at the C5 position of cytosine, frequently but not exclusively within 'CpG' dinucleotides (cytosine preceding guanine). The primary modification at C5 is methylation, resulting in 5-methylcytosine (5mC), and is catalyzed by a family of enzymes, the **DNA M**ethyl**t**ransferases (DNMTs). 5mC can be further oxidized by the **T**en-**e**lven **t**ranslocation (TET) family of dioxygenases, sequentially, to 5-hydroxymethyl cytosine (5hmC), 5-formyl cytosine (5fC), and lastly 5-carboxyl cytosine (5caC), which can be viewed as secondary, tertiary, and quaternary modifications at C5. All four DNA marks carry distinct epigenetic information and functional implications, and are central to driving development, differentiation, and maintaining cellular homeostasis. In fact, aberrant patterns of these C5 modifications are associated with the initiation and progression of several cancers. Misregulation of the molecular components of the DNA methylation pathway forms the basis of most, if not all cancers. This chapter will provide an overview on how the molecular components of the DNA methylation pathway are deregulated to facilitate cancer initiation and progression, and their mechanistic contribution to achieving the hallmarks of cancerous cells.

1.1 Molecular Components of the DNA Epigenetic Pathway: Establishment, Interpretation, and Turnover of DNA Modifications

As in all epigenetic pathways, the DNA methylation pathway has three major components – writers, readers, and erasers. The DNMTs, which include three cata-lytically active enzymes, DNMT1, 3A, and 3B, and a catalytically inactive DNMT3L (3-Like), function as the 'writers' of the DNA epigenetic pathway. The structurally homologous de novo DNMT3A/3B, along with the accessory DNMT3L, establish 5mC patterns during early embryonic development and are implicated in develop-ment [1], differentiation, and lineage commitment [2–4] while the maintenance DNMT1 faithfully maintains and propagates established 5mC patterns during DNA replication in somatic cells [5]. Both DNMTs 3A and 3B possess a variable N-terminal domain with a proline-tryptophan rich – PWWP domain, followed by the ATRX–DNMT3–DNMT3L (ADD) domain, which contains a CXXC zinc finger and an atypical plant homeodomain (PHD) finger domain, and lastly a catalytic methyltransferase (MTase) domain at their C-terminal end [6]. DNMTs 3A and 3B are highly expressed during early embryonic development and in differentiating cells, but are generally lowly expressed in terminally differentiated somatic cells. However, somatic cells do express catalytically inactive isoforms of the DNMT3 enzymes [7], suggesting their pivotal role in non-epigenetic mechanisms. DNMT1 has similar structural organization as the DNMT3s, with a C-terminal catalytic and N-terminal regulatory domain, but shares very little homology with the DNMT3s. DNMT1 has a 30- to 40-fold higher preference for hemi methylated DNA [8], and is recruited at the replication fork via its interactions with PCNA [9, 10] and UHRF1 [11, 12], where it functions to copy and maintain DNA methylation patterns during replication.

DNA methylation patterns are interpreted by 'readers', which thereby affect local chromatin structure by recruiting histone modifying enzymes and chromatin remodeling complexes at these sites. The Methyl Binding Domain (MBD) family of proteins and the zinc-finger proteins ZBTB4, 33, and 38 are currently known to function as readers of DNA methylation [13–15]. The mammalian MBD-family has five members which recognize 5mC using a similar mechanism but with differing specificities. MeCP2, the first of the members to be identified, is highly expressed in neuronal tissue [16] and recognizes 5mC at specific genomic loci [17], whereas the other members are expressed more ubiquitously and exhibit a more general rec-ognition pattern. All MBD family members act as transcriptional repressors by recruiting repressive epigenetic complexes at the 5mC sites recognized by them. The ZBTB readers belong to the BTB-POZ family of zinc-finger proteins, currently composed of 49 structurally homologous members, most of which are implicated in driving B-cell and T-cell function, primarily through transcriptional repression. All ZBTB family members possess an N-terminal BTB domain, which mediates interactions with other transcriptional co-regulators, (e.g. N-CoR, SMRT, HDACs, SIN3), C-terminal C2H2-type zinc fingers (2-14 in number) which enable sequence-specific DNA binding, and in some cases an AT-hook domain that mediates binding by non-specific interactions with the minor groove in A-T rich DNA sequence binding, which include centromeric satellite repeats [18]. Of the entire family, just three members, ZBTB4, 33, and 38 are known to function as 5mC readers. Of these, Kaiso (ZBTB33) has been widely studied and is capable of recognizing both unmethylated and methylated Cs, at different recognition motifs [19, 20], however, its ability to recognize 5mC in vivo has been questioned [21].

Finally, the TET family of O_2, Fe^{2+}, and α-ketoglutarate dependent demethylases, TETs 1, 2, and 3, erase 5mC through step-wise oxidation to 5hmC, 5fC, and 5caC which are diluted during replication passively diminishing epigenetic marks on DNA, or are actively replaced by the base-excision repair pathway, specifically by thymine DNA glycosylase (TDG), to cytosine [22, 23]. The TET genes are believed to have arisen from segmental duplication of a single gene. The three family members share a great degree of homology at their carboxyl terminal catalytic domain, which consists of a cysteine-rich region and a His-Xaa-Asp/Glu signature motif in the double stranded B-helix (DSHB) fold. However, the TETs differ at their amino-terminal ends, with TET1 and TET3 possessing the CXXC motif, which is absent in the TET2 enzyme [22, 23]. The TET2 associated CXXC domain is carried on a separate gene, owing to an evolutionary gene inversion event, the IDAX (CXXC4) gene. The CXXC domains are capable of binding DNA and their function in the TETs is speculatively to direct the enzymes to their target sites [23, 24], though the catalytic domain is capable of non-specific DNA binding by itself [23].

DNA methylation signatures are cell type and cell stage specific, and are established by regulated cross-talk between the writers, readers, and erasers of the DNA methylation pathway, while integrating instructions from epigenetic pathways acting on different components of chromatin. The functional implication of DNA methylation is positional and context dependent, i.e. it shows variations in interpretation across the genome.

1.2 Genome-Wide Variation in DNA Modifications, How They Are Achieved, and Their Functional Interpretation

Initially, DNA methylation was largely studied at CpG sites (mCG) in the context of promoters of repressed genes, and it was largely perceived as a repressive epigenetic mark. However, recent advances have led to a transformation of this view on

DNA methylation. Firstly, methylation occurs at cytosines outside of CpG sites. This non-CpG methylation, termed 'CH' methylation (H = Adenosine/Thymine/Cytosine), is abundant in oocytes [25], embryonic stem cells, and a subset of neurons [26], and present in small amounts in other human cell types and tissues [27]. Secondly, mCG sites are not abundant in promoters alone, but show 'mosaicism' with respect to genome-wide distribution. The occurrence of 5mC, and thereby its functional impact, is dependent on the density of CpGs at a locus, the underlying genomic sequence, and the surrounding chromatin environment [28].

Across the genome, CpG sites are unequally distributed. Sites of high CpG density (at least 200 bps long with a GC content greater than 50 percent) are termed CpG islands (CGIs), and are largely exempt from DNA methylation. CGIs are by and large abundant in promoter elements. Surrounding the CGIs, 2 kb on either side of the island, are CGI shores, regions with relatively lower CG frequency. 2 kb on either side of the CGI shores are termed CGI shelves [29]. Very recently, the term CG canyons (or valleys) was coined to describe large regions of low methylation, distinct from CGIs, and frequently associated with transcription factor binding sites [30]. Additionally, isolated CG sites are seen across the genome, and these are mostly methylated. It is a general observation that CGIs in active promoters are devoid of 5mC, while CGIs are heavily methylated in repressed promoters. Isolated CG sites across the genome show a cell type specific methylation pattern, thus defining the associated active transcriptome, and the CpG sites within repeat elements, including centromeric and telomeric repeats, are largely methylated to maintain them in a constitutively repressed state thereby preventing spurious expansion of these elements [28]. A consequence of demethylation of repeat elements is genome instability [31], frequently observed in cancer, as is aberrant methylation patterns across the genome. Since irregularities in 5mC patterns across genomic features can have profound deleterious effects on cellular function, understanding the molecular pathways involved in establishing and regulating these patterns is of utmost importance.

Members of both families, DNMT and TET, show some degree of non-redundant function in regulating DNA methylation patterns, as observed by various selective knockdown and over-expression studies [32–34]. One mechanism by which distinct, cell-type specific, 5mC patterns are established, is by selectively targeting the DNMTs at particular genomic loci. How selective targeting is achieved across the genome, has been a deeply investigated question in the field of DNA methylation. Interaction with sequence-specific DNA-binding proteins mediating locus-specific recruitment of the DNMTs has been one school of thought [35]. These DNA-binding proteins can be selectively expressed, or post-translationally regulated, in a cell-type and cell-stage specific manner to establish differential methylation patterns. Several studies have isolated unique and common interactors of each of the DNMTs. For instance, DNMT3B is recruited by the transcription factor E2F6 to mediate silencing of the germ-line genes, Slc25a31, Syce1, Tex11, and Ddx41. DNMTs also cooperate with histone marks and chromatin complexes to achieve locus-specific targeting [36]. Interactions with the H3K9 methylating enzymes, Suv39h1, Setdb1 and G9a, target DNMTs to heterochromatin to establish 5mC [37]. Specifically, DNMT3B is recruited to centromeric and pericentromeric repeat regions via interactions with CENP-C, an essential core component of the centromere, where it establishes DNA methylation and coordinates with other epigenetic components to mediate constitutive heterochromatization of the centromeric region [38].

2   Cancer: The Result of a Deregulated DNA Methylation Pathway

As DNA methylation pathways are fundamental to normal progression of several biological processes, dysregulation in its molecular pathway inevitably results in deleterious effects on cellular function. One of the most widely studied consequences of altered methylation patterns is cancer. It has been known for sometime that cancers are associated with globally hypomethylated genomes, accompanied by local hypermethylation events [39]. The local hypermethylation events generally accumulate at promoters of tumor suppressor genes (TSGs), enabling transcriptional silencing of these genes, consequently promoting tumor initiation and facilitating tumor progression. Aberrant DNA methylation patterns, in addition to distorting the normal transcriptome, also promote genomic instability, a significant contributor to tumor progression. Several studies have reported altered DNA methylation patterns to be the effector interface between a driver genetic mutation in a non-epigenetic gene and the resulting cancer associated transcriptome. However, cancers driven purely by epimutations with no associated genetic alterations are being identified. Ependymomas, a recurrent pediatric brain tumor, are driven by epigenetic events and are associated with very low recurring frequencies of somatic mutations and chromosomal aberrations [40].

Epimutations refer to non-genetic, heritable, aberrant lesions in the expression of a gene, arising from DNA modifications or other epigenetic modifications on local chromatin. Epimutations are typically not associated with base changes in DNA, either in -cis or -trans, but show transgenerational inheritance by mitotic transmission of the epigenetic mark. Epimutations can be classified into 'somatic' or 'constitutional' depending on whether it originated in differentiated cells and is thus contained in a specific tissue type (somatic), or it originated in germ-line cells and is thus present in all of the organisms' cells (constitutional) [41]. Evidence in several tumor types suggests the association of a particular DNA methylation signature with tumor progression, signifying its aggressiveness and having a diagnostic and prognostic value. Such specific 5mC signatures are more widely seen in, but not restricted to, promoter elements, and are termed CpG Island Methylator Phenotype (CIMP) [42].

Tumorigenic epigenetic events driven by CIMP can be attributed to deregulation of individual molecular components of the DNA methylation pathway by various mechanisms;

(i) Inactivating or hyper activating mutations in the DNMTs or TETs.

(ii) Mutations in co-factors of DNMTs/TETs altering their catalytic activity

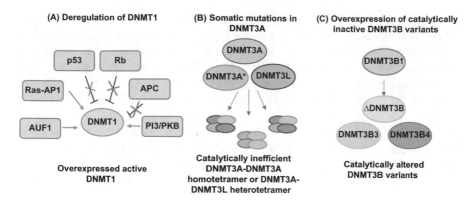

Fig. 1 Mechanisms deregulating the DNMT family to promote cancer. (**a**) DNMT1 is deregulated by hyperactivated signaling pathways. (**b**) DNMT3A is mainly inactivated by somatic mutations. (**c**) DNMT3B function is compromised by overexpression of catalytically inactive, truncated variants (DNMTΔ3B), or alternative splice variants (DNMT3B3/4). (* = mutant)

(iii) Mutations in mediators of signaling pathways regulating the DNMTs/TETs transcriptionally, post-transcriptionally, and post-translationally.

(iv) Mutational disruption of the DNMT/TET functional interactome resulting in their inappropriate targeting across the genome

Each of the above mentioned strategies can be employed by cancer cells to generate aberrant DNA methylation patterns subsequently facilitating tumorigenesis.

2.1   Compromised Writers and Their Contribution to Cancer

DNMTs are frequently deregulated in cancer to achieve an altered DNA methylome. Of the three, DNMT1 and DNMT3B function as oncogenes, and are frequently activated in cancer, whereas DNMT3A functions as a tumor suppressor gene, and is functionally inactivated to promote cancer. Mechanisms targeting each of the DNMTs and their role in tumorigenesis are briefly described in this section (Fig. 1).

2.1.1   DNMT1

Single base mutations disrupting the entire DNMT1 catalytic domain were first defined in a small population of colorectal cancers (7%) [43]. Typically, DNMT1 has high affinity for hemimethylated DNA, and acts as a maintenance methyltransferase with little or no de novo methyltransferase activity. This preference for hemimethylated DNA is explained by an auto-inhibition model of the DNMT1 enzyme. Structural studies on DNMT1 have shown that the mammalian enzyme is a multimodular protein, composed of a replication foci-targeting sequence domain (RFTS domain), a DNA-binding CXXC domain, a pair of bromo-adjacent homology (BAH) domains, and a C-terminal catalytic domain. A stretch of acidic amino acid residues, termed the autoinhibitory linker region, lies between the CXXC and BAH domains and functions to prevent methylation at unmethylated CpGs, thus conserving the preference of the MTase domain for hemimethylated CpGs. Unmethylated CpG is recognized and bound by the CXXC domain, which prevents the catalytic domain from binding to it [44]. Additionally the RFTD mediates autoinhibitory effects by occulding unmethylated CpG binding at the catalytic domain [45]. Mutations in the autoinhibitory linker region as well as the RFTD evidently affect the catalytic efficiency of DNMT1 at unmethylated CpGs in vitro [44, 46]. Although both gain of function and loss of function mutations are proto-oncogenic in vitro, genetic mutations in DNMT1 are not a frequent event in tumorigenesis. However, deregulation of DNMT1 activity is central to tumor progression, suggesting alternative mechanisms targeting DNMT1 to be the underlying oncogenic phenomenon. DNMT1 levels are elevated in lung, hepatocellular, acute and chronic myelogenous leukemia, colorectal, gastric, and breast cancers [47–52], suggesting that DNMT1 is a transcriptional target of several oncogenic signaling pathways.

One of the pathways positively regulating DNMT1 expression is the Ras-AP1 pathway. AP1 (activating-protein 1), is a collective term for a group of basic leucine-zipper (bZIP) transcription factors, and constitutes proteins belonging to the Jun, Fos, Maf and ATF sub-families. AP-1 functions as a dimeric transcription factor recognizing either 12-O-tetradecanoylphorbol-13-acetate response elements (TPA, 5'-TGAG/CTCA-3') or cAMP response elements (CRE, 5'-TGACGTCA-3'). Functionally, AP1 regulates cellular proliferation, survival, death, and differentiation, mostly by promoting gene expression, although cases of gene repression have also been reported [53]. Evidence suggests that neoplastic transformation relying on AP1-mediated mechanisms exert their effects in part through increased DNMT1 levels, which thereby methylate and represses expression of negative regulators of cell growth, conferring an advantage on cell growth. The 5' regulatory region in the DNMT1 gene has three AP1 response elements, which are heavily methylated in early embryonic stem cells and normal somatic cells (preventing AP1 binding), but lose methylation in transformed cells allowing binding and induction by AP1 [54]. Cellular transformation by continuous c-Fos expression, which heterodimerizes with c-Jun to form a functional AP1 bZIP, subsequently induces DNMT1 expression to drive and maintain neoplastic transformation. cFos-mediated transformation can be reverted by direct abrogation of cFos, or through DNMT1 depletion, suggesting cFos relies significantly on DNMT1 to functionally disrupt cell growth regulation [55].

The APC/β-catenin/TCF pathway, which is critical to maintaining homeostasis in the gastrointestinal system, also regulates DNMT1 transcriptionally. APC, which functions as a tumor suppressor gene, is frequently mutated in cancers of the GI tract. Mutational inactivation of APC leads to upregulation of the Wnt/β-catenin/TCF pathway, conferring growth advantage on cancer cells and facilitating metastasis by promoting epithelial to mesenchymal transition (EMT). DNMT1 is transcriptionally inhibited by APC, and inactivating mutations in APC lead to overexpression of DNMT1, facilitating tumor initiation [56]. DNMT1 is also the transcriptional target of the p53 and Rb pathways. Pathways involving both p53 and Rb negatively regulate DNMT1 expression levels, and are frequently deregulated in several cancers, allowing overexpression of DNMT1 and hypermethylation of tumor suppressor genes. In some tumors, p53 acquires mutations in its DNA-binding domain, disrupting its ability to bind to the p53 consensus sequence in the promoters of its target genes. Over-expression of Wild-type p53, but not mutant p53 (Mut R248L or Mut R273H), could bind at the DNMT1 promoter and repress it transcriptionally in lung cancer cell lines – A549 and H1299 [57]. The p53 binding site within the DNMT1 promoter was mapped to the exon 1 region (−19 to +317), which contains putative Sp1, p53, and E2F binding sites. p53 binding at the DNMT1 promoter is Sp1 dependent. Sp1, p53, HDAC1, and HDAC6 form a complex at the DNMT1 promoter, and p53 cannot suppress DNMT1 in the absence of Sp1 [57]. However, Sp1 can function as a transcriptional activator of DNMT1, and the stoichiometric ratio of p53 and Sp1 determines the effect of Sp1 on DNMT1 transcription. Sp1 levels regulate p53 nuclear-cytoplasmic distribution thereby modulating MDM2 mediated ubiquitination and degradation of p53. At high levels of Sp1, p53 is degraded in the cytoplasm and its inhibitory effect on DNMT1 is released, resulting in DNMT1 transcriptional activation and hypermethylation of tumor suppressor genes – p16INK4a, RARβ, FHIT, RASSF1A, and hRAB37, which are frequently hypermethylated in lung cancer [57]. Rb plays a crucial role in regulating cell cycle progression, especially passage through the restriction point, and is inactivated by several mechanisms to promote tumor progression. Increased DNMT1 is invariably associated with Rb inactivation. The increase in DNMT1 is attributable to enhanced E2F1 activity in the absence of Rb, which directly binds at the DNMT1 promoter activating it to bring about methylation-mediated silencing of tumor suppressor genes [58].

In addition to modulating DNMT1 transcript levels, post-transcriptional and post-translational modifications also serve as mechanistic modulators of DNMT1. AUF1, the RNA binding protein, regulates DNMT1 mRNA stability in a cell cycle specific manner and functions to regulate the epigenetic integrity of the cell during cell division [59]. DNMT1 protein stability is regulated by the PI3K/PKB (phosphatidylinositol 3-kinase/protein kinaseB) pathway, mainly responsible for cell growth, viability, and metabolism. PI3K/PKB pathway inhibits Gsk3β (glycogen synthase kinase 3β) mediated DNMT1 proteasomal degradation contributing to elevated DNMT1 protein levels [60]. DNMT1 levels are also regulated by its replication fork-targeting factor, UHRF1, an E3 ubiquitin ligase, which ubiquitinates and directs DNMT1 degradation [61]. In vitro mutational analysis suggests that UHRF1 also stimulates DNMT1 catalytic activity [62], suggesting a dual role for UHRF1 in DNMT1 regulation. Mutations disrupting the DNMT1/UHRF1/PCNA complex result in loss of DNMT1 recruitment to the replication fork and global DNA hypomethylation, thereby promoting initiation of tumorigenesis [63, 64].

2.1.2 DNMT3A

DNMT3A is frequently mutated in several hematological malignancies. Mutations are generally heterozygous and span various domains of the enzymes, but the most frequently mutated site is R882 [65]. This mutation results in formation of a hypomorphic enzyme which impedes catalytic activity by functioning in a dominant negative fashion [66]. DNMT3A functions by forming homotetramers with itself and heterotetramers with DNMT3L [67, 68], and the R882 mutant competes with WT DNMT3A encoded by the non-mutant allele, to form a dysfunctional homo- or hetero-tetramer, which exhibits reduced DNA binding and catalytic activity [66]. The R882 mutation is highly prevalent in de novo Acute Myeloid Leukemia (AML) patients (frequency of 22%) as compared to its occurrence in other hematological malignancies, including myelodysplastic syndrome (MDS), myeloproliferative neoplasms (MPNs) and chronic myelomonocytic leukemia (CMML). Other catalytically inactivating mutations, and truncating mutations (missense, non-sense, frame-shift, and splicing mutations), have also been mapped across functional domains of DNMT3A [65]. Most of these mutations have been biochemically characterized in vitro, and their effect on disrupting de novo methylation by DNMT3A can be explained by reduced catalytic activity (e.g. R664), reduced DNA binding (e.g. R831), loss of co-factor – S-adenosyl-L-methionine (AdoMet) binding (e.g. C710) [69], and loss of interactions with locus-specific recruiting histone marks (e.g. Q308) [70, 71]. How do these mutations affect cellular biology to facilitate tumorigenesis? In hematopoietic malignancies, loss of DNMT3A function alters the differentiation potential of hematopoietic stem cells while preserving their self-renewal and expansion properties, thus presumably creating a pool of stem cells predisposed to tumorigenesis upon acquisition of additional mutagenic insults. This presumption is partially substantiated by studies in murine models. Conditional genetic ablation of Dnmt3a in HSCs hampers their differentiation potential while favoring stem cell renewal. Paradoxically, loss of Dnmt3a results in hypermethylation of CGIs associated with the Basp1, Pdxdc1, and Wbscr17 genes, presumably through aberrant activity of DNMT1 and/or DNMT3b [3]. HSC fingerprint genes, which are repressed in differentiated cells, become overexpressed upon Dnmt3a ablation while differentiation specific genes are silenced, conferring the cells with a stem cell phenotype while blocking their differentiation. However, no leukemia was observed, suggesting functional disruption of Dnmt3a is a pre-leukemic event and is not sufficient to initiate tumorigenesis by itself [3].

Indeed, DNMT3A mutated HSCs acquire secondary mutations that induce tumorigenesis resulting in several blood malignancies. Mutations in the nucleophosmin gene (NPM1) and tandem duplication of the receptor tyrosine kinase FLT3 gene (FLT3ITD) [65], are the two mutations most frequently co-occurring with DNMT3A. The interactive contribution of these co-occurring mutations to leukemia is not completely understood and warrants further investigation. Mutations in DNMT3A show a strong association with mutations in the spliceosome factor SF3B1 (splicing factor 3b, subunit 1), in MDS patients. Positive association with mutations in the spliceosome factor U2AF1 (U2 small nuclear RNA auxiliary factor 1), and negative association with mutations in serine/arginine-rich splicing factor 2 (SRSF2) have been reported [71]. Interestingly, DNMT3A mutations co-occur with IDH1/2 mutations in AML derived from MDS, suggesting a possible interactive mechanism in progression of AML from MDS [72].

DNMT3A is also inactivated by mechanisms other than mutations. UHRF1, known to regulate DNMT1 mediated methylation, along with UHRF2, negatively regulates DNMT3A by functioning as E3 ligases to promote DNMT3A degradation [73]. Both UHRF1 and UHRF2 are overexpressed in cancer. UHRF1 is exclusively involved in regulation of maintenance methylation, by directly controlling DNMT1 levels and its catalytic activity. UHRF2, however, is not associated with maintenance methylation, but is evidently involved in degrading DNMT3A, thus providing an explanation for the global hypomethylation associated with UHRF2 overexpressing tumors. DNMT3A is also subject to regulation by the MDM2/Rb pathway. In lung cancers, it was reported by Tang et al. that, depleted Rb levels, owing to overexpression of the Rb regulating E3 ubiquitin ligase MDM2, resulted in transcriptional activation of DNMT3A thereby resulting in downstream silencing of tumor suppressor genes by promoter methylation, thus promoting lung cancer [74]. The DNMT3A promoter possesses E2F binding sites, and is transcriptionally silenced by a repressive Rb-E2F complex formed at these sites. MDM2 attenuates DNMT3A repression by degrading Rb, allowing de novo methylation and silencing of multiple TSGs [74]. In this scenario, DNMT3A functions like an oncogene as opposed to its tumor suppressor role in myeloid malignancies. However, a mouse model of lung cancer contradicts the oncogenic role DNMT3A, since genetic ablation of DNMT3A promoted lung cancer progression, pointing again toward a tumor suppressor role for DNMT3A [75].

2.1.3 DNMT3B

Mutations in DNMT3B have not been observed in cancers. However, polymorphisms in the DNMT3B promoter are associated with cancer risk. The C to T polymorphism (C46359 > T) -149 bps upstream to the DNMT3B start site enhances promoter activity resulting in increased DNMT3B levels [76], potentially contributing to CIMP events occurring at tumor suppressor genes. This polymorphism, also represented as −149 C > T, is associated with an increased risk for lung cancer [77] and carcinoma of the head and neck [78]. The C46359T SNP positively correlates with age dependent Hereditary Nonpolyposis Colorectal Cancer [79], but shows no co-relation in breast cancers [80]. In fact, two DNMT3B polymorphisms, −283 T > C and −579 G > T, are associated with reduced cancer risk [81], although these results have been disputed [82].

Though mutations in DNMT3B are not associated with tumors, deregulation of DNMT3B expression levels, catalytic activity, and targeting across the genome are essential epigenomic driver events in tumorigenesis. To achieve DNMT3B mediated aberrant methylation patterns, tumors may rely on several mechanisms. One mechanism is expressing truncated DNMT3B variants generated by aberrant splicing, to bring about redistribution of methylation patterns. A family of truncated variants, termed ΔDNMT3B, are overexpressed in non-small cell lung carcinoma (NSCLC) [83] and contribute to lung tumorigenesis by modulating DNA methylation at the promoters of tumor suppressor genes, p16INK4a and RASSF1A [84]. The ΔDNMT3B family is produced by non-conventional pre-mRNA splicing and consists of seven members, ΔDNMT3B1-4 lacking the N-terminal domain while preserving the PWWP and catalytic domains, and ΔDNMT3B5-7, which lack enzymatic activity. In NSCLC, the ΔDNMT3B1, ΔDNMT3B2, and ΔDNMT3B4 variants are highly expressed. ΔDNMT3B2/4 regulate promoter methylation of RASSF1A but not p16INK4a, suggesting a non-redundant function in regulating de novo methylation by the different truncated DNMT3B isoforms [84].

A separate family of DNMT3B splice variants, resulting again in truncated variants exhibiting absence, or varying degrees of catalytic activity, is responsible for global DNA methylation changes associated with cancer progression [85]. One such catalytically inactive splice variant, DNMT3B7, is overexpressed in several cancer cell lines of diverse origin [86]. In breast cancers, DNMT3B7 expression leads to promoter hypermethylation and silencing of the E-cadherin gene, activating the β-catenin pathway and conferring growth advantage. DNMT3B7 expression increases between stages I and II, implying its role in facilitating tumor progression [87]. In neuroblastoma cells, however, DNMT3B7 shows an anti-tumorigenic effect. Neuroblastoma cell lines express DNMT3B7 as well as other truncated DNMT3B variants, but the more aggressive forms show depleted DNMT3B7 levels and its forced overexpression results in inhibition of growth and increased global methylation. This suggests that a finely regulated interplay between the DNMT3B variants drives tumorigenesis. In hepatocellular carcinoma (HCC), overexpression of the variant DNMT3B4, lacking conserved methyltransferase motifs IX and X is associated with demethylation of pericentromeric satellite DNA, thus contributing to heterochromatin instability and promoting tumorigenesis [88]. DNMT3B4 overexpression in chronic myeloid leukemia (CML) is associated with demethylation of LINE-1 elements. In both, HCC and CML, the catalytically inactive DNMT3B3 is also expressed, and an increased DNMT3B4 to DNMT3B3 ratio promotes tumorigenic demethylation events. Although both isoforms lack MTase activity, the two have different effects on the catalytic activity of the functional heterodimer formed with DNMT3A. DNMT3B3 enhances DNMT3A activity, while DNMT3B4 attenuates DNMT3A, thus functioning in a dominant negative fashion [85].

In contrast to DNMT3A, DNMT3B functions like an oncogene and is often overexpressed in cancer. Analysis of an array of breast cancer cell lines showed that DNMT3B overexpression is positively associated with the hypermethylator phenotype characterized by silencing of the tumor suppressor genes CDH1, CEACAM6, CST6, ESR1, LCN2, and SCNN1A [89]. Cell lines not showing a robust CIMP, did not exhibit DNMT3B overexpression. DNMT3B is also overexpressed in lung cancer and is regulated by MDM2/FOXO3. As in the case of DNMT3A, which is regulated by MDM2/Rb, DNMT3B is negatively regulated by FOXO3, typically an activating transcription factor. The DNMT3B promoter contains two FOXO3 binding sites which when occupied by FOXO3, leads to transcriptional silencing. FOXO3 is a target for degradation by MDM2 mediated ubiqitination, and is thus repressed in MDM2 overexpressing lung cancer cell lines relieving its inhibitory control on DNMT3B [90].

2.1.4 DNMT3L

The catalytically inactive DNMT3L, though incapable of depositing 5mC by itself, plays a crucial role in establishing 5mC patterns through its influence on DNMT3A and DNMT3B activity. DNMT3L directly binds DNMT3A and enhances its catalytic activity by enhancing its binding affinity for the co-factor AdoMet, and increasing its catalytic processivity [91–93]. A similar enhancement of DNMT3B activity by interaction with DNMT3L has also been reported [94]. Additionally, DNMT3L mediates locus-specific recruitment of the de novo DNMTs, through interactions with unique sequence specific transcription factors. For instance, DNMT3L forms a complex with p65-NFkB and DNMT3B, recruiting DNMT3B to specific genomic loci to mediate their methylation [95]. DNMT3L is highly expressed in germ cells and undifferentiated pluripotent stem cells, and plays an essential role in gametogenesis. Recent evidences suggest DNMT3L may have an oncogenic role in tumors arising from early developmental stages, involving germ cells. Both seminomatous and nonseminomatous testicular germ cell tumors (TGCTs), associated with a unique 5mC profile, showed an overexpression of DNMT3L [96]. Hypomethylation of the DNMT3L promoter is observed in cervical cancer [97] and in ocular surface squamous neoplasia [98], although the biological significance of this is yet to be elucidated. DNMT3L was also reported to affect promoter methylation, and therefore expression, of the thymine DNA glycosylase (TDG) gene in an array of human gastric cancer cell lines [99]. These findings point toward a pro-oncogenic function of DNMT3L.

2.2 Dysregulated Erasers

The TET proteins are involved in actively recycling the 5mC marks, and in the process produce additional functional epigenetic marks. The three mammalian TET proteins are non-redundant, share structural homology, and function via similar mechanisms. However, they show distinct expression patterns and are associated with a unique set of interacting proteins. TET proteins play a crucial role in embryonic development, hematopoiesis, and neurogenesis, and mutations in the TETs are observed in several solid tumors as well as leukemia. Mutations in metabolic genes, especially IDH1/IDH2, are also frequent in tumors, and manifest their effects through deregulation of TET activity. In general, the TETs are oncoprotective, and

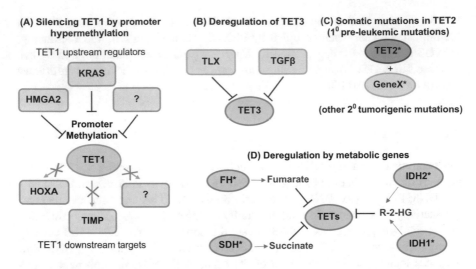

Fig. 2 Mechanisms deregulating the TET family to promote cancer. (**a**) TET1 is transcriptionally silenced by KRAS/ERK- or HMGA2-mediated promoter methylation. (**b**) TET3 levels are transcriptionally regulated by TLX and TGF β, and post-translationally regulated by IDAX. (**c**) TET2 is inactivated by somatic mutations, and upon acquisition of secondary mutations facilitates tumorigenesis. (**d**) Mutations in metabolic genes produces oncometabolites, which inhibit TET catalytic activity. (1^0 –primary, 2^0 –secondary, * = mutant, red font = oncometabolites)

TET2 is a bona fide tumor suppressor gene. Tumorigenic mutations in TET or their associated factors generally target a reduction in TET demethylation activity, thus preserving and allowing 5mC deposition and promoting the hypermethylator phenotype underlying tumorigenesis. The epigenetic basis of several cancers has been traced to deregulated activity of each of the TETs (Fig. 2).

2.2.1   TET1

The pluripotency factors, OCT4, NANOG, and SOX2, transcriptionally regulate TET1 [100], to promote high expression in embryonic stem cells where TET1 functions to maintain pluripotency by contributing to active demethylation. TET1 is also expressed in some neuronal cells and differentiated adult cell types, where it functions as a maintenance demethylase, by occupying hypomethylated CGIs via its CXXC domain, hydroxymethylating the CGI boundaries, and preventing 5mC spreading by occluding DNMTs [101]. Since TET1 was first identified as a fusion partner of MLL1 in AML, it was suspected to play an oncogenic role. However, evidence suggests otherwise. Cimmono et al., demonstrated that genetic ablation in a mouse model promotes lymphomagenesis, particularly the formation of follicular lymphoma (FL) and diffuse large B cell lymphoma (DLBCL) suggesting that the presence of TET1 is oncoprotective and loss of its function promotes B cell lymphoma. Human FL and DLBCL samples showed no associated TET1 loss of function mutations, though a small percentage were associated with mutations in TET2. All FL and DLBCL samples unassociated with TET1 mutations, exclusively showed diminished TET1 expression as a result of promoter hypermethylation. This is indicative of transcriptional, post-transcriptional and post-translational mechanisms acting to diminish functional TET1 as an oncogenic event in the absence of loss-of-function genetic mutations in TET1 [102].

In vitro knockdown studies imply an inhibitory effect of TET1 on cell proliferation [103], explaining why it is downregulated in several cancers. Analysis of adenocarcinomas originating from lung, colon, breast, and rectum, at stages I to IV, showed that TET1, but not TET2/3, was downregulated in stage1 adenocarcinoma, suggesting repression of TET1 is an early event in tumorigenesis [104]. As in FL and DLBCL, hypermethylation of the TET1 promoter results in transcriptional silencing, and is a significant contributor to CIMP associated with colorectal cancers [105]. In primary colorectal cancer cells, TET1 inhibition facilitates tumorigenesis via activation of the Wnt signaling pathway, mainly a result of repression of negative regulators of Wnt, DKK3 and DKK4, which are TET1 transcriptional targets, and in its absence are repressed by promoter methylation [104]. In addition to controlling proliferation, TET1 also negatively regulates invasion and metastatic potential. Members of the Tissue inhibitors of metalloproteases (TIMP) family, TIMP2 and TIMP3, are directly bound by and regulated by TET1-mediated demethylation. Suppression of TET1 in invasive cancers results in repression of the TIMPs, thereby resulting in derepression of matix metalloproteinases (MMPs), an essential step towards gaining invasiveness and promoting metastasis [106]. This mechanism of MMP reactivation through TET1 inhibition was also observed in breast cancers dependent on HDAC-mediated epigenetic events [107]. Breast cancer metastasis has also been attributed to inhibition of HOXA (HOXA7 and HOXA9), which is targeted by TET1-mediated promoter demethylation to bring about transcriptional activation. Overexpression of the tumorigeneic architectural transcription factor, HMGA2, in breast cancer cells, results in transcriptional silencing of TET1 and thereby its downstream targets - HOXA7 and HOXA9. TET1, which autoregulates itself by preventing 5mC deposition at its promoter, is silenced by promoter methylation in HMGA2-overexpressing breast cancer cells, thus implying the involvement of an HMGA2/TET1/HOXA signaling pathway in promoting breast cancer metastasis [103]. Another signaling pathway dependent on TET1 repression to promote TSG repression is the KRAS-ERK signaling pathway. KRAS overexpression is oncogenic, results in cellular transformation, and is observed in numerous cancers. KRAS overexpression is concomitant with reduced 5hmC levels and increased 5mC levels, particularly at the promoters of TSGs. Of these, DAPK, MGMT, and DUOX1 are direct targets of TET1, and KRAS overexpression results in reduced TET1 occupancy at the promoters of these TSGs resulting in their silencing by hypermethylation [108]. TET1 activity is also affected by hypoxic conditions, and will be discussed in Sect. 4.

2.2.2   TET2

This family member lacking the N-terminal CXXC domain plays an essential role in myelopoiesis, and is highly expressed in normal myeloid progenitor cells, granulocytes, and erythroid cells. TET2 is an established tumor suppressor of myeloid malignancies and is frequently mutated in myelodysplastic syndromes and myeloproliferative disorders, including AML. The first reported mutations in the TET2 gene were myeloid cancer associated chromosomal aberrations-microdeletions and uniparental disomy involving the chromosomal region 4q24, where the human TET2 gene is located [109]. Thereafter, several TET2 point mutations were identified across several blood malignancies, including MDS, CMML, primary AML, blastic plasmacytoid dendritic neoplasm, myeloproliferative neoplasms (MPNs) such as polycythemia vera, primary myelofibrosis, and B- and T-cell lymphomas. These somatic mutations, encompassing insertions, deletions, missense, nonsense, and frameshift mutations, were heterozygous and mapped to the TET2 catalytic domain, potentially resulting in TET2 enzymatic deficiency [110]. However, TET2 mutations are only pre-leukemic, potentiating tumor initiation, but not causative on their own. Evidence suggests that TET2 mutations are acquired at an early stage in the onset of hematological malignancies. Analysis of HSCs from MDS patients show accumulation of monoallelic TET2 mutations with progressive accumulation of secondary mutations at the MDS stage, suggesting that TET2 inactivation creates a clonal population of HSCs poised for oncogenesis upon accumulation of secondary mutations. This notion is supported by studies in different models of Tet2 knockout mice. Disrupting Tet2 in HSCs or hematopoietic progenitor cells (HPCs) led to decreased 5hmC levels, an increase in self-renewal capacity, and expansion of the stem cell compartment with concordant blockage in myeloid differentiation. Interestingly, lymphoid differentiation remains unaffected [111]. A similar effect was seen when the Tet2 catalytic domain was selectively ablated. The HSC and HPC compartments exhibited enhanced self-renewal and expansion in serial transplantation assays, with impaired differentiation down the myeloid lineage [112]. The enhanced self-renewal capacity and antagonistic differentiation can be attributed to increased expression of self-renewal factors, Meis1 and Evi1 with concomitant decrease in differentiation/myeloid specific factors [111]. To further support the idea that acquisition of TET2 mutations is an early event in hematological malignancies, Zhao et al. specifically disrupted TET2 in different compartments of the hematopoietic system, and showed that mutations in the HSC/HPC, but not the more differentiated cell types, led to myeloid malignancies [113]. TET2 mutations have been shown to accumulate in healthy ageing individuals showing clonal hematopoiesis, predisposing them to developing hematological malignancies [114].

In order to initiate tumorigenesis, TET2 mutated hematopoietic clones acquire a second hit. Several genes are co-mutated with TET2 across different cancer types. In MDS, TET2 mutations are associated with the splicing factor, SF3B1. Additionally, mutations in SRSR2, EZH2, and ASXL1, also reportedly co-exist with TET2 mutations in MDS [110]. Mouse models with co-mutations in TET2 and

EZH2/ASXLI recapitulate the MDS phenotype [115, 116]. The gene encoding the small GTPase of the Rho family, RHOA, is exclusively co-mutated with TET2 in peripheral T-cell lymphoma (PTCL) [117], while DNMT3A co-mutations are observed in angioimmunoblastic T-cell lymphoma (AITL) [118]. Mutations in IDH2 have been reported to co-occur with TET2 mutations in MDS [119], but IDH1 and TET2 mutations are still believed to be mutually exclusive.

While inactivating mutations in TET2 seem to be the major route towards achieving oncogenic potential, alternate mechanisms affecting TET2 function have also been reported. The TET2 associated CXXC domain is carried as a separate gene, IDAX, which binds promoters and CpG islands in the genome. IDAX directly interacts with TET2, and mediates TET2 degradation in a caspase-dependent manner [120]. By negatively regulating TET2 protein levels, IDAX abrogates TET2's tumor suppressor function, to promote cancer initiation and/or progression. TET protein levels are also regulated by the calcium dependent cysteine proteases, calpains (Calpain1 – Tet1/2, Calpain2-Tet3) [121], which are overexpressed in cancers [122], providing an additional mechanism by which TET2 can be negatively controlled to facilitate and sustain cancer.

Lastly, loss of TET2 targeting across the genome could result in the hypermethylator phenotype underlying tumor progression. Mutations in a TET2 interacting transcription factor, Wilms Tumor 1 (WT1), occur in AML and are mutually exclusive of TET2, IDH1, and IDH2 mutations. WT1 recruits TET2 to specific target sites to mediate transcriptional activation. AML associated mutations in TET2 disrupting its interaction with WT1 result in loss of transcriptional activation of WT1 target genes, signifying the dependence of WT1 on TET2 to mediate transcriptional activation [123].

2.2.3 TET3

TET3 is highly expressed in oocytes and has been functionally implicated in regulating methylation patterns in the male pronucleus. Like TET1, mutations in TET3 contributing to cancer development are rare. Nonetheless, a tumor suppressor function has been attributed to TET3 in a few tumor types. Inhibition of TET3 is critical to maintaining self-renewal and tumorigenic potential in glioblastoma stem cells (GSCs), and is achieved by repression by the transcription factor TLX. TLX binds to the TET3 promoter to transcriptionally silence it and promote GSC tumorigenecity, possibly through repression of the tumor suppressor genes, BTG2, TUSC1, BAK1, LATS2, FZD6 and PPP2R1B. The TLX-TET3 inverse regulatory axis, if disrupted, results in reduced oncogenic potential of GSCs [124]. The tumor suppressor role of TET3 was further elucidated in ovarian cancer cells. TET3 was targeted for repression by TGFβ1-induced EMT, and EMT was blocked upon overexpression of TET3 in ovarian cancer cell lines. TET3 mediates its oncoprotective function in ovarian cancer by regulating promoter demethylation and hence activation of miR-30d, a proven inhibitor of EMT [125].

3 Modulation of DNA Methylation Regulators by Metabolic Mechanisms

3.1 IDH1/IDH2

The genes coding for the enzyme isocitrate dehydrogenase (IDH) are frequently mutated in myeloid malignancies (AML, MDS, and MPN), neural malignancies (astrocytoma, oligodendrocytoma, and glioblastoma), and less frequently in other solid tumors (cholangiocarcinoma, chondrosarcoma, colorectal cancer, esophageal cancer, bladder cancer, melanoma, prostate carcinoma, and breast adenocarcinoma). The IDH family converts isocitrate to αKG via oxidative decarboxylation and consists of three active enzymes, IDH1 which localizes to the cytosol and peroxisomes, and IDH2 and 3, which localize to the mitochondria. IDH1 and IDH2 function as homodimers and use nicotinamide adenine dinucleotide phosphate (NADP+) as a cofactor, whereas IDH3 functions as a heterotetramer (consisting of two alpha, one beta and one gamma subunit) in the TCA cycle, utilizing nicotinamide adenine dinucleotide (NAD+) as a cofactor. However, somatic mutations in IDH1/2, but not IDH3 have been attributed to promoting tumorigenesis by altering metabolism, specifically α-ketoglutarate levels, thereby inhibiting the function of α-KG dependent dioxygenases which include the TET family, JmjC domain-containing histone demethylases, and EglN prolyl-4-hydroxylases.

Somatic mutations, mostly missense mutations, in IDH1/2, are restricted to one of three arginine residue in the catalytic pocket of the enzyme essential for isocitrate binding. In IDH1, this residue is invariably R132, while in IDH2, the R172 and R140 residues are targets for somatic mutations. As opposed to inactivating enzymatic mutations, frequently underlying mechanisms promoting cancer, IDH1/2 mutations are activating and produce a neomorphic enzyme that catalyzes the reduction of α-ketoglutarate (α-KG) to the R-enantiomer of 2-hydroxyglutarate (R-2-HG), an oncometabolite [126]. Accumulation of R-2-HG promotes proliferation while inhibiting differentiation, and competitively inhibits the dioxygenase activity of the α-KG and Fe^{2+} dependent TET enzymes [127]. The consequence of inhibiting TET activity in this manner is DNA hypermethylation, and in fact IDH mutant tumors exhibit CIMP. Expression of the mutant IDH1 in an in vitro system redefines the methylome to recapitulate the hypermethylator phenotype observed in IDH1 mutant tumors. This was independently shown in isogenic human primary astrocytes and an isogenic colorectal cancer cell line, HCT116, both genetically engineered to express IDH1 (R132H) [128].

IDH mutations have been suggested to be causative, rather than simply contributing, to CIMP. Studies involving low grade glioma (LGG) showed that the G-CIMP+, but not the G-CIMP- LGGs were associated with IDH1 mutations. G-CIMP+ tumors are associated with hypermethylation at CGIs and shores at loci enriched for PRC2 targets, and indeed showed deposition of H3K27me3, a histone mark positively correlating with/permissive to 5hmC deposition [129]. Hypermethylation in IDH mutant primary gliomas also show a loss in CTCF-binding, disrupting the organization of topologically associated domains (TADs), resulting in aberrant expression of oncogenes. The term TAD refers to the three-dimentional subdomain arising from spatially favourable conformations of locally interacting chromatin. Boundaries between TADs ensure maintenace of the environment within them, and are maintained by the insulator binding protein - CTCF. PDGFRA, an established glioma associated oncogene, is activated by this mechanism. G-CIMP associated with IDH1 mutation results in disruption of the boundary between PDGFRA and FIP1L1 (from an adjacent TAD) leading to association of the PDGFRA promoter with a constitutive enhancer, resulting its constitutive expression and oncogenic signaling [130]. How does IDH1 mutation lead to CIMP? Inhibition of TET catalytic activity is one explanation, however, loss of TET recruitment has also been reported. Chondrosarcomas driven by IDH1 and IDH2 mutations exhibit a CIMP in regulatory regions, including promoter associated transcription start sites and CpG islands and shores at genes enriched to function in the retinoic acid pathway. These genes were co-bound by EBF1 and TET2, suggesting the hypermethylation was a result of altered TET2 targeting by EBF1 at these sites. Recruitment of both EBF1 and TET2 was altered at three of the most differentially hypermethylated loci – CCND2, FABP3 and FBRSL1, as determined by ChIP-seq. EBF1 and TET2 co-immunoprecipitate in the chondrosarcoma cell line SW1353 [131].

3.2 Hypoxia

Hypoxia is a cancer prevalent microenvironment promoting tumor growth by influencing cellular processes that confer upon cells aggressive pro-survival phenotypes of uncontrolled proliferation, invasion, evasion from apoptosis, while also facilitating angiogenesis. The adaptive response to hypoxic conditions is mediated by the oxygen tension-dependent hypoxia inducible factor-1 (HIF-1). HIF1 functions as a heterodimeric transcription factor, and regulates expression of genes containing a 5'-ACGTG-3' hypoxia-response element (HRE) in their associated promoters or enhancers [132]. The active transcription factor consists of a hypoxia inducible HIF-1α subunit and a ubiquitously expressed HIF-1β subunit. HIF1α levels are regulated by targeted degradation by O_2, Fe^{2+}, and α-ketoglutarate-dependent prolyl hydroxylases, which have reduced activity under hypoxia, resulting in HIF1α accumulation. It is well-accepted that hypoxia is accompanied by global hypomethylation events, which have been attributed to induction of TET enzymes, direct transcriptional targets of HIF1. In N-type neuroblastoma cells, TET1 is directly bound and activated by HIF1 at the HRE within its proximal promoter, resulting in transcriptional activation and a concordant increase in 5hmC levels. Studies suggest that TET1 is specifically bound by HIF2α, and not HIF1α, and HIF1 interaction with TET1 enhances its transcriptional activity, independent of catalytic activity [133], and functions as a co-activator to regulate expression of genes involved in glucose metabolism (glucose transporter 3 (GLUT3), hexokinase 1 (HK1), phosphoglycerate kinase 2 (PGK2), pyruvate kinase M (PKM), and lactate dehydrogenase A (LDHA)). An important mediator of the Hypoxia/HIF1/TET1 gene regulation is INSIG (insulin induced gene 1), which is activated under hypoxic conditions by promoter demethylation to regulate glucose metabolism [134]. Hypoxia induced cellular proliferation and invasion, properties responsible for achieving EMT, can be abrogated by TET1 depletion, demonstrating its central role in the process [134]. In addition to TET1, TET3 (but not TET2) was also shown to be a transcriptional target of HIF1, and is induced under hypoxic conditions along with TET1 to regulate cancer phenotypes in breast cancer cells [135]. It is surprising that TET1 functions as an oncogene and is transcriptionally activated in hypoxic conditions, but is a tumor suppressor gene that is inactivated to promote tumorigenesis in other instances (myeloid malignancies). In addition to activating TET enzymes, demethylation under hypoxia is also achieved by silencing of the DNMT family of enzymes, as shown in colorectal cancer cells, which results in demethylation of the p16INK4a gene promoter [136].

3.3   Fumarate Hydratase (FH) and Succinate Dehydrogenase (SDH)

Two enzymes acting at consecutive steps in the TCA cycle, succinate dehydrogenase (SDH), and fumarate hydratase (FH), are mutated in familial paraganglioma (PGL), pheochromocytoma (PCC), uterine and skin leiomyoma, and papillary renal cell carcinoma [137]. FH and SDH are tumor suppressors, and inactivating mutations in these enzymes result in an accumulation of their substrates, fumarate and succinate, which act as oncometabolites [138]. Since fumarate and succinate are structurally similar to α-KG, they effectively inhibit α-KG dependent enzymes, including the TET family, through competitive inhibition [139]. Studies have reported a global loss of 5hmC, resulting from inhibition of TET enzymatic activity in tumors carrying FH and SDH mutations [137]. Loss of genomic 5hmC can facilitate hypermethylation events contributing to CIMP. This has been reported in paraganglioma driven by SDH mutations [140]. Additionally, fumarate and succinate function as oncometabolites by inhibiting the α-KG dependent HIF prolyl hydroxylases, which leads to increased HIF1α stabilization, creating a 'pseudohypoxic' condition, augmenting angiogenesis and anaerobic respiration [141].

4   Summary, Conclusions, and Perspectives

The epigenomic contribution to promoting cancerous events is being increasingly appreciated, and in this chapter we have covered mechanisms by which aberrant epigenetic information on DNA may occur, and its role in tumorigenesis. Two major components of the DNA methylation pathway, the writers – DNMTs and the erasers -TETs, are frequently deregulated by multiple mechanisms during tumorigenesis. A recurring theme in cancer is global genomic hypomethylation accompanied by

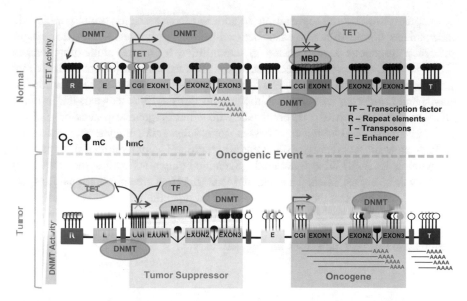

Fig. 3 Overview of how a CpG island hypermethylator phenotype is inactivates tumor suppressor genes. DNMTs in general act as oncogenes and are overexpressed/activated in tumors, whereas the TETs act as tumor suppressors and are functionally silenced or inactivated. The net outcome of these deregulation events result is CIMP, most prominently observed at promoters of TSGs. Tumors are also associated with global hypomethylation that results in demethylation of regulatory features associated with oncogenes, leading to their activation. Additionally, demethylation of repeat elements is frequently observed in cancers, resullting in spurious transcription from these elements which contibutes to genome instability

local hypermethylation events, giving rise to a 'hypermethylator phenotype' termed CIMP (Fig. 3). Since these two components are functionally antagonistic, the DNMTs are hyperactivated, while the TETs are functionally inactivated to promote CIMP in tumors. To establish tumorigenic aberrant DNA methylation patterns, the molecular components of the DNA methylation pathway are functionally intervened with somatic mutations, transcriptional regulation, mRNA stability, and protein turnover. Figure 3 gives an overview of how different genomic features undergo a switch in their DNA epigenetic marks to promote oncogenesis. This chapter addresses the pro-cancer modifications of the components directly affecting deposition (DNMTs) and erasure (TETs) of DNA methylation patterns. However, DNA methylation patterns exert their functional effects through a cascade involving other components of the chromatin-histones, nucleosomes, and larger chromosomal domains-which feedback onto DNA. This intricate cross-talk is particularly evident at the centromeric repeats, which form a part of the constitutive heterochromatin compartment silenced by DNA methylation, repressive histone modifications, specifically H3K9me3, and macromolecular repressive factors like the HP1 family. DNMT3A/3B localize to, and methylate pericentromeric repeats, and closely interact with H3K9me3 and HP1 to form a reinforcing feedback loop to ensure complete heterochromatization and structural maintenance of the centromere which is essential for preventing chromosomal aberrations like aneuploidies arising from incomplete chromosome segregation. In addition to cooperation among epigenetic mechanisms, cooperation also exists between cellular processes. Metabolic changes influence epigenetic modifications, as exemplified by tumors with mutations in IDH/FH/SDH, and local epigenetic changes influence cellular properties including proliferation, adhesion, migratory, and invasive potential, disturbing cellular homeostasis, and promoting metastasis. Although our current knowledge of the intricate DNA methylation process, its cross talk with other epigenetic processes, and the molecular impact on biological processes seems substantial, many lose ends remain. (i) How are writers and erasers preferentially recruited to, or excluded from particular genomic loci? (ii) What functional epigenetic boundaries exist at the DNA level and how these are established and maintained? (iii) How are epimutational hotspots generated, and how can these be exploited for therapeutic intervention or early cancer detection? Addressing these questions will provide additional insights into how the DNA methylation pathway is deregulated to facilitate cancer, and may lead to identification of new molecules for targeted therapy.

Glossary

CpG site Linear sequence of DNA where a cytosine is followed by guanine in the 5' to 3' direction.
CpG methylation (mCG) Cytosine within a CpG site, methylated by the DNMTs at the C5 position, represented as mCG.
Non CpG methylation (mCH) Methylation occurring outside of CpG sites, where H could be adenine, cytosine or thymine.
CpG Islands (CGI) Short interspersed sequence of DNA, around 200 base-pairs long, with high CpG fequency, and GC content greater than 50%.
CpG shores and shelves 2 kb on either side of CpG islands are termed CpG shores, and 2 kb on either side of the CGI shores are termed CGI shelves.
CpG Canyons Regions of low methylation, distinct from CGIs, and frequently associated with transcription factor binding sites.
Epimutations Non-genetic, heritable, aberrant lesions in the expression of a gene, arising from epigenetic DNA modifications or other epigenetic modifications on local chromatin.
CpG hypermethylator phenotype (CIMP) Hypermethylated CpG islands forming a diagnostic/prognostic tumor specific DNA methylation signature.

References

1. Okano M et al (1999) DNA methyltransferases Dnmt3a and Dnmt3b are essential for de novo methylation and mammalian development. Cell 99(3):247–257
2. Bai S et al (2005) DNA methyltransferase 3b regulates nerve growth factor-induced differentiation of PC12 cells by recruiting histone deacetylase 2. Mol Cell Biol 25(2):751–766

3. Challen GA et al (2012) Dnmt3a is essential for hematopoietic stem cell differentiation. Nat Genet 44(1):23–31
4. Challen GA et al (2014) Dnmt3a and Dnmt3b have overlapping and distinct functions in hematopoietic stem cells. Cell Stem Cell 15(3):350–364
5. Leonhardt H et al (1992) A targeting sequence directs DNA methyltransferase to sites of DNA replication in mammalian nuclei. Cell 71(5):865–873
6. Denis H, Ndlovu MN, Fuks F (2011) Regulation of mammalian DNA methyltransferases: a route to new mechanisms. EMBO Rep 12(7):647–656
7. Robertson KD et al (1999) The human DNA methyltransferases (DNMTs) 1, 3a and 3b: coordinate mRNA expression in normal tissues and overexpression in tumors. Nucleic Acids Res 27(11):2291–2298
8. Goyal R, Reinhardt R, Jeltsch A (2006) Accuracy of DNA methylation pattern preservation by the Dnmt1 methyltransferase. Nucleic Acids Res 34(4):1182–1188
9. Chuang LS et al (1997) Human DNA-(cytosine-5) methyltransferase-PCNA complex as a target for p21WAF1. Science 277(5334):1996–2000
10. Iida T et al (2002) PCNA clamp facilitates action of DNA cytosine methyltransferase 1 on hemimethylated DNA. Genes Cells 7(10):997–1007
11. Bostick M et al (2007) UHRF1 plays a role in maintaining DNA methylation in mammalian cells. Science 317(5845):1760–1764
12. Sharif J et al (2007) The SRA protein Np95 mediates epigenetic inheritance by recruiting Dnmt1 to methylated DNA. Nature 450(7171):908–912
13. Fatemi M, Wade PA (2006) MBD family proteins: reading the epigenetic code. J Cell Sci 119(Pt 15):3033–3037
14. Spruijt CG, Vermeulen M (2014) DNA methylation: old dog, new tricks? Nat Struct Mol Biol 21(11):949–954
15. Bogdanovic O, Veenstra GJ (2009) DNA methylation and methyl-CpG binding proteins: developmental requirements and function. Chromosoma 118(5):549–565
16. Shahbazian MD et al (2002) Insight into Rett syndrome: MeCP2 levels display tissue- and cell-specific differences and correlate with neuronal maturation. Hum Mol Genet 11(2):115–124
17. Klose RJ et al (2005) DNA binding selectivity of MeCP2 due to a requirement for A/T sequences adjacent to methyl-CpG. Mol Cell 19(5):667–678
18. Lee SU, Maeda T (2012) POK/ZBTB proteins: an emerging family of proteins that regulate lymphoid development and function. Immunol Rev 247(1):107–119
19. Prokhortchouk A et al (2001) The p120 catenin partner Kaiso is a DNA methylation-dependent transcriptional repressor. Genes Dev 15(13):1613–1618
20. Daniel JM et al (2002) The p120(ctn)-binding partner Kaiso is a bi-modal DNA-binding protein that recognizes both a sequence-specific consensus and methylated CpG dinucleotides. Nucleic Acids Res 30(13):2911–2919
21. Blattler A et al (2013) ZBTB33 binds unmethylated regions of the genome associated with actively expressed genes. Epigenetics Chromatin 6(1):13
22. Lu X, Zhao BS, He C (2015) TET family proteins: oxidation activity, interacting molecules, and functions in diseases. Chem Rev 115(6):2225–2239
23. Pastor WA, Aravind L, Rao A (2013) TETonic shift: biological roles of TET proteins in DNA demethylation and transcription. Nat Rev Mol Cell Biol 14(6):341–356
24. Duncan DS, Pennings S, Meehan RR (2013) The CXXC-TET bridge--mind the methylation gap! Cell Res 23(8):973–974
25. Tomizawa S et al (2011) Dynamic stage-specific changes in imprinted differentially methylated regions during early mammalian development and prevalence of non-CpG methylation in oocytes. Development 138(5):811–820
26. Lister R et al (2013) Global epigenomic reconfiguration during mammalian brain development. Science 341(6146):1237905
27. Ziller MJ et al (2011) Genomic distribution and inter-sample variation of non-CpG methylation across human cell types. PLoS Genet 7(12):e1002389

28. Jones PA (2012) Functions of DNA methylation: islands, start sites, gene bodies and beyond. Nat Rev Genet 13(7):484–492
29. Illingworth RS, Bird AP (2009) CpG islands—'a rough guide'. FEBS Lett 583(11):1713–1720
30. Jeong M et al (2014) Large conserved domains of low DNA methylation maintained by Dnmt3a. Nat Genet 46(1):17–23
31. Dion V et al (2008) Genome-wide demethylation promotes triplet repeat instability independently of homologous recombination. DNA Repair (Amst) 7(2):313–320
32. Choi SH et al (2011) Identification of preferential target sites for human DNA methyltransferases. Nucleic Acids Res 39(1):104–118
33. Tiedemann RL et al (2014) Acute depletion redefines the division of labor among DNA methyltransferases in methylating the human genome. Cell Rep 9(4):1554–1566
34. Liao J et al (2015) Targeted disruption of DNMT1, DNMT3A and DNMT3B in human embryonic stem cells. Nat Genet 47(5):469–478
35. Hervouet E, Vallette FM, Cartron PF (2009) Dnmt3/transcription factor interactions as crucial players in targeted DNA methylation. Epigenetics 4(7):487–499
36. Velasco G et al (2010) Dnmt3b recruitment through E2F6 transcriptional repressor mediates germ-line gene silencing in murine somatic tissues. Proc Natl Acad Sci U S A 107(20):9281–9286
37. Rose NR, Klose RJ (2014) Understanding the relationship between DNA methylation and histone lysine methylation. Biochim Biophys Acta 1839(12):1362–1372
38. Gopalakrishnan S et al (2009) DNMT3B interacts with constitutive centromere protein CENP-C to modulate DNA methylation and the histone code at centromeric regions. Hum Mol Genet 18(17):3178–3193
39. Ehrlich M (2009) DNA hypomethylation in cancer cells. Epigenomics 1(2):239–259
40. Mack SC et al (2014) Epigenomic alterations define lethal CIMP-positive ependymomas of infancy. Nature 506(7489):445–450
41. Oey H, Whitelaw E (2014) On the meaning of the word 'epimutation'. Trends Genet 30(12):519–520
42. Issa JP (2004) CpG island methylator phenotype in cancer. Nat Rev Cancer 4(12):988–993
43. Kanai Y et al (2003) Mutation of the DNA methyltransferase (DNMT) 1 gene in human colorectal cancers. Cancer Lett 192(1):75–82
44. Song J et al (2011) Structure of DNMT1-DNA complex reveals a role for autoinhibition in maintenance DNA methylation. Science 331(6020):1036–1040
45. Syeda F et al (2011) The replication focus targeting sequence (RFTS) domain is a DNA-competitive inhibitor of Dnmt1. J Biol Chem 286(17):15344–15351
46. Bashtrykov P et al (2014) Targeted mutagenesis results in an activation of DNA methyltransferase 1 and confirms an autoinhibitory role of its RFTS domain. Chembiochem 15(5):743–748
47. Tang M et al (2009) Potential of DNMT and its epigenetic regulation for lung cancer therapy. Curr Genomics 10(5):336–352
48. Fang QL et al (2015) Mechanistic and biological significance of DNA methyltransferase 1 upregulated by growth factors in human hepatocellular carcinoma. Int J Oncol 46(2):782–790
49. Mizuno S et al (2001) Expression of DNA methyltransferases DNMT1, 3A, and 3B in normal hematopoiesis and in acute and chronic myelogenous leukemia. Blood 97(5):1172–1179
50. Yang J et al (2011) Clinical significance of the expression of DNA methyltransferase proteins in gastric cancer. Mol Med Rep 4(6):1139–1143
51. Wang H et al (2011) MicroRNA-342 inhibits colorectal cancer cell proliferation and invasion by directly targeting DNA methyltransferase 1. Carcinogenesis 32(7):1033–1042
52. Agoston AT et al (2005) Increased protein stability causes DNA methyltransferase 1 dysregulation in breast cancer. J Biol Chem 280(18):18302–18310
53. Shaulian E, Karin M (2002) AP-1 as a regulator of cell life and death. Nat Cell Biol 4(5):E131–E136
54. Rouleau J, MacLeod AR, Szyf M (1995) Regulation of the DNA methyltransferase by the Ras-AP-1 signaling pathway. J Biol Chem 270(4):1595–1601

55. Bakin AV, Curran T (1999) Role of DNA 5-methylcytosine transferase in cell transformation by fos. Science 283(5400):387–390
56. Campbell PM, Szyf M (2003) Human DNA methyltransferase gene DNMT1 is regulated by the APC pathway. Carcinogenesis 24(1):17–24
57. Lin RK et al (2010) Dysregulation of p53/Sp1 control leads to DNA methyltransferase-1 overexpression in lung cancer. Cancer Res 70(14):5807–5817
58. McCabe MT, Davis JN, Day ML (2005) Regulation of DNA methyltransferase 1 by the pRb/E2F1 pathway. Cancer Res 65(9):3624–3632
59. Torrisani J et al (2007) AUF1 cell cycle variations define genomic DNA methylation by regulation of DNMT1 mRNA stability. Mol Cell Biol 27(1):395–410
60. Sun L et al (2007) Phosphatidylinositol 3-kinase/protein kinase B pathway stabilizes DNA methyltransferase I protein and maintains DNA methylation. Cell Signal 19(11):2255–2263
61. Qin W, Leonhardt H, Spada F (2011) Usp7 and Uhrf1 control ubiquitination and stability of the maintenance DNA methyltransferase Dnmt1. J Cell Biochem 112(2):439–444
62. Bashtrykov P et al (2014) The UHRF1 protein stimulates the activity and specificity of the maintenance DNA methyltransferase DNMT1 by an allosteric mechanism. J Biol Chem 289(7):4106–4115
63. Pacaud R et al (2014) The DNMT1/PCNA/UHRF1 disruption induces tumorigenesis characterized by similar genetic and epigenetic signatures. Sci Rep 4:4230
64. Hervouet E et al (2010) Disruption of Dnmt1/PCNA/UHRF1 interactions promotes tumorigenesis from human and mice glial cells. PLoS One 5(6):e11333
65. Ley TJ et al (2010) DNMT3A mutations in acute myeloid leukemia. N Engl J Med 363(25):2424–2433
66. Russler-Germain DA et al (2014) The R882H DNMT3A mutation associated with AML dominantly inhibits wild-type DNMT3A by blocking its ability to form active tetramers. Cancer Cell 25(4):442–454
67. Jia D et al (2007) Structure of Dnmt3a bound to Dnmt3L suggests a model for de novo DNA methylation. Nature 449(7159):248–251
68. Jurkowska RZ et al (2008) Formation of nucleoprotein filaments by mammalian DNA methyltransferase Dnmt3a in complex with regulator Dnmt3L. Nucleic Acids Res 36(21):6656–6663
69. Gowher H et al (2006) Mutational analysis of the catalytic domain of the murine Dnmt3a DNA-(cytosine C5)-methyltransferase. J Mol Biol 357(3):928–941
70. Li BZ et al (2011) Histone tails regulate DNA methylation by allosterically activating de novo methyltransferase. Cell Res 21(8):1172–1181
71. Yang L, Rau R, Goodell MA (2015) DNMT3A in haematological malignancies. Nat Rev Cancer 15(3):152–165
72. Lin CC et al (2014) IDH mutations are closely associated with mutations of DNMT3A, ASXL1 and SRSF2 in patients with myelodysplastic syndromes and are stable during disease evolution. Am J Hematol 89(2):137–144
73. Jia Y et al (2016) Negative regulation of DNMT3A de novo DNA methylation by frequently overexpressed UHRF family proteins as a mechanism for widespread DNA hypomethylation in cancer. Cell Discov 2:16007
74. Tang YA et al (2012) MDM2 overexpression deregulates the transcriptional control of RB/E2F leading to DNA methyltransferase 3A overexpression in lung cancer. Clin Cancer Res Off J Am Assoc Cancer Res 18(16):4325–4333
75. Gao Q et al (2011) Deletion of the de novo DNA methyltransferase Dnmt3a promotes lung tumor progression. Proc Natl Acad Sci U S A 108(44):18061–18066
76. Wang L et al (2004) Functional relevance of C46359T in the promoter region of human DNMT3B6. Cancer Res 64(7 Supplement):672–672
77. Shen H et al (2002) A novel polymorphism in human cytosine DNA-methyltransferase-3B promoter is associated with an increased risk of lung cancer. Cancer Res 62(17):4992–4995
78. Liu Z et al (2008) Polymorphisms of the DNMT3B gene and risk of squamous cell carcinoma of the head and neck: a case-control study. Cancer Lett 268(1):158–165

79. Jones JS et al (2006) DNMT3b polymorphism and hereditary nonpolyposis colorectal cancer age of onset. Cancer Epidemiol Biomark Prev 15(5):886–891
80. Montgomery KG et al (2004) The DNMT3B C-->T promoter polymorphism and risk of breast cancer in a British population: a case-control study. Breast Cancer Res 6(4):R390–R394
81. Zhu S et al (2012) DNMT3B polymorphisms and cancer risk: a meta analysis of 24 case-control studies. Mol Biol Rep 39(4):4429–4437
82. Xia Z et al (2015) Quantitative assessment of the association between DNMT3B-579G>T polymorphism and cancer risk. Cancer Biomark 15(5):707–716
83. Wang L et al (2006) A novel DNMT3B subfamily, DeltaDNMT3B, is the predominant form of DNMT3B in non-small cell lung cancer. Int J Oncol 29(1):201–207
84. Wang J et al (2006) Expression of Delta DNMT3B variants and its association with promoter methylation of p16 and RASSF1A in primary non-small cell lung cancer. Cancer Res 66(17):8361–8366
85. Gordon CA, Hartono SR, Chedin F (2013) Inactive DNMT3B splice variants modulate de novo DNA methylation. PLoS One 8(7):e69486
86. Ostler KR et al (2007) Cancer cells express aberrant DNMT3B transcripts encoding truncated proteins. Oncogene 26(38):5553–5563
87. Brambert PR et al (2015) DNMT3B7 expression promotes tumor progression to a more aggressive phenotype in breast cancer cells. PLoS One 10(1):e0117310
88. Saito Y et al (2002) Overexpression of a splice variant of DNA methyltransferase 3b, DNMT3b4, associated with DNA hypomethylation on pericentromeric satellite regions during human hepatocarcinogenesis. Proc Natl Acad Sci U S A 99(15):10060–10065
89. Roll JD et al (2008) DNMT3b overexpression contributes to a hypermethylator phenotype in human breast cancer cell lines. Mol Cancer 7:15
90. Yang YC et al (2014) DNMT3B overexpression by deregulation of FOXO3a-mediated transcription repression and MDM2 overexpression in lung cancer. J Thorac Oncol 9(9):1305–1315
91. Suetake I et al (2004) DNMT3L stimulates the DNA methylation activity of Dnmt3a and Dnmt3b through a direct interaction. J Biol Chem 279(26):27816–27823
92. Holz-Schietinger C, Reich NO (2010) The inherent processivity of the human de novo methyltransferase 3A (DNMT3A) is enhanced by DNMT3L. J Biol Chem 285(38):29091–29100
93. Chedin F, Lieber MR, Hsieh CL (2002) The DNA methyltransferase-like protein DNMT3L stimulates de novo methylation by Dnmt3a. Proc Natl Acad Sci U S A 99(26):16916–16921
94. Van Emburgh BO, Robertson KD (2011) Modulation of Dnmt3b function in vitro by interactions with Dnmt3L, Dnmt3a and Dnmt3b splice variants. Nucleic Acids Res 39(12):4984–5002
95. Pacaud R et al (2014) DNMT3L interacts with transcription factors to target DNMT3L/DNMT3B to specific DNA sequences: role of the DNMT3L/DNMT3B/p65-NFkappaB complex in the (de-)methylation of TRAF1. Biochimie 104:36–49
96. Minami K et al (2010) DNMT3L is a novel marker and is essential for the growth of human embryonal carcinoma. Clin Cancer Res 16(10):2751–2759
97. Gokul G et al (2007) DNA methylation profile at the DNMT3L promoter: a potential biomarker for cervical cancer. Epigenetics 2(2):80–85
98. Manderwad GP et al (2010) Hypomethylation of the DNMT3L promoter in ocular surface squamous neoplasia. Arch Pathol Lab Med 134(8):1193–1196
99. Kim H et al (2010) DNA methyltransferase 3-like affects promoter methylation of thymine DNA glycosylase independently of DNMT1 and DNMT3B in cancer cells. Int J Oncol 36(6):1563–1572
100. Neri F et al (2015) TET1 is controlled by pluripotency-associated factors in ESCs and down-modulated by PRC2 in differentiated cells and tissues. Nucleic Acids Res 43(14):6814–6826
101. Jin C et al (2014) TET1 is a maintenance DNA demethylase that prevents methylation spreading in differentiated cells. Nucleic Acids Res 42(11):6956–6971
102. Cimmino L et al (2015) TET1 is a tumor suppressor of hematopoietic malignancy. Nat Immunol 16(6):653–662

103. Sun M et al (2013) HMGA2/TET1/HOXA9 signaling pathway regulates breast cancer growth and metastasis. Proc Natl Acad Sci U S A 110(24):9920–9925
104. Neri F et al (2015) TET1 is a tumour suppressor that inhibits colon cancer growth by derepressing inhibitors of the WNT pathway. Oncogene 34(32):4168–4176
105. Ichimura N et al (2015) Aberrant TET1 methylation closely associated with CpG island methylator phenotype in colorectal cancer. Cancer Prev Res (Phila) 8(8):702–711
106. Hsu CH et al (2012) TET1 suppresses cancer invasion by activating the tissue inhibitors of metalloproteinases. Cell Rep 2(3):568–579
107. Lu HG et al (2014) TET1 partially mediates HDAC inhibitor-induced suppression of breast cancer invasion. Mol Med Rep 10(5):2595–2600
108. Wu BK, Brenner C (2014) Suppression of TET1-dependent DNA demethylation is essential for KRAS-mediated transformation. Cell Rep 9(5):1827–1840
109. Jankowska AM et al (2009) Loss of heterozygosity 4q24 and TET2 mutations associated with myelodysplastic/myeloproliferative neoplasms. Blood 113(25):6403–6410
110. Delhommeau F et al (2009) Mutation in TET2 in myeloid cancers. N Engl J Med 360(22):2289–2301
111. Moran-Crusio K et al (2011) Tet2 loss leads to increased hematopoietic stem cell self-renewal and myeloid transformation. Cancer Cell 20(1):11–24
112. Ko M et al (2011) Ten-eleven-translocation 2 (TET2) negatively regulates homeostasis and differentiation of hematopoietic stem cells in mice. Proc Natl Acad Sci U S A 108(35):14566–14571
113. Zhao Z et al (2016) The catalytic activity of TET2 is essential for its myeloid malignancy-suppressive function in hematopoietic stem/progenitor cells. Leukemia 30(8):1784–1788
114. Busque L et al (2012) Recurrent somatic TET2 mutations in normal elderly individuals with clonal hematopoiesis. Nat Genet 44(11):1179–1181
115. Muto T et al (2013) Concurrent loss of Ezh2 and Tet2 cooperates in the pathogenesis of myelodysplastic disorders. J Exp Med 210(12):2627–2639
116. Abdel-Wahab O et al (2013) Deletion of Asxl1 results in myelodysplasia and severe developmental defects in vivo. J Exp Med 210(12):2641–2659
117. Sakata-Yanagimoto M et al (2014) Somatic RHOA mutation in angioimmunoblastic T cell lymphoma. Nat Genet 46(2):171–175
118. Couronne L, Bastard C, Bernard OA (2012) TET2 and DNMT3A mutations in human T-cell lymphoma. N Engl J Med 366(1):95–96
119. Wang C et al (2015) IDH2R172 mutations define a unique subgroup of patients with angio-immunoblastic T-cell lymphoma. Blood 126(15):1741–1752
120. Ko M et al (2013) Modulation of TET2 expression and 5-methylcytosine oxidation by the CXXC domain protein IDAX. Nature 497(7447):122–126
121. Wang Y, Zhang Y (2014) Regulation of TET protein stability by calpains. Cell Rep 6(2):278–284
122. Lakshmikuttyamma A et al (2004) Overexpression of m-calpain in human colorectal adenocarcinomas. Cancer Epidemiol Biomark Prev 13(10):1604–1609
123. Wang Y et al (2015) WT1 recruits TET2 to regulate its target gene expression and suppress leukemia cell proliferation. Mol Cell 57(4):662–673
124. Cui Q et al (2016) Downregulation of TLX induces TET3 expression and inhibits glioblastoma stem cell self-renewal and tumorigenesis. Nat Commun 7:10637
125. Ye Z et al (2016) TET3 inhibits TGF-beta1-induced epithelial-mesenchymal transition by demethylating miR-30d precursor gene in ovarian cancer cells. J Exp Clin Cancer Res 35(1):72
126. Dang L, Yen K, Attar EC (2016) IDH mutations in cancer and progress toward development of targeted therapeutics. Ann Oncol 27(4):599–608
127. Losman JA, Kaelin WG Jr (2013) What a difference a hydroxyl makes: mutant IDH, (R)-2-hydroxyglutarate, and cancer. Genes Dev 27(8):836–852
128. Duncan CG et al (2012) A heterozygous IDH1R132H/WT mutation induces genome-wide alterations in DNA methylation. Genome Res 22(12):2339–2355

129. Turcan S et al (2012) IDH1 mutation is sufficient to establish the glioma hypermethylator phenotype. Nature 483(7390):479–483
130. Flavahan WA et al (2016) Insulator dysfunction and oncogene activation in IDH mutant gliomas. Nature 529(7584):110–114
131. Guilhamon P et al (2013) Meta-analysis of IDH-mutant cancers identifies EBF1 as an interaction partner for TET2. Nat Commun 4:2166
132. Fukasawa M et al (2004) Identification and characterization of the hypoxia-responsive element of the human placental 6-phosphofructo-2-kinase/fructose-2,6-bisphosphatase gene. J Biochem 136(3):273–277
133. Mariani CJ et al (2014) TET1-mediated hydroxymethylation facilitates hypoxic gene induction in neuroblastoma. Cell Rep 7(5):1343–1352
134. Tsai YP et al (2014) TET1 regulates hypoxia-induced epithelial-mesenchymal transition by acting as a co-activator. Genome Biol 15(12):513
135. Wu MZ et al (2015) Hypoxia drives breast tumor malignancy through a TET-TNFalpha-p38-MAPK signaling axis. Cancer Res 75(18):3912–3924
136. Skowronski K et al (2010) Ischemia dysregulates DNA methyltransferases and p16INK4a methylation in human colorectal cancer cells. Epigenetics 5(6):547–556
137. Hoekstra AS et al (2015) Inactivation of SDH and FH cause loss of 5hmC and increased H3K9me3 in paraganglioma/pheochromocytoma and smooth muscle tumors. Oncotarget 6(36):38777–38788
138. Yang M, Soga T, Pollard PJ (2013) Oncometabolites: linking altered metabolism with cancer. J Clin Invest 123(9):3652–3658
139. Laukka T et al (2016) Fumarate and succinate regulate expression of hypoxia-inducible genes via TET enzymes. J Biol Chem 291(8):4256–4265
140. Letouze E et al (2013) SDH mutations establish a hypermethylator phenotype in paraganglioma. Cancer Cell 23(6):739–752
141. MacKenzie ED et al (2007) Cell-permeating alpha-ketoglutarate derivatives alleviate pseudohypoxia in succinate dehydrogenase-deficient cells. Mol Cell Biol 27(9):3282–3289

Part II
Histone Methylation and Cancer

The Molecular Basis of Histone Methylation

Lidong Sun and Jia Fang

Abstract As an integrated part of the complex array of post-translational modifications on histone, methylation mainly occurs on histone lysine and arginine residues and plays pivotal roles in the regulation of chromatin organization and function. Histone methylation is catalyzed by different groups of methyltransferases while methylation marks on different residues as well as different methylation states on the same residue serve as docking sites to recruit a variety of binding proteins harboring specific recognition domains. These methyl-histone binding proteins further recruit additional chromatin modifiers and other proteins to transduce methylation signals into diverse functional outcomes. Here we summarize histone methyltransferases and discuss their specificities and regulations for different methylation reactions. We also discuss specific methyl-histone recognition by different families of binding proteins at multiple molecular layers. Given that the disruption of histone methylation and recognition has been associated with altered gene function in various diseases and human malignancy, understanding the regulation of histone methylation and recognition will also provide molecular basics for therapeutics.

Keywords Epigenetics • Chromatin • Histone methylation • Histone methyltransferase • Methyl-histone binding domain • Structure and function

1 Introduction

In eukaryotes, about 147 bp DNA wraps around a histone octamer (assembled from H3-H4 tetramer and two H2A-H2B dimers) to form the nucleosome core-particle. This structure is stabilized by histone H1 and can be further folded into higher-order chromatin structures [1]. It has been demonstrated that histone molecules are subject to diverse modifications, including methylation, acetylation, phosphorylation, ubiquitination and many others, which constitute a unique "code" for the regulation

L. Sun • J. Fang (✉)
Department of Tumor Biology, H. Lee Moffitt Cancer Center and Research Institute,
MRC-4072H, 12902 Magnolia Drive, Tampa, FL 33612, USA
e-mail: Lidong.Sun@moffitt.org; Jia.Fang@moffitt.org

© Springer International Publishing AG 2017   127
A. Kaneda, Y.-i. Tsukada (eds.), *DNA and Histone Methylation as Cancer Targets*,
Cancer Drug Discovery and Development, DOI 10.1007/978-3-319-59786-7_6

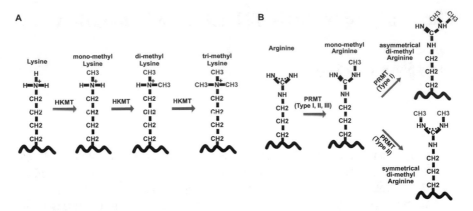

Fig. 1 Lysine and arginine methylation. (**a**) Catalyzed by different histone KMTs, lysine residues can be mono-, di-, and tri-methylated. (**b**) Arginine residue in histones can be mono-methylated by type I, II, III PRMTs. Type I and II PRMTs can further introduce asymmetric and symmetric di-methylation, respectively

of chromatin function and dynamics [2, 3]. Histone methylation was discovered in 1964 [4, 5], however, its regulation and functional significance were revealed in the past 15 years. Through reactions catalyzed by different families of enzymes, histone lysine residues can be mono-, di- or tri-methylated [6] whereas arginines can be mono- or di-methylated (symmetrically or asymmetrically) [7] (Fig. 1). While most methylation occurs on the flexible histone N-terminal tails, several methylations were also detected within the globular domain. It has been well-documented that histone methylation at different residues as well as different methylation states within the same residue can confer a variety of biological functions. Table 1 summarized validated histone methylation sites together with their catalyzing enzymes and the functional outcomes. In this Chapter, we discuss several major histone methyltransferases (HMTases) and molecular mechanisms underlying methylation reactions. In most cases, the addition of methyl groups to histones does not directly affect chromatin structure. It is believed that diverse functions of different histone methylations are mediated through binding proteins harboring specific motifs. Therefore, we also discuss different methyl-histone binding domains and their recognition mechanisms.

2 Histone Methyltransferase

Methylation is one of the most common protein modifications on multiple amino acids, which is catalyzed by protein methyltransferases (MTases) using S-Adenosyl methionine (SAM) as the cofactor and methyl-donor [65]. Histone methylation main occurs on lysine and arginine residues, although glutamine (H2AQ104) methylation has been recently reported which is catalyzed by a nucleolus specific rRNA 2'-O-methyltransferase [66]. Histone lysine and arginine methylations are catalyzed

Table 1 Methylated sites on histone

Modification	Enzyme	Function
Histone H3		
H3R2me2a	PRMT6 [8–10], PRMT4 [11]	Transcription repression
H3R2me2s	PRMT5 [12], PRMT7 [12]	Euchromatin maintenance
H3K4me	MLL1-MLL4, hSET1A(SETD1A) [13], SETD1B [14], SETD7 [15], SETMAR [16], PRDM7 [17], PRDM9 [18, 19], SMYD1 [20], SMYD2, SMYD3 [21, 22]	Transcription activation
H3R8me2a	PRMT2 [23]	Poised chromatin architecture
H3R8me2s	PRMT5 [24],	Gene inactivation
H3K9me	SUV39H1 [25], SUV39H2 [26], GLP [27], G9A [28], SETDB1[29], SETDB2 [30], RIZ1(PRDM2) [31], PRDM3 [32], PRDM16 [32], PRDM8 [33]	Heterochromatin, gene silencing
H3R17me2a	PRMT4 [11, 34]	Transcription activation
H3R26me2a	PRMT4 [11]	Transcription activation
H3K27me	EZH1,EZH2,G9A [35]	Gene silence
H3K36me	NSD1 [36], NSD2(MMSET) [37, 38], NDS3 [39], SMYD2 [40], SETD2 [41], SETD3 [42, 43], ASH1L [44, 45], SETMAR [16], PRDM9 [46]	Transcription elongation, DNA damage repair
H3K56me1	G9A [47]	DNA replication
H3R42me2a	PRMT4 [48], PRMT6 [48]	Promote transcription in vitro
H3K79me	DOT1L [49, 50]	Gene activation
Histone H4		
H4R3me2a	PRMT1 [51],PRMT6 [9]	Gene activation
H4R3me2s	PRMT5 [24],	Gene inactivation
H4R3me	PRMT7 [52]	Gene inactivation
H4K5me	SMYD3 [22]	Unknown
H4R17me	PRMT7 [53, 54]	Unknown
H4R19me	PRMT7 [53, 54]	Unknown
H4K20me	SUV420H1/2 [55], SETD8 [56, 57], SMYD3 [58]	Cell cycle regulation, gene silencing, DNA damage repair
Histone H2A		
H2AR3me2a	PRMT6 [9]	Unknown
H2AR3me2s	PRMT5 [59]	Gene repression
H2AR3me2	PRMT7 [52]	Gene repression
H2AR11me1	PRMT1 PRMT6 [60]	Unknown
H2AR29me2a	PRMT6 [60]	Transcriptional repression
H2AZ-K7	SETD6 [61]	Cell differentiation
Histone H2B		
H2BR29me1	PRMT7 [54]	Unknown
H2BR31me1	PRMT7 [54]	Unknown
H2BR33me1	PRMT7 [54]	Unknown
H2BK120me	EZH2 [62]	Inhibiting H2BK120ub

(continued)

Table 1 (continued)

Modification	Enzyme	Function
Histone H1		
H1K26me	EZH2 [63]	Gene silencing
H1.2K187me1	GLP/G9A [64]	Unknown

by two major types of MTases, lysine methyltransferase (KMT) and protein argi-nine methyltransferase (PRMT). While most KMTs catalyze methyl transfer mainly onto histones, PRMTs methylate histones and a wide range of non-histone sub-strates. These two types of enzymes share little similarity in primary and tertiary structures and reaction mechanisms which are discussed separately in different categories.

2.1 Lysine Methyltransferases (KMTs)

SUV39H1 is the first characterized de novo histone KMT, containing a conserved catalytic motif (~120aa) which was initially identified in three drosophila proteins, Suppressor of variegation [Su(var)3–9], Enhancer of zeste [E(z)]and Trithorax (Trx) [67] and thereafter named as the SET domain [25]. While sequence alignment identi-fied ~50 SET domain-containing proteins in human genome [68], many of them have been shown to possess histone KMT activities. Among the characterized KMTs, human DOT1-like (DOT1L) does not harbor a SET domain but processes the robust catalytic activity [49]. SET domain often localizes in the C-terminus of histone KMTs while this bifurcated motif can be divided into the conserved SET-N, SET-C and a highly variable insertion (SET-I) in the middle. These enzymes also harbor dif-ferent sets of other domains and can be briefly classified into seven families, includ-ing SUV39, SET1, SET2, EZH, SMYD, PRDM, SUV420 and others (Fig. 2).

The SET domain of SUV39 family KMTs are encompassed by two conserved cysteine-rich pre-SET and post-SET domains. These KMTs mainly catalyze H3K9 methylation with the exception of SETMAR which methylates H3K4 and H3K36 [16]. The SET1 and SET2 families KMTs comprise different groups of large enzymes which specifically methylate H3K4 and H3K36 respectively. The SET1 family KMTs lack the pre-SET domain and their enzymatic activities require the formation of complexes with other proteins including RBBP5 and ASH2L [69]. In contrast, the pre-SET domain is replaced by a AWS (Associated with SET) domain in the SET2 family KMTs. This unique AWS-SET-postSET configuration is believed to confer the specific methyl transfer onto H3K36 [42]. In the EZH family KMTs, both pre-SET and post-SET domains are absent. However, these enzymes harbor a conserved CXC domain which is located upstream of the SET domain and is critical for their activity. EZH1/2 also have no detectable activity unless they form the

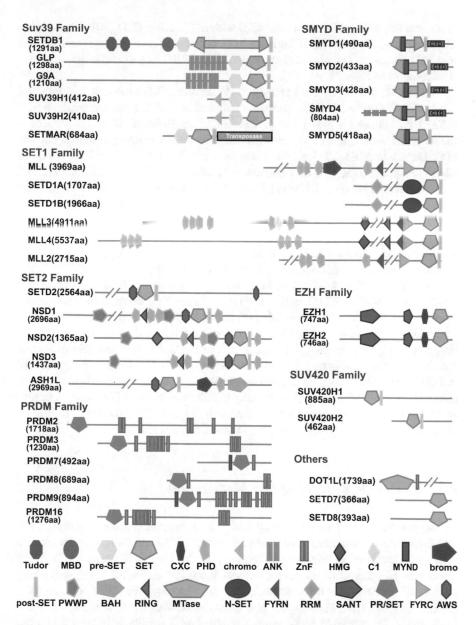

Fig. 2 Human histone lysine methyltransferases. 35 active human histone lysine methyltransferases (KMTs) are grouped into eight families according to their domain organization

Polycomb Repressive Complex 2 (PRC2) with SUZ12 and EED [70]. Unlike other KMT families, the SUV420H family KMTs only contain the conserved SET and post-SET domains but no other domains. SUV420H1/H2 are able to introduce H4K20me2/3 to H4K20me1 [55].

The SET domain in the SMYD and PRDM families KMTs has unique configurations. SMYD family of KMTs contain a long interposed sequence composed by a MYND domain and a SET-I motif. The MYND domain of SMYD1/2 has been shown to interact with the proline-rich motif in their binding partners while the MYND domain of SMYD3 is believed to bind to DNA [71]. The SMYD family of KMTs also contain the post-SET domain and a conserved C-terminal domain (CTD) with unknown function. Different from other KMT families, SMYDs display diverse substrate specificity [40, 58]. The PRDM family of KMTs harbor a catalytic PR/SET domain which only shares 20% similarity with the SET domain in sequence but displays a similar tertiary structure. Most PRDMs contain multiple zinc-fingers while some also have a zinc knuckle motif. The human PRDM family has 17 members in which six have histone KMT activities [31–33, 46].

Other human KMTs do not fit into above categories are SETD7, SETD8 and DOT1L. SETD7 and SETD8 only contain the catalytic SET domain and specifically mediate mono-methylation on H3K4 [72] and H4K20 [73] respectively. DOT1L is a non-SET domain-containing KMT which specifically catalyzes H3K79 methylation. The catalytic domain of DOT1L is similar to the catalytic domain of PRMT which utilizes a Rossmann fold for SAM binding [74, 75]. Furthermore, in vitro methylation catalyzed by DOT1L is a non-processive reaction whereas the reaction mediated by most SET domain-containing KMTs is processive [76]. Although several other proteins have also been reported to possess KMT activities [77, 78], the molecular details underlying these reactions still remain elusive.

2.2   Molecular Basis of Lysine Methylation

The representative SET domains of all KMT family members have been crystalized and their tertiary structures reveal several common features which are critical to confer efficient methyl transfer reaction [79]. Overall the SET domain is a highly interwined globular structure with extensive intra-domain interactions, suggesting each motif is critical for the structural integrity. The conserved SET-N and SET-C motifs form three beta-sheets and two beta-sheets with a pseudo-knot structure respectively. The variable SET-I motif also displays a similar structural fold, containing two anti-parallel β-strands and a short α-helix. Together with SET-C, SET-I motif is directly involved in substrate and SAM bindings and thus contributes to the substrate specificity [79]. Furthermore, zinc-chelating was observed in several structures. For example, the pre-SET domain of SUV39H family chelates three zinc ions [80, 81] and the AWS domain of SET2 family chelates two [36, 44], whereas the Zinc-Knuckle domain of PRDM9 chelate one zinc ion [82] and the CXC domain of EZH2 binds to six [70]. These domains do not contact substrate but pack against the SET domain to facilitate its structure stability and enzymatic activity [79]. Zinc-chelating was missing in SU420H1, SETD7 and SETD8 structures, however, a α-helix bundle, a beta-sheet and a long alpha-helix were observed respectively [72, 73, 83], suggesting that they may exert the similar function without zinc binding. Additionally, three cysteines in the post-SET domain of many KMTs chelate one zinc ion together with a conserved cysteine in the SET-C motif and this structure is also critical for the enzymatic activity [84]. Without zinc- chelating, the C-terminal sequences of the SET domain in SETD7 [72] and SETD8 [73] also form the similar structural fold for substrate and SAM binding.

Furthermore, the SET domain interacts with histone substrate and SAM through opposite surfaces. While SAM fits into an open concave pocket, histone peptide exhibits an extended conformation and extensively interactions with the binding groove. In this way, the target lysine is precisely positioned and its side chain can go through a narrow channel to meet with SAM [79, 85]. Different SET domains form different interactions with the backbone of their substrates to specifically define the methylation site. For instance, DIM-5, a neurospora SUV39 family KMT methylates H3K9 (QARK$_9$ST) but not H3K27 (AARK$_{27}$SA) due to its specific interaction with the side chain of T11 [81]. Moreover, the alkyl component of the lysine side-chain inhibits a hydrophobic environment while the ε-Nitrogen is stabilized by hydrogen bonds with surrounding carbonyl groups and hydroxyl-group [85]. In SETD7 structure, one ε-nitrogen on the side chain of H3K4 forms a hydrogen bond with a conserved Y245 and another with a tightly bound water molecule to prohibit the rotation of the εC-N bond for additional methylation. Accordingly, Y245A mutation enables SETD7 to catalyze H3K4me2/3 [72]. Mutation of another the target lysine binding tyrosine (Y305F) also results in H3K4me2 [84]. While the same Y-to-F mutation in SETD8 [73], MLL [86], G9A [70, 71] leads to similar effects on methylation, the F281Y mutation in DIM-5 disables the catalyzed H3K9me3 [84]. Intriguingly, the ε-N on the target lysine side chain forms a critical hydrogen-bond with S161 in the SET domain of mouse Suv420h2, which makes the enzyme inefficient for trimethylation [83, 87]. Disabling this hydrogen-bond by S161A mutation greatly increases H4K20me3 [83]. Together, the substrate specificity of KMTs is determined by extensive substrate-SET domain interactions whereas the methylation states rely on the accommodation of the ammonium group on the target lysine side chain in the structure.

SMYD proteins share a conserved bilobal structure in which the catalytic core is located in the middle of the N-terminal lobe with the MYND domain and CTD around. While the MYND domain is dispensable for methylation, the SET and post-SET domains form a surface pocket for cofactor binding and a deep pocket of the interface between the SET domain and CTD binds to substrate [71]. Although the overall structures are similar, SMYD1-3 display substantial differences in the size and surrounding structure of the substrate binding pocket, which could be responsible for divergent specificities on substrate and methylation states [88]. In the PRDM family KMTs, the SET domain signature motifs are poorly conserved. However, the overall structure of the PR/SET domain corresponds to the SET domains, in which the central SET domain fold is flanked by pre-SET and post-SET regions. The bindings of cofactor and substrate peptide to the PR/SET domain of Prdm9 are also similar to the SET domains [82]. These findings suggest that the structural similarity to the SET domain confers the lysine methylation activity of both SMYD and PR/SET domains. In contrast, the catalytic domain of DOT1L forms an open α/β structure which is comprised of a seven-stranded β sheet. This structure is distinct from the SET, SMYD or PR/SET domain but similar to several class I SAM-dependent MTases [89]. The active core of DOT1L has an elongated structure, containing a SAM binding pocket and a lysine binding channel. While the SAM binding pocket is critical for methylation, the lysine binding channel allows the accommodation of all three methylation states. The positive charged C-terminal region of the catalytic domain is also critical for the enzymatic activity, likely through binding to negatively charged nucleosomal DNA [75]. Despite of the structure similarity between DOT1L and PRMTs, arginine methylation by DOT1L was not detected.

2.3 Protein Arginine Methyltransferase

Human genome harbors eleven protein arginine methyltransferases (PRMTs), eight of them are able to methylate different histones. Based on methylation products, PRMTs are classified into four different types [7]. Type I enzymes, including PRMT1, 3, 4, 6 and 8 introduce monomethylation on arginine and further proceed to asymmetrical di-methylation (aDMA). PRMT5, 7 and 9 are type II PRMTs which generate the symmetrical dimethylated products (sDMA) after the initial monomethylation. Type III enzymes only catalyze monomethylation but do not proceed. Different from methylation on the terminal guanidine nitrogen atoms catalyzed by above PRMTs, Type IV PRMTs introduce monomethylation of δ-nitrogen. Most PRMTs catalyze aDMA on arginine, which is likely attributed to the higher energetically challenging with sDMA [90]. The characterized PRMTs and their function are also summarized in Table 1.

2.4 Molecular Basis of Arginine Methylation

Different from the SET domain, the conserved 310-aa catalytic core of PRMTs shares a similar structure with a Rossmann-fold domain and a C-terminal β-barrel domain and functions in a homo-dimer [91]. The methylation occurs at the interface of the catalytic core where SAM is accommodated in the Rossmann-fold, whereas the substrate peptide binds to an acidic groove with the side chain of target arginine inserted into a narrow tunnel to meet SAM [92]. Two notable structures were observed at the interface, a double-E loop from the Rossmann fold and a THW loop from the beta-barrel, which are important for methylation. It has been shown that E181D mutation in the double-E loop of Trypanosoma brucei PRMT7 converts this type III enzyme to a type I enzyme to catalyze asymmetric dimethylarginine (aDMA) [93]. Another critical motif for the SAM and target arginine binding is in the N-terminal helix of Rossmann-fold. F379M mutation in this motif of *C. elegans* PRMT5 partially shifts the reaction towards aDMA. This mutation likely opens up the active site to allow more bulky asymmetrical di-methyl groups [94]. To corroborate the importance of this residue, M48F mutation of rat PRMT1 enables its ability to catalyze symmetrical di-methylation [90], suggesting the Phe or Met residue in the N-terminal helix of Rossmann-fold could define the type of the methylation. However, type II PRMT9 contains a Met at the exact is position. Therefore, this proposed F/M switch could only be the part of the underlying mechanism [91]. In general, the size of the target arginine binding pocket significantly affects the product specificity catalyzed by different PRMTs.

3   Regulation of Histone Methylation

The enzymatic activity of HMTs is often evaluated in an in vitro assay in which the enzyme is incubated with SAM and substrate to catalyze methylation. In this reaction, several HMTases, including EZH2 and MLL failed to show robust activity unless their core protein complexes were used [95, 96]. Different substrates have also been used in this assay, including histone peptides, recombinant histones, histone octamers and nucleosomes [56]. While several KMTs prefer nucleosomes, such as SETD8 [56], SUV420H1/2 [55] and DOT1L [49], many enzymes predominantly methylate recombinant histones or octamers, such as SETD7 [15], G9A and GLP [97]. These observations suggest that the intact catalytic domain is necessary but not sufficient for histone methylation. Therefore, we discuss several regulatory mechanisms at different molecular layers.

3.1   Regulation by Interacting Proteins

The structure of EZH2 SET domain uncovers an inappropriate position of the SET-I and post-SET domains, which prohibits their interactions with substrate peptide and SAM [98, 99]. Recently, the crystal structures of PRC2 reveal that the extensive protein interactions with EED and SUZ12 optimize the structure of EZH2's SET-I to form an active catalytic moiety for H3K27 methylation [70]. In the SET domain of MLL, the SET-I motif is highly dynamic. After forming the protein complex with the RBP5-ASH2L heterodimer, extensive protein interactions significantly reduce this inherent flexibility and lock the SET domain in an active conformation to enable efficient methyl transfer [69]. Intriguingly, the intermolecular β-sheet interactions between MLL SET-I and RBBP5(330–344aa) was also observed in the structure of other KMTs. In SUV39 and SET2 family KMTs, the similar interactions are formed intramolecularly between the SET-I and a short fragment upstream of the pre-SET domain. This fragment also exists in EZH2 and functions as SET activation loop (SAL) [70], suggesting it is a conserved structural configuration for the functional SET domain. Together, these novel advances in structure demonstrate that the inherent imperfection of certain SET domains can be corrected through interactions with their binding partners.

Furthermore, interacting proteins can regulate HMTases' activity through different mechanisms. In the in vitro assays, PRMT5 equally catalyzes symmetrical methylation on both H3R8 and H4R3. However, it preferentially methylates H4R3 after binding to COPR5 [100], suggesting this regulatory protein fine-tunes PRMT5's substrate specificity. HSP90α, the binding partner of SMYD2 stimulates methylation on H3K4 but not H3K36 [101]. Similarly, the substrate specificity of EZH2 on either H1K26 or H3K27 is modulated by a PRC2 core component EED [63]. A Polycomb-like protein PHF1 also facilitates PRC2-mediated H3K27me3 without affecting H3K27me1/2 [102, 103]. Additionally, SETDB1's binding partner ATF7IP/AM, an ATFα-associated factor not only augments SETDB1's enzymatic activity, but also facilitates the conversion of H3K9me2 to H3K9me3 in vitro and in vivo [104]. However, the similar effects were not observed when peptide substrates were used in the in vitro assays [105]. The molecular mechanisms underlying these regulations are largely unknown.

3.2   Regulation by Post-Translational Modifications

Several HMTases are subjected to different post-translational modifications which could also regulate their catalytic activity. For example, PKB/AKT phosphorylate EZH2-Ser21 and this phosphorylation inhibits EZH2 binding to H3 and thus reduces H3K27me3 in vitro and in vivo [106]. In glioblastoma stem-like cells, EZH2 interacts with and methylates STAT3, while the Ser21 phosphorylation facilitates PRC2-catalyzed STAT3-K180 methylation to activate STAT3 signaling [107]. In response to DNA damage, SETD7 has been shown to interact with and methylate SUV39H1 at K105 and K123, leading to a dramatically reduced enzymatic activity of SUV39H1. Since these lysines are close to the chromodomain which is critical for chromatin binding, these methylations could weaken the SUV39H1-substrate interaction [108]. While SUV39H1-K266 acetylation within the SET domain reduces its catalytic activity, SIRT1-mediated deacetylation can restore it by facilitating the interaction between the SET and post-SET domains [109].

Moreover, bacteria-purified SETDB1 failed to methylate histones in the in vitro assays but 293T or Sf9 cell-purified enzymes displayed robust activity [110], indicating post-translational modifications could regulate SETDB1's activity. Recently we demonstrate that SETDB1 is monoubiquitinated at K867 (K867ub1) within its unique SET-I motif via an E3-independent mechanism. The conjugated-ubiquitin is protected from active deubiquitination, likely through multiple intramolecular interactions. Importantly, the resulting constitutive monoubiquitination is required for SETDB1's enzymatic activity and function. While most post-translational modifications are dynamically regulated, our findings highlight the constitutive role of K867Ub1 in regulating enzymatic activity of KMTs [97].

3.3 Regulation by Histone Modification

It is well-documented that histone methylation is also modulated by other histone modifications. On the same molecule, H3S10 phosphorylation blocks the access of the adjacent H3K9 for methylation [111]. The similar regulation also exists on different histones and one good example is that H2A and H2B ubiquitination affects H3K4 and H3K79 methylation. Site-specific installation of H2BK120ub1 causes the allosteric regulation of nucleosomes to facilitate DOT1L binding and thus increases the intranucleosomal H3K79me1/2 [112]. H2BK120ub1 also interacts with the N-terminal winged helix motif of ASH2L and promotes H3K4 methylation catalyzed by ASH2L-MLL-RBP5 complex [113]. However, H2AK119ub1 inhibits PRC2-catalyzed H3K27 methylation, suggesting that ubiquitination at different sites trans-regulates different histone methylations [114]. Similarly, the internucleosomal regulations have also been reported. While the SET domain of GLP and G9A preferentially methylates histone octamer, the full-length proteins efficiently catalyze oligonucleosomal methylation because G91/GLP bind to methyl-H3K9 binding on adjacent nucleosomes through their Ankyrin repeats domain [115]. Similarly, PRC2-catalzyed H3K27 methylation is stimulated by EED which binds to methyl-H3K27 on adjacent nucleosomes [116, 117]. In the PRC2 structure, H3K27me3 binding also stabilizes the conformation of EZH2 N-terminal SRM motif and affects the SET-I conformation to facilitate H3K27 methylation [70]. Similar to G9A/GLP, the chromodomain of SUV39H1 recognizes H3K9me3 and this methyl-binding anchors the enzyme to chromatin allosterically to allow further spreading of H3K9me3 [118]. Therefore, pre-existing modifications on histones could dramatically modulate methylation through different mechanisms.

4 Recognition of Histone Methylation

Although histone methylation does not neutralize the positive charge of DNA, several methylations could affect nucleosome structure to facilitate transcription [119]. For example, H3R42 locates at the DNA entry-exit region of nucleosome and addition of asymmetric dimethylation by CARM1 and PRMT6 could reduce nucleosome stability [48]. Structural study reveals that H3K79me2 leads to a subtle reorientation of the surrounding region in nucleosome [120]. Moreover, H3R17me2a and H3K4me1 have been shown to reduce chromatin association of NuRD complex, suggesting that these methylation marks could indirectly regulate accessibility of chromatin [121, 122]. In most cases, however, histone methylation serves as docking site for specific binding proteins which in turn recruit additional chromatin modifiers for diverse functional outcomes [119]. So far at least nine domains have been characterized as methyl-histone binding motifs that are briefly summarized in Table 2 together with their recognition sites.

Table 2 Histone methylation binding protein

Chromodomain		PWWP domain	
CBX1/3/5 (HP1β/γ/α)	H3K9me2/3 [123]	BRPF1	H3K36me3 [124]
MPP8	H3K9me2/3 [125]	ZMYND11	H3K36Me3 [126]
CBX2(PC1)	H3K9me3, H3K27me3 [127]	DNMT3A	H3K36me3 [128], H4R3me2s [129]
CBX7	H3K9me3, H3K27me3 [127]	**PHD domain**	
CBX4(PC2)	H3K9me3 [127]	ING1/2/3/4/5	H3K4me2/3 [130–134]
CBX6	H3K27me3 [127]	CHD4	H3K9me [135]
CBX8(PC3)	H3K27me3 [127]	MLL1	H3K4me2/3 [136]
CHD1	H3K4me2/3 [137]	UHRF1	H3K9me2/3 [138]
CDY1	H3K9me2/3 [139]	JARID1A	H3K4me2/3 [140]
TIP60	H3K9me3 [141]	JARID1C	H3K9me3 [142]
MRG15	H3K36me [143]	PHF2	H3K4me2/3 [144]
MSL3	H4K20me1 [145, 146]	PHF8	H3K4me2/3 [147]
Tudor domain		TAF3	H3K4me3 [148]
53BP1	H4K20me1/2 [149]	BPTF	H3K4me2/3 [150, 151]
UHRF1	H3K9me3 [152]	RAG2	H3K4me3 [153]
PHF1	H3K36me3 [154]	Pygo	H3K4me2/3 [155]
JMJD2A	H3K4me3 [156], H4K20me3 [157]	**Ankyrin repeats**	
PHF19	H3K36me3 [158, 159]	G9a/GLP	H3K9me1/2 [160]
PHF20	H4K20me2, H3K9me2 [161]	**ZF-CW domain**	
LBR	H4K20me2 [162]	ZCWPW1/2	H3K4me3 [163, 164]
SGF29	H3K4me3 [165]	MORC3/4	H3K4me3 [164]
TDRD3	H3R17me2a, H4R3me2a [166]	**BAH domain**	
Spindlin1	H3K4me3 [167]	ORC1	H4K20me2 [168]
MBT domain		BAHD1	H3K27me3 [169]
L3MBTL1	H4K20me1/2 [170], H1bK26me1/2 [170]	**WD repeats**	
L3MBTL2	H3K4me, H3K9me1/2, H3K27me1/2, H4K20me1/2 [171]	EED	H3K27me3, H1K26me3, H3K9me3, H4K20me3 [116, 117]
MBTD1	H3K20me1/2 [172]		
SFMBT	H3K9me1/2 [131], H4K20me1/2 [131]		

4.1 The Royal Family of Domains

Several methyl-histone binding motifs, including chromodomain, Tudor, MBT and PWWP belong to the Royal family of domains that are descended from a common ancestor [173]. These domains share a similar structure of barrel-like three-strand β-sheet with a short helix and bind to different methyl-lysines [174]. Existing in ~31 human proteins [175], the chromodomain recognizes methyl-lysines using an aromatic cage formed by three highly conserved residue [176]. The binding site specificity is determined by specific interactions between amino acids around the methyl-lysine and the chromodomain. For example, the chromodomains of HP1 [176, 177] and MPP8 [125, 178, 179] preferentially recognize H3K9me3 [176, 177] while the same domain in PC binds to H3K27me3 [180, 181]. Intriguingly, the CHD family proteins contain tandem chromodomains which bind to a single H3K4me3 mark in a coordinated manner [182, 183]. In most cases, the aromatic cage of chromodomain accommodates trimethylation and binds to mono- or di-methylation with a lower affinity due to less optimal van der Waals and cation-π interaction [149, 184].

The Tudor domain forms four- or five β-strands and bind to methyl-lysine with a similar aromatic cage. The tandem Tudor domains of JMJD2A specifically recognize H3K4me3 [156]. In the Tudor domains of 53BP1, the carboxylate group of Asp1521 forms a hydrogen bond with the nitrogen group of dimethyl-amine to confer stable binding to H4K20me2 but causes a steric hindrance for the trimethyl-amine [149]. Therefore, binding specificity to different methylation states is precisely regulated in different Tudor domains. Although the tandem Tudor domains are often observed, only one of the tandem domains interacts with methyl-lysine, leaving another free of binding.

The MBT domain is a larger motif (~100aa) containing 2–4 repeats and exists in nine human proteins. All human MBT domains harbor the conserved aromatic residues, indicating they can bind to methyl-lysines. However, the MBT domain preferentially recognizes mono- and di-methylated lysines [185] with poor site specificity. It is likely due to the lack of interactions with amino acids around the methyl-lysine [186, 187]. The PWWP domain (100–150aa) folds into a five-strand β-sheet packed against a helical bundle with significant variations in β2 and β3 while many have the conserved aromatic cage [188]. It has been shown that the PWWP domains of Pdp1 and DNMT3A/3B specifically recognize H4K20me [189] and H3K36me3 [128, 190] respectively.

4.2 Other Methyl-Lysine Binding Domains

In addition to the Royal family of domains, several other motifs can recognize different methyl-lysines as well, including PHD finger, CW, Ankyrin repeat, WD repeat and BAH. The PHD finger domain forms two anti-parallel beta strands and one C-terminal alpha-helix, which are stabilized by two zinc ions chelated by a consensus C4HC3 sequence [191]. This motif exists in multiple chromatin-associated proteins and many have been shown to recognize methylated histones [130, 192]. Due to a favorable accommodation of H3R2, most PHD finger domains bind to methyl-H3K4 [150, 151]. For example, the PHD domains of BPTF and ING2 recognize

H3K4me3 through an aromatic cage similar to the Royal family domains [150, 151]. Similarly, CW domain also centers two anti-parallel beta-strands and chelates one Zinc ion with the consensus C4 sequence [164]. The CW domain of ZCWPW1 preferentially recognizes H3K4me3 [163] through an aromatic cage. Among the seven human CW domain-containing proteins, four contain at least two conserved aromatic residues and can bind to H3K4me3 peptide in vitro [164].

The Ankyrin repeat domain is a widely distributed motif for protein-protein interactions. Intriguingly, the Ankyrin repeat domains of G9a and GLP can bind to H3K9me2 [160]. Similar to the chromodomain, three aromatic residues and a Glu are involved in the binding. However, the size of the aromatic cage cannot accommodate trimethyl groups. Distinctly, the WD repeats form a seven-bladed β-propeller, in which three scattered aromatic residues are responsible for methyl-lysine binding. It has been shown that the WD40 repeat domain of a PRC2 component EED recognizes multiple methyl-lysines, including H1K26me3, H3K9me3, H3K27me3 and H4K20me3 with similar affinity [116, 117]. The MLL complex subunit WDR5 contains seven WD40 repeats which have been reported to bind to methyl-H3K4 [193]. Existing in many chromatin-associated proteins, the BAH domain folds into a beta-rich structure. It has been demonstrated that the BAH domain of a DNA replication protein ORC1 specifically recognizes H4K20me2 through a four aromatic residues cage [168]. Due to a hydrogen bond between methyl-ammonium and side carboxylate chain of a nearby Glu, this binding favors H4K20me2 over H4K20me3 [168]. The BAH domain in BAHD1 has also been reported to recognize H3K27me3 [169].

4.3   Recognition of Arginine Methylation

Among methyl-histone binding domains, multiple Tudor domain-containing proteins also bind to methyl-arginine in various proteins, suggesting they can recognize methyl-arginine in histones [194]. The extended Tudor domain of SND1 has been shown to interact with peptides harboring H4R3 methylation [195]. Similar to methyl-lysine recognition, methyl-H4R3 binding also involves the aromatic cage of the Tudor domain of SND1. However, two aromatic residues pack to the guanidium planar in parallel, whose distance to the ammonium group is shorter than methyl-lysine binding [195]. While some Tudor domains recognize aDMA and sDMA on histones with comparable affinity, others display clear preference. In a peptide pull-down assay, the Tudor domain of TDRD3 preferentially recognizes aDMA on histone H3 tail [166]. Structural study reveals that such selectivity is rendered by a unique hydrogen bond between the unmodified amino group and the hydroxyl group of a Tyr in the aromatic cage [196]. Unexpectedly, the Glu-rich region in PELP1 has also been shown to bind to H3K4me2, H3K9me2 [197] and arginine methylated in vitro [198], suggesting there are more unidentified methyl-histone binding motifs.

4.4 Modulation of Methyl-Histone Binding

The methyl-histone binding by different domains is also subject to multiple regulations. Because of the extensive interaction between the binding domain and amino acids adjacent to the methylated residue, post-translational modifications on these amino acids could have drastic effects. For example, H3S10 phosphorylation, one of the most prominent modification on mitotic chromosome, inhibits HP1 binding to H3K9me3 [199, 200]. Similarly, H3K4me3 binding by different domains are blocked when H3R2 is asymmetrically dimethylated [10]. Intriguingly, modification adjacent to the methyl-lysine has also been shown to facilitate the recognition by binding domains. For example, the structure of RAG2 PHD finger domain complexed with H3K4me3 peptide uncovers an additional binding pocket. Therefore, H3K4me3 binding is increased when H3R2 is symmetrically methylated on the same molecule [201]. Furthermore, methyl-histone binding are regulated by other interacting partners. The structure of the ternary complex of Pygo PHD finger, the BCL9/Legless HD1 domain and H3K4me peptides demonstrates that the efficient H3K4me2 recognition requires the PHD-HD1 complex in instead of the PHD domain alone [155]. In addition to interacting proteins, ncRNA TUG1 can switch H3K9me3 binding by the PC2 chromodomain to H4R3me2s and H3K27me2. Through unknown mechanisms, another ncRNA NEAT2 can convert PC2's H3K9me3 binding to H2AK5ac and H2AK13ac binding [202].

5 Conclusion Remark

As a key component of the proposed "histone code", histone methylation is precisely regulated in cells and plays pivotal roles in the regulation of all chromatin-based processes. Histone methylation "code" is introduced by different groups of HMTases and recognized by various methyl-histone binding proteins. These proteins coordinate with various transcription factors, chromatin modifying proteins, signal pathway cascades and non-coding RNAs to constitute a large sophisticated network for diverse functional outcomes. It has been acknowledged that many histone methylating and binding proteins are altered in human diseases, including various cancers. Accordingly, numerous small molecule modulators have been developed and characterized for the pharmaceutical intervention of these diseases [203]. Multiple inhibitors targeting different HMTases have also been applied to various clinical trials. Therefore, a thorough understanding of the molecular basics underlying histone methylation and recognition will not only shed lights on their physiological functions, but also facilitate the development of therapeutic strategies for human diseases.

Acknowledgements This work was supported by grant from the National Cancer Institute (R01CA172774) to Jia Fang. This work was also supported in part by Core Facilities at the H. Lee Moffitt Cancer Center & Research Institute, an NCI designated Comprehensive Cancer Center.

References

1. Woodcock CL, Ghosh RP (2010) Chromatin higher-order structure and dynamics. Cold Spring Harb Perspect Biol 2:a000596
2. Strahl BD, Allis CD (2000) The language of covalent histone modifications. Nature 403:41–45
3. Ruthenburg AJ, Li H, Patel DJ, Allis CD (2007) Multivalent engagement of chromatin modifications by linked binding modules. Nat Rev Mol Cell Biol 8:983–994
4. Allfrey VG, Faulkner R, Mirsky AE (1964) Acetylation and methylation of histones and their possible role in the regulation of RNA synthesis. Proc Natl Acad Sci U S A 51:786–794
5. Murray K (1964) The occurrence of epsilon-N-methyl lysine in histones. Biochemistry 3:10–15
6. Strahl BD, Ohba R, Cook RG, Allis CD (1999) Methylation of histone H3 at lysine 4 is highly conserved and correlates with transcriptionally active nuclei in Tetrahymena. Proc Natl Acad Sci U S A 96:14967–14972
7. Bedford MT (2007) Arginine methylation at a glance. J Cell Sci 120:4243–4246
8. Guccione E et al (2007) Methylation of histone H3R2 by PRMT6 and H3K4 by an MLL complex are mutually exclusive. Nature 449:933–937
9. Hyllus D et al (2007) PRMT6-mediated methylation of R2 in histone H3 antagonizes H3 K4 trimethylation. Genes Dev 21:3369–3380
10. Iberg AN et al (2008) Arginine methylation of the histone H3 tail impedes effector binding. J Biol Chem 283:3006–3010
11. Schurter BT et al (2001) Methylation of histone H3 by coactivator-associated arginine methyltransferase 1. Biochemistry 40:5747–5756
12. Migliori V et al (2012) Symmetric dimethylation of H3R2 is a newly identified histone mark that supports euchromatin maintenance. Nat Struct Mol Biol 19:136–144
13. Wysocka J, Myers MP, Laherty CD, Eisenman RN, Herr W (2003) Human Sin3 deacetylase and trithorax-related Set1/Ash2 histone H3-K4 methyltransferase are tethered together selectively by the cell-proliferation factor HCF-1. Genes Dev 17:896–911
14. Lee JH, Tate CM, You JS, Skalnik DG (2007) Identification and characterization of the human Set1B histone H3-Lys4 methyltransferase complex. J Biol Chem 282:13419–13428
15. Wang H et al (2001) Purification and functional characterization of a histone H3-lysine 4-specific methyltransferase. Mol Cell 8:1207–1217
16. Lee SH et al (2005) The SET domain protein Metnase mediates foreign DNA integration and links integration to nonhomologous end-joining repair. Proc Natl Acad Sci U S A 102:18075–18080
17. Blazer LL et al (2016) PR domain-containing protein 7 (PRDM7) is a histone 3 lysine 4 trimethyltransferase. J Biol Chem 291:13509–13519
18. Powers NR et al (2016) The meiotic recombination activator PRDM9 trimethylates both H3K36 and H3K4 at recombination hotspots in vivo. PLoS Genet 12:e1006146
19. Hayashi K, Yoshida K, Matsui Y (2005) A histone H3 methyltransferase controls epigenetic events required for meiotic prophase. Nature 438:374–378
20. Tan X, Rotllant J, Li H, De Deyne P, Du SJ (2006) SmyD1, a histone methyltransferase, is required for myofibril organization and muscle contraction in zebrafish embryos. Proc Natl Acad Sci U S A 103:2713–2718
21. Hamamoto R et al (2004) SMYD3 encodes a histone methyltransferase involved in the proliferation of cancer cells. Nat Cell Biol 6:731–740

22. Van Aller GS et al (2012) Smyd3 regulates cancer cell phenotypes and catalyzes histone H4 lysine 5 methylation. Epigenetics 7:340–343

23. Blythe SA, Cha SW, Tadjuidje E, Heasman J, Klein PS (2010) Beta-catenin primes organizer gene expression by recruiting a histone H3 arginine 8 methyltransferase, Prmt2. Dev Cell 19:220–231

24. Pal S, Vishwanath SN, Erdjument-Bromage H, Tempst P, Sif S (2004) Human SWI/SNF-associated PRMT5 methylates histone H3 arginine 8 and negatively regulates expression of ST7 and NM23 tumor suppressor genes. Mol Cell Biol 24:9630–9645

25. Rea S et al (2000) Regulation of chromatin structure by site-specific histone H3 methyltransferases. Nature 406:593–599

26. O'Carroll D et al (2000) Isolation and characterization of Suv39h2, a second histone H3 methyltransferase gene that displays testis-specific expression. Mol Cell Biol 20:9423–9433

27. Ogawa H, Ishiguro K, Gaubatz S, Livingston DM, Nakatani Y (2002) A complex with chromatin modifiers that occupies E2F- and Myc-responsive genes in G0 cells. Science 296:1132–1136

28. Tachibana M, Sugimoto K, Fukushima T, Shinkai Y (2001) Set domain-containing protein, G9a, is a novel lysine-preferring mammalian histone methyltransferase with hyperactivity and specific selectivity to lysines 9 and 27 of histone H3. J Biol Chem 276:25309–25317

29. Yang L et al (2002) Molecular cloning of ESET, a novel histone H3-specific methyltransferase that interacts with ERG transcription factor. Oncogene 21:148–152

30. Falandry C et al (2010) CLLD8/KMT1F is a lysine methyltransferase that is important for chromosome segregation. J Biol Chem 285:20234–20241

31. Kim KC, Geng L, Huang S (2003) Inactivation of a histone methyltransferase by mutations in human cancers. Cancer Res 63:7619–7623

32. Pinheiro I et al (2012) Prdm3 and Prdm16 are H3K9me1 methyltransferases required for mammalian heterochromatin integrity. Cell 150:948–960

33. Eom GH et al (2009) Histone methyltransferase PRDM8 regulates mouse testis steroidogenesis. Biochem Biophys Res Commun 388:131–136

34. Bauer UM, Daujat S, Nielsen SJ, Nightingale K, Kouzarides T (2002) Methylation at arginine 17 of histone H3 is linked to gene activation. EMBO Rep 3:39–44

35. Wu H et al (2011) Histone methyltransferase G9a contributes to H3K27 methylation in vivo. Cell Res 21:365–367

36. Qiao Q et al (2011) The structure of NSD1 reveals an autoregulatory mechanism underlying histone H3K36 methylation. J Biol Chem 286:8361–8368

37. Kuo AJ et al (2011) NSD2 links dimethylation of histone H3 at lysine 36 to oncogenic programming. Mol Cell 44:609–620

38. Asangani IA et al (2012) Characterization of the EZH2-MMSET histone methyltransferase regulatory axis in cancer. Mol Cell 49:80–93

39. Li Y et al (2009) The target of the NSD family of histone lysine methyltransferases depends on the nature of the substrate. J Biol Chem 284:34283–34295

40. Brown MA, Sims RJ 3rd, Gottlieb PD, Tucker PW (2006) Identification and characterization of Smyd2: a split SET/MYND domain-containing histone H3 lysine 36-specific methyltransferase that interacts with the Sin3 histone deacetylase complex. Mol Cancer 5:26

41. Sun XJ et al (2005) Identification and characterization of a novel human histone H3 lysine 36-specific methyltransferase. J Biol Chem 280:35261–35271

42. Kim DW, Kim KB, Kim JY, Seo SB (2011) Characterization of a novel histone H3K36 methyltransferase setd3 in zebrafish. Biosci Biotechnol Biochem 75:289–294

43. Eom GH et al (2011) Histone methyltransferase SETD3 regulates muscle differentiation. J Biol Chem 286:34733–34742

44. An S, Yeo KJ, Jeon YH, Song JJ (2011) Crystal structure of the human histone methyltransferase ASH1L catalytic domain and its implications for the regulatory mechanism. J Biol Chem 286:8369–8374

45. Tanaka Y, Katagiri Z, Kawahashi K, Kioussis D, Kitajima S (2007) Trithorax-group protein ASH1 methylates histone H3 lysine 36. Gene 397:161–168
46. Eram MS et al (2014) Trimethylation of histone H3 lysine 36 by human methyltransferase PRDM9 protein. J Biol Chem 289:12177–12188
47. Yu Y et al (2012) Histone H3 lysine 56 methylation regulates DNA replication through its interaction with PCNA. Mol Cell 46:7–17
48. Casadio F et al (2013) H3R42me2a is a histone modification with positive transcriptional effects. Proc Natl Acad Sci U S A 110:14894–14899
49. Feng Q et al (2002) Methylation of H3-lysine 79 is mediated by a new family of HMTases without a SET domain. Curr Biol 12:1052–1058
50. Ng HH et al (2002) Lysine methylation within the globular domain of histone H3 by Dot1 is important for telomeric silencing and Sir protein association. Genes Dev 16:1518–1527
51. Wang H et al (2001) Methylation of histone H4 at arginine 3 facilitating transcriptional activation by nuclear hormone receptor. Science 293:853–857
52. Karkhanis V et al (2012) Protein arginine methyltransferase 7 regulates cellular response to DNA damage by methylating promoter histones H2A and H4 of the polymerase delta catalytic subunit gene, POLD1. J Biol Chem 287:29801–29814
53. Tweedie-Cullen RY et al (2012) Identification of combinatorial patterns of post-translational modifications on individual histones in the mouse brain. PLoS One 7:e36980
54. Feng Y et al (2013) Mammalian protein arginine methyltransferase 7 (PRMT7) specifically targets RXR sites in lysine- and arginine-rich regions. J Biol Chem 288:37010–37025
55. Schotta G et al (2004) A silencing pathway to induce H3-K9 and H4-K20 trimethylation at constitutive heterochromatin. Genes Dev 18:1251–1262
56. Fang J et al (2002) Purification and functional characterization of SET8, a nucleosomal histone H4-lysine 20-specific methyltransferase. Curr Biol 12:1086–1099
57. Nishioka K et al (2002) PR-Set7 is a nucleosome-specific methyltransferase that modifies lysine 20 of histone H4 and is associated with silent chromatin. Mol Cell 9:1201–1213
58. Foreman KW et al (2011) Structural and functional profiling of the human histone methyltransferase SMYD3. PLoS One 6:e22290
59. Ancelin K et al (2006) Blimp1 associates with Prmt5 and directs histone arginine methylation in mouse germ cells. Nat Cell Biol 8:623–630
60. Waldmann T et al (2011) Methylation of H2AR29 is a novel repressive PRMT6 target. Epigenetics Chromatin 4:11
61. Binda O et al (2013) SETD6 monomethylates H2AZ on lysine 7 and is required for the maintenance of embryonic stem cell self-renewal. Epigenetics 8:177–183
62. Kogure M et al (2013) The oncogenic polycomb histone methyltransferase EZH2 methylates lysine 120 on histone H2B and competes ubiquitination. Neoplasia 15:1251–1261
63. Kuzmichev A, Jenuwein T, Tempst P, Reinberg D (2004) Different EZH2-containing complexes target methylation of histone H1 or nucleosomal histone H3. Mol Cell 14:183–193
64. Weiss T et al (2010) Histone H1 variant-specific lysine methylation by G9a/KMT1C and Glp1/KMT1D. Epigenetics Chromatin 3:7
65. Polevoda B, Sherman F (2007) Methylation of proteins involved in translation. Mol Microbiol 65:590–606
66. Tessarz P et al (2014) Glutamine methylation in histone H2A is an RNA-polymerase-I-dedicated modification. Nature 505:564–568
67. Jenuwein T, Laible G, Dorn R, Reuter G (1998) SET domain proteins modulate chromatin domains in eu- and heterochromatin. Cell Mol Life Sci 54:80–93
68. Cheng X, Collins RE, Zhang X (2005) Structural and sequence motifs of protein (histone) methylation enzymes. Annu Rev Biophys Biomol Struct 34:267–294
69. Li Y et al (2016) Structural basis for activity regulation of MLL family methyltransferases. Nature 530:447–452
70. Jiao L, Liu X (2015) Structural basis of histone H3K27 trimethylation by an active polycomb repressive complex 2. Science 350:aac4383

71. Spellmon N, Holcomb J, Trescott L, Sirinupong N, Yang Z (2015) Structure and function of SET and MYND domain-containing proteins. Int J Mol Sci 16:1406–1428
72. Xiao B et al (2003) Structure and catalytic mechanism of the human histone methyltransferase SET7/9. Nature 421:652–656
73. Couture JF, Collazo E, Brunzelle JS, Trievel RC (2005) Structural and functional analysis of SET8, a histone H4 Lys-20 methyltransferase. Genes Dev 19:1455–1465
74. Sawada K et al (2004) Structure of the conserved core of the yeast Dot1p, a nucleosomal histone H3 lysine 79 methyltransferase. J Biol Chem 279:43296–43306
75. Min J, Feng Q, Li Z, Zhang Y, Xu RM (2003) Structure of the catalytic domain of human DOT1L, a non-SET domain nucleosomal histone methyltransferase. Cell 112:711–723
76. Chen X, Liu H, Shim AH, Focia PJ, He X (2008) Structural basis for synaptic adhesion mediated by neuroligin-neurexin interactions. Nat Struct Mol Biol 15:50–56
77. Cao F et al (2010) An Ash2L/RbBP5 heterodimer stimulates the MLL1 methyltransferase activity through coordinated substrate interactions with the MLL1 SET domain. PLoS One 5:e14102
78. Patel A, Vought VE, Dharmarajan V, Cosgrove MS (2011) A novel non-SET domain multi-subunit methyltransferase required for sequential nucleosomal histone H3 methylation by the mixed lineage leukemia protein-1 (MLL1) core complex. J Biol Chem 286:3359–3369
79. Xiao B, Wilson JR, Gamblin SJ (2003) SET domains and histone methylation. Curr Opin Struct Biol 13:699–705
80. Wu H et al (2010) Structural biology of human H3K9 methyltransferases. PLoS One 5:e8570
81. Zhang X et al (2002) Structure of the Neurospora SET domain protein DIM-5, a histone H3 lysine methyltransferase. Cell 111:117–127
82. Wu H et al (2013) Molecular basis for the regulation of the H3K4 methyltransferase activity of PRDM9. Cell Rep 5:13–20
83. Southall SM, Cronin NB, Wilson JR (2014) A novel route to product specificity in the Suv4-20 family of histone H4K20 methyltransferases. Nucleic Acids Res 42:661–671
84. Zhang X et al (2003) Structural basis for the product specificity of histone lysine methyltransferases. Mol Cell 12:177–185
85. Dillon SC, Zhang X, Trievel RC, Cheng X (2005) The SET-domain protein superfamily: protein lysine methyltransferases. Genome Biol 6:227
86. Southall SM, Wong PS, Odho Z, Roe SM, Wilson JR (2009) Structural basis for the requirement of additional factors for MLL1 SET domain activity and recognition of epigenetic marks. Mol Cell 33:181–191
87. Wu H et al (2013) Crystal structures of the human histone H4K20 methyltransferases SUV420H1 and SUV420H2. FEBS Lett 587:3859–3868
88. Xu S, Zhong C, Zhang T, Ding J (2011) Structure of human lysine methyltransferase Smyd2 reveals insights into the substrate divergence in Smyd proteins. J Mol Cell Biol 3:293–300
89. Nguyen AT, Zhang Y (2011) The diverse functions of Dot1 and H3K79 methylation. Genes Dev 25:1345–1358
90. Gui S et al (2014) A remodeled protein arginine methyltransferase 1 (PRMT1) generates symmetric dimethylarginine. J Biol Chem 289:9320–9327
91. Fuhrmann J, Clancy KW, Thompson PR (2015) Chemical biology of protein arginine modifications in epigenetic regulation. Chem Rev 115:5413–5461
92. Zhang X, Zhou L, Cheng X (2000) Crystal structure of the conserved core of protein arginine methyltransferase PRMT3. EMBO J 19:3509–3519
93. Debler EW et al (2016) A glutamate/aspartate switch controls product specificity in a protein arginine methyltransferase. Proc Natl Acad Sci U S A 113:2068–2073
94. Sun L et al (2011) Structural insights into protein arginine symmetric dimethylation by PRMT5. Proc Natl Acad Sci U S A 108:20538–20543
95. Kuzmichev A, Nishioka K, Erdjument-Bromage H, Tempst P, Reinberg D (2002) Histone methyltransferase activity associated with a human multiprotein complex containing the enhancer of Zeste protein. Genes Dev 16:2893–2905

96. Cao R et al (2002) Role of histone H3 lysine 27 methylation in polycomb-group silencing. Science 298:1039–1043
97. Sun L, Fang J (2016) E3-independent constitutive monoubiquitination complements histone methyltransferase activity of SETDB1. Mol Cell 62:958–966
98. Wu H et al (2013) Structure of the catalytic domain of EZH2 reveals conformational plasticity in cofactor and substrate binding sites and explains oncogenic mutations. PLoS One 8:e83737
99. Antonysamy S et al (2013) Structural context of disease-associated mutations and putative mechanism of autoinhibition revealed by X-ray crystallographic analysis of the EZH2-SET domain. PLoS One 8:e84147
100. Lacroix M et al (2008) The histone-binding protein COPR5 is required for nuclear functions of the protein arginine methyltransferase PRMT5. EMBO Rep 9:452–458
101. Abu-Farha M et al (2008) The tale of two domains: proteomics and genomics analysis of SMYD2, a new histone methyltransferase. Mol Cell Proteomics 7:560–572
102. Cao R et al (2008) Role of hPHF1 in H3K27 methylation and Hox gene silencing. Mol Cell Biol 28:1862–1872
103. Sarma K, Margueron R, Ivanov A, Pirrotta V, Reinberg D (2008) Ezh2 requires PHF1 to efficiently catalyze H3 lysine 27 trimethylation in vivo. Mol Cell Biol 28:2718–2731
104. Wang H et al (2003) mAM facilitates conversion by ESET of dimethyl to trimethyl lysine 9 of histone H3 to cause transcriptional repression. Mol Cell 12:475–487
105. Basavapathruni A et al (2016) Characterization of the enzymatic activity of SETDB1 and its 1:1 complex with ATF7IP. Biochemistry 55:1645–1651
106. Cha TL et al (2005) Akt-mediated phosphorylation of EZH2 suppresses methylation of lysine 27 in histone H3. Science 310:306–310
107. Kim E et al (2013) Phosphorylation of EZH2 activates STAT3 signaling via STAT3 methylation and promotes tumorigenicity of glioblastoma stem-like cells. Cancer Cell 23:839–852
108. Wang D et al (2013) Methylation of SUV39H1 by SET7/9 results in heterochromatin relaxation and genome instability. Proc Natl Acad Sci U S A 110:5516–5521
109. Vaquero A et al (2007) SIRT1 regulates the histone methyl-transferase SUV39H1 during heterochromatin formation. Nature 450:440–444
110. Schultz DC, Ayyanathan K, Negorev D, Maul GG, Rauscher FJ 3rd (2002) SETDB1: a novel KAP-1-associated histone H3, lysine 9-specific methyltransferase that contributes to HP1-mediated silencing of euchromatic genes by KRAB zinc-finger proteins. Genes Dev 16:919–932
111. Duan Q, Chen H, Costa M, Dai W (2008) Phosphorylation of H3S10 blocks the access of H3K9 by specific antibodies and histone methyltransferase. Implication in regulating chromatin dynamics and epigenetic inheritance during mitosis. J Biol Chem 283:33585–33590
112. McGinty RK, Kim J, Chatterjee C, Roeder RG, Muir TW (2008) Chemically ubiquitylated histone H2B stimulates hDot1L-mediated intranucleosomal methylation. Nature 453:812–816
113. Wu L et al (2013) ASH2L regulates ubiquitylation signaling to MLL: trans-regulation of H3 K4 methylation in higher eukaryotes. Mol Cell 49:1108–1120
114. Whitcomb SJ et al (2012) Histone monoubiquitylation position determines specificity and direction of enzymatic cross-talk with histone methyltransferases Dot1L and PRC2. J Biol Chem 287:23718–23725
115. Liu N et al (2015) Recognition of H3K9 methylation by GLP is required for efficient establishment of H3K9 methylation, rapid target gene repression, and mouse viability. Genes Dev 29:379–393
116. Margueron R et al (2009) Role of the polycomb protein EED in the propagation of repressive histone marks. Nature 461:762–767
117. Xu C et al (2010) Binding of different histone marks differentially regulates the activity and specificity of polycomb repressive complex 2 (PRC2). Proc Natl Acad Sci U S A 107:19266–19271

118. Muller MM, Fierz B, Bittova L, Liszczak G, Muir TW (2016) A two-state activation mechanism controls the histone methyltransferase Suv39h1. Nat Chem Biol 12:188–193
119. Tessarz P, Kouzarides T (2014) Histone core modifications regulating nucleosome structure and dynamics. Nat Rev Mol Cell Biol 15:703–708
120. Lu X et al (2008) The effect of H3K79 dimethylation and H4K20 trimethylation on nucleosome and chromatin structure. Nat Struct Mol Biol 15:1122–1124
121. Wu J, Cui N, Wang R, Li J, Wong J (2012) A role for CARM1-mediated histone H3 arginine methylation in protecting histone acetylation by releasing corepressors from chromatin. PLoS One 7:e34692
122. Nishioka K et al (2002) Set9, a novel histone H3 methyltransferase that facilitates transcription by precluding histone tail modifications required for heterochromatin formation. Genes Dev 16:479–489
123. Lachner M, O'Carroll D, Rea S, Mechtler K, Jenuwein T (2001) Methylation of histone H3 lysine 9 creates a binding site for HP1 proteins. Nature 410:116–120
124. Vezzoli A et al (2010) Molecular basis of histone H3K36me3 recognition by the PWWP domain of Brpf1. Nat Struct Mol Biol 17:617–619
125. Kokura K, Sun L, Bedford MT, Fang J (2010) Methyl-H3K9-binding protein MPP8 mediates E-cadherin gene silencing and promotes tumour cell motility and invasion. EMBO J 29:3673–3687
126. Wen H et al (2014) ZMYND11 links histone H3.3K36me3 to transcription elongation and tumour suppression. Nature 508:263–268
127. Bernstein E et al (2006) Mouse polycomb proteins bind differentially to methylated histone H3 and RNA and are enriched in facultative heterochromatin. Mol Cell Biol 26:2560–2569
128. Dhayalan A et al (2010) The Dnmt3a PWWP domain reads histone 3 lysine 36 trimethylation and guides DNA methylation. J Biol Chem 285:26114–26120
129. Zhao Q et al (2009) PRMT5-mediated methylation of histone H4R3 recruits DNMT3A, coupling histone and DNA methylation in gene silencing. Nat Struct Mol Biol 16:304–311
130. Shi X et al (2006) ING2 PHD domain links histone H3 lysine 4 methylation to active gene repression. Nature 442:96–99
131. Klymenko T et al (2006) A polycomb group protein complex with sequence-specific DNA-binding and selective methyl-lysine-binding activities. Genes Dev 20:1110–1122
132. Kim S et al (2016) Mechanism of histone H3K4me3 recognition by the plant homeodomain of inhibitor of growth 3. J Biol Chem 291:18326–18341
133. Hung T et al (2009) ING4 mediates crosstalk between histone H3 K4 trimethylation and H3 acetylation to attenuate cellular transformation. Mol Cell 33:248–256
134. Champagne KS et al (2008) The crystal structure of the ING5 PHD finger in complex with an H3K4me3 histone peptide. Proteins 72:1371–1376
135. Musselman CA et al (2009) Binding of the CHD4 PHD2 finger to histone H3 is modulated by covalent modifications. Biochem J 423:179–187
136. Chang PY et al (2010) Binding of the MLL PHD3 finger to histone H3K4me3 is required for MLL-dependent gene transcription. J Mol Biol 400:137–144
137. Sims RJ 3rd et al (2005) Human but not yeast CHD1 binds directly and selectively to histone H3 methylated at lysine 4 via its tandem chromodomains. J Biol Chem 280:41789–41792
138. Karagianni P, Amazit L, Qin J, Wong J (2008) ICBP90, a novel methyl K9 H3 binding protein linking protein ubiquitination with heterochromatin formation. Mol Cell Biol 28:705–717
139. Fischle W, Franz H, Jacobs SA, Allis CD, Khorasanizadeh S (2008) Specificity of the chromodomain Y chromosome family of chromodomains for lysine-methylated ARK(S/T) motifs. J Biol Chem 283:19626–19635
140. Wang GG et al (2009) Haematopoietic malignancies caused by dysregulation of a chromatin-binding PHD finger. Nature 459:847–851
141. Sun Y et al (2009) Histone H3 methylation links DNA damage detection to activation of the tumour suppressor Tip60. Nat Cell Biol 11:1376–1382

142. Iwase S et al (2007) The X-linked mental retardation gene SMCX/JARID1C defines a family of histone H3 lysine 4 demethylases. Cell 128:1077–1088
143. Zhang P et al (2006) Structure of human MRG15 chromo domain and its binding to Lys36-methylated histone H3. Nucleic Acids Res 34:6621–6628
144. Wen H et al (2010) Recognition of histone H3K4 trimethylation by the plant homeodomain of PHF2 modulates histone demethylation. J Biol Chem 285:9322–9326
145. Moore SA, Ferhatoglu Y, Jia Y, Al-Jiab RA, Scott MJ (2010) Structural and biochemical studies on the chromo-barrel domain of male specific lethal 3 (MSL3) reveal a binding preference for mono- or dimethyllysine 20 on histone H4. J Biol Chem 285:40879–40890
146. Kim D et al (2010) Corecognition of DNA and a methylated histone tail by the MSL3 chromodomain. Nat Struct Mol Biol 17:1027–1029
147. Feng W, Yonezawa M, Ye J, Jenuwein T, Grummt I (2010) PHF8 activates transcription of rRNA genes through H3K4me3 binding and H3K9me1/2 demethylation. Nat Struct Mol Biol 17:445–450
148. Vermeulen M et al (2007) Selective anchoring of TFIID to nucleosomes by trimethylation of histone H3 lysine 4. Cell 131:58–69
149. Botuyan MV et al (2006) Structural basis for the methylation state-specific recognition of histone H4-K20 by 53BP1 and Crb2 in DNA repair. Cell 127:1361–1373
150. Li H et al (2006) Molecular basis for site-specific read-out of histone H3K4me3 by the BPTF PHD finger of NURF. Nature 442:91–95
151. Wysocka J et al (2006) A PHD finger of NURF couples histone H3 lysine 4 trimethylation with chromatin remodelling. Nature 442:86–90
152. Nady N et al (2011) Recognition of multivalent histone states associated with heterochromatin by UHRF1 protein. J Biol Chem 286:24300–24311
153. Liu Y, Subrahmanyam R, Chakraborty T, Sen R, Desiderio S (2007) A plant homeodomain in RAG-2 that binds Hypermethylated lysine 4 of histone H3 is necessary for efficient antigen-receptor-gene rearrangement. Immunity 27:561–571
154. Musselman CA et al (2012) Molecular basis for H3K36me3 recognition by the Tudor domain of PHF1. Nat Struct Mol Biol 19:1266–1272
155. Fiedler M et al (2008) Decoding of methylated histone H3 tail by the Pygo-BCL9 Wnt signaling complex. Mol Cell 30:507–518
156. Huang Y, Fang J, Bedford MT, Zhang Y, Xu RM (2006) Recognition of histone H3 lysine-4 methylation by the double tudor domain of JMJD2A. Science 312:748–751
157. Lee J, Thompson JR, Botuyan MV, Mer G (2008) Distinct binding modes specify the recognition of methylated histones H3K4 and H4K20 by JMJD2A-tudor. Nat Struct Mol Biol 15:109–111
158. Brien GL et al (2012) Polycomb PHF19 binds H3K36me3 and recruits PRC2 and demethylase NO66 to embryonic stem cell genes during differentiation. Nat Struct Mol Biol 19:1273–1281
159. Ballare C et al (2012) Phf19 links methylated Lys36 of histone H3 to regulation of polycomb activity. Nat Struct Mol Biol 19:1257–1265
160. Collins RE et al (2008) The ankyrin repeats of G9a and GLP histone methyltransferases are mono- and dimethyllysine binding modules. Nat Struct Mol Biol 15:245–250
161. Badeaux AI et al (2012) Loss of the methyl lysine effector protein PHF20 impacts the expression of genes regulated by the lysine acetyltransferase MOF. J Biol Chem 287:429–437
162. Hirano Y et al (2012) Lamin B receptor recognizes specific modifications of histone H4 in heterochromatin formation. J Biol Chem 287:42654–42663
163. He F et al (2010) Structural insight into the zinc finger CW domain as a histone modification reader. Structure 18:1127–1139
164. Liu Y et al (2016) Family-wide characterization of histone binding abilities of human CW domain-containing proteins. J Biol Chem 291:9000–9013
165. Bian C et al (2011) Sgf29 binds histone H3K4me2/3 and is required for SAGA complex recruitment and histone H3 acetylation. EMBO J 30:2829–2842

166. Yang Y et al (2010) TDRD3 is an effector molecule for arginine-methylated histone marks. Mol Cell 40:1016–1023
167. Wang W et al (2011) Nucleolar protein Spindlin1 recognizes H3K4 methylation and stimulates the expression of rRNA genes. EMBO Rep 12:1160–1166
168. Kuo AJ et al (2012) The BAH domain of ORC1 links H4K20me2 to DNA replication licensing and Meier-Gorlin syndrome. Nature 484:115–119
169. Zhao D et al (2016) The BAH domain of BAHD1 is a histone H3K27me3 reader. Protein Cell 7:222–226
170. Trojer P et al (2007) L3MBTL1, a histone-methylation-dependent chromatin lock. Cell 129:915–928
171. Guo Y et al (2009) Methylation-state-specific recognition of histones by the MBT repeat protein L3MBTL2. Nucleic Acids Res 37:2204–2210
172. Jacquet K et al (2016) The TIP60 complex regulates bivalent chromatin recognition by 53BP1 through direct H4K20me binding and H2AK15 acetylation. Mol Cell 62:409–421
173. Maurer-Stroh S et al (2003) The Tudor domain 'Royal Family': Tudor, plant agenet, chromo, PWWP and MBT domains. Trends Biochem Sci 28:69–74
174. Yap KL, Zhou MM (2010) Keeping it in the family: diverse histone recognition by conserved structural folds. Crit Rev Biochem Mol Biol 45:488–505
175. Yap KL, Zhou MM (2011) Structure and mechanisms of lysine methylation recognition by the chromodomain in gene transcription. Biochemistry 50:1966–1980
176. Nielsen PR et al (2002) Structure of the HP1 chromodomain bound to histone H3 methylated at lysine 9. Nature 416:103–107
177. Jacobs SA, Khorasanizadeh S (2002) Structure of HP1 chromodomain bound to a lysine 9-methylated histone H3 tail. Science 295:2080–2083
178. Chang Y, Horton JR, Bedford MT, Zhang X, Cheng X (2011) Structural insights for MPP8 chromodomain interaction with histone H3 lysine 9: potential effect of phosphorylation on methyl-lysine binding. J Mol Biol 408:807–814
179. Li J et al (2011) Structural basis for specific binding of human MPP8 chromodomain to histone H3 methylated at lysine 9. PLoS One 6:e25104
180. Fischle W et al (2003) Molecular basis for the discrimination of repressive methyl-lysine marks in histone H3 by Polycomb and HP1 chromodomains. Genes Dev 17:1870–1881
181. Min J, Zhang Y, Xu RM (2003) Structural basis for specific binding of Polycomb chromodomain to histone H3 methylated at Lys 27. Genes Dev 17:1823–1828
182. Pray-Grant MG, Daniel JA, Schieltz D, Yates JR 3rd, Grant PA (2005) Chd1 chromodomain links histone H3 methylation with SAGA- and SLIK-dependent acetylation. Nature 433:434–438
183. Flanagan JF et al (2005) Double chromodomains cooperate to recognize the methylated histone H3 tail. Nature 438:1181–1185
184. Kamps JJ et al (2015) Chemical basis for the recognition of trimethyllysine by epigenetic reader proteins. Nat Commun 6:8911
185. Nady N et al (2012) Histone recognition by human malignant brain tumor domains. J Mol Biol 423:702–718
186. Li H et al (2007) Structural basis for lower lysine methylation state-specific readout by MBT repeats of L3MBTL1 and an engineered PHD finger. Mol Cell 28:677–691
187. Min J et al (2007) L3MBTL1 recognition of mono- and dimethylated histones. Nat Struct Mol Biol 14:1229–1230
188. Qin S, Min J (2014) Structure and function of the nucleosome-binding PWWP domain. Trends Biochem Sci 39:536–547
189. Wang Y et al (2009) Regulation of Set9-mediated H4K20 methylation by a PWWP domain protein. Mol Cell 33:428–437
190. Baubec T et al (2015) Genomic profiling of DNA methyltransferases reveals a role for DNMT3B in genic methylation. Nature 520:243–247

191. Sanchez R, Zhou MM (2011) The PHD finger: a versatile epigenome reader. Trends Biochem Sci 36:364–372
192. Pena PV et al (2006) Molecular mechanism of histone H3K4me3 recognition by plant homeodomain of ING2. Nature 442:100–103
193. Wysocka J et al (2005) WDR5 associates with histone H3 methylated at K4 and is essential for H3 K4 methylation and vertebrate development. Cell 121:859–872
194. Gayatri S, Bedford MT (2014) Readers of histone methylarginine marks. Biochim Biophys Acta 1839:702–710
195. Liu K et al (2010) Structural basis for recognition of arginine methylated Piwi proteins by the extended Tudor domain. Proc Natl Acad Sci U S A 107:18398–18403
196. Sikorsky T et al (2012) Recognition of asymmetrically dimethylated arginine by TDRD3. Nucleic Acids Res 40:11748–11755
197. Nair SS et al (2010) PELP1 is a reader of histone H3 methylation that facilitates oestrogen receptor-alpha target gene activation by regulating lysine demethylase 1 specificity. EMBO Rep 11:438–444
198. Mann M, Cortez V, Vadlamudi R (2013) PELP1 oncogenic functions involve CARM1 regulation. Carcinogenesis 34:1468–1475
199. Hirota T, Lipp JJ, Toh BH, Peters JM (2005) Histone H3 serine 10 phosphorylation by Aurora B causes HP1 dissociation from heterochromatin. Nature 438:1176–1180
200. Fischle W et al (2005) Regulation of HP1-chromatin binding by histone H3 methylation and phosphorylation. Nature 438:1116–1122
201. Yuan CC et al (2012) Histone H3R2 symmetric dimethylation and histone H3K4 trimethylation are tightly correlated in eukaryotic genomes. Cell Rep 1:83–90
202. Yang L et al (2011) ncRNA- and Pc2 methylation-dependent gene relocation between nuclear structures mediates gene activation programs. Cell 147:773–788
203. Arrowsmith CH, Bountra C, Fish PV, Lee K, Schapira M (2012) Epigenetic protein families: a new frontier for drug discovery. Nat Rev Drug Discov 11:384–400

The Molecular Basis of Histone Demethylation

John R. Horton, Molly Gale, Qin Yan, and Xiaodong Cheng

Abstract The methylation of lysine residues on histone tails--and their subsequent demethylation--is among some of the most important covalent post-translational modifications controlling gene expression. When gene expression goes awry, disease ensues and often this disease is some form of cancer. Thus, an understanding of histone tail modification in nucleosomes is critical in mankind's attempts to eradicate cancers. This chapter examines our present knowledge of the enzymes that demethylate the lysine residues on histone tails, known as KDMs. The substrate-binding specificities of KDMs are quite diverse. The determinants of their specificity goes beyond just the amino acids involved in recognition and catalysis as observed in KDM crystal structures of their catalytic domains but extend to interactions of their many domains to each other and with other proteins in multicomponent complexes. These aspects of all seven known KDM families are reviewed as well as our present knowledge of their involvement in cancers. Control of their aberrant behavior by design of chemical inhibitors, that have the potential to be powerful cancer fighting drugs, is an expanding human endeavor and is chronicled at the end of the chapter.

Keywords Epigenetics • Histone lysine methylation • Histone lysine demethylation • KDM family • Fe(II)- and α-ketoglutarate-dependent dioxygeneses • Flavin adenine dinucleotide (FAD)-dependent LSD • Mono/di/tri-methylation • Protein arginine methylation • Jumonji domain Jmj • Combinatorial readout of multiple covalent histone modifications

J.R. Horton (✉) • X. Cheng
Department of Molecular and Cellular Oncology, The University of Texas -
MD Anderson Cancer Center, Houston, TX 77030, USA
e-mail: jrhorton@mdanderson.org

M. Gale • Q. Yan
Department of Pathology, Yale School of Medicine, New Haven, CT 06520, USA

© Springer International Publishing AG 2017   151
A. Kaneda, Y.-i. Tsukada (eds.), *DNA and Histone Methylation as Cancer Targets*,
Cancer Drug Discovery and Development, DOI 10.1007/978-3-319-59786-7_7

1 Introduction

Methylation occurs on arginine and lysine residues in histones and is involved in a wide range of biological processes such as gene expression, chromatin organization, dosage compensation, and epigenetic memory. Unlike acetylation, where positive charges on histones are removed, relaxing chromatin and activating genes, methylation or its removal does not affect charges on histones. Histone methylation can be transcriptionally repressive or activating, depending on the position of the methylated residue and the extent of methylation. Histone lysine residues can be monomethylated, dimethylated, or trimethylated [1], while arginine residues can be monomethylated or dimethylated symmetrically or asymmetrically [2]. The methylation of lysines 4, 36, or 79 of histone H3 is typically associated with active transcription, while the methylation of lysines 9 or 27 on histone H3 and lysine 20 on histone H4 contributes to repressed transcription. Methylation with the overall combination of other histone "marks," such as acetylation, phosphorylation, and ubiquitination, as well as the presence of other regulatory factors and DNA methylation ultimately determine chromatin conformation and expression level of the associated gene.

In order to change chromatin structure and gene expression level, histone modifications have to be altered, which can include a reversal of methylation *i.e.* demethylation. Unlike phosphorylation and acetylation, histone methylation was long regarded as irreversible partially because of the stable nature of the carbon-nitrogen bond and lack of evidence for its role in dynamic regulation of gene expression [3]. In addition, in a number of early studies, the half-life of histones and methyl-lysine residues within them appeared to be the same, implying histone methylation was not reversible [4, 5]. However, other studies seemed to show that active turnover of methyl groups did occur at a low but detectable level [6, 7]. Furthermore, in many documented cases, it appeared that different histone methylation patterns were necessary for regulation of gene expression [8].

As early as the 1960s, protein extracts containing lysine demethylase activity were identified and partially purified [9–11]. Decades later, in 2004, as evidence was mounting that histone methylation was dynamic and reversible, the first histone demethylase, a flavin-containing amine oxidase, was finally identified. Lysine-Specific Demethylase 1 (LSD1, also known as KDM1A) provided the first experimental evidence for enzymatic histone demethylation [12]. It was shown to mediate oxidative demethylation on monomethylated or dimethylated H3K4, but not trimethylated H3K4 because the enzymatic mechanism requires a protonated nitrogen [13]. Subsequently, a second and larger class of demethylases containing what was called a Jumonji C (JmjC) domain was theorized [14] and then independently identified through biochemical purification in 2005 [15]. Within a year, more JmjC demethylases were discovered in rapid succession [16–19] and even a crystal structure of a JmjC catalytic domain was published [20]. Unlike KDM1A, the JmjC proteins do not require a protonated nitrogen allowing some JmjC family members to act on trimethylated H3K4 as well [13].

Arginine methylation is also a very stable mark, but unlike lysine methylation, it is still unclear if this modification can be enzymatically reversed. Arginine residues can be monomethylated or asymmetrically or symmetrically dimethylated on R3, R8, R17, and R26 on H3, and R3 on both histones H2A and H4 [21]. A putative arginine demethylase JMJD6, a JmjC domain-containing protein, was reported to demethylate both asymmetric and symmetric H3R2me2 and H4R3me2 substrates [22]. However, others have not been able to replicate this observation and have found JMJD6 to be a lysine-hydroxylase, catalyzing C-5 hydroxylation of lysine residues in mRNA splicing-regulatory proteins and in histones with no demethylase activity on either H3R2me2 or H4R3me2 peptides [23–25]. Additionally, mutational and structural analysis of JMJD6 suggests that it is not an arginine demethylase and has a novel substrate binding groove and two positively charged surfaces with a stack of aromatic residues located near the active center not found in any JmjC oxygenase family member and may even interact with ssRNA [26, 27]. While it appears JMJD6 may play some role in regulating gene expression, there is still no clear consensus what that role is [25]. Interestingly, it has very recently reported that some JmjC demethylases are also able to demethylate histone and non-histone arginine residues *in vitro* albeit not as efficiently as histone lysine residues; a crystal structure of a known JmjC lysine demethylase (KDM4A) with an H4R3me2s containing-peptide (PDB code 5FWE) was also determined [28].

Arginine residues are not only substrates for methylation, but can also be converted to citrulline by deimination through the action of peptidylarginine deiminases [29]. Deimination has been suggested as a path for arginine demethylation but it appears that these deiminases act only on unmethylated arginines, and not on methylated arginine [30, 31]. As no enzyme has been found that converts citrulline back to arginine, methylation of arginine can only be antagonized by this modification [32].

Thus, since there are no verifiable *in vivo* arginine demethylases at this time, this chapter will only discuss histone lysine (K) demethylases (KDMs). Over the last decade, over 20 KDMs have been discovered representing two distinct classes: the KDM1 family containing two lysine-specific demethylase (LSD) enzymes, and the KDM2–7 families consisting of the JmjC domain-containing enzymes (Table 1). Each KDM demethylates only certain methylated histone residues and sometimes only certain methylated states (mono-, di-, tri) of those residues. The demethylases that primarily act on methylated H3K4 (KDM1 and KDM5) belong to the two different enzyme families; those that primarily act on other histone methylated lysines belong only to the second JmjC family.

The substrate-binding specificities of KDMs are quite diverse. The most prevalent histone lysine substrates are H3K4, H3K9, H3K27, H3K36, H4K20, and H1.4K26. In part, substrate specificity of each demethylase depends on the histone peptide sequence surrounding target lysine residues. However, another important component of KDM specificity is mediated by combinations of additional conserved "helper" domains within KDMs which can include combinations of such "helpers" as the plant homeodomain (PHD) [33], Tudor [34, 35], zinc fingers (such as zf-CXXC and zf-C2HC4) [36–38], F-box [39], AT-rich interactive domain (ARID) [40], tetratricopeptide repeat (TPR) [41] and leucine-rich region (LRR) domains [42, 43]. In addition, selectivity can be conferred by the composition and character of "linker" sequences between the catalytic and neighboring helper domain [44]. Furthermore, KDMs are part of large multimeric and dynamic complexes that contribute yet another level of specificity for gene localization and histone targeting. Finally, alternative splicing of mRNA of JmjC demethylases can lead to different isoforms. These isoforms could have different specificities and/or form different protein complexes.

Table 1 Lysine demethylase families and their histone substrates

Lysine demethylase family	Human family homologs	Common alternative homolog name(s)	Histone substrates
KDM1	KDM1A	LSD1	H3K4me2/1
	KDM1B	AOF1, LSD2	H3K4me2/1
KDM2	KDM2A	JHDM1A, FBXL11	H3K36me2/1,
	KDM2B	JHDM1B, FBXL10	H3K4me3
			H3K36me2/1
KDM3	KDM3A	JHDM2A, JMJD1A	H3K9me2/me1
	KDM3B	JHDM2B, JMJD1B	H3K9me2/me1
	KDM3C	JMJD1C	H3K9me2/me1
KDM4	KDM4A	JMJD2, JMJD2A	H3K9me3/me2,
	KDM4B	JMJD2B	H3K36me3/me2
	KDM4C	JMJD2C	H3K36me3/me2
	KDM4D	JMJD2D	H3K36me3/me2
	KDM4E	JMJD2E, KDM4DL	H3K9me3/me2,
			H3K36me3/me2/me1,
			H3K56me3
KDM5	KDM5A	JARID1A, RBP2	H3K4me3/me2
	KDM5B	JARID1B, PLU1	H3K4me3/me2
	KDM5C	JARID1C, SMCX	H3K4me3/me2
	KDM5D	JARID1D, SMCY	H3K4me3/me2
KDM6	KDM6A	UTX	H3K27me3/me2
	KDM6B	JMJD3	H3K27me3/me2
	KDM6C	UTY	H3K27me3/me2
KDM7	KDM7A	JHDM1D,	H3K9me2/me1,
	KDM7B	KIAA1718	H3K27me2/me1
	KDM7C	PHF8	H4K20me1
		PHF2	

Each of these topics must be discussed to understand our limited knowledge of the molecular basis of histone demethylation. Aberrant histone methylation caused by mutation or misregulation of histone demethylases and histone methyltransferases has been observed in several human diseases, particularly cancer. Modulation of histone methylation status for aberrant gene expression in cancers offers medicinal potential for the treatment of cancers via the development of molecular inhibitors of histone demethylases.

2   KDM1 Family Architecture and Mechanism

Unlike other KDMs, the KDM1 family utilizes the cofactor flavin adenine dinucleotide (FAD) to demethylate the methylated lysine substrate via a redox reaction (Fig. 1). The catalytic domain of the KDM1 family, the amine oxidase-like (AOD) domain, is related to the large superfamily of flavin-dependent monoamine oxidases, with MAO-A and MAO-B being the closest homologues [12]. Like other members of this

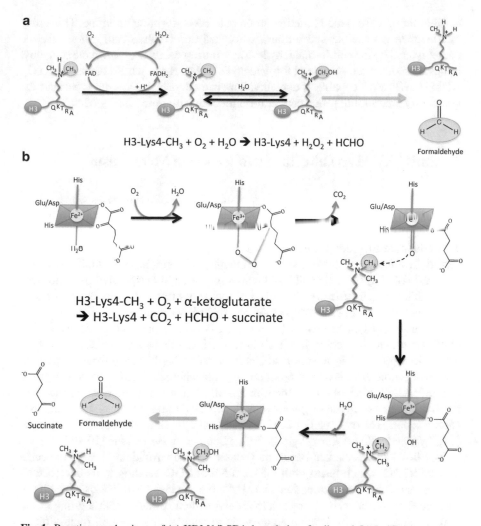

Fig. 1 Reaction mechanisms of (**a**) KDM1/LSD1 demethylase family and (**b**) JmjC demethylases

superfamily, the AOD of the two KDM1 family members can be further subdivided into two separate subdomains, with one subdomain involved in substrate binding and the other forming an expanded Rossmann fold used to bind the cofactor FAD. Each of these subdomains is formed from sequence components spread throughout the primary structure. The substrate-binding subdomain is composed of a six-stranded mixed β-sheet flanked by six α-helices. The two subdomains create a big cavity that defines the demethylase catalytic center at their interface [20, 45–47].

The FAD cofactor, binding to the KDM1A protein, undergoes two-electron reduction by substrate oxidation (Fig. 1a). The oxidized form of FAD is restored by molecular oxygen to generate hydrogen peroxide. The coupled oxidation of methyl-lysine forms a hydrolytically labile imine and $FADH_2$. Molecular oxygen is used as the electron acceptor, and methyl group oxidation is then followed via hydride transfer from the N-methyl group onto FAD, forming an imine. This imine intermediate is unstable and further hydrolyzed non-enzymatically to release the demethylated lysine and formaldehyde. Thus, during catalysis, each cycle of methyl removal produces a molecule of formaldehyde and of H_2O_2, while consuming an O_2. KDM1/LSDs are incapable of demethylating trimethyl-lysine residues, because the quaternary ammonium group cannot form the requisite imine intermediate.

3   JmjC KDM Architecture and Reaction Mechanism

The JmjC KDM family belongs to a larger superfamily of oxygenases which utilize 2-oxoglutarate (2OG) (also referred to as α-ketoglutarate or α-KG) as a co-substrate and Fe(II) as a cofactor, and couples substrate oxidation to the decarboxylation of 2-oxoglutarate to produce succinate and CO_2 (Fig. 1b). These enzymes are conserved in eukaryotes from yeast to humans [15], and have a double-stranded β-helical (DSBH) or "jelly-roll" fold consisting of eight antiparallel β-strands that form a β-sandwich structure comprised of two four-stranded antiparallel β-sheets. This structure is often referred to as the Jmj or JmjC domain.

The distorted/squashed barrel-like structure is open at one end where the octahedrally coordinated catalytic iron resides in a funnel-shaped active site with three interactions provided by a conserved His-X-Asp/Glu-X_N-His triad from the protein. The co-substrate 2OG is in a compact binding site where its 2-oxo carboxylate group also bidentately binds the iron; the iron ion also has a water molecule at the sixth position where a catalytic oxygen species is expected to reside during the demethylation reaction. The other end of 2OG interacts with the side-chain of a basic residue (Arg/Lys) and with a hydroxyl group from a Ser/Thr or Tyr residue [20, 48].

The JmjC KDM reaction begins by generating a superoxide radical by the complex Fe^{2+}/2OG, which reacts with the C2 atom of 2OG, leading to its decarboxylation to succinate and formation of a Fe^{4+}-oxo species. Afterwards, the highly reactive Fe^{4+}-oxo species abstracts a hydrogen from a lysine ζ-methyl group as the iron is reduced to Fe^{3+}, forming an unstable carbinolamine that will rapidly break down, leading to the release of formaldehyde and loss of a methyl group from the methylated lysine residue. Unlike the KDM1 family, JmjC KDMs do not require lone pair electrons on the target nitrogen atom and thereby can demethylate trimethylated as well as di- and monomethylated lysines.

JmjC demethylases bind methyl-lysine in a highly conserved pocket in the active site through the formation of a network of C–H•••O hydrogen bonds between the methyl groups and the oxygen atoms from the backbone and side chain of active-site residues. Many crystallographic studies have revealed that substrate binding often involves residues from the first and second β-strand of the DSBH, together with strands and loops that extend the JmjC domain. In contrast, "reader" domains such as PHD bind methyl-lysine through cation–π interactions between the methylammonium ion and a cage formed by multiple aromatic residues [49–51].

An additional N-terminal interaction element has been identified in many JmjC KDMs that resides at varying distances away from the JmjC domain and is referred to as the JmjN domain [20]. In KDM2A and the KDM4 and KDM5 families, it interacts extensively with the catalytic JmjC domain and provides structural integrity without participating in active site formation [17, 52–54]. However, modeling and other recent analysis suggests that the JmjN-like fold exists in all KDM families [54, 55]. Thus, the JmjN domain is not a "domain" per se, but an integral part of the catalytic core. Therefore, it should be considered that the JmjC domain in several KDM families has had additional insertions over evolution, and in one case, in the KDM5 family, other domains have been included in the insertion.

In the following sections, each KDM family is discussed individually. First, a general description of the family and its members is given which includes our present knowledge of their relationship to cancers. A table containing all known NMR and crystal structures containing a family's one or more domains, with cofactors and sometimes peptide substrates, is supplied at the end of each section. It is important to remember that a demethylase's catalytic and other domains do not act in isolation but interact with each other and many other proteins. In fact, there are three main components that confer specificity to a demethylase: the active site of its catalytic domain, the other domains that the demethylase contains, and the other proteins with which the demethylase participates in multicomponent complexes. Therefore, secondly, each of these attributes for each family will be discussed. At the end of the chapter, there will be a short review that highlights the discovery of KDM inhibitors for which the information acquired could aid in drug development.

4 The KDM1 Family

KDM1A was shown to be a histone demethylase by the Shi group in 2004 [12]. At the same time, a second human flavin-dependent histone demethylase, KDM1B, was identified through a domain homology search of genomic databases [12]. In 2009, the Mattevi laboratory isolated and confirmed the flavin-dependent demethylation activity of KDM1B, noting specificity for H3K4me1/2, despite the relatively low sequence identity to KDM1A of less than 25% [56].

The KDM1 family primarily demethylates H3K4me2 and H3K4me1. H3K4 methylation is a gene activation marker [57]. These epigenetic marks are located in open chromatin, primarily in transcription factor binding regions, including promoters and enhancers that positively regulate expression of genes and can be located many thousands of base pairs down- or upstream of a gene [58–60]. These genomic loci are commonly devoid of H3K4me3 [61]. KDM1A appears to regulate histone methylation at promoters, while KDM1B is found in transcriptional elongation complexes and removes H3K4 methyl markings in gene bodies, thereby facilitating gene expression by reducing spurious transcriptional initiation outside of promoters [62]. KDM1B is highly expressed in oocytes and is required for *de novo* DNA methylation of some imprinted genes, a function dependent on its H3K4 demethylase activity [63].

While KDM1A and KDM1B each share a SWIRM domain and a C-terminal catalytic AOD domain, these demethylases have distinct functions and domains that mediate interactions with other biomolecules (Fig. 2) [64]. The N-terminal regions

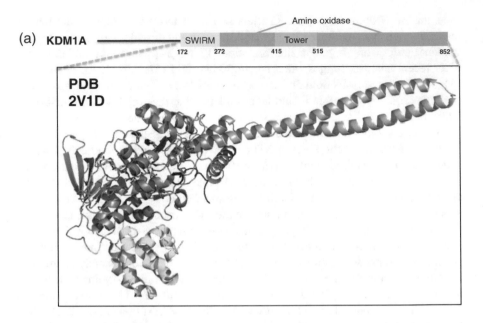

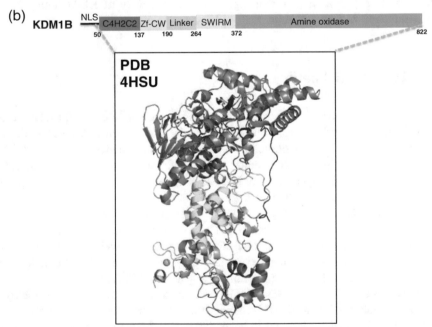

Fig. 2 Representative crystal and domain structures of (**a**) KDM1A and (**b**) KDM1B

of the KDM1 proteins have no predicted conserved structural elements, but do contain nuclear localization signals for nuclear import [63, 65, 66].

There are isoforms of KDM1A resulting from alternative splicing events [67] in which some KDM1A isoforms acquire a new substrate specificity. One of these isoforms, LSD1n, targets H4K20 methylation, both *in vitro* and *in vivo*, and is involved in neuronal activity–regulated transcription that is necessary for long-term memory formation [68]. Another isoform, LSD1 + 8a, functions as a co-activator by demethylating the repressive H3K9me2 mark. LSD1 + 8a interacts with supervillin; the LSD1 + 8a/supervillin-containing complex demethylates H3K9me2 and thereby regulates neuronal differentiation [69].

KDM1A is overexpressed and/or correlated to poor outcomes such as shorter survival, relapse, high tumor grade, and metastasis in several cancers including prostate cancer [70, 71], bladder cancer [72], neuroblastoma [73], breast cancer [74, 75], non-small cell lung cancer [76], hepatocellular cancer [77], oral cancer [78], colon cancer [79], and sarcomas [80, 81]. Knockdown or inhibition of KDM1A decreased cell growth [71–73, 77–79, 82–86] and migration/invasion [76, 78, 87, 88], as well as increased differentiation [73, 82, 83] in multiple cancer types, both solid and non-solid. The oncogenic activities of KDM1A have been studied extensively in hematological malignancies, and KDM1A was found to be a major contributor to stemness [82, 83]. KDM1A inhibitors are currently in clinical trials for the treatment of particular leukemia subtypes [89]. In contrast to other studies, one report indicates that KDM1A restrains invasion and metastasis in triple-negative breast cancer [90].

Any roles KDM1B may be playing in cancer are just beginning to be elucidated [91, 92]. KDM1B directly ubiquitylates and promotes proteasome-dependent degradation of O-GlcNAc transferase (OGT), and inhibits A549 lung cancer cell growth in a manner dependent on this E3 ligase activity, but not its demethylase activity [92].

4.1 KDM1 Active Site

It has been shown that KDM1A requires a sufficiently long peptide consisting of the first 20 N-terminal amino acids of the H3 histone tail for productive binding [93]. In contrast to many other H3K4 binding proteins where the peptide has an extended conformation, several crystal structures of KDM1A with H3 peptide show that the peptide is severely compressed and has a serpentine shape in a deep active site cavity of KDM1A [94]. The peptide binds in a funnel-shaped pocket adopting a folded conformation in which three structural elements were identified: a helical turn (residues 1–5) located in front of the flavin molecule, a sharp bend (residues 6–9), and a more extended stretch (residues 10–16) that remains partially solvent-exposed on the rim of the binding pocket. The H3 polar residues Arg2, Thr6, Arg8, Lys9 and Thr11, in addition to the N-terminal amino group, lie in well- defined pockets, forming specific and extensive electrostatic and hydrogen- bonding interactions with the surrounding KDM1A residues. The Arg2 residue of the histone H3 tail is essential for stabilization of this tail conformation in the binding site of KDM1A, due to the formation of intrapeptide hydrogen bonds with the side chain of Ser10, and main chain of Gly12 and Gly13. Any disruption of these precise interactions explains the negative effect that nearly all epigenetic modifications (away from H3K4) have on KDM1A–H3 binding [93–95].

In a KDM1B-H3K4me1(1–26) crystal structure, the H3K4me1 peptide extends away from the catalytic cavity and interacts with KDM1B at a second binding site composed of two loops within the linker region of KDM1B [46]. Biochemical analyses indicate that this second binding site is important for substrate recognition and essential for the demethylase activity of KDM1B. KDM1A lacks this second binding site.

4.2 KDM1 Helper Domains

The SWIRM domain was first found in and named after the protein subunits Swi3, Rsc8 and Moira of SWI/SNF-family chromatin remodeling complexes. SWIRM has a compact fold composed of 6 α helices, in which a 20 amino acid long helix (α4) is surrounded by 5 other short helices. The SWIRM domain structure can be divided into the N-terminal part (α1–α3) and the C-terminal part (α4–α6), which are connected to each other by a salt bridge. SWIRM domains are highly conserved amongst chromatin associating proteins and have been shown to bind DNA [96, 97]. However, the residues that compose the typical DNA-binding interface are not conserved and are partially blocked by their interaction in KDM1 proteins with the AOD [45, 98, 99]. This ~85 amino acid domain is believed to help maintain the structural integrity of KDM1 AOD and acts as an anchor site for a histone tail.

In KDM1A, the AOD domain is interrupted with the inclusion of the Tower domain that is absent from KDM1B. KDM1A was originally identified as a component of transcriptional repressor complexes [100, 101] and many of these complexes are formed through this domain. Tower is an ~100 amino acid α-helical, antiparallel coiled-coil domain. This domain is infrequently found in eukaryotic proteins, but is in many prokaryotic proteins involved with intermolecular protein recruitment, membrane docking, and membrane translocation functions [102].

KDM1B lacks a Tower domain, but does contain a novel C4H2C2-type zinc finger (ZnF) and a CW-type zinc finger (Zf-CW) [46, 47]. The ZnF domain is required for KDM1B enzymatic activity through its interaction with the SWIRM domain [103, 104]. Mutations which disrupt the ZnF domains or relays of interactions among the ZnF-SWIRM-AOD may lead to subtle conformational alterations in the AOD that in turn impair the incorporation of FAD, and consequently its enzymatic activity [104]. The surface of the C4H2C2- type zinc finger shows a marked concentration of basic residues, and thus may impact demethylase substrate specificity or positioning within nucleosomal DNA. Additionally, these residues may facilitate interactions with coregulatory molecules or serve to recruit transcriptional machinery, such as phosphorylated RNA polymerase II [62, 104].

4.3 KDM1 in Multicomponent Complexes

The Tower domain of KDM1A forms a complex with the C-terminal domain of CoREST [105], the corepressor for the transcriptional repressor RE1-Silencing Transcription factor (REST) [106–108]. KDM1A is typically associated with CoREST and required for it to demethylate nucleosome substrates. This subcomplex is found in combination with histone deacetylase (HDAC) 1 or 2, forming a stable larger core complex recruited by many chromatin remodeling multiprotein complexes [100, 101, 109–111]. The CoREST corepressor is necessary for maintaining a repressive chromatin environment in important physiological contexts like neural cell differentiation [105, 112–114].

While structural studies of KDM1A co-crystalized with an H3 substrate peptide revealed that the enzyme active site cannot productively accommodate more than three residues on the N-terminal side of the methylated K4, there is evidence *in vivo* that KDM1A demethylates other substrates. For instance, when associated with the androgen receptor (AR), KDM1A appears to remove repressive methyl groups from H3K9, thereby enhancing AR-dependent gene transcription and resulting in prostate tumor cell proliferation [71]. KDM1A may do this by binding factors that dictate its substrate specificity. Protein kinase C beta 1 (PKCB1)-mediated phosphorylation of H3 threonine-6 also has been proposed as a mechanism to block the H3K4 site and shift the specificity of KDM1A to H3K9 [115]. Recently, EHMT2 (euchromatic histone-lysine N-methyltransferase 2 or G9a) was found to methylate KDM1A at Lys114. KDM1A K114me2, but not unmethylated KDM1A peptide, specifically interacts with the CHD1 (chromodomain-helicase- DNA-binding protein 1) double chromodomain, thus indicating that CHD1 is a reader of KDM1A K114me2. Methylation of KDM1A at Lys114 by EHMT2 and recruitment of CHD1 to AR-binding regions are key events controlling chromatin binding of AR. Thus, the dimethylation of KDM1A at Lys114 appears to ultimately control AR-dependent gene expression [116].

KDM1A appears to be recruited by many CoREST-like and other proteins to form complexes that perform coregulatory or scaffolding functions [64]. In one instance, KDM1A is an integral component of the Mi-2/nucleosome remodeling and deacetylase (NuRD) complex, adding histone demethylation activity to this complex [90]. The NuRD complex contains two other catalytic subunits, the deacetylase HDAC1 and the CHD4 ATPase, both of which are essential for the regulation of gene expression and chromatin remodeling [117]. KDM1A/NuRD complexes regulate several cellular signaling pathways including TGFβ1 signaling pathway that are critically involved in cell proliferation, survival, and epithelial-to-mesenchymal transition [90].

Temporal expression patterns of specific components of KDM1A complexes modulate gene regulatory programs in mammalian development [63, 67, 118, 119]. Any interruption of these patterns, their transcriptional control and/or mutation of components can lead to cancer [64, 120] and other disease [121]. KDM1A is overexpressed in a variety of tumors, and its inactivation or downregulation can inhibit cancer progression [122, 123]. KDM1A targeting inhibitors are an avenue for anticancer drug discovery and will be discussed in a later section of this chapter.

Compared to KDM1A, there is much less known about the multicomponent complexes of KDM1B. In highly transcribed, H3K36me3-enriched coding regions downstream of gene promoters, KDM1B aids in the maintenance of H3K4 and H3K9 methylation by associating with a larger complex that includes Pol II and other elongation factors, as well as the SET-family histone methyltransferases NSD3 and G9a, which methylate histone H3K36 and H3K9 sites, respectively [62]. In addition, the H3K36me3 reader NPAC/ GLYR1 is likely part of this complex as well, which augments the KDM1B demethylation of H3K4me1/2 by binding at its AOD/SWIRM interface [47].

A recent kinetic study showed there is a tight-binding interaction between full-length unmodified histone H3 and KDM1A, which suggests the existence of a secondary binding site on the demethylase surface available for complex formation. The contact between H3 and KDM1A likely occurs through an extensive interaction interface that contributes significantly to its recognition of substrates and products [124]. Apparently, there is still much to discover about KDM1 demethylase function and its control (Table 2).

5   The KDM2 Family

The KDM2 family (Fig. 3) contains the first JmjC KDMs to be discovered and to be established as conserved in eukaryotes from yeast to humans [15]. KDM2 specifically demethylates H3K36me2, and to a lesser extent H3K36me1, which are histone modifications that are associated with transcriptional repression. There have been some indications that KDM2B is also a H3K4me3 demethylase [121], but this observation has only been made *in vivo* and not *in vitro* [135]. In some instances, one could imagine that KDM2B is in a complex with a KDM5 family member, as suggested by one study [136].

KDM2A is over-expressed and correlated to poor prognosis in breast [137, 138], non-small cell lung [139], and gastric cancer [140]. Several studies show that knockdown of KDM2A decreases cell growth [138–140], angiogenesis [138], invasion/migration [139, 140] and metastasis [140]. KDM2A promotes tumorigenicity through upregulation of target genes such as *JAG1* in breast cancer [138] and *DUSP3* in lung cancer [139]. In contrast, one study found that KDM2A knockdown had an opposite effect in breast cancer, increasing invasion, migration, and angiogenesis [141].

KDM2B is implicated in the pathology of breast cancer [142], pancreatic cancer [136], myelodysplastic syndromes [143], and acute myeloid leukemia [144]. Knockdown of KDM2B reduced cancer cell growth [136, 142, 144], as well as impaired stem cell self-renewal [142, 145] and transformation [135, 145, 146]. It is linked to senescence [135, 142, 147] and metabolism [146, 148] control. KDM2B has been shown to regulate cell cycle and senescence associated genes such as *p15* and *p16* [135, 144, 147].

5.1   KDM2 Active Site

Crystal structures of KDM2A with H3K36me2/1 peptides [53] (Table 3) reveal a narrow binding channel that can perfectly fit the specific peptide sequence H3G33 and H3G34 close to H3K36 mark. Any larger side chain in these positions would result in steric hindrance. A pocket binds Pro38 and stabilizes a sharp turn in the H3 backbone. The side chain of Tyr41 binds in a pocket on the demethylase surface through van der Waals interactions and hydrogen binding. Residues Gly33, Gly34,

Table 2 Structures containing domains of KDM1 demethylases

PDB ID	Structure title	Dep. date	Resolution (Å)	Reference
KDM1A/LSD1				
2COM	The solution structure of the SWIRM domain of human LSD1	5/18/05		[99]
2H94	Crystal structure and mechanism of human Lysine-Specific Demethylase-1	6/8/06	2.9	[45]
2IW5	Structural basis for CoREST-dependent demethylation of nucleosomes by the human LSD1 histone demethylase	6/26/06	2.57	[45]
2HKO	Crystal structure of LSD1	7/5/06	2.8	[98]
2DW4	Crystal structure of human LSD1 at 2.3 A resolution	8/2/06	2.3	[125]
2EJR	LSD1-tranylcypromine complex	3/20/07	2.7	[125]
2UXN	Structural basis of histone demethylation by LSD1 revealed by suicide inactivation	3/28/07	2.72	[126]
2UXN	Structural basis of histone demethylation by LSD1 revealed by suicide inactivation	3/28/07	2.72	
2UXX	Human LSD1 histone demethylase-CoREST in complex with an FAD- tranylcypromine adduct	3/30/07	2.74	[126]
2V1D	Structural basis of lsd1-corest selectivity in histone H3 recognition	5/23/07	3.1	[95]
2X0L	Crystal structure of a neuro-specific splicing variant of human histone lysine demethylase LSD1	12/15/09	3	[67]
3ABT	Crystal structure of LSD1 in complex with trans-2-pentafluorophenylcyclopropylamine	12/21/09	3.2	[127]
3ABU	Crystal structure of LSD1 in complex with a 2-PCPA derivative, S1201	12/21/09	3.1	[127]
2XAF	Crystal structure of LSD1-CoREST in complex with para-bromo-(+)-cis-2-phenylcyclopropyl-1-amine	3/31/10	3.25	[128]
2XAG	Crystal structure of LSD1-CoREST in complex with para-bromo-(−)-trans-2-phenylcyclopropyl-1-amine	3/31/10	3.1	[128]
2XAH	Crystal structure of LSD1-CoREST in complex with (+)-trans-2-phenylcyclopropyl-1-amine	3/31/10	3.1	[128]
2XAJ	Crystal structure of LSD1-CoREST in complex with (−)-trans-2-phenylcyclopropyl-1-amine	3/31/10	3.3	[128]
2XAQ	Crystal structure of LSD1-CoREST in complex with a tranylcypromine derivative (mc2584, 13b)	3/31/10	3.2	[128]
2XAS	Crystal structure of LSD1-CoREST in complex with a tranylcypromine derivative (mc2580, 14e)	3/31/10	3.2	[128]
2L3D	The solution structure of the short form SWIRM domain of LSD1	9/13/10		
2Y48	Crystal structure of LSD1-CoREST in complex with a n-terminal snail peptide	1/5/11	3	[129]
4BAY	Phosphomimetic mutant of LSD1-8a splicing variant in complex with CoREST	9/17/12	3.1	[119]

(continued)

Table 2 (continued)

PDB ID	Structure title	Dep. date	Resolution (Å)	Reference
3ZMS	LSD1-CoREST in complex with INSM1 peptide	2/12/13	2.96	[130]
3ZMT	LSD1-CoREST in complex with PRSFLV peptide	2/12/13	3.1	[130]
3ZMU	LSD1-CoREST in complex with PKSFLV peptide	2/12/13	3.2	[130]
3ZMV	LSD1-CoREST in complex with PLSFLV peptide	2/12/13	3	[130]
3ZMZ	LSD1-CoREST in complex with PRSFAV peptide	2/13/13	3	[130]
3ZN0	LSD1-CoREST in complex with PRSFAA peptide	2/13/13	2.8	[130]
3ZN1	LSD1-CoREST in complex with PRLYLV peptide	2/13/13	3.1	[130]
4KUM	Structure of LSD1-CoREST-Tetrahydrofolate complex	5/22/13	3.05	[131]
4CZZ	Histone demethylase LSD1(KDM1A)-CoREST3 Complex	4/23/14	3	[132]
4UV8	LSD1(KDM1A)-CoREST in complex with 1-Benzyl-Tranylcypromine	8/5/14	2.3	[133]
4UV9	LSD1(KDM1A)-CoREST in complex with 1-Ethyl-Tranylcypromine	8/5/14	3	[133]
4UVA	LSD1(KDM1A)-CoREST in complex with 1-Methyl-Tranylcypromine (1R,2S)	8/5/14	2.9	[133]
4UVB	LSD1(KDM1A)-CoREST in complex with 1-Methyl-Tranylcypromine (1S,2R)	8/5/14	2.8	[133]
4UVC	LSD1(KDM1A)-CoREST in complex with 1-Phenyl-Tranylcypromine	8/5/14	3.1	[133]
4UXN	LSD1(KDM1A)-CoREST in complex with Z-Pro derivative of MC2580	8/27/14	2.85	[133]
4XBF	Structure of LSD1:CoREST in complex with ssRNA	12/16/14	2.8	
5AFW	Assembly of methylated LSD1 and CHD1 drives AR-dependent transcription and translocation	1/26/15	1.6	[116]
5IT3	Swirm domain of human Lsd1 (A Tlx-interacting peptide)	3/16/16	1.4	
5L3B	Human LSD1/CoREST: LSD1 D556G mutation	4/6/16	3.3	[134]
5L3C	Human LSD1/CoREST: LSD1 E379K mutation	4/6/16	3.31	[134]
5L3D	Human LSD1/CoREST: LSD1 Y761H mutation	4/6/16	2.6	[134]

KDM1B/LSD2

4FWE	Native structure of LSD2 /AOF1/KDM1b in space group of C2221 at 2.13A	7/1/12	2.13	[104]
4FWF	Complex structure of LSD2/AOF1/KDM1b with H3K4 mimic	7/1/12	2.7	[104]
4FWJ	Native structure of LSD2/AOF1/KDM1b in spacegroup of I222 at 2.9A	7/1/12	2.9	[104]
4GU0	Crystal structure of LSD2 with H3	8/29/12	3.1	[46]
4GU1	Crystal structure of LSD2	8/29/12	2.94	[47]
4GUR	Crystal structure of LSD2-NPAC with H3 in space group P21	8/29/12	2.51	[47]
4GUS	Crystal structure of LSD2-NPAC with H3 in space group P3221	8/29/12	2.23	[47]
4GUT	Crystal structure of LSD2-NPAC	8/29/12	2	[47]
4GUU	Crystal structure of LSD2-NPAC with tranylcypromine	8/29/12	2.3	[47]
4HSU	Crystal structure of LSD2-NPAC with H3(1–26)in space group P21	10/30/12	1.99	[46]

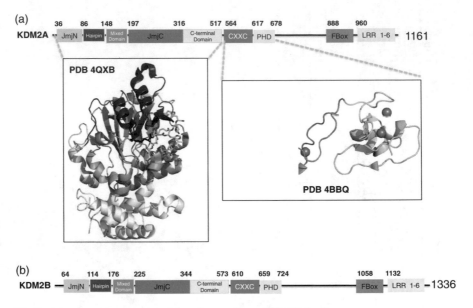

Fig. 3 Representative crystal and domain structures of KDM2 family

Table 3 Structures containing domains of KDM2 demethylases

PDB ID	Structure title	Dep. date	Resolution(Å)	Reference
KDM2A				
4BBQ	Crystal structure of the CXXC and PHD domain of human lysine-specific demethylase 2A (KDM2A)(FBXL11)	9/27/12	2.24	
4TN7	Crystal structure of mouse KDM2A-H3K36ME-NO complex with succinic acid	6/3/14	2.2	[53]
4QWN	Histone demethylase KDM2A-H3K36ME1-alpha-KG complex structure	7/16/14	2.1	[53]
4QX7	Crystal structure of histone demethylase KDM2A-H3K36me2 with alpha-KG	7/18/14	2.34	[53]
4QX8	Crystal structure of histone demethylase KDM2A-H3K36me3 complex with alpha-KG	7/19/14	1.65	[53]
4QXB	crystal structure of histone demethylase KDM2A-H3K36ME3 with NOG	7/19/14	1.6	[53]
4QXC	Crystal structure of histone demethylase KDM2A-H3K36ME2 with NOG	7/19/14	1.75	[53]
4QXH	Crystal structure of histone demethylase KDM2A-H3K36ME1 with NOG	7/20/14	2.2	[53]
KDM2B				
4O64	Human CXXC and PHD domain of KDM2B	4/16/14	2.13	–

Pro38, and Tyr41 are only found near H3K36 and such residues do not flank any other lysine methylation sites on histone H3 or H4.

Surprisingly, KDM2A bound with H3K36me3 peptide, the inactive substrate for KDM2A, could be crystallized. Comparison of structures with H3K36me3 peptide with those with substrate H3K36me2/1 peptide and/or different cofactors suggests that a third methyl group on H3K36me2 may sterically hinder an axial-to-in-plane conversion of the 2OG positioning required for catalysis [149].

5.2   KDM2 Helper Domains and Multicomponent Complexes

Both KDM2 homologs contain a zinc finger CXXC domain that specifically recognizes non-methylated CpG dinucleotides [150], seemingly targeting these histone demethylases to the so-called genomic regions known as CpG islands (CGIs; these contain a high density of CpG dinucleotides where the cytosine nucleotide is primarily not methylated) that are associated with ~70% of mammalian gene promoters and gene regulatory units [151–154]. When KDM2B recognizes non-methylated DNA in CGIs, it recruits the polycomb repressive complex 1 (PRC1) that then contributes to histone H2A Lys119 ubiquitylation (H2AK119ub1) and gene repression [155, 156]. KDM2B associates with a noncanonical PRC1 to regulate adipogenesis [157]. Furthermore, KDM2B, via its F-box domain, functions as a subunit of the CUL1-RING ubiquitin ligase (CRL1/SCF^{KDM2B}) complex where SCF is an acronym for combination of $\underline{S}$kp, $\underline{C}$ullin, $\underline{F}$-box proteins. KDM2B targets c-Fos for polyubiquitylation and regulates c-Fos protein levels [158]. Another paper suggests KDM2B has unexpected E3 ubiquitin ligase activity. The F-box in KDM2B shows E3 ligase activity *in vitro*, but has not been characterized further *in vivo* [159].

The F-box domains encoded by KDM2A and KDM2B have 78% protein sequence identity. This suggests that KDM2A may also recognize CpG through its CXXC domain and is likely to form a functional SCF E3 ligase [137]. Interestingly, KDM2A and KDM5B had the highest frequency of genetic amplification and overexpression in breast cancer among 24 KDM genes tested [137]. KDM2A had the highest correlation between copy number and mRNA expression, and high mRNA levels of KDM2A were significantly associated with shorter survival of breast cancer patients. KDM2A has two isoforms: the long isoform that is the whole protein and a short form that lacks the N-terminal JmjC domain but contains all other motifs, including the CXXC and F-box domains. It is this short form of KDM2A that has oncogenic potential and functions as an oncogenic isoform in a subset of breast cancers [137].

6   The KDM3 Family

The KDM3 family (Fig. 4) contains three members in humans, but only two, KDM3A and KDM3B, are fully verified demethylases, which act upon H3K9me2/1. The domains of the KDM3 family encompass a C2HC4 zinc finger followed by a

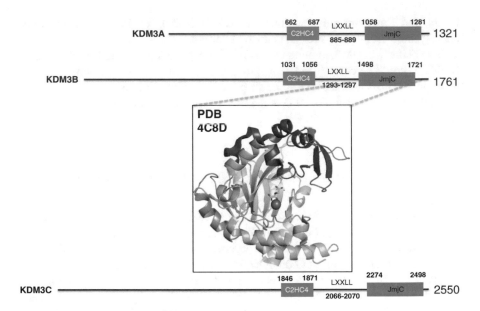

Fig. 4 Representative crystal and domain structures of KDM3 family

~225-residue long JmjC domain which shows 86% similarity between KDM3A and KDM3B. In between these domains lies a LXXLL motif known to be involved in nuclear hormone-receptor interactions [160, 161].

KDM3A is a crucial regulator of spermatogenesis, embryonic stem cell self-renewal, and metabolic gene expression. Both KDM3A and KDM3B may have roles in sex determination [162–168]. KDM3A expression is upregulated in lung cancer [169, 170], gastric cancer [171], neuroblastoma [172], Ewing sarcoma [173], bladder cancer [170], renal cell carcinoma [174], and hepatocellular carcinoma [175]. Additionally, it is implicated in the tumorigenesis of multiple myeloma [176], prostate cancer [177], and colon carcinoma [178, 179]. Knockdown or inhibition of KDM3A inhibited growth [169–171, 173, 174, 176–181] as well as migration or invasion [169, 172, 174, 179] in several tumor cell types. KDM3A was shown to control expression of several well-known proto-oncogenes including *c-Myc* [177], *HOXA1* and *CCND1* [170]. It has been shown to be regulated by hypoxia in cancers [175, 178] and to play a role in angiogenesis [180], further supported by a report that expression of KDM3A is higher in hypoxic environments and near blood vessels in renal cell carcinoma [174]. Contradictorily, one study reports that KDM3A acts as a tumor suppressor in human germ cell-derived tumors like embryonal carcinomas, seminomas, and yolk sac tumors [182].

The biological functions of KDM3B are not as well characterized. The human gene for KDM3B is located at 5q31, a chromosomal area that is often deleted in malignant myeloid disorders, including acute myeloid leukemia and myelodysplasia [183]. The enforced expression of this demethylase in a cell line carrying a 5q deletion inhibits clonogenic growth, indicating that loss of KDM3B may be involved in the pathogenesis of these cancers and that KDM3B may have tumor suppressor activities. Further strengthening its role as a tumor suppressor, high KDM3B expression was correlated to better disease-free survival after mastectomy in breast cancer patients [184]. However, contrary to the above studies, KDM3B is overexpressed in acute lymphoblastic leukemia and displays specific activity *in vitro* and *in vivo* in leukemogenesis. In this setting, it acts as a transcriptional coactivator to repress differentiation [185]. KDM3B is amplified in non-small cell lung cancer [186].

A third member of the family, KDM3C, has no verifiable demethylase activity on H3K9 peptides *in vitro*, but seems to in cells [187–189]. KDM3C inhibits the neuronal differentiation of human embryonic stem cells and has been found mutated in intracranial germline tumors [188, 190, 191]. KDM3C is reported to play a role in the maintenance of leukemias by functioning as a coactivator for key transcription factors, where its knockdown resulted in apoptosis and impaired growth of cancer cells [189, 190].

6.1   KDM3 Activity and Helper Domains

The C2HC4 zinc finger domain is required for enzymatic activity of KDM3A [192] and the demethylase appears to dimerize through interactions between this domain and the JmjC domain [193]. In addition, if one active site in the KDM3A dimer is mutated, the enzymatic activity of two-step demethylation is significantly decreased. For this KDM family, it appears that the initial conversion of H3K9me2 into H3K9me1 occurs at one active site of the dimer. After the first demethylation step is finished, allosteric regulation of substrate channeling occurs, the monomethylated substrate binds, and conversion of H3K9me1 into H3K9me0 takes place at the second site [193]. Another observation is that one residue, Thr667, contributes to the H3K9me1/2 substrate specificity of wild-type KDM3A: a T667A mutation alters specificity towards H3K9me2 [187]. Thr667 may aid in aligning the methyl group of monomethylated H3K9 correctly in the active site center, presumably bringing it in close proximity to the iron so that the reaction can be catalyzed.

While no papers discussing KDM3 crystal structures have been published, one KDM3 crystal structure has been deposited in the PDB databank (PDB: 4C8D) of the catalytic region of KDM3B (residues 1380–1720) illustrating an unusual JmjC architecture (Table 4). An N-terminal motif proceeding the JmjC domain comprises several α-helices and two three-stranded anti-parallel β-sheets that form β-extension motifs that buttress each side of the central JmjC β-barrel. One of the three-stranded β-sheets is located near the entrance of the active site, implicating it in recognizing the H3 peptide substrate.

Table 4 Structures containing domains of KDM3 demethylases

PDB ID	Structure title	Dep. date	Resolution (Å)	Reference
KDM3B				
4C8D	Crystal structure of JmjC domain of human histone 3 lysine-specific demethylase 3B (KDM3B)	9/30/13	2.18	

6.2 KDM3 in Multicomponent Complexes

Several studies have indicated that KDM3A has a role in regulating hypoxia-inducible genes through interaction with transcription factors that are targeted to KDM3A under hypoxic conditions [178, 194–197]. Hypoxic conditions have been linked to enhanced tumor growth [194]. Hypoxia is commonly found in solid tumors where the access of anticancer drugs is restricted, and the hypoxia allows for a selective environment for aggressive cancer cells [196, 198]. KDM3A has been shown to maintain some demethylase activity even under severe hypoxic conditions [199]. KDM3A exhibits hormone-dependent recruitment to androgen-receptor target genes through interaction with the androgen receptor (AR) to upregulate AR target gene expression [192].

7 The KDM4 Family

This demethylase family (Fig. 5) is probably the most examined of all the JmjC demethylase families, especially KDM4A; presently, there are over 55 crystal structures of this enzyme deposited in the PDB which includes complex structures with >20 inhibitors (Table 5, discussed below). There are many excellent published reviews [52, 200–202]. The KDM4 family has specificity for two regions of H3 with different sequences. Members act on H3K9me3/me2 and, in some cases, H3K36me3/

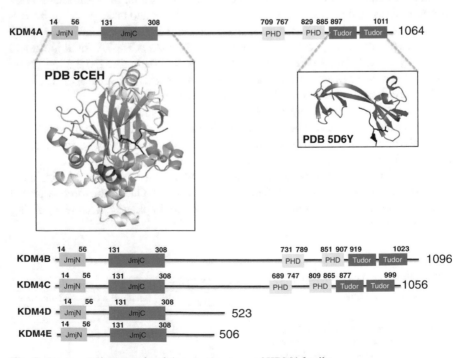

Fig. 5 Representative crystal and domain structures of KDM4 family

Table 5 Structures containing domains of KDM4 demethylases

PDB ID	Structure title	Dep. date	Resolution (Å)	Reference
KDM4A				
2GF7	Double Tudor domain structure	3/21/06	2.2	[206]
2GFA	Double Tudor domain complex structure	3/21/06	2.1	[206]
2QQR	JMJD2A hybrid Tudor domains	7/26/07	1.8	[256]
2QQS	JMJD2A tandem Tudor domains in complex with a trimethylated histone H4-K20 peptide	7/26/07	2.82	[256]
5D6W	Crystal structure of double Tudor domain of human lysine demethylase KDM4A	8/13/15	1.99	
5D6X	Crystal structure of double Tudor domain of human lysine demethylase KDM4A	8/13/15	2.15	
5D6Y	Crystal structure of double Tudor domain of human lysine demethylase KDM4A complexed with histone H3K23me3	8/13/15	2.29	
2OX0	Crystal structure of JMJD2A complexed with histone H3 peptide dimethylated at Lys9	2/19/07	1.95	[253]
2P5B	The complex structure of JMJD2A and trimethylated H3K36 peptide	3/14/07	1.99	[261]
2PXJ	The complex structure of JMJD2A and monomethylated H3K36 peptide	5/14/07	2.00	[261]
2Q8C	Crystal structure of JMJD2A in ternary complex with an histone H3K9me3 peptide and 2-oxoglutarate	6/10/07	2.05	[254]
2Q8D	Crystal structure of JMJD2A in ternary complex with histone H3-K36me2 and succinate	6/10/07	2.29	[254]
2Q8E	Specificity and mechanism of JMJD2A, a trimethyllysine-specific histone demethylase	6/10/07	2.05	[254]
2VD7	Crystal structure of JMJD2A complexed with inhibitor pyridine-2,4- dicarboxylic acid	10/1/07	2.25	[262]
2WWJ	Structure of JMJD2A complexed with inhibitor 10A	10/23/09	2.6	[263]
3NJY	Crystal structure of JMJD2A complexed with 5-carboxy-8-hydroxyquinoline	6/18/10	2.6	[264]
3PDQ	Crystal structure of JMJD2A complexed with bipyridyl inhibitor	10/23/10	1.99	[265]
2YBK	JMJD2A complexed with R-2-hydroxyglutarate	3/8/11	2.4	[266]
2YBP	JMJD2A complexed with R-2-hydroxyglutarate and histone H3K36me3 peptide (30–41)	3/9/11	2.02	[266]
2YBS	JMJD2A complexed with S-2-hydroxyglutarate and histone H3K36me3 peptide (30–41)	3/10/11	2.32	[266]
3RVH	Crystal structure of JMJD2A complexed with inhibitor 8-hydroxy-3-(piperazin-1-yl) quinoline-5-carboxylic acid	5/6/11	2.25	

(continued)

Table 5 (continued)

PDB ID	Structure title	Dep. date	Resolution (Å)	Reference
3U4S	Histone lysine demethylase JMJD2A in complex with T11C peptide substrate crosslinked to N-oxalyl-D-cysteine	10/10/11	2.15	[267]
4AI9	JMJD2A complexed with daminozide	2/8/12	2.25	[268]
4GD4	Crystal structure of JMJD2A complexed with inhibitor, 2-(1H-pyrazol-3-yl)pyridine-4-carboxylic acid	7/31/12	2.33	
4BIS	JMJD2A complexed with 8-hydroxyquinoline-4-carboxylic acid	4/12/13	2.49	[269]
4URA	Crystal structure of human JMJD2A in complex with compound 14a	6/27/14	2.23	
4V2V	JMJD2A complexed with Ni(II), NOG and histone H3K27me3 peptide (25–29) ARK(me3)SA	10/15/14	2	[270]
4V2W	JMJD2A complexed with Ni(II), NOG and histone H3K27me3 peptide (16–35)	10/15/14	1.81	[270]
5A7N	Crystal structure of human JMJD2A in complex with compound 43	7/9/15	2.39	[271]
5A7O	Crystal structure of human JMJD2A in complex with compound 42	7/9/15	2.15	[271]
5A7P	Crystal structure of human JMJD2A in complex with compound 36	7/9/15	2.28	[271]
5A7Q	Crystal structure of human JMJD2A in complex with compound 30	7/9/15	2	[271]
5A7S	Crystal structure of human JMJD2A in complex with compound 44	7/9/15	2.2	[271]
5A7W	Crystal structure of human JMJD2A in complex with compound 35	7/10/15	2.27	[271]
5A80	Crystal structure of human JMJD2A in complex with compound 40	7/11/15	2.28	[271]
5ANQ	Inhibitors of JumonjiC domain-containing histone demethylases	9/7/15	2	[272]
5F2S	Crystal structure of human KDM4A in complex with compound 15	12/2/15	2.08	[273]
5F2W	Crystal structure of human KDM4A in complex with compound 16	12/2/15	2.6	[273]
5F32	Crystal structure of human KDM4A in complex with compound 40	12/2/15	2.05	[273]
5F37	Crystal structure of human KDM4A in complex with compound 58	12/2/15	2.22	[273]
5F39	Crystal structure of human KDM4A in complex with compound 37	12/2/15	2.65	[273]
5F3C	Crystal structure of human KDM4A in complex with compound 52d	12/2/15	2.06	[273]
5F3E	Crystal structure of human KDM4A in complex with compound 54a	12/2/15	2.16	[273]
5F3G	Crystal structure of human KDM4A in complex with compound 53a	12/2/15	2.5	[273]
5F3I	Crystal structure of human KDM4A in complex with compound 54j	12/2/15	2.24	[273]
5FPV	Crystal structure of human JMJD2A in complex with compound KDOAM20A	12/3/15	2.44	[274]

5F5I	Crystal structure of human JMJD2A complexed with KDOOA011340	12/4/15	2.63	[273]
5FWE	JMID2A complexed with Ni(II), NOG and histone H4(1–15)R3me2s peptide	2/15/16	2.05	
5FY8	Crystal structure of human JMJD2A in complex with D-threo-isocitrate	3/4/16	2.34	
5FYC	Crystal structure of human JMJD2A in complex with succinate	3/7/16	2.26	
5FYH	Crystal structure of human JMJD2A in complex with fumarate	3/7/16	2.35	
5FYI	Crystal structure of human JMJD2A in complex with pyruvate	3/7/16	2.1	
KDM4B				
4LXL	Crystal structure of JMJD2B complexed with pyridine-2,4-dicarboxylic acid and H3K9me3	7/30/13	1.87	
4UC4	Crystal structure of hybrid Tudor domain of human lysine demethylase KDM4B	8/13/14	2.56	
KDM4C				
2XDP	Crystal structure of the Tudor domain of human JMJD2C	5/6/10	1.56	
2XML	Crystal structure of human JMJD2C catalytic domain	7/28/10	2.55	[252]
4XDO	Crystal structure of human KDM4C catalytic domain with OGA	12/19/14	1.97	[275]
4XDP	Crystal structure of human KDM4C catalytic domain bound to tris	12/19/14	2.07	[275]
5FJH	Crystal structure of human JMJD2C catalytic domain in complex with epitheraputic compound 2-(((2-((2-(dimethylamino)ethyl) (ethyl)amino) -2-oxoethyl)amino)methyl)isonicotinic acid	10/9/15	2.1	
5FJK	Crystal structure of human JMJD2C catalytic domain in complex 6-ethyl- 5-methyl-7-oxo-4,7-dihydropyrazolo(1,5-a)pyrimidine-3-carbonitrile			
KDM4D				
3DXT	Crystal structure of the catalytic core domain of JMJD2D	7/25/08	1.8	
3DXU	The crystal structure of core JMJD2D complexed with FE and N-oxalylglycine	7/25/08	2.2	
4HON	Crystal structure of human JMJD2D/KDM4D in complex with an H3K9me3 peptide and 2-oxoglutarate	10/22/12	1.8	[276]
4HOO	Crystal structure of human JMJD2D/KDM4D apoenzyme	10/22/12	2.49	[276]
4D6Q	Crystal structure of human JMJD2D in complex with 2,4-PDCA	11/14/14	1.29	
4D6R	Crystal structure of human JMJD2D in complex with N-oxalylglycine and bound o-toluenesulfonamide	11/14/14	1.4	
4D6S	Crystal structure of human JMJD2D in complex with N-oxalylglycine and bound 5,6-dimethylbenzimidazole	11/14/14	1.4	
5F5A	Crystal structure of human JMJD2D complexed with KDOAM16	12/4/15	1.41	[273]
5F5C	Crystal structure of human JMJD2D complexed with KDOPP7	12/4/15	1.88	[273]

(continued)

Table 5 (continued)

PDB ID	Structure title	Dep. date	Resolution (Å)	Reference
5FP3	Crystal structure of human JMJD2D complexed with 3-(4-phenylbutanamido)pyridine-4-carboxylic acid	11/27/15	2.05	[277]
5FP4	Crystal structure of human KDM4D in complex with 3-(4- phenylbutanamido)pyridine-4-carboxylic acid	11/27/15	2	[277]
5FP8	Crystal structure of human KDM4D in complex with 3-4-methylthiophen-2- ylmethylaminopyridine-4- carboxylic acid	11/27/15	1.98	[277]
5FP9	Crystal structure of human KDM4D in complex with 3-aminopyridine-4- carboxylic acid(w/S-oxy cysteine)	11/27/15	2	[277]
5FPA	Crystal structure of human KDM4D in complex with 3H,4H-pyrido-3,4-d- pyrimidin-4-one	11/27/15	1.96	[277]
5FPB	Crystal structure of human KDM4D in complex with 2-1H-pyrazol-4-yloxy- 3H,4H-pyrido-3,4-d-pyrimidin-4-one	11/27/15	1.91	[277]

me2. H3K9me3 demethylation promotes an open chromatin state, contributing to the transcriptional activation of promoter regions [200]. KDM4A and KDM4B occupancy is fairly evenly distributed across different genomic regions, while KDM4C localizes predominantly to H3K4me3-containing promoter regions [203–205].

In humans, this family contains five known members. The KDM4A-C proteins share more than 50% sequence identity; each contains JmjN, JmjC, two plant homeodomains (PHD) and two hybrid Tudor domains that form a bilobal structure, with each lobe resembling a normal Tudor domain. KDM4D and KDM4E, in contrast, are considerably shorter proteins that lack the C-terminal region, including the PHD and Tudor domains [17, 52]. Biochemical studies indicate that KDM4A-C catalyze the removal of H3K9 and H3K36 di- and trimethyl marks. However, *in vivo*, KDM4A seems to demethylate only trimethylated residues [19] and has a greater affinity for H3K9me3 over H3K36me3 [16, 20, 206]. KDM4D can only demethylate H3K9me3/me2 [17, 52]. KDM4E meanwhile, catalyzes the removal of two methyl groups from H3K9me3 and also H3K56me3 [207, 208].

The KDM4 family members are associated with cancer in several ways, summarized for most family members below (reviewed in [52, 200, 201, 209]). Several members are involved in hypoxia [210, 211] and DNA mismatch repair [212]. KDM4A, B, and C are required for the survival of acute myeloid leukemia cells [213].

KDM4A expression is upregulated and/or correlates to poor outcomes in many cancers including breast [214, 215], prostate [17, 216, 217], lung [218–220], bladder [220], gastric [221], and endometrial carcinoma [222, 223]. KDM4A overexpression led to the development of prostatic intraepithelial neoplasia, and combined overexpression of KDM4A and ETV1 resulted in prostate carcinoma formation in *Pten*[+/−] mice [217]. Furthermore, overexpression of KDM4A has been shown to cause localized copy gains and DNA re-replication in tumor cells [224]. Knockdown or knockout of KDM4A inhibits growth [217, 221–223, 225–228], migration/invasion [222, 223, 227], and metastasis [87] in several cancer models, and provokes apoptosis [218, 221, 226] and senescence [219]. KDM4A regulates target genes such as *p27* [223], *YAP1* (*yes-associated protein 1*) [217], *ARHI* (*aplasia Ras homolog member I*) [215], *CHD5* (*chromodomain helicase DNA-binding domain 5*), and activating protein 1 (AP1) family genes [87]. It is associated with cancer-related proteins such as the androgen receptor (AR) [223], p53 [226], and SIRT2 (sirtuin 2) [228].

KDM4B is overexpressed and correlates to adverse outcomes in many cancers including endometrial cancer [223], luminal breast cancer [214], colorectal cancer [229], bladder [230], lung [230], prostate [17, 231], gastric [232–234], hepatocellular carcinoma [235], and osteosarcoma [236]. Knockdown of KDM4B inhibits growth [211, 225, 229, 230, 232, 237–239], migration/invasion [223, 229, 233], and metastasis [233], and induced DNA damage [239] and apoptosis [232, 239, 240]. It is known to associate with nuclear receptors to drive cancers such as AR [223, 231] and ERα (estrogen receptor α) [211, 237, 238], regulating target genes such as *c-Myc* [223], *CDK6* (*cyclin-dependent kinase 6*) [230], and ERα target genes such as *CCND1* [211, 237].

KDM4C is amplified in basal-like breast cancer [214, 241], esophageal squamous cell carcinomas [242], sarcomatoid lung carcinoma [243], lymphomas [244], and medulloblastoma [245, 246]. Likewise, it is overexpressed and/or associated with negative patient outcomes in basal-like breast cancer [214], esophageal squamous cell carcinoma [242], prostate cancer [17], osteosarcoma [236], and esophageal squamous cell carcinoma [247]. KDM4C knockdown or inhibition prevents growth of several cancer types [17, 210, 244, 248], as well as breast cancer metastasis to the lung [210]. Overexpression of KDM4C was able to transform normal-like breast epithelial cells [241]. KDM4C was reported to interact with HIF1α (hypoxia inducible factor 1 α) [210] and FGF2 (fibroblast growth factor 2) [236], as well as to target p53 pathway gene *MDM2* (mouse double minute 2 homolog) [249]. In contrast, one study reports that KDM4C expression is associated with improved breast cancer survival and response to therapy [250]. KDM4D is overexpressed in basal-like breast cancer [214]. KDM4D knockdown blocked the proliferation of colon cancer cells, but surprisingly, KDM4D was shown to bind p53 and activate *p21* expression [251].

7.1   KDM4 Active Site

Binding specificity in KDM4 members originates from amino acids surrounding lysines 9 and 36 on histone H3, whereas space and electrostatic environment in the methyl group–binding pocket of these enzymes allow for di- and trimethyl and not the monomethylated lysine residues to position a methyl group productively toward the Fe^{2+} atom in the catalytic center. Crystal structures and modeling punctuates the importance of certain residues in KDM4 demethylases for defining H3K36me3 recognition [225]. In KDM4A and KDM4B, residues Ile71, Asn86, and Asp135 engage in van der Waals interactions or hydrogen bonds with H3 residues H39 and R40 on the C-terminal side of H3K36me3 while the side chains of Leu75, His90, and Asp139 in KDM4D cannot avoid steric clashes with H39 and R40. The crystal structure of the KDM4D-peptide complex also shows that the R42 side chain of H3 lies in close proximity to Lys91 and Lys92 on the surface of KDM4D, resulting in potential electrostatic repulsion between the enzyme and H3K36me3 peptide. In KDM4A, the corresponding residues, Ile87 and Gln88, possess uncharged side chains, alleviating this electrostatic repulsion. Ile71, Asn86, Ile87, and Gln88 in KDM4A are strictly conserved in KDM4B and KDM4C and mutations of these residues to the corresponding amino acids in KDM4D and KDM4E (i.e., I71L, N86H, I87K, and Q88K) disrupt H3K36me3 demethylation *in vitro* and *in vivo* [252].

In KDM4A-C, the C–H•••O hydrogen-bonding network in the active site places one of the three methyl groups of the trimethylated lysine close to the Fe^{2+} and in an ideal position for catalysis. When dimethylated or monomethylated lysines bind at the active site, the methyl groups are sequestered away from the metal ion by C–H•••O hydrogen bonds. Therefore, the catalysis-competent methyl position is energetically disfavored. For a dimethylated lysine, a rotational movement could allow one of the methyl groups to gain access to Fe^{2+} for catalysis, probably with less efficiency than a trimethylated lysine [253, 254]. A monomethylated lysine would be completely sequestered and cannot reach the proper positioning for catalysis. Ser288 (whose hydroxyl group forms C–H•••O hydrogen bonds with methyl groups) is frequently substituted by Ala in other JmjC demethylases, such as KDM4D and KDM6A (A1238). The substitution of Ser288 in KDM4A with Ala enhances its activity, especially on dimethylated substrates, indicative of this residue's role in the determination of the methylation state specificity [20, 254].

7.2   KDM4 Helper Domains

The functions of the two PHD domains in KDM4A-C remain unknown. However, it appears that differential tandem Tudor domain (TTD) binding properties across the KDM4 demethylase family may distinguish the targets of the KDM4 family in the genome. The TTD domain has two shared β-strands that interdigitate to form a bilobal structure, with each lobe resembling a normal Tudor domain. The KDM4A TTD recognizes both H3K4me3 and H4K20me3 [206, 255, 256], while the KDM4B TTD binds methylated H4K20 [257], and the KDM4C TTD is specialized to recognize only methylated H3K4 [203, 258]. In the crystal structure of the KDM4A TTD, the second Tudor domain uses a cluster of aromatic residues, Phe932, Trp967 and Tyr973, to establish an open cage pocket for binding the side chain of H3K4me3 or H4K20me3 while the side chains of the other Tudor domain form intermolecular contacts [206]. However, the H3 and H4 peptides contact the Tudor domains in opposite orientations and at different surfaces of the second hybrid Tudor domain, while the side chains of the other Tudor domain form intermolecular contacts [35, 259].

7.3   KDM4 in Multicomponent Complexes

Recall that H3K4 trimethylation is a hallmark of active promoters that are usually devoid of H3K9 trimethylation, a mark of inactive chromatin. Through its Tudor domain, KDM4A could be recruited to active gene promoters where it would demethylate H3K9 ensuring amplification of gene transcription. As one example of a KDM4 family member in an epigenetic modifying complex, KDM4B is physically associated with and an integral component of the H3K4 methyltransferase mixed-lineage leukemia 2 (MLL2) complex [238]. This complex could potentially be a Tudor domain-independent instance (possibly through PHD) in which KDM4B can simultaneously demethylate H3K9 while H3K4 becomes trimethylated. This KDM4B/MLL2 complex co-purifies with estrogen receptor α (ERα) and is required for ERα-regulated transcription [238]. ERα exhibits greater stability when KDM4B is overexpressed, and ERα can upregulate KDM4B. This creates a positive feedback loop between these two molecules to amplify the estrogen signal [260]. A similar mechanism has been proposed for AR signaling [231]. In this manner, KDM4B has an oncogenic role in both breast and prostate cancers. Another report finds KDM4B and KDM4C work distinctly and combinatorially in different multicomponent complexes in embryonic stem cells that affect their differentiation [204].

8   The KDM5 Family

The human KDM5 family (Fig. 6 and Table 6), specific for the demethylation of
H3K4me3/2, encompasses four enzymes: KDM5A/JARID1A/RBP2 (retinoblas-
toma-binding protein 2), KDM5B/JARID1B/PLU-1, KDM5C/JARID1C/SMCX
(selected mouse cDNA on the X), and KDM5D/JARID1D/SMCY (selected mouse
cDNA on the Y) [278]. KDM5 members show a high degree of homology in
sequence and domain organization [54, 279]. In addition to the catalytic JmjC
domain, each contains a JmjN domain, an ARID DNA-binding motif, two or three
PHD finger domains and a C5CH2-type zinc finger domain. The KDM5 family is
unique among JmjC-containing histone demethylases in that there are identifiable
domains, the ARID and PHD, between the JmjN and JmjC. Despite the fact that all
members of KDM5 catalyze the demethylation of the same histone mark, they
appear to have exclusive functional properties probably because of their different
expression profiles and presence in distinct protein complexes [278, 279].

   This family of KDMs is the only one to demethylate the H3K4me3 mark.
In genome-wide studies, this mark broadly correlates with RNA polymerase II occupancy at sites of active gene expression, and is thought to provide an additional layer
of transcriptional regulation. H3K4me3 is known to be associated with transcriptionally active genes or in combination with repressive histone marks [280], such as
H3K27me3, at the promoters and transcriptional start sites at the 5′-end of important
developmental genes [280, 281], keeping them in the "poised for activation" state.

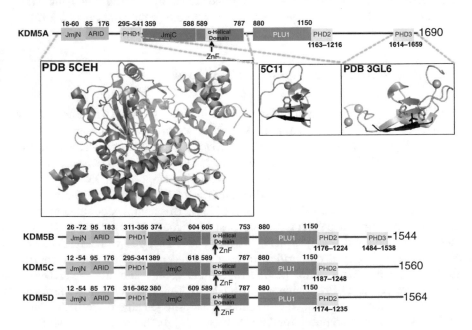

Fig. 6 Representative crystal and domain structures of KDM5 family

Table 6 Structures containing domains of KDM5 demethylases

PDB ID	Structure title	Dep. date	Resolution (Å)	Reference
KDM5A				
2JXJ	NMR structure of the ARID domain from the histone H3K4 demethylase RBP2	11/20/07		
2KGG	Crystal structure of JARID1A-PHD3 complexed with H3(1–9)K4me3 peptide	3/11/09	1.9	[325]
2KGI	Solution structure of JARID1A C-terminal PHD finger in complex with H3(1–9)K4me3	3/12/09		[325]
3GL6	Crystal structure of JARID1A-PHD3 complexed with H3(1–9)K4me3 peptide	3/11/09	1.9	[325]
5C11	Crystal Structure of JARID1A PHD finger bound to histone H3C4me3 peptide	6/12/15	2.8	
5CEH	Structure of histone lysine demethylase KDM5A in complex with selective inhibitor	7/6/15	3.14	[283]
5E6H	A linked Jumonji domain of the KDM5A lysine demethylase	10/9/15	2.24	[54]
5IVJ	Linked KDM5A Jmj domain bound to the inhibitor N11 [3-({1-[2-(4,4-difluoropiperidin-1-yl)ethyl]-5-fluoro-1H-indazol-3-yl}amino)pyridine-4-carboxylic acid]			[282]
5IVV	Linked KDM5A Jmj domain bound to the inhibitor N12 [3-((1-methyl-1H-pyrrolo[2,3-b]pyridin-3-yl)amino)isonicotinic acid]			[282]
5IVY	Linked KDM5A Jmj domain bound to the inhibitor N16 [3-(2-(4-chlorophenyl)acetamido)isonicotinic acid]			[282]
5IW0	Linked KDM5A Jmj domain bound to the inhibitor N19 [2-(5-((4-chloro-2-methylbenzyl)oxy)-1H-pyrazol-1-yl)isonicotinic acid]			[282]
5IVB	A high resolution structure of a linked KDM5A Jmj domain with alpha-ketoglutarate			[282]
5IVC	Linked KDM5A Jmj domain bound to the inhibitor N3 (4'-[(2-phenylethyl)carbamoyl][2,2'-bipyridine]-4-carboxylic acid)			[282]
5IVE	Linked KDM5A Jmj domain bound to the inhibitor N8 (5-methyl-7-oxo-6-(propan-2-yl)-4,7-dihydropyrazolo[1,5-a]pyrimidine-3-carbonitrile)			[282]
5IVF	Linked KDM5A Jmj domain bound to the inhibitor N10 8-(1-methyl-1H-imidazol-4-yl)-2-(4,4,4-trifluorobutoxy)pyrido[3,4-d]pyrimidin-4-ol			[282]
KDM5B				
2EQY	Solution structure of the ARID domain of Jarid1b protein	03/30/07		
2MA5	Solution NMR structure of PHD type zinc finger domain of lysine-specific demethylase 5B (PLU-1/ JARID1B) from *Homo sapiens*, Northeast Structural Genomics Consortium (NESG) Target HR7375C	6/28/13		
2MNY	NMR structure of KDM5B PHD1 finger	4/16/14		[322]

Table 6 (continued)

PDB ID	Structure title	Dep. date	Resolution (Å)	Reference
2MNZ	NMR structure of KDM5B PHD1 finger in complex with H3K4me0(1-10aa)	4/16/14		[322]
5A1F	Crystal structure of the catalytic domain of PLU1 in complex with N-oxalylglycine	4/29/15	2.1	[274]
5A3N	Crystal structure of human PLU-1 (JARID1B) in complex with KDOAM25a	6/2/15	2	
5A3P	Crystal structure of the catalytic domain of human PLU1 (JARID1B)	6/2/15	2.01	[274]
5A3T	Crystal structure of human PLU-1 (JARID1B) in complex with KDM5-C49 (2-(((2-((2-(dimethylamino) ethyl)(ethyl)amino)-2-oxoethyl)amino)methyl) isonicotinic acid)	6/2/15	1.9	[274]
5A3W	Crystal structure of human PLU-1 (JARID1B) in complex with pyridine-2, 6-dicarboxylic acid (PDCA)	6/3/15	2	[274]
5FPL	Crystal structure of human JARID1B in complex with CCT363901	12/2/15	2.35	[274]
5FPU	Crystal structure of human JARID1B in complex with GSKJ1	12/3/15	2.24	[274]
5FUN	Crystal structure of human JARID1B in complex with GSK467	1/28/16	2.5	[274]
5FUP	Crystal structure of human JARID1B in complex with 2-oxoglutarate	1/28/16	2.15	[274]
5FV3	Crystal structure of human JARID1B construct c2 in complex with N- oxalylglycine	2/2/16	2.37	[274]
5FYT	Crystal structure of the catalytic domain of human JARID1B in complex with 3D fragment (5-fluoro-2-oxo-2,3-dihydro-1H-indol-3-yl)acetic acid (N09996a)	3/9/16	1.87	
5FYU	Crystal structure of the catalytic domain of human JARID1B in complex with 3D fragment 3-amino-4-methyl-1,3-dihydro-2H-indol-2-one (N10042a)	3/9/16	2.06	
5FYY	Crystal structure of the catalytic domain of human JARID1B in complex with N05798a	3/10/16	2.18	
5FYZ	Crystal structure of the catalytic domain of human JARID1B in complex with 3D fragment 2-(2-oxo-2,3-dihydro-1H-indol-3-yl)acetonitrile (N10063a)	3/10/16	1.75	
5FZ0	Crystal structure of the catalytic domain of human JARID1B in complex with N11213a	3/10/16	2.42	
5FZ1	Crystal structure of the catalytic domain of human JARID1B in complex with Maybridge fragment 2,4-dichloro-N-pyridin-3-ylbenzamide (E481115b) (ligand modeled based on PANDDA event map)	3/10/16	2.39	
5FZ3	Crystal structure of the catalytic domain of human JARID1B in complex with Maybridge fragment 3,6-Dihydroxybenzonorbornane (N087776b) (ligand modelled based on PANDDA event map)	3/10/16	2.5	
5FZ4	Crystal structure of the catalytic domain of human JARID1B in complex with 3D fragment (3R)-1-[(3-phenyl-1,2,4-oxadiazol-5-yl)methyl]pyrrolidin-3-ol (N10057a) (ligand modelled based on PANDDA event map, SGC - Diamond I04-1 fragment screening)	3/10/16	2.07	

5FZ6	Crystal structure of the catalytic domain of human JARID1B in complex with Maybridge fragment N05859b (ligand modelled based on PANDDA event map, SGC - Diamond I04-1 fragment screening)	3/11/16	2.33	
5FZ7	Crystal structure of the catalytic domain of human JARID1B in complex with Maybridge fragment ethyl 2-amino-4-thiophen-2-ylthiophene-3- carboxylate (N06131b) (ligand modelled based on PANDDA event map, SGC - Diamond I04-1 fragment screening)	3/11/16	2.3	
5FZ9	Crystal structure of the catalytic domain of human JARID1B in complex with Maybridge fragment thieno(3,2-b)thiophene-5-carboxylic acid (N06263b) (ligand modelled based on PANDDA event map, SGC - Diamond I04-1 fragment screening)	3/12/16	2.06	
5FZA	Crystal structure of the catalytic domain of human JARID1B in complex with 3D fragment 2-piperidin-4-yloxy-5-(trifluoromethyl)pyridine (N10072a) (ligand modelled based on PANDDA event map)	3/12/16	2.1	
5FZB	Crystal structure of the catalytic domain of human JARID1B in complex with Maybridge fragment 4-Pyridylthiourea (N06275b) (ligand modelled based on PANDDA event map, SGC - Diamond I04-1 fragment screening)	3/12/16	2.18	
5FZC	Crystal structure of the catalytic domain of human JARID1B in complex with Maybridge fragment 4,5-dihydronaphtho(1,2-b)thiophene-2- carboxylicacid (N11181a) (ligand modelled based on PANDDA event map, SGC - Diamond I04-1 fragment screening)	3/14/16	2.05	
5FZH	Crystal structure of the catalytic domain of human JARID1B in complex with Maybridge fragment 4,5-dihydronaphtho(1,2-b)thiophene-2- carboxylicacid (N11181a) (ligand modelled based on PANDDA event map, SGC - Diamond I04-1 fragment screening)	3/14/16	2.09	
5FZK	Crystal structure of the catalytic domain of human JARID1B in complex with 3D fragment N,3-dimethyl-N-(pyridin-3-ylmethyl)-1,2-oxazole-5- carboxamide (N10051a) (ligand modelled based on PANDDA event map, SGC - Diamond I04-1 fragment screening)	3/14/16	2.05	
5FZL	Crystal structure of the catalytic domain of human JARID1B in complex with 3D fragment 3-methyl-N-pyridin-4-yl-1,2-oxazole-5-carboxamide (N09954a) (ligand modelled based on PANDDA event map, SGC - Diamond I04-1 fragment screening)	3/14/16	2.55	
KDM5C				
2JRZ	Solution structure of the Bright/ARID domain from the human JARID1C protein	07/10/2007		[329]
5FWJ	Crystal structure of human JARID1C in complex with KDM5-C49	2/17/16	2.1	[274]
KDM5D				
2E6R	Solution structure of the PHD domain in SmcY protein	07/03/2007		
2YQE	Solution structure of the ARID domain of JARID1D protein	04/01/2008		

Recently, crystal structures of truncated KDM5A, KDM5B, and KDM5C proteins have been determined [54, 274, 282, 283]. In truncated KDM5 proteins, the ARID and PHD1 domains between JmjN and JmjC are dispensable to activity, while the C5HC2 zinc finger motif is required for its *in vivo* [284] and *in vitro* activity [54, 274]. The active KDM5A and KDM5B structures showed that the domain arrangement of this KDM family most closely resembles that of KDM6, despite the fact that the catalytic domain shares the greatest sequence identity with the KDM4 family (33%). The fold of the catalytic JmjC domain is highly conserved with that of KDM6A (PDB ID 3AVS; r.m.s. deviation = 0.46 Å over 107 Cα) and other JmjC demethylases, despite the fact that this region retains only 16% sequence identity with KDM6A. There is a C-terminal helical domain composed of four helices, and a zinc finger C5HC2 motif was found, similar to the GATA-like motif in the KDM6 family (see below).

KDM5 family enzymes have been studied in several types of cancer and cancer processes (for reviews, please see [278, 279]). KDM5A and KDM5B are reported to be amplified or overexpressed in many cancers, and have been shown to play key roles in cancer cell proliferation, drug resistance and metastasis. KDM5A is amplified or over-expressed in several cancers including breast [285], lung [286, 287], hepatocellular [288], and gastric [289, 290] cancers. It is linked to proliferation and senescence control by antagonizing the functions of retinoblastoma protein (pRB) [291–293] and suppressing the expression of cyclin-dependent kinase inhibitor genes such as *p21*, *p27*, and *p16* [286, 288, 289]. In three different genetically-engineered mouse tumor models, knockout of KDM5A significantly prolonged survival [293, 294]. KDM5A has also been shown to play a role in epithelial-mesenchymal transition [287, 295], invasion [286, 294], and metastasis [294, 296]. Additionally, expression of KDM5A is implicated in anti-cancer drug resistance in lung cancer [297], breast cancer [285], and glioblastoma [298].

KDM5B is reported to be overexpressed in breast [284, 299], lung [300], bladder [301], diffuse large B-cell lymphoma [302], prostate [303], colorectal [304], glioma [305], ovarian [306], and hepatocellular [307, 308] cancers. KDM5B has been shown to repress expression of tumor suppressor genes such as *BRCA1* and *HOXA5*, as well as cell cycle checkpoint genes such as *p15*, *p27*, and *p21* [284, 305, 307, 309]. Furthermore, KDM5B expression is linked to stem cell-like properties and resistance to a targeted therapy in melanoma [310, 311]. Many recent studies link expression of KDM5B to poor prognosis, chemoresistance, and metastasis in a variety of cancers [306, 308, 312–315].

Several studies indicate that KDM5 enzymes may have tumor suppressive functions in particular contexts. Breast cancer patients with high expression of KDM5A had a better response to docetaxel [184]. Migration and invasion are suppressed in triple negative breast cancer cells when KDM5B is artificially overexpressed [316]. Finally, KDM5C and KDM5D are inactivated or deleted in renal cell carcinoma [317] and prostate cancer [318], respectively. KDM5C knockdown significantly increased growth of renal cell carcinoma cells in a xenograft model [319].

8.1 KDM5 Active Site

Modeling places a trimethylated lysine residue in the active site of KDM5A, surrounded on four sides by Trp470, Tyr472, Asn585, and the metal-ligand water molecule. The aromatic indole ring of Trp470 would be in parallel with the hydrophobic portion of the target lysine. The side chains of Tyr472 and Asn585 would each coordinate one methyl group, whereas the third methyl group would be in close proximity to a metal ligand-coordinated water molecule. During the catalytic cycle, this site would be occupied by the dioxygen O_2 molecule that initiates the demethylation reaction by abstracting a hydrogen atom from the substrate.

8.2 KDM5 Helper Domains

The ARID domain binds double-stranded DNA and may be involved in anchoring KDM5 proteins onto linear or nucleosome-wrapped nucleic acid [303, 320, 321]. In the KDM5A structure containing an ARID domain [283], the domain adopts the canonical fold but differs slightly in its loop conformations compared to the NMR structure of the isolated KDM5A ARID domain [320] and may block part of the substrate binding site, suggesting that ARID-PHD1 may interfere with substrate binding until interaction with nucleosome.

The PHD1 domains of both KDM5A and KDM5B have been shown to bind to unmodified H3K4me0 [316, 322–324], whereas both of their PHD3 domains have been shown to bind to H3K4me3 [316, 325]. Though KDM5B's PHD3 domain favors binding to H3K4me3, it will also bind to lower methylation states of H3K4 [316, 325]. The PHD2 domain of KDM5B apparently does not recognize histone [316]. Of note, binding of the PHD1 domain of KDM5D to H3K4me0 is ~30X weaker than that of KDM5B, even though their sequences are very similar. This is likely because the Leu326 residue in the KDM5B sequence is replaced by a phenylalanine in KDM5D, where this bulky side chain may cause steric hindrance and obstruct this interaction with a peptide [316]. The binding of these PHD domains to both the substrate and the product of KDM5 demethylases may seem unusual. Yet, binding of PHD1 to H3K4me0 may provide an anchoring mechanism for KDM5A/B to sense H3K4me3 through PHD3 and slide along the H3K4me3-enriched promoters, demethylating other nearby methylated H3K4 and further spreading the transcriptionally inactive state of chromatin. Interestingly, such a model was proposed in one of the first papers to identify that a KDM5 family member is capable of erasing methyl groups of trimethylated H3K4 [326].

As mentioned above, the C5HC2 zinc finger motif is required for activity. In KDM6A, the interaction of a similar zinc finger domain with the KDM6 JmjC domain is required for activity, and in a KDM6A crystal structure with peptide, the zinc finger domain undergoes rearrangement and aids in recognition of a portion of histone H3 around the substrate H3K27 [327]. A future structure of a KDM5 demethylase with peptide may reveal something similar.

8.3   KDM5 in Multicomponent Complexes

KDM5A interacts with the Sin3B/HDAC complex, and KDM5A and Sin3B/HDAC cooperate in transcriptional repression of a subset of E2F4 target genes through deacetylation, demethylation, and nucleosome repositioning [328]. Similarly, KDM5B copurifies and colocalizes with components of the NuRD complex, indicating that KDM5B and NuRD may cooperate in transcriptional repression [316]. The NuRD complex contains two catalytic subunits, the deacetylase HDAC1 and the CHD4 ATPase, both of which are essential for the regulation of gene expression and chromatin remodeling.

9   The KDM6 Family

This KDM family contains three human demethylases (Fig. 7). KDM6A consists of 1401 amino acids and contains a JmjC catalytic domain and 6 tetratricopeptide repeat (TPR) protein-protein interaction domains [41, 330]. KDM6B consists of 1679 amino acids, but it does not appear to contain any characterized domains other than the JmjC domain [331]; however, sequence analysis suggests that it

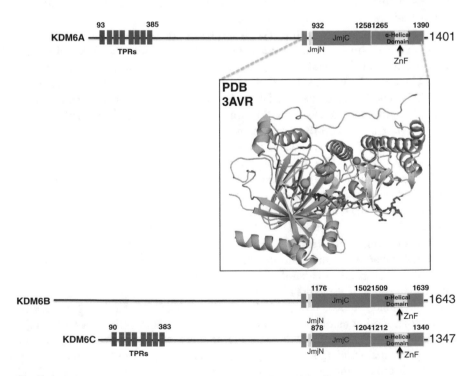

Fig. 7 Representative crystal and domain structures of KDM6 family

may also contain similar TPR domains as KDM6A. These two enzymes have 84% sequence similarity in the JmjC domain [330]. KDM6C consists of 1347 amino acids [332] and shares 83% amino acid identity with KDM6A throughout its sequence [333]. It was once thought to be enzymatically inactive [330, 334], but minimal demethylase activity was later demonstrated and appears to be due to a subtle sequence divergence in the JmjC catalytic domain [332]. KDM6C is located on the Y chromosome and partially compensates for some KDM6A functions, some which may be demethylase-independent, as it was demonstrated using knockout mouse models [335]. KDM6C may activate transcription in a gene-specific manner, as there has been no observation of a decrease in global levels of H3K27me3 upon overexpression of KDM6C in HEK 293 T cells. It is thought that this demethylase may be required in male sex determination during development [332].

KDM6 family members have both pro- and anti-oncogenic roles in cancer, depending on the cell type (reviewed in [336–338]). KDM6A is often classified as a tumor suppressor. Inactivating mutations have been reported in medulloblastoma [339], bladder cancer [340, 341], T-cell acute lymphoblastic leukemia (T-ALL) [342, 343], acute lymphoblastic leukemia [344], renal cell carcinoma [317], chronic myeloamonocytic leukemia [345], and in many other solid and non-solid tumors [346]. Its expression was necessary and sufficient to arrest the cell cycle in human fibroblasts by targeting genes encoding Rb-binding proteins, and depleting KDM6A increased proliferation [347]. Re-expression of KDM6A in KDM6A-null esophageal carcinoma cell lines slowed proliferation [346], and knockdown of KDM6A enhanced *in vitro* and *in vivo* growth of bladder cancer cells [341].

KDM6A knockout in T-ALL cells increased T-ALL kinetics and decreased lifespan of recipient mice. Overexpression of KDM6A in T-ALL cell lines decreased growth and induced apoptosis [343]. Similarly, knockdown of KDM6A boosted development of T-ALL in mice and sensitized cells to treatment with the EZH2 inhibitor 3-DZNep [342]. In the TAL1-positive subgroup of T-ALL, however, KDM6A is oncogenic, and its knockdown attenuated cell growth and induced apoptosis, while overexpression increased cell growth [348].

There are divergent reports of KDM6A's role in breast cancer as well. While one study reports that low KDM6A expression predicts poor survival in breast cancer [347], another reports that high KDM6A expression is associated with poor prognosis in breast cancer [349]. The latter is supported by a study that finds KDM6A is overexpressed in breast cancer and correlated to tumor grade [350]. Additionally, knockdown of KDM6A decreased breast cancer cell proliferation, invasion, and lung colonization [349].

KDM6B can act as a tumor suppressor through interactions with p53 [351, 352] and activation of *p16* [351, 353, 354], promoting senescence after oncogene induction [353, 354] and differentiation of cancer stem cells [351]. In support, KDM6B expression is reduced in several cancer types [353, 355]. KDM6B knockdown decreased p15 expression, with a concurrent increase in proliferation and decrease in apoptosis in colorectal cancer cells, where low expression predicts poor patient prognosis [355].

On the other hand, KDM6B expression is increased in melanoma [356]. Depletion of KMD6B in melanoma boosted self-renewal, trans-endothelial migration, metastasis, angiogenesis, and macrophage recruitment [356]. Similarly, knockdown of KDM6B reduced tumor growth and induced apoptosis in diffuse large B-cell lymphoma cells [357]. In T-ALL, KDM6B was critical for tumor initiation and maintenance through control of NOTCH1 target genes like *HEY1*, *HES1*, and *NRARP* [343]. Treatment with the pan-KDM6/5 inhibitor GSK-J4 [358] has anti-tumor effects on K27 M H3.3 mutants in brainstem gliomas [359], ovarian cancer cells [360], T-ALL cells [343], and TAL1-positive T-ALL patient derived xenografts [348]. KDM6C may play a role in prostate cancer tumorigenesis [361, 362], but its roles have yet to be fully elucidated.

9.1   KDM6 Helper Domains

A domain lies C-terminal to the JmjC domain of KDM6 demethylases that contains a four α-helix bundle which is bisected between the third and fourth helices by a Zn^{2+}-coordinated GATA-like domain of novel topology [363] containing four conserved cysteine residues that coordinate a zinc ion to stabilize the structure. The JmjC and GATA-like zinc-binding domains in KDM6 proteins pack against each other with a large buried surface area (~ 4000 Å^2). This zinc-binding domain is required for optimal stability and the catalytic competence of the truncated KDM6 proteins observed in crystal structures.

Of note, this zinc-binding domain is involved in recognizing an N-terminal portion (H3A17 to H3T22) of the histone H3 target site [327] (Table 7). The zinc-binding domain undergoes a significant conformational change upon binding to the N-terminal portion of histone H3, and this change exposes a hydrophobic patch composed of His1320, His1329, Leu1342, and Val1356 by displacing Tyr1354, which was masking this hydrophobic patch. Among the residues in the N-terminal portion of histone H3, H3A17 and H3L20 exhibit extensive interactions with this hydrophobic patch. Because H3L20 is found only in the context of the H3K27 target, the zinc-binding domain is likely to serve as a substrate determinant for KDM6A. Thus, KDM6A recognizes a relatively large portion of histone H3 with two domains and this contributes to the highly specific activity of KDM6A toward H3K27.

It is noted here that possible "cross-talk" can exist between different epigenetic marks on a histone molecule. Histone H3A17 and H3A26 can be methylated by CARM1/PRMT4, and the zinc-binding domain and the JmjC domain of KDM6A interact with Arg17 and Arg26, respectively. Because KDM6A tightly holds the charged side chains of the histone H3A17 and H3A26 residues, methylation of Arg17 and Arg26 would decrease or block H3 peptide binding and subsequent KDM6A demethylase activity.

Table 7 Structures containing domains of KDM6

PDB ID	Structure title	Dep. date	Resolution (Å)	Reference
KDM6A				
3AVR	Catalytic fragment of UTX/KDM6A bound with histone H3K27me3 peptide, N-oxalylglycine, and Ni(II)	3/7/11	1.8	[327]
3AVS	Catalytic fragment of UTX/KDM6A bound with N-oxalylglycine, and Ni(II)	3/7/11	1.85	[327]
KDM6B				
2XUE	Crystal structure of JMJD3	10/19/10	2	[358]
2XXZ	Crystal structure of the human JMJD3 Jumonji domain	11/12/10	1.8	
4ASK	Crystal structure of JMJD3 with GSK-J1	5/1/12	1.86	[358]
4EYU	The free structure of the mouse C-terminal domain of KDM6B	5/1/12	2.3	[358]
4EZ4	Free KDM6B structure	5/2/12	2.99	[358]
4EZH	The crystal structure of KDM6B bound with H3K27me3 peptide	5/2/12	2.52	[358]
5FP3	Cell penetrant inhibitors of the JMJD2 (KDM4) and JARID1 (KDM5) families of histone lysine demethylases	11/27/15	2.05	[277]
KDM6C				
3ZLI	Crystal structure of JmjC domain of human histone demethylase UTY	1/31/13	1.8	[332]
3ZPO	Crystal structure of JmjC domain of human histone demethylase UTY with bound GSK J1	2/28/13	2	[332]

9.2 KDM6 in Multicomponent Complexes

Protein-protein interaction residues in KDM6 demethylases have not been identified, although the TPR repeats are suspected. Similar to the H3K9me3 epigenetic mark, H3K27me3 is tightly associated with inactive gene promoters and acts in opposition to H3K4me3. Like KDM4A-C, KDM6A and B are part of the MLL2 complex [364, 365] and appear to be involved in differentiation, development, and disease [338, 342, 366, 367].

10 The KDM7 Family

The KDM7 family consists of three members (Fig. 8). Each member harbors two domains in its respective N-terminal half: a PHD domain that binds H3K4me3 and a JmjC domain that demethylates H3K27me2/1 via KDM7A, H3K9me2/1 and H4K20me1 via KDM7B, and H3K9me1 via KDM7C [44, 368]. However, KDM7C

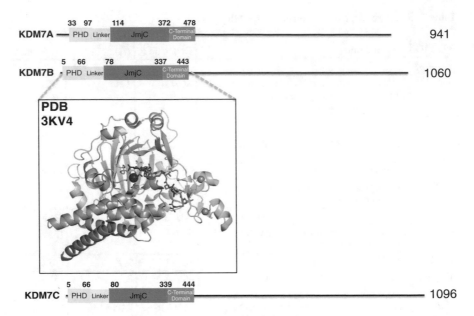

Fig. 8 Representative crystal and domain structures of KDM7 family

activity has not been observed *in vitro* [369]. However, *in vivo*, KDM7C becomes active through a protein kinase A (PKA)-dependent histone lysine demethylase complex, PHF2–ARID5B [370, 371]. KDM7 family members have been implicated as both oncogenic and tumor suppressive. KDM7A expression was upregulated by nutrient starvation, and under those conditions its expression suppressed xenograft tumor growth by restraining angiogenesis [372].

KDM7B is overexpressed in prostate cancer [216, 373], breast cancer [374], laryngeal and hypopharyngeal cancer [375], non-small cell lung cancer [376], and esophageal cancer [377]. It was shown to target and promote expression of onco-miRs miR-21 [376] and miR-125b [373]. Knockdown of KDM7B in cancer cells attenuates growth [216, 373, 376, 377] as well as migration/invasion [216, 377], and induces apoptosis [216, 373, 376]. In contrast, KDM7B expression and activity is critical for response to all-*trans* retinoic acid treatment by acute promyelocytic leukemia cells [378].

KDM7C expression is increased in esophageal squamous cell carcinoma and associated with poor overall survival [379]. However, most studies point to a tumor suppressor function for KDM7C in cancer. It is deleted and/or downregulated in breast cancer [380], head and neck squamous cell carcinoma [381], as well as colon and stomach cancers [382]. KDM7C was shown to associate with p53, and knockdown of KDM7C in p53 competent cells led to decreased sensitivity to genotoxic drugs, as well as reduced drug-induced expression of p21 [382]. Finally, KDM7C was shown to be necessary for treatment-induced mesenchymal to epithelial transition (MET) in breast cancer cells, which led to loss of their tumor initiating ability [383].

10.1 KDM7 Active Site

In the structure of KDM7B with histone peptide, the target H3K9me2 lies in the active site right next to the Fe^{2+} and the 2OG inactive analog N-oxalylglycine (NOG) [44] (Table 8). One of its terminal $N-CH_3$ groups projects toward the aromatic ring of Tyr234, and the other methyl group points toward Asp249 and Asn333, forming two hydrogen bonds of C–H•••O type. The dimethylated terminal nitrogen atom carrying the lone pair of electrons forms a hydrogen bond with one of the oxygen atoms of NOG. The active site cannot accommodate a trimethylated lysine because the third methyl group would cause repulsive tension with NOG. Phe279 makes van der Waals contacts with Ile248 and Ile318, forming a hydrophobic core supporting the backbone of Fe^{2+}-coordinating residues His247, Asp249, and His319. Substitution of Phe279 to serine is associated with inherited X-linked mental retardation [384–387].

In *C. elegans* KDM7A, NOG is stabilized by residues Asn421, Thr492, and Tyr505 [388]. The methylated side chain of H3K9me2 (or H3K27me2) is checked by Phe482 and Phe498 through hydrophobic interactions. One of the methyl groups of dimethylated lysine interacts with the side chains of Asp497 and Asn581 through two C–H•••O hydrogen bonds.

KDM7C appears to be an inactive demethylase. The metal binding site in KDM7C closely resembles the Fe^{2+} sites in other JmjC domains [369]. However, KDM7C contains a tyrosine (Tyr321) in the place of the fifth ligand, and the longer side chain of Tyr321 makes the Fe^{2+} move away from the corresponding binding site in KDM7B, an active demethylase. The small movement of the ferrous iron, induced by the presence of Tyr321, could position the reactive oxygen in a non-reactive mode.

10.2 KDM7 Helper Domains

KDM7A/B structures provided one of the first examples of how helper domains can both upregulate and/or downregulate JmjC demethylase activity through contributions associated with steric effects. The presence of H3K4me3 on the same peptide as H3K9me2 makes the doubly methylated peptide a significantly better substrate of KDM7B, resulting in a 12-fold increase in enzymatic activity as revealed by activity assays [44, 389–391]. By contrast, the presence of H3K4me3 diminishes the H3K9me2 demethylase activity of KDM7A with no adverse effect on its H3K27me2 activity, because the distance between the H3K4me3 and H3K27me2 marks is long enough for occupation of the PHD and JmjC domain pockets simultaneously [44, 388]. Differences in substrate specificity between the two enzymes are explained by a bent conformation of KDM7B, allowing each of its domains to engage their respective targets, and an extended conformation of KDM7A, which prevents its JmjC domain from accessing H3K9me2 when its PHD domain engages H3K4me3. Thus, the structural linkage between the PHD domain binding to H3K4me3 and the placement of the catalytic JmjC domains relative to this 'on' H3K4me3 epigenetic mark determine which repressive marks are removed by both

Table 8 Structures containing domains of KDM7

PDB ID	Structure title	Dep. date	Resolution (Å)	Reference
KDM7A				
3KV5	Structure of KIAA1718, human Jumonji demethylase, in complex with N-oxalylglycine	11/29/09	2.39	[44]
3KV6	Structure of KIAA1718, human Jumonji demethylase, in complex with alpha-ketoglutarate	11/29/09	2.89	[44]
3KV9	Structure of KIAA1718 Jumonji domain	11/29/09	2.29	[44]
3KVA	Structure of KIAA1718 Jumonji domain in complex with alpha-ketoglutarate	11/29/09	2.79	[44]
3KVB	Structure of KIAA1718 Jumonji domain in complex with N-oxalylglycine	11/29/09	2.69	[44]
3N9L	ceKDM7A from C.elegans, complex with H3K4me3 peptide and NOG	05/31/10	2.80	[388]
3N9M	ceKDM7A from C.elegans, alone	05/31/10	2.49	[388]
3N9N	ceKDM7A from C.elegans, complex with H3K4me3K9me2 peptide and NOG	05/31/10	2.30	[388]
3N9O	ceKDM7A from C.elegans, complex with H3K4me3 peptide, H3K9me2 peptide and NOG	05/31/10	2.31	[388]
3N9P	ceKDM7A from C.elegans, complex with H3K4me3K27me2 peptide and NOG	05/31/10	2.39	[388]
3N9Q	ceKDM7A from C.elegans, complex with H3K4me3 peptide, H3K27me2 peptide and NOG	05/31/10	2.30	[388]
3PUQ	CEKDM7A from C.Elegans, complex with alpha-KG	12/06/10	2.25	[395]
3PUR	CEKDM7A from C.Elegans, complex with D-2-HG	12/06/10	2.10	[395]
3U78	E67-2 selectively inhibits KIAA1718, a human histone H3 lysine 9 Jumonji demethylase	10/13/11	2.69	[396]

1WEP	Solution structure of PHD domain in PHF8	05/25/04		
3K3N	Crystal structure of the catalytic core domain of human PHF8	10/03/09	2.40	[397]
3K3O	Crystal structure of the catalytic core domain of human PHF8 complexed with alpha-ketoglutarate	10/03/09	2.10	[397]
2WWU	Crystal structure of the catalytic domain of PHD finger protein 8	10/29/09	2.15	[398]
3KV4	Structure of PHF8 in complex with histone H3	11/29/09	2.19	[44]
4DO0	Crystal structure of human PHF8 in complex with daminozide	02/09/12	2.55	
KDM7C				
3KQI	Crystal structure of PHF2 PHD domain complexed with H3K4me3 peptide	11/17/09	1.78	[399]
3PTR	PHF2 Jumonji domain	12/03/10	1.95	[369]
3PU3	PHF2 Jumonji domain-NOG complex	12/03/10	1.95	[369]
3PU8	PHF2 Jumonji-NOG-Fe(II) complex	12/03/10	1.94	[369]
3PUA	PHF2 Jumonji-NOG-Ni(II)	12/03/10	1.89	[369]
3PUS	PHF2 Jumonji-NOG-Ni(II)	12/06/10	2.08	[369]

demethylases. Thus, the KDM7A and KDM7B JmjC domains on their own are promiscuous enzymes; it is the associated PHD domains and linker—a determinant for the relative positioning of the two domains—that are mainly responsible for substrate specificity. It should also be noted that KDM helper domains can affect the orientation of peptide binding: a peptide in complex with a KDM6 demethylase has an opposite orientation across the JmjC domain compared to a peptide in complex with a KDM7 demethylase [44, 327, 388].

A structural study on *C. elegans* KDM7A suggested that the extended conformation between the PHD and Jumonji domains might enable a trans-histone peptide-binding mechanism, in which H3K4me3 associated with the PHD domain and the H3K9me2 bound to the Jumonji domain could be coming from two separate histone H3 molecules of the same nucleosome or two neighboring nucleosomes [388]. However, this trans-binding mechanism can be excluded for human KDM7A because the presence of an H3K4me3 *in trans* or *in cis* with H3K9me2 substrate peptide strongly inhibits KDM7A activity toward H3K9me2 [44]. Nevertheless, the trans-binding mechanism is an attractive model for KDM7B if the flexible loop between the PHD and JmjC enables the enzyme to adopt an extended conformation to allow binding of two peptides simultaneously. The trans-binding mechanism could explain the finding that KDM7B also functions *in vivo* as an H4K20me1 demethylase while its PHD domain interacts with H3K4me3/me2 in the context of nucleosome [392, 393]. However, if this were the case, an explanation would be needed as to why KDM7B is only active on monomethylated H4K20, whereas it is active on mono- and dimethylated H3K9 and H3K27. One possibility is that only H4K20me1 co-exists with H3K4me3/me2 *in vivo*.

10.3   KDM7 in Multicomponent Complexes

The C-terminal halves show little homology among the family members and do not contain any known domains. Nonetheless, C-terminal parts of members are essential for their gene regulatory functions. For example, it was found that KDM7B binds to RNA polymerase I/II, KMT2, HCF1, E2F1, ZNF711 and RAR, under the control of the C-terminal portion of KDM7B [389, 390, 392, 394]. In addition, KDM7C is associated with p53 through its C-terminal region [382]. It appears probable that the variability of the C-terminal halves of KDM7 members provides functional diversity by choosing different histone demethylase partners for transcription.

11   Molecular Basis of KDM Inhibition and Development of Inhibitors into Drugs

At present, current epigenetic therapies primarily involve inhibitors of DNA demethylation and histone deacetylation [400]. Considering the significant implication of KDMs in the development of various diseases, a thorough understanding of their molecular mechanism and effective therapeutic inhibition is of considerable interest, but at its infancy. Further characterization of many demethylases is proceeding through both functional studies and the development of small molecule inhibitors targeted against them. These studies will be invaluable for our understanding and treatment of cancer. There are two possible ways by which a demethylase-inhibiting drug may be able to halt or even prevent cancers. It can repress oncogenes and/or activate tumor-suppressor genes that are deregulated by methylation processes [401, 402] or overcome resistance to chemotherapy [283, 403, 404]. Transient and reversible drug resistance develops in certain cancer cell populations during treatment with cancer drugs. KDM5A is as at least one chromatin-modifying enzyme required for establishing a drug-tolerant subpopulation [297]. Reduced methylation of H3K4 has also been linked to poor prognosis in cancer patients [405].

The many crystal structures of demethylases have revealed substantially con served Fe^{2+} and 2OG binding sites; yet, differences in Fe^{2+} and 2OG binding sites are idiosyncratic to each KDM family and may be able to be exploited for the development of selective inhibitors. For instance, N198 in KDM4A and N1156 in KDM6A establish a hydrogen bond at the back of the pocket with the carboxylic moiety of 2OG, while in KDM2A and KDM7 family members, the asparagine is replaced by a tyrosine that causes a different Fe^{2+} coordination of the carboxylic moiety of the cofactor and a loss of the hydrogen bond. In a KDM4A-inhibitor structure [263], a π-π stacking interaction with F185 at the front part of the pocket can be observed; this phenylalanine is only conserved within the KDM4 and KDM5 families [406]. KDM2A/6A/7 show a threonine at this location that would prohibit a π-ring system at this position. Another example is the invariant cysteine in the active site of the KDM5 family (Cys-481 in KDM5A), which spatially replaces residues in other KDMs (i.e. Pro-1388 of KDM6B). Exploring the interaction between this noncatalytic cysteine and studied inhibitors could provide an avenue for improved potency, selectivity, and prolonged on-target residence times of inhibitors specific for the KDM5 family. For example, an approach of using reversible covalent inhibitors that target noncatalytic cysteine residues to achieve prolonged and tunable residence time has recently been demonstrated with protein kinases [407]. Both reversible [408] and irreversible inhibitors [122, 123, 409, 410] have been made against KDM1A, and some of these inhibitors have entered into clinical trials as drugs for cancers such as acute myeloid leukemia [411] and small cell lung carcinoma [412, 413].

The pace of inquiry in the KDM inhibitor field is accelerating: the number of papers published and applications for patents in the last several years are a testament to the presupposition that study in this area will lead to great discovery of KDM chemical probes and drug candidates [122, 273, 277, 411, 414–416]. A comprehensive review is beyond the scope of this chapter. A few highlights in this area will be discussed.

11.1   Inhibitors of KDM1 Demethylases

There are many compounds that are KDM1 inhibitors (Fig. 9a). The AOD catalytic domain of KDM1 is homologous to those of the monoamine oxidases (MAOs) A and B and this has facilitated studies for this KDM family. Consequently, several

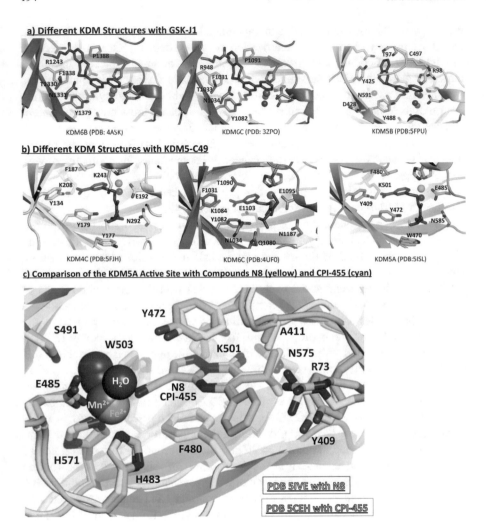

Fig. 9 Crystal structures containing (**a**) GSK-J1, (**b**) KDM5-C49 and (**c**) compounds N8 and CPI-455

well-studied MAO inhibitors, including phenelzine and tranylcypromine (TCP), an FDA-approved treatment for psychological disorders [417], have been demonstrated to also inhibit KDM1A [418, 419]. A mechanism-based irreversible inhibitor, TCP forms a covalent adduct with the FAD cofactor within the active site of the enzyme [94, 126, 419]. The application of TCP as an inhibitor of KDM1A has provided promising proof-of-principle data in mouse models and leukemia cell lines [82, 83]. However, such non-selective amine oxidase inhibitors could obviously have adverse effects and are not ideal solutions for KDM1 inhibitors. Therefore, derivatives of tranylcypromine have been made, and the first structures with enhanced potency and target selectivity for KDM1A were obtained through modification of the phenyl group of TCP using crystal structures of KDM1A with TCP or a KDM1-selective peptide-based inhibitor [127, 420].

Since KDM1 can specifically recognize the twenty-one amino acids from the N-terminal tail of histone H3, inhibitors containing these twenty-one amino acid long peptides from the histone H3 N-terminal tail with modifications on target lysine have been synthesized; a propargyl-Lys-derivatized peptide functions as a potent and selective time-dependent inactivator of KDM1A [421]. However, even a H3 peptide with methionine replacement for the target lysine appears to be a good inhibitor ($K_i = 40$ nM) and a structure was determined [95]. Peptides derived from SNAIL1 and INSM1 sequences could also act as KDM1A inhibitors [130]. SNAIL1 is a transcription factor that binds to the KDM1A active site through its SNAG (Snail/GFI) domain with the N-terminal 21 residues adopting a similar conformation to the H3 substrate and acts as a competitive inhibitor. INSM1 (insulinoma-associated protein) is another member of the same family of transcription factors as SNAIL1 and binds to KDM1A with similar affinity. However, crystal structures showed that only the first nine and eight residues of the two transcription factor peptides, respectively, bind in an ordered conformation. Several such small peptides exhibited competitive inhibition and crystal structures of both of these with KDM1A were determined (see Table 2). In addition, novel and potent cyclic peptide inhibitors of KDM1A have been developed [422]; an advantage of cyclic peptides is their significant stability to hydrolysis in plasma.

11.2   Inhibitors of JmjC Demethylases

Many different types of compounds inhibit the JmjC demethylases (Fig. 9b). The majority of JmjC KDM inhibitors identified to date incorporate carboxylic acids/carboxylic acid analogs, leading to use of pro-drug ester forms for sufficient cellular activity. The inhibitors occupy the 2OG binding site and may contain moieties that occupy other potential binding sites such as the region where the methyl-lysine binds. There has been a rapid increase in reports of JmjC KDM inhibitors both in the scientific literature and in patents in the last few years; several excellent reviews and reports of new molecular inhibitor scaffolds have appeared recently [271, 277, 414, 423–426]. However, many of these KDM inhibitors lack the desired selectivity, potency and pharmacokinetic properties (particularly cell permeability) necessary to be considered as probe molecules for the investigation of individual KDM function in cancer or for development as cancer drugs. There are basically three types of JmjC demethylase inhibitors: 2OG mimetics, compounds that target peptide binding sites, and compounds that interfere with the action of helper domains. We discuss select compounds from each category below, as well as some of the challenges associated with their use.

11.3   TCA Cycle Intermediates and 2OG Mimetics

The development of JmjC demethylase inhibitors is likely to pose challenges with respect to reaching sufficient potency, given the intracellular competition by excess cofactor and cofactor-like compounds. Cancer-associated mutations in tricarboxylic acid (TCA) cycle enzymes lead to abnormal accumulation of TCA cycle metabolites that have been linked to oncogenic transformation. These metabolites are themselves inhibitors of KDMs when they exist in a cell at high concentrations. Mutations to these enzymes are common in tumors and can result in very substantial increases in the concentrations of succinate, fumarate, or 2-hydroxyglutarate (2HG) [427–430]. 2HG is a five-carbon dicarboxylic acid with a chiral center at the second carbon atom; therefore, there are two possible enantiomers of 2HG: ((S/R)-2HG). Mutations cause isocitrate dehydrogenase (IDH) 1 and 2 to convert 2OG into 2HG, as well as produce 2OG from isocitrate [431]. IDH mutants exclusively produce the (R) enantiomer of 2HG, and the levels of (R)-2HG in IDH mutant tumors can be extremely elevated, ranging from 1 mM to as high as 35 mM [432–434]. Succinate, a co-product of the JmjC demethylase reaction, fumarate, and 2HG all inhibit JmjC demethylases, though rather weakly (in the µM to mM range for KDM2A, KDM4A, KDM4C and KDM5B, as shown with isolated proteins and in cells [266, 395, 435]), via competition with 2OG [254, 436]. A number of KDM4A and KDM6C crystal structures with these compounds have been solved (see Tables 5 and 7).

The 2OG analog NOG has generally been used as an inhibitor for *in vitro* studies [17]. In NOG, the C-3 methylene group of 2OG is replaced with an NH group to give an N-oxalyl amide derivative that likely stalls the catalytic reaction by hindering oxygen binding to the active site iron. NOG has been utilized in many crystallizations of JmjC demethylases, especially those in which peptide is present. Often structures also include a non-catalytic metal ion such as Ni^{2+}, Co^{2+}, or Mg^{2+} as a substitute for Fe^{2+}. Metal chelating compounds such as diols can also inhibit JmjC KDMs at high concentration. For example, the common buffer TRIS inhibits KDM4C with a $K_i = 11$ mM and a crystal structure with TRIS has been solved with the compound clearly in the active site when the crystal was grown in the absence of 2OG [275].

Analysis of the X-ray crystal structure of KDM4A in complex with NOG and a trimethylated peptide [253] led to the design and synthesis of NOG derivatives substituted with an alkyl-linked dimethylaniline group in order to mimic the interactions of the trimethylated peptide with the protein [437]. These derivatives maintained the inhibitory action of NOG against KDM4A, and illustrate a strategy of linking the 2OG and peptide substrate binding sites to further increase JmjC KDM inhibition.

11.4   Daminozide and Hydroxamic Acid-Based JmjC KDM Inhibitors

Daminozide is selective for the KDM2/7 families over other members of the human JmjC KDMs [KDM2A ($IC_{50} = 1.5$ µM) and KDM7B ($IC_{50} = 0.55$ µM)] [268]. Crystallographic studies revealed that daminozide chelates the active site iron via its dimethylamino nitrogen lone pair and C-4 carbonyl group, with its C-1 carbonyl occupying the same site as the 2OG C-5 carboxylate. This selectivity may be engendered by the more hydrophobic region created by the Tyr257, Val255 and Ile191 residues adjacent to the iron ion in the KDM2/7 families compared to the more hydrophobic residues in the corresponding regions in KDM4A and other JmjC demethylases.

11.5   Pyridine Derivatives

A screen using known inhibitors of other 2OG dependent oxygenases identified 2,4-pyridinedicarboxylic acid (2,4-PDCA), which showed potent inhibitory activity on KDM4E ($IC_{50} = 1.4$ μM) [262]. The structure of KDM4A (and later other KDMs see Tables 5 and 6) with bound 2,4-PDCA showed that 2,4-PDCA functions in a 2OG competitive manner. 2,4-PDCA binds the Ni^{2+} cation in a bidentate manner via its N-atom and 2-carboxylate, whereas the 4-carboxylate mimics 2OG binding by forming two hydrogen bonds with a Lys and a Tyr in the active site. Many compounds have a similar binding mechanism; however, the minimal binding requirements in the 2OG site appear to one atom binding to metal and one binding to the Lys residue in JmjC demethylase binding sites [282].

There are two other inhibitors that are pyridine derivatives and have been studied in greater detail, both biochemically and structurally, than other inhibitors amongst several KDM families: GSK-J1/J4 (4) and KDM5-C49/C70. GSK-J4 and KDM5-C70 are cell permeable prodrug ethyl esters that are hydrolyzed by an esterase within the cell to generate GSK-J1 and KDM5-C49, respectively. GSK-J1 is a potent inhibitor of the H3K27 histone demethylases KDM6A and KDM6B with *in vitro* IC_{50} values of 56 and 18 μM, respectively [358]. However, GSK-J1 is a good inhibitor for other KDM families as well, particularly KDM5 [438, 439]. GSK-J1 contains a propanoic acid moiety that mimics 2OG binding, and a pyridyl-pyrimidine biaryl chelates the active site Fe^{2+}, inducing a shift in its position. GSK-J4 is still one of the few inhibitors revealed to have cell activity. GSK-J4 has anticancer effects against acute lymphoblastic leukemia and pediatric brainstem glioma [343, 359], as well as the ability to target ovarian cancer stem cells [360]. GSK-J1 has been crystalized with members of the KDM5 and KDM6 families (Tables 6 and 7).

KDM5-C49/C70 is reported to be a potent and selective inhibitor for the KDM5 family, but is a good inhibitor for the KDM4 and KDM6 families as well [274, 282]. KDM5-C49 is a 2,4-PDCA analog and shows nanomolar inhibitory potencies in enzymatic assays across several JmjC families. KDM5-C70 also lead to cell cycle arrest in a multiple myeloma cells and breast cancer cell lines with an observed increase in global H3K4me3 levels [274, 282].

A pan-inhibitor, JIB-04, was identified in an unbiased cellular screen, and shown to effectively and specifically inhibit several KDM families' activity *in vivo* as well as *in vitro* [440]. Furthermore, JIB-04 could specifically inhibit KDM function in cancer cells, as well as in tumors *in vivo*. JIB-04 is not a competitive inhibitor of 2OG, and the exact molecular mechanism is unclear. There is relative selectivity of

JIB-04 toward KDM5B *versus* KDM5C *in vitro*, which correlated with an increased cellular potency overall *in vivo* and a propensity for cell type specificity not observed with GSK-J4 in one study [54]. High-throughput screening also identified 2,4-PDCA-related 8-hydroxyquinoline compounds as inhibitors of KDM demethylases that were further developed [264, 269, 414]. Natural products such as flavonoids and catechols have been demonstrated to inhibit a number of 2OG oxygenases, including the JmjC KDMs [416, 441].

11.6   A Compound Showing Some Selectivity

Two similar compounds have been crystallized with variant truncated constructs of KDM5A [282, 283]. One compound, CPI-455, is cell permeable while the other, N8, is not. However, both are amongst the most effective KDM5 inhibitors *in vitro* and are more selective for the KDM5 family than other KDM families. The only difference between the two compounds is a substitution of a methyl group in N8 with a phenyl group in CPI-455 (Fig. 9b). Interestingly, the addition of a methyl group to the phenyl group of CPI-455 to produce CPI-4203 makes this inhibitor less cell permeable and an inactive or very weak control for cell assays [283]. Our lack of understanding of how these small changes make compounds less or more cell permeable reflect our present lack of knowledge of the characteristics required to endow compounds with properties for permeability.

The position occupied by these inhibitors (Fig. 10c) completely overlaps the binding site of 2OG, demonstrating a competitive mode of action, as suggested by biochemical assays [282, 283]. The nitrile group of these KDM5 inhibitors makes a single interaction with the active-site metal ion, while a ring nitrogen atom forms a hydrogen bond with the side chain of Lys501. The carbonyl oxygen off the ring is within hydrogen bonding distance to the side chains of Asn575, as well as Lys501. In the KDM5 structure with 2OG, the side chain Asn575 bridges between Lys501 and Tyr409, which form hydrogen bonds with the carboxylic group of 2OG. In contrast to the structure with 2OG, the side chain of Tyr409 is pushed away by the bulky pyrazolopyrimidine ring and is rotated nearly 90° from that of the 2OG-bound form, resulting in a van der Waals contact with the isopropyl substituent on these compounds [54]. In the CPI-455 structure, Tyr409 as well as Arg73 is pushed even further away from the active site because of the phenyl ring substitution of the methyl group in N8. In both structures, the central pyrimidine ring sandwiches between the aromatic rings of Tyr472 and Phe480. The phenyl group in CPI-455 forms an edge-to-face aromatic contact with Tyr409 and points toward solvent.

All amino acids within 4 Å of the inhibitor are conserved in the KDM5 family; hence, N8 and CPI-455 inhibit all KDM5 family members. The selectivity of these compounds for KDM5 versus KDM2, KDM3 and KDM6 proteins derives from conformational and sequence differences within their active sites. For

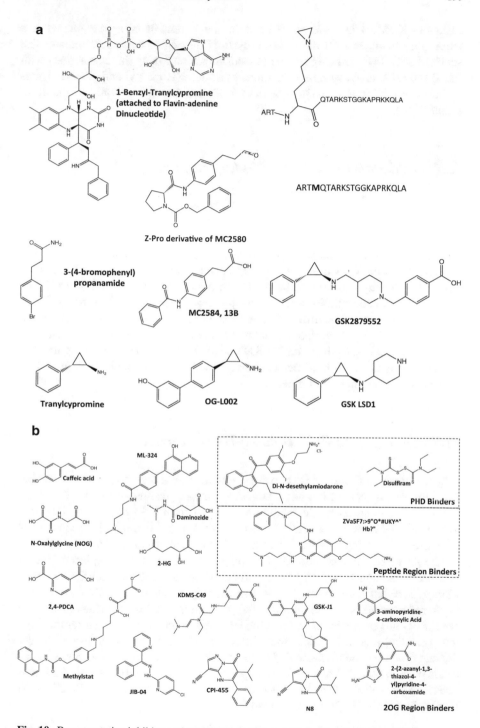

Fig. 10 Representative inhibitors of (**a**) KDM1 family and (**b**) JmjC demethylase families

instance, KDM6B is more constricted in the region flanking the phenyl and isopropyl substituents off the pyrazolopyrimidine ring of these compounds. The scaffold of CPI-455 is being further developed by improving the interactions with the Tyr409 side chain with modifications of both the isopropyl and phenyl groups to improve inhibition of KDM5 demethylases and the cell potency of the compound [442].

11.7 Inhibitors to Substrate Binding Regions

An inhibitor of G9a methyltransferase (BIX-01294) and its analog E67 also inhibited the human H3K9me2 demethylase KDM7A [396]. These compounds act as H3 substrate analogues and therefore, both enzymes can recognize methyl-lysine residues either as product or as substrate. Compound E67 was shown to inhibit KDM7A and KDM7B with IC_{50} values in the low-micromolar range in an *in vitro* mass spectrometric demethylation assay, but was inactive against KDM5C. E67 exhibited cytotoxicity at concentrations around 50 μM against mouse and human primary fibroblasts. A crystal structure confirmed binding of this compound to the active site of the enzyme [396]. A compound that mimics both Lys and 2OG was synthesized which appeared to selectively inhibit KDMs [443]. In addition, its prodrug methylstat selectively inhibited JmjC demethylases in cells and could inhibit cell growth of an esophageal carcinoma cell line.

11.8 Inhibitors to PHD Binding Helper Domains

Helper domains of JmjC KDMs can be tractable targets and provide promising leads for development of inhibitors targeting noncatalytic domains of JmjC KDMs. For instance, small molecule inhibitors targeting the PHD3 domain of KDM5A were identified through application of an assay that uses 96-well polystyrene plates activated with synthetic ligand for covalent and oriented capture of a protein fusion to KDM5A PHD3 which allowed screening for molecules that displaced histone H3K4me3 binding to PHD3 [444]. Screening of the NIH Clinical Collection 1 library identified compounds such as disulfiram, phenothiazine, aminodarone, and tegaserod maleate as inhibitors (Fig. 10a). Disulfiram inhibits KDM5A PHD3 and other PHD fingers not by acting as a ligand, but through ejection of structural zinc, thus revealing a general susceptibility specific to PHD fingers as a histone reader domain. The compounds were further tested through affinity pull-downs, fluorescence polarization, and histone reader specificity studies. Inhibitors based on aminodarone derivatives were identified to be potent against KDM5A-PHD3, with IC50 values in the 25–40 μM range [444].

12 Conclusions

Crystal structures of catalytic domains exist for every human KDM family. Additionally, there is a quickly growing number of structures of these domains with inhibitors containing different chemical moieties in the active site. However, there is a substantial need for developing new types of inhibitors, likely aided by improving our understanding of all of these structures. Because we know that some catalytic domains are inactive when expressed alone, these structures need to be further supplemented by solution studies and greater biochemical analysis of KDM selectivity.

There are still much to learn about these demethylases. For instance, very little is known about large parts of some KDM demethylases, such as the second half of the KDM5 and KDM7 families. Discovery is just beginning on how KDM domains interact with each other and how these domains interact with other proteins in multicomponent complexes. Recent advances in single-particle cryo-electron microscopy (cryo-EM) may aide in this regard [445]. These advances are enabling generation of numerous near-atomic resolution structures for well-ordered protein complexes with sizes ≥ 200 kDa. Cryo-EM should allow structure determination of the large KDMs with all their domains, complexes with their interacting proteins and nucleosomes as well as information about the dynamic conformational states of these domains and complexes.

Future detailed structural information from both X-ray crystallography and cryo-EM will offer further understanding about the molecular basis of histone demethylation, *i.e.* how demethylases exert their substrate specificities and function in histone regulation. In turn, this will allow better development of inhibitors, which may potentially be utilized as drugs in mankind's battle against various cancers where demethylases play a substantial role.

Acknowledgements The work in the Cheng laboratory is supported by NIH grant GM114306-02; the work in the Yan laboratory is supported by American Cancer Society Research Scholar Grant (RSG-13-384-01-DMC) and DoD Breast Cancer Research Program Award (W81XWH-14-1-0308). National Science Foundation Graduate Research Fellowship (DGE-1122492) supports M.G. in the Yan laboratory. X.C. is a Georgia Research Alliance Eminent Scholar.

References

1. Bannister AJ, Kouzarides T (2004) Histone methylation: recognizing the methyl mark. Methods Enzymol 376:269–288
2. Bedford MT, Richard S (2005) Arginine methylation an emerging regulator of protein function. Mol Cell 18(3):263–272
3. Jenuwein T, Allis CD (2001) Translating the histone code. Science 293(5532):1074–1080
4. Lee CT, Duerre JA (1974) Changes in histone methylase activity of rat brain and liver with ageing. Nature 251(5472):240–242
5. Byvoet P et al (1972) The distribution and turnover of labeled methyl groups in histone fractions of cultured mammalian cells. Arch Biochem Biophys 148(2):558–567

6. Borun TW, Pearson D, Paik WK (1972) Studies of histone methylation during the HeLa S-3 cell cycle. J Biol Chem 247(13):4288–4298
7. Annunziato AT, Eason MB, Perry CA (1995) Relationship between methylation and acetylation of arginine-rich histones in cycling and arrested HeLa cells. Biochemistry 34(9):2916–2924
8. Bannister AJ, Schneider R, Kouzarides T (2002) Histone methylation: dynamic or static? Cell 109(7):801–806
9. Kim S, Benoiton L, Paik WK (1964) Epsilon-alkyllysinase. Purification and properties of the enzyme. J Biol Chem 239:3790–3796
10. Paik WK, Kim S (1973) Enzymatic demethylation of calf thymus histones. Biochem Biophys Res Commun 51(3):781–788
11. Paik WK, Kim S (1974) Epsilon-alkyllysinase. New assay method, purification, and biological significance. Arch Biochem Biophys 165(1):369–378
12. Shi Y et al (2004) Histone demethylation mediated by the nuclear amine oxidase homolog LSD1. Cell 119(7):941–953
13. Shi Y, Whetstine JR (2007) Dynamic regulation of histone lysine methylation by demethylases. Mol Cell 25(1):1–14
14. Trewick SC, McLaughlin PJ, Allshire RC (2005) Methylation: lost in hydroxylation? EMBO Rep 6(4):315–320
15. Tsukada Y et al (2006) Histone demethylation by a family of JmjC domain-containing proteins. Nature 439(7078):811–816
16. Whetstine JR et al (2006) Reversal of histone lysine trimethylation by the JMJD2 family of histone demethylases. Cell 125(3):467–481
17. Cloos PA et al (2006) The putative oncogene GASC1 demethylates tri- and dimethylated lysine 9 on histone H3. Nature 442(7100):307–311
18. Fodor BD et al (2006) Jmjd2b antagonizes H3K9 trimethylation at pericentric heterochromatin in mammalian cells. Genes Dev 20(12):1557–1562
19. Klose RJ et al (2006) The transcriptional repressor JHDM3A demethylates trimethyl histone H3 lysine 9 and lysine 36. Nature 442(7100):312–316
20. Chen Z et al (2006) Structural insights into histone demethylation by JMJD2 family members. Cell 125(4):691–702
21. Di Lorenzo A, Bedford MT (2011) Histone arginine methylation. FEBS Lett 585(13):2024–2031
22. Chang B et al (2007) JMJD6 is a histone arginine demethylase. Science 318(5849):444–447
23. Webby CJ et al (2009) Jmjd6 catalyses lysyl-hydroxylation of U2AF65, a protein associated with RNA splicing. Science 325(5936):90–93
24. Unoki M et al (2013) Lysyl 5-hydroxylation, a novel histone modification, by Jumonji domain containing 6 (JMJD6). J Biol Chem 288(9):6053–6062
25. Bottger A et al (2015) The oxygenase Jmjd6 – a case study in conflicting assignments. Biochem J 468(2):191–202
26. Mantri M et al (2010) Crystal structure of the 2-oxoglutarate- and Fe(II)-dependent lysyl hydroxylase JMJD6. J Mol Biol 401(2):211–222
27. Hong X et al (2010) Interaction of JMJD6 with single-stranded RNA. Proc Natl Acad Sci U S A 107(33):14568–14572
28. Walport LJ et al (2016) Arginine demethylation is catalysed by a subset of JmjC histone lysine demethylases. Nat Commun 7:11974
29. Thompson PR, Fast W (2006) Histone citrullination by protein arginine deiminase: is arginine methylation a green light or a roadblock? ACS Chem Biol 1(7):433–441
30. Hidaka Y, Hagiwara T, Yamada M (2005) Methylation of the guanidino group of arginine residues prevents citrullination by peptidylarginine deiminase IV. FEBS Lett 579(19):4088–4092
31. Raijmakers R et al (2007) Methylation of arginine residues interferes with citrullination by peptidylarginine deiminases in vitro. J Mol Biol 367(4):1118–1129
32. Cuthbert GL et al (2004) Histone deimination antagonizes arginine methylation. Cell 118(5):545–553
33. Musselman CA, Kutateladze TG (2011) Handpicking epigenetic marks with PHD fingers. Nucleic Acids Res 39(21):9061–9071

34. Pek JW, Anand A, Kai T (2012) Tudor domain proteins in development. Development 139(13):2255–2266
35. Lu R, Wang GG (2013) Tudor: a versatile family of histone methylation 'readers'. Trends Biochem Sci 38(11):546–555
36. Laity JH, Lee BM, Wright PE (2001) Zinc finger proteins: new insights into structural and functional diversity. Curr Opin Struct Biol 11(1):39–46
37. Klug A (2010) The discovery of zinc fingers and their applications in gene regulation and genome manipulation. Annu Rev Biochem 79:213–231
38. Gamsjaeger R et al (2007) Sticky fingers: zinc-fingers as protein-recognition motifs. Trends Biochem Sci 32(2):63–70
39. Wang Z et al (2014) Roles of F-box proteins in cancer. Nat Rev Cancer 14(4):233–247
40. Wilsker D et al (2002) ARID proteins: a diverse family of DNA binding proteins implicated in the control of cell growth, differentiation, and development. Cell Growth Differ 13(3):95–106
41. Blatch GL, Lassle M (1999) The tetratricopeptide repeat: a structural motif mediating protein-protein interactions. BioEssays 21(11):932–939
42. Ng A, Xavier RJ (2011) Leucine-rich repeat (LRR) proteins: integrators of pattern recognition and signaling in immunity. Autophagy 7(9):1082–1084
43. Ng AC et al (2011) Human leucine-rich repeat proteins: a genome-wide bioinformatic categorization and functional analysis in innate immunity. Proc Natl Acad Sci U S A 108(Suppl 1):4631–4638
44. Horton JR et al (2010) Enzymatic and structural insights for substrate specificity of a family of Jumonji histone lysine demethylases. Nat Struct Mol Biol 17(1):38–43
45. Stavropoulos P, Blobel G, Hoelz A (2006) Crystal structure and mechanism of human lysine-specific demethylase-1. Nat Struct Mol Biol 13(7):626–632
46. Chen F et al (2013) Structural insight into substrate recognition by histone demethylase LSD2/KDM1b. Cell Res 23(2):306–309
47. Fang R et al (2013) LSD2/KDM1B and its cofactor NPAC/GLYR1 endow a structural and molecular model for regulation of H3K4 demethylation. Mol Cell 49(3):558–570
48. Hou H, Yu H (2010) Structural insights into histone lysine demethylation. Curr Opin Struct Biol 20(6):739–748
49. Musselman CA et al (2012) Perceiving the epigenetic landscape through histone readers. Nat Struct Mol Biol 19(12):1218–1227
50. Taverna SD et al (2007) How chromatin-binding modules interpret histone modifications: lessons from professional pocket pickers. Nat Struct Mol Biol 14(11):1025–1040
51. Kamps JJ et al (2015) Chemical basis for the recognition of trimethyllysine by epigenetic reader proteins. Nat Commun 6:8911
52. Berry WL, Janknecht R (2013) KDM4/JMJD2 histone demethylases: epigenetic regulators in cancer cells. Cancer Res 73(10):2936–2942
53. Cheng Z et al (2014) A molecular threading mechanism underlies Jumonji lysine demethylase KDM2A regulation of methylated H3K36. Genes Dev 28(16):1758–1771
54. Horton JR et al (2016) Characterization of a linked Jumonji domain of the KDM5/JARID1 family of histone H3 lysine 4 demethylases. J Biol Chem 291(6):2631–2646
55. Pilka ES, James T, Lisztwan JH (2015) Structural definitions of Jumonji family demethylase selectivity. Drug Discov Today 20(6):743–749
56. Karytinos A et al (2009) A novel mammalian flavin-dependent histone demethylase. J Biol Chem 284(26):17775–17782
57. Sims RJ 3rd, Nishioka K, Reinberg D (2003) Histone lysine methylation: a signature for chromatin function. Trends Genet 19(11):629–639
58. Barski A et al (2007) High-resolution profiling of histone methylations in the human genome. Cell 129(4):823–837
59. Maston GA et al (2012) Characterization of enhancer function from genome-wide analyses. Annu Rev Genomics Hum Genet 13:29–57
60. Wang Y, Li X, Hu H (2014) H3K4me2 reliably defines transcription factor binding regions in different cells. Genomics 103(2–3):222–228
61. Heintzman ND et al (2009) Histone modifications at human enhancers reflect global cell-type-specific gene expression. Nature 459(7243):108–112

62. Fang R et al (2010) Human LSD2/KDM1b/AOF1 regulates gene transcription by modulating intragenic H3K4me2 methylation. Mol Cell 39(2):222–233
63. Ciccone DN et al (2009) KDM1B is a histone H3K4 demethylase required to establish maternal genomic imprints. Nature 461(7262):415–418
64. Burg JM et al (2015) KDM1 class flavin-dependent protein lysine demethylases. Biopolymers 104(4):213–246
65. Jin Y et al (2014) Nuclear import of human histone lysine-specific demethylase LSD1. J Biochem 156(6):305–313
66. Kubicek S, Jenuwein T (2004) A crack in histone lysine methylation. Cell 119(7):903–906
67. Zibetti C et al (2010) Alternative splicing of the histone demethylase LSD1/KDM1 contributes to the modulation of neurite morphogenesis in the mammalian nervous system. J Neurosci 30(7):2521–2532
68. Wang J et al (2015) LSD1n is an H4K20 demethylase regulating memory formation via transcriptional elongation control. Nat Neurosci 18(9):1256–1264
69. Laurent B et al (2015) A specific LSD1/KDM1A isoform regulates neuronal differentiation through H3K9 demethylation. Mol Cell 57(6):957–970
70. Kahl P et al (2006) Androgen receptor coactivators lysine-specific histone demethylase 1 and four and a half LIM domain protein 2 predict risk of prostate cancer recurrence. Cancer Res 66(23):11341–11347
71. Metzger E et al (2005) LSD1 demethylates repressive histone marks to promote androgen-receptor-dependent transcription. Nature 437(7057):436–439
72. Kauffman EC et al (2011) Role of androgen receptor and associated lysine-demethylase coregulators, LSD1 and JMJD2A, in localized and advanced human bladder cancer. Mol Carcinog 50(12):931–944
73. Schulte JH et al (2009) Lysine-specific demethylase 1 is strongly expressed in poorly differentiated neuroblastoma: implications for therapy. Cancer Res 69(5):2065–2071
74. Serce N et al (2012) Elevated expression of LSD1 (Lysine-specific demethylase 1) during tumour progression from pre-invasive to invasive ductal carcinoma of the breast. BMC Clin Pathol 12:13
75. Lim S et al (2010) Lysine-specific demethylase 1 (LSD1) is highly expressed in ER-negative breast cancers and a biomarker predicting aggressive biology. Carcinogenesis 31(3):512–520
76. Lv T et al (2012) Over-expression of LSD1 promotes proliferation, migration and invasion in non-small cell lung cancer. PLoS One 7(4):e35065
77. Zhao ZK et al (2013) Overexpression of LSD1 in hepatocellular carcinoma: a latent target for the diagnosis and therapy of hepatoma. Tumour Biol 34(1):173–180
78. Wang Y et al (2016) The histone demethylase LSD1 is a novel oncogene and therapeutic target in oral cancer. Cancer Lett 374(1):12–21
79. Ding J et al (2013) LSD1-mediated epigenetic modification contributes to proliferation and metastasis of colon cancer. Br J Cancer 109(4):994–1003
80. Schildhaus HU et al (2011) Lysine-specific demethylase 1 is highly expressed in solitary fibrous tumors, synovial sarcomas, rhabdomyosarcomas, desmoplastic small round cell tumors, and malignant peripheral nerve sheath tumors. Hum Pathol 42(11):1667–1675
81. Bennani-Baiti IM et al (2012) Lysine-specific demethylase 1 (LSD1/KDM1A/AOF2/BHC110) is expressed and is an epigenetic drug target in chondrosarcoma, Ewing's sarcoma, osteosarcoma, and rhabdomyosarcoma. Hum Pathol 43(8):1300–1307
82. Harris WJ et al (2012) The histone demethylase KDM1A sustains the oncogenic potential of MLL-AF9 leukemia stem cells. Cancer Cell 21(4):473–487
83. Schenk T et al (2012) Inhibition of the LSD1 (KDM1A) demethylase reactivates the all-trans-retinoic acid differentiation pathway in acute myeloid leukemia. Nat Med 18(4):605–611
84. Yatim A et al (2012) NOTCH1 nuclear interactome reveals key regulators of its transcriptional activity and oncogenic function. Mol Cell 48(3):445–458
85. Theisen ER et al (2016) Therapeutic opportunities in Ewing sarcoma: EWS-FLI inhibition via LSD1 targeting. Oncotarget 7(14):17616–17630
86. Sankar S et al (2014) Reversible LSD1 inhibition interferes with global EWS/ETS transcriptional activity and impedes Ewing sarcoma tumor growth. Clin Cancer Res 20(17):4584–4597

87. Ding X et al (2013) Epigenetic activation of AP1 promotes squamous cell carcinoma metastasis. Sci Signal 6(273):ra28 1–13, S0–15
88. Lin T et al (2010) Requirement of the histone demethylase LSD1 in Snai1-mediated transcriptional repression during epithelial-mesenchymal transition. Oncogene 29(35):4896–4904
89. Morera L, Lubbert M, Jung M (2016) Targeting histone methyltransferases and demethylases in clinical trials for cancer therapy. Clin Epigenetics 8:57
90. Wang Y et al (2009) LSD1 is a subunit of the NuRD complex and targets the metastasis programs in breast cancer. Cell 138(4):660–672
91. Katz TA et al (2014) Inhibition of histone demethylase, LSD2 (KDM1B), attenuates DNA methylation and increases sensitivity to DNMT inhibitor-induced apoptosis in breast cancer cells. Breast Cancer Res Treat 146(1):99–108
92. Yang Y et al (2015) Histone demethylase LSD2 acts as an E3 ubiquitin ligase and inhibits cancer cell growth through promoting proteasomal degradation of OGT. Mol Cell 58(1):47–59
93. Forneris F et al (2005) Human histone demethylase LSD1 reads the histone code. J Biol Chem 280(50):41360–41365
94. Yang M et al (2007) Structural basis of histone demethylation by LSD1 revealed by suicide inactivation. Nat Struct Mol Biol 14(6):535–539
95. Forneris F et al (2007) Structural basis of LSD1-CoREST selectivity in histone H3 recognition. J Biol Chem 282(28):20070–20074
96. Da G et al (2006) Structure and function of the SWIRM domain, a conserved protein module found in chromatin regulatory complexes. Proc Natl Acad Sci U S A 103(7):2057–2062
97. Qian C et al (2005) Structure and chromosomal DNA binding of the SWIRM domain. Nat Struct Mol Biol 12(12):1078–1085
98. Yang M et al (2006) Structural basis for CoREST-dependent demethylation of nucleosomes by the human LSD1 histone demethylase. Mol Cell 23(3):377–387
99. Tochio N et al (2006) Solution structure of the SWIRM domain of human histone demethylase LSD1. Structure 14(3):457–468
100. Ballas N et al (2001) Regulation of neuronal traits by a novel transcriptional complex. Neuron 31(3):353–365
101. Shi Y et al (2003) Coordinated histone modifications mediated by a CtBP co-repressor complex. Nature 422(6933):735–738
102. Barta ML et al (2012) The structures of coiled-coil domains from type III secretion system translocators reveal homology to pore-forming toxins. J Mol Biol 417(5):395–405
103. Yang Z et al (2010) AOF1 is a histone H3K4 demethylase possessing demethylase activity-independent repression function. Cell Res 20(3):276–287
104. Zhang Q et al (2013) Structure-function analysis reveals a novel mechanism for regulation of histone demethylase LSD2/AOF1/KDM1b. Cell Res 23(2):225–241
105. Andres ME et al (1999) CoREST: a functional corepressor required for regulation of neural-specific gene expression. Proc Natl Acad Sci U S A 96(17):9873–9878
106. Chong JA et al (1995) REST: a mammalian silencer protein that restricts sodium channel gene expression to neurons. Cell 80(6):949–957
107. Schoenherr CJ, Anderson DJ (1995) Silencing is golden: negative regulation in the control of neuronal gene transcription. Curr Opin Neurobiol 5(5):566–571
108. Schoenherr CJ, Anderson DJ (1995) The neuron-restrictive silencer factor (NRSF): a coordinate repressor of multiple neuron-specific genes. Science 267(5202):1360–1363
109. You A et al (2001) CoREST is an integral component of the CoREST- human histone deacetylase complex. Proc Natl Acad Sci U S A 98(4):1454–1458
110. Hakimi MA et al (2002) A core-BRAF35 complex containing histone deacetylase mediates repression of neuronal-specific genes. Proc Natl Acad Sci U S A 99(11):7420–7425
111. Humphrey GW et al (2001) Stable histone deacetylase complexes distinguished by the presence of SANT domain proteins CoREST/kiaa0071 and Mta-L1. J Biol Chem 276(9):6817–6824
112. Abrajano JJ et al (2009) REST and CoREST modulate neuronal subtype specification, maturation and maintenance. PLoS One 4(12):e7936

113. Qureshi IA, Gokhan S, Mehler MF (2010) REST and CoREST are transcriptional and epigenetic regulators of seminal neural fate decisions. Cell Cycle 9(22):4477–4486

114. Lakowski B, Roelens I, Jacob S (2006) CoREST-like complexes regulate chromatin modification and neuronal gene expression. J Mol Neurosci 29(3):227–239

115. Metzger E et al (2010) Phosphorylation of histone H3T6 by PKCbeta(I) controls demethylation at histone H3K4. Nature 464(7289):792–796

116. Metzger E et al (2016) Assembly of methylated KDM1A and CHD1 drives androgen receptor-dependent transcription and translocation. Nat Struct Mol Biol 23(2):132–139

117. Basta J, Rauchman M (2015) The nucleosome remodeling and deacetylase complex in development and disease. Transl Res 165(1):36–47

118. Wang J et al (2007) Opposing LSD1 complexes function in developmental gene activation and repression programmes. Nature 446(7138):882–887

119. Toffolo E et al (2014) Phosphorylation of neuronal lysine-specific demethylase 1LSD1/KDM1A impairs transcriptional repression by regulating interaction with CoREST and histone deacetylases HDAC1/2. J Neurochem 128(5):603–616

120. McGrath J, Trojer P (2015) Targeting histone lysine methylation in cancer. Pharmacol Ther 150:1–22

121. Pedersen MT, Helin K (2010) Histone demethylases in development and disease. Trends Cell Biol 20(11):662–671

122. Zheng YC et al (2015) A systematic review of histone lysine-specific demethylase 1 and its inhibitors. Med Res Rev 35(5):1032–1071

123. Zheng YC et al (2016) Irreversible LSD1 inhibitors: application of tranylcypromine and its derivatives in cancer treatment. Curr Top Med Chem 16(19):2179–2188

124. Burg JM et al (2016) Lysine-specific demethylase 1A (KDM1A/LSD1): product recognition and kinetic analysis of full-length histones. Biochemistry 55(11):1652–1662

125. Mimasu S et al (2008) Crystal structure of histone demethylase LSD1 and tranylcypromine at 2.25 A. Biochem Biophys Res Commun 366(1):15–22

126. Yang M et al (2007) Structural basis for the inhibition of the LSD1 histone demethylase by the antidepressant trans-2-phenylcyclopropylamine. Biochemistry 46(27):8058–8065

127. Mimasu S et al (2010) Structurally designed trans-2-phenylcyclopropylamine derivatives potently inhibit histone demethylase LSD1/KDM1. Biochemistry 49(30):6494–6503

128. Binda C et al (2010) Biochemical, structural, and biological evaluation of tranylcypromine derivatives as inhibitors of histone demethylases LSD1 and LSD2. J Am Chem Soc 132(19):6827–6833

129. Baron R et al (2011) Molecular mimicry and ligand recognition in binding and catalysis by the histone demethylase LSD1-CoREST complex. Structure 19(2):212–220

130. Tortorici M et al (2013) Protein recognition by short peptide reversible inhibitors of the chromatin-modifying LSD1/CoREST lysine demethylase. ACS Chem Biol 8(8):1677–1682

131. Luka Z et al (2014) Crystal structure of the histone lysine specific demethylase LSD1 complexed with tetrahydrofolate. Protein Sci 23(7):993–998

132. Barrios AP et al (2014) Differential properties of transcriptional complexes formed by the CoREST family. Mol Cell Biol 34(14):2760–2770

133. Vianello P et al (2014) Synthesis, biological activity and mechanistic insights of 1-substituted cyclopropylamine derivatives: a novel class of irreversible inhibitors of histone demethylase KDM1A. Eur J Med Chem 86:352–363

134. Pilotto S et al (2016) LSD1/KDM1A mutations associated to a newly described form of intellectual disability impair demethylase activity and binding to transcription factors. Hum Mol Genet 25(12):2578–2587

135. He J et al (2008) The H3K36 demethylase Jhdm1b/Kdm2b regulates cell proliferation and senescence through p15(Ink4b). Nat Struct Mol Biol 15(11):1169–1175

136. Tzatsos A et al (2013) KDM2B promotes pancreatic cancer via Polycomb-dependent and -independent transcriptional programs. J Clin Invest 123(2):727–739

137. Liu H et al (2016) Integrated genomic and functional analyses of histone demethylases identify oncogenic KDM2A isoform in breast cancer. Mol Carcinog 55(5):977–990

138. Chen JY et al (2016) Lysine demethylase 2A promotes stemness and angiogenesis of breast cancer by upregulating Jagged1. Oncotarget 7(19):27689–27710
139. Wagner KW et al (2013) KDM2A promotes lung tumorigenesis by epigenetically enhancing ERK1/2 signaling. J Clin Invest 123(12):5231–5246
140. Huang Y et al (2015) Histone demethylase KDM2A promotes tumor cell growth and migration in gastric cancer. Tumour Biol 36(1):271–278
141. Rizwani W et al (2014) Mammalian lysine histone demethylase KDM2A regulates E2F1-mediated gene transcription in breast cancer cells. PLoS One 9(7):e100888
142. Kottakis F et al (2014) NDY1/KDM2B functions as a master regulator of polycomb complexes and controls self-renewal of breast cancer stem cells. Cancer Res 74(14):3935–3946
143. Karoopongse E et al (2014) The KDM2B- let-7b -EZH2 axis in myelodysplastic syndromes as a target for combined epigenetic therapy. PLoS One 9(9):e107817
144. Nakamura S et al (2013) JmjC-domain containing histone demethylase 1B-mediated p15(Ink4b) suppression promotes the proliferation of leukemic progenitor cells through modulation of cell cycle progression in acute myeloid leukemia. Mol Carcinog 52(1):57–69
145. He J, Nguyen AT, Zhang Y (2011) KDM2b/JHDM1b, an H3K36me2-specific demethylase, is required for initiation and maintenance of acute myeloid leukemia. Blood 117(14):3869–3880
146. Ueda T et al (2015) Fbxl10 overexpression in murine hematopoietic stem cells induces leukemia involving metabolic activation and upregulation of Nsg2. Blood 125(22):3437–3446
147. Tzatsos A et al (2009) Ndy1/KDM2B immortalizes mouse embryonic fibroblasts by repressing the Ink4a/Arf locus. Proc Natl Acad Sci U S A 106(8):2641–2646
148. Yu X et al (2015) A systematic study of the cellular metabolic regulation of Jhdm1b in tumor cells. Mol BioSyst 11(7):1867–1875
149. Hausinger RP (2004) FeII/alpha-ketoglutarate-dependent hydroxylases and related enzymes. Crit Rev Biochem Mol Biol 39(1):21–68
150. Zhou JC et al (2012) Recognition of CpG island chromatin by KDM2A requires direct and specific interaction with linker DNA. Mol Cell Biol 32(2):479–489
151. Blackledge NP, Klose R (2011) CpG island chromatin: a platform for gene regulation. Epigenetics 6(2):147–152
152. Blackledge NP et al (2010) CpG islands recruit a histone H3 lysine 36 demethylase. Mol Cell 38(2):179–190
153. Long HK, Blackledge NP, Klose RJ (2013) ZF-CxxC domain-containing proteins, CpG islands and the chromatin connection. Biochem Soc Trans 41(3):727–740
154. Blackledge NP, Thomson JP, Skene PJ (2013) CpG island chromatin is shaped by recruitment of ZF-CxxC proteins. Cold Spring Harb Perspect Biol 5(11):a018648
155. Farcas AM et al (2012) KDM2B links the polycomb repressive complex 1 (PRC1) to recognition of CpG islands. elife 1:e00205
156. Wu X, Johansen JV, Helin K (2013) Fbxl10/Kdm2b recruits polycomb repressive complex 1 to CpG islands and regulates H2A ubiquitylation. Mol Cell 49(6):1134–1146
157. Inagaki T et al (2015) The FBXL10/KDM2B scaffolding protein associates with novel polycomb repressive complex-1 to regulate adipogenesis. J Biol Chem 290(7):4163–4177
158. Han XR et al (2016) KDM2B/FBXL10 targets c-Fos for ubiquitylation and degradation in response to mitogenic stimulation. Oncogene 35(32):4179–4190
159. Janzer A et al (2012) The H3K4me3 histone demethylase Fbxl10 is a regulator of chemokine expression, cellular morphology, and the metabolome of fibroblasts. J Biol Chem 287(37):30984–30992
160. Heery DM et al (1997) A signature motif in transcriptional co-activators mediates binding to nuclear receptors. Nature 387(6634):733–736
161. Plevin MJ, Mills MM, Ikura M (2005) The LxxLL motif: a multifunctional binding sequence in transcriptional regulation. Trends Biochem Sci 30(2):66–69
162. Kuroki S et al (2013) Epigenetic regulation of mouse sex determination by the histone demethylase Jmjd1a. Science 341(6150):1106–1109
163. Liu Z et al (2015) Knockout of the histone demethylase Kdm3b decreases spermatogenesis and impairs male sexual behaviors. Int J Biol Sci 11(12):1447–1457

164. Okada Y et al (2007) Histone demethylase JHDM2A is critical for Tnp1 and Prm1 transcription and spermatogenesis. Nature 450(7166):119–123
165. Loh YH et al (2007) Jmjd1a and Jmjd2c histone H3 Lys 9 demethylases regulate self-renewal in embryonic stem cells. Genes Dev 21(20):2545–2557
166. Tateishi K et al (2009) Role of Jhdm2a in regulating metabolic gene expression and obesity resistance. Nature 458(7239):757–761
167. Inagaki T et al (2009) Obesity and metabolic syndrome in histone demethylase JHDM2a-deficient mice. Genes Cells 14(8):991–1001
168. Kuroki S et al (2013) JMJD1C, a JmjC domain-containing protein, is required for long-term maintenance of male germ cells in mice. Biol Reprod 89(4):93
169. Zhan M et al (2016) JMJD1A promotes tumorigenesis and forms a feedback loop with EZH2/let-7c in NSCLC cells. Tumour Biol 37(8):11237–11247
170. Cho HS et al (2012) The JmjC domain-containing histone demethylase KDM3A is a positive regulator of the G1/S transition in cancer cells via transcriptional regulation of the HOXA1 gene. Int J Cancer 131(3):E179–E189
171. Yang H et al (2015) Elevated JMJD1A is a novel predictor for prognosis and a potential therapeutic target for gastric cancer. Int J Clin Exp Pathol 8(9):11092–11099
172. Tee AE et al (2014) The histone demethylase JMJD1A induces cell migration and invasion by up-regulating the expression of the long noncoding RNA MALAT1. Oncotarget 5(7):1793–1804
173. Parrish JK et al (2015) The histone demethylase KDM3A is a microRNA-22-regulated tumor promoter in Ewing sarcoma. Oncogene 34(2):257–262
174. Guo X et al (2011) The expression of histone demethylase JMJD1A in renal cell carcinoma. Neoplasma 58(2):153–157
175. Yamada D et al (2012) Role of the hypoxia-related gene, JMJD1A, in hepatocellular carcinoma: clinical impact on recurrence after hepatic resection. Ann Surg Oncol 19(Suppl 3):S355–S364
176. Ohguchi H et al (2016) The KDM3A-KLF2-IRF4 axis maintains myeloma cell survival. Nat Commun 7:10258
177. Fan L et al (2016) Regulation of c-Myc expression by the histone demethylase JMJD1A is essential for prostate cancer cell growth and survival. Oncogene 35(19):2441–2452
178. Krieg AJ et al (2010) Regulation of the histone demethylase JMJD1A by hypoxia-inducible factor 1 alpha enhances hypoxic gene expression and tumor growth. Mol Cell Biol 30(1):344–353
179. Uemura M et al (2010) Jumonji domain containing 1A is a novel prognostic marker for colorectal cancer: in vivo identification from hypoxic tumor cells. Clin Cancer Res 16(18):4636–4646
180. Osawa T et al (2013) Inhibition of histone demethylase JMJD1A improves anti-angiogenic therapy and reduces tumor-associated macrophages. Cancer Res 73(10):3019–3028
181. Park SJ et al (2013) The histone demethylase JMJD1A regulates adrenomedullin-mediated cell proliferation in hepatocellular carcinoma under hypoxia. Biochem Biophys Res Commun 434(4):722–727
182. Ueda J et al (2014) The hypoxia-inducible epigenetic regulators Jmjd1a and G9a provide a mechanistic link between angiogenesis and tumor growth. Mol Cell Biol 34(19):3702–3720
183. Hu Z et al (2001) A novel nuclear protein, 5qNCA (LOC51780) is a candidate for the myeloid leukemia tumor suppressor gene on chromosome 5 band q31. Oncogene 20(47):6946–6954
184. Paolicchi E et al (2013) Histone lysine demethylases in breast cancer. Crit Rev Oncol Hematol 86(2):97–103
185. Kim JY et al (2012) KDM3B is the H3K9 demethylase involved in transcriptional activation of lmo2 in leukemia. Mol Cell Biol 32(14):2917–2933
186. Baik SH et al (2009) DNA profiling by array comparative genomic hybridization (CGH) of peripheral blood mononuclear cells (PBMC) and tumor tissue cell in non-small cell lung cancer (NSCLC). Mol Biol Rep 36(7):1767–1778
187. Brauchle M et al (2013) Protein complex interactor analysis and differential activity of KDM3 subfamily members towards H3K9 methylation. PLoS One 8(4):e60549
188. Wang J et al (2014) Epigenetic regulation of miR-302 by JMJD1C inhibits neural differentiation of human embryonic stem cells. J Biol Chem 289(4):2384–2395

189. Chen M et al (2015) JMJD1C is required for the survival of acute myeloid leukemia by functioning as a coactivator for key transcription factors. Genes Dev 29(20):2123–2139
190. Sroczynska P et al (2014) shRNA screening identifies JMJD1C as being required for leukemia maintenance. Blood 123(12):1870–1882
191. Wang L et al (2014) Novel somatic and germline mutations in intracranial germ cell tumours. Nature 511(7508):241–245
192. Yamane K et al (2006) JHDM2A, a JmjC-containing H3K9 demethylase, facilitates transcription activation by androgen receptor. Cell 125(3):483–495
193. Goda S et al (2013) Control of histone H3 lysine 9 (H3K9) methylation state via cooperative two-step demethylation by Jumonji domain containing 1A (JMJD1A) homodimer. J Biol Chem 288(52):36948–36956
194. Lim S et al (2010) Epigenetic regulation of cancer growth by histone demethylases. Int J Cancer 127(9):1991–1998
195. Pollard PJ et al (2008) Regulation of Jumonji-domain-containing histone demethylases by hypoxia-inducible factor (HIF)-1alpha. Biochem J 416(3):387–394
196. Sar A et al (2009) Identification and characterization of demethylase JMJD1A as a gene upregulated in the human cellular response to hypoxia. Cell Tissue Res 337(2):223–234
197. Wellmann S et al (2008) Hypoxia upregulates the histone demethylase JMJD1A via HIF-1. Biochem Biophys Res Commun 372(4):892–897
198. Lin Q, Yun Z (2010) Impact of the hypoxic tumor microenvironment on the regulation of cancer stem cell characteristics. Cancer Biol Ther 9(12):949–956
199. Beyer S et al (2008) The histone demethylases JMJD1A and JMJD2B are transcriptional targets of hypoxia-inducible factor HIF. J Biol Chem 283(52):36542–36552
200. Guerra-Calderas L et al (2015) The role of the histone demethylase KDM4A in cancer. Cancer Genet 208(5):215–224
201. Labbe RM, Holowatyj A, Yang ZQ (2013) Histone lysine demethylase (KDM) subfamily 4: structures, functions and therapeutic potential. Am J Transl Res 6(1):1–15
202. Del Rizzo PA, Trievel RC (2014) Molecular basis for substrate recognition by lysine methyltransferases and demethylases. Biochim Biophys Acta 1839(12):1404–1415
203. Pack LR, Yamamoto KR, Fujimori DG (2016) Opposing Chromatin Signals Direct and Regulate the Activity of Lysine Demethylase 4C (KDM4C). J Biol Chem 291(12):6060–6070
204. Das PP et al (2014) Distinct and combinatorial functions of Jmjd2b/Kdm4b and Jmjd2c/Kdm4c in mouse embryonic stem cell identity. Mol Cell 53(1):32–48
205. Zhang X et al (2009) Genome-wide analysis of mono-, di- and trimethylation of histone H3 lysine 4 in Arabidopsis thaliana. Genome Biol 10(6):R62
206. Huang Y et al (2006) Recognition of histone H3 lysine-4 methylation by the double tudor domain of JMJD2A. Science 312(5774):748–751
207. Yu Y et al (2012) Histone H3 lysine 56 methylation regulates DNA replication through its interaction with PCNA. Mol Cell 46(1):7–17
208. Jack AP et al (2013) H3K56me3 is a novel, conserved heterochromatic mark that largely but not completely overlaps with H3K9me3 in both regulation and localization. PLoS One 8(2):e51765
209. Young LC, Hendzel MJ (2013) The oncogenic potential of Jumonji D2 (JMJD2/KDM4) histone demethylase overexpression. Biochem Cell Biol 91(6):369–377
210. Luo W et al (2012) Histone demethylase JMJD2C is a coactivator for hypoxia-inducible factor 1 that is required for breast cancer progression. Proc Natl Acad Sci U S A 109(49):E3367–E3376
211. Yang J et al (2010) The histone demethylase JMJD2B is regulated by estrogen receptor alpha and hypoxia, and is a key mediator of estrogen induced growth. Cancer Res 70(16):6456–6466
212. Awwad SW, Ayoub N (2015) Overexpression of KDM4 lysine demethylases disrupts the integrity of the DNA mismatch repair pathway. Biol Open 4(4):498–504
213. Agger K et al (2016) Jmjd2/Kdm4 demethylases are required for expression of Il3ra and survival of acute myeloid leukemia cells. Genes Dev 30(11):1278–1288
214. Ye Q et al (2015) Genetic alterations of KDM4 subfamily and therapeutic effect of novel demethylase inhibitor in breast cancer. Am J Cancer Res 5(4):1519–1530

215. Li LL et al (2014) JMJD2A contributes to breast cancer progression through transcriptional repression of the tumor suppressor ARHI. Breast Cancer Res 16(3):R56
216. Bjorkman M et al (2012) Systematic knockdown of epigenetic enzymes identifies a novel histone demethylase PHF8 overexpressed in prostate cancer with an impact on cell proliferation, migration and invasion. Oncogene 31(29):3444–3456
217. Kim TD et al (2016) Histone demethylase JMJD2A drives prostate tumorigenesis through transcription factor ETV1. J Clin Invest 126(2):706–720
218. Xu W et al (2016) Jumonji domain containing 2A predicts prognosis and regulates cell growth in lung cancer depending on miR-150. Oncol Rep 35(1):352–358
219. Mallette FA, Richard S (2012) JMJD2A promotes cellular transformation by blocking cellular senescence through transcriptional repression of the tumor suppressor CHD5. Cell Rep 2(5):1233–1243
220. Kogure M et al (2013) Deregulation of the histone demethylase JMJD2A is involved in human carcinogenesis through regulation of the G(1)/S transition. Cancer Lett 336(1):76–84
221. Hu CE et al (2014) JMJD2A predicts prognosis and regulates cell growth in human gastric cancer. Biochem Biophys Res Commun 449(1):1–7
222. Wang HL et al (2014) Expression and effects of JMJD2A histone demethylase in endometrial carcinoma. Asian Pac J Cancer Prev 15(7):3051–3056
223. Qiu MT et al (2015) KDM4B and KDM4A promote endometrial cancer progression by regulating androgen receptor, c-myc, and p27kip1. Oncotarget 6(31):31702–31720
224. Black JC et al (2013) KDM4A lysine demethylase induces site-specific copy gain and rereplication of regions amplified in tumors. Cell 154(3):541–555
225. Chu CH et al (2014) KDM4B as a target for prostate cancer: structural analysis and selective inhibition by a novel inhibitor. J Med Chem 57(14):5975–5985
226. Kim TD et al (2012) The JMJD2A demethylase regulates apoptosis and proliferation in colon cancer cells. J Cell Biochem 113(4):1368–1376
227. Li BX et al (2011) Effects of RNA interference-mediated gene silencing of JMJD2A on human breast cancer cell line MDA-MB-231 in vitro. J Exp Clin Cancer Res 30:90
228. Xu W et al (2015) SIRT2 suppresses non-small cell lung cancer growth by targeting JMJD2A. Biol Chem 396(8):929–936
229. Liu Y et al (2013) An epigenetic role for PRL-3 as a regulator of H3K9 methylation in colorectal cancer. Gut 62(4):571–581
230. Toyokawa G et al (2011) The histone demethylase JMJD2B plays an essential role in human carcinogenesis through positive regulation of cyclin-dependent kinase 6. Cancer Prev Res (Phila) 4(12):2051–2061
231. Coffey K et al (2013) The lysine demethylase, KDM4B, is a key molecule in androgen receptor signalling and turnover. Nucleic Acids Res 41(8):4433–4446
232. Li W et al (2011) Histone demethylase JMJD2B is required for tumor cell proliferation and survival and is overexpressed in gastric cancer. Biochem Biophys Res Commun 416(3–4):372–378
233. Zhao L et al (2013) JMJD2B promotes epithelial-mesenchymal transition by cooperating with beta-catenin and enhances gastric cancer metastasis. Clin Cancer Res 19(23):6419–6429
234. Han F et al (2016) JMJD2B is required for Helicobacter pylori-induced gastric carcinogenesis via regulating COX-2 expression. Oncotarget 7(25):38626–38637
235. Lu JW et al (2015) JMJD2B as a potential diagnostic immunohistochemical marker for hepatocellular carcinoma: a tissue microarray-based study. Acta Histochem 117(1):14–19
236. Li X, Dong S (2015) Histone demethylase JMJD2B and JMJD2C induce fibroblast growth factor 2: mediated tumorigenesis of osteosarcoma. Med Oncol 32(3):53
237. Kawazu M et al (2011) Histone demethylase JMJD2B functions as a co-factor of estrogen receptor in breast cancer proliferation and mammary gland development. PLoS One 6(3):e17830
238. Shi L et al (2011) Histone demethylase JMJD2B coordinates H3K4/H3K9 methylation and promotes hormonally responsive breast carcinogenesis. Proc Natl Acad Sci U S A 108(18):7541–7546
239. Chen L et al (2014) Jumonji domain-containing protein 2B silencing induces DNA damage response via STAT3 pathway in colorectal cancer. Br J Cancer 110(4):1014–1026

240. Sun BB et al (2014) Silencing of JMJD2B induces cell apoptosis via mitochondria-mediated and death receptor-mediated pathway activation in colorectal cancer. J Dig Dis 15(9):491–500
241. Liu G et al (2009) Genomic amplification and oncogenic properties of the GASC1 histone demethylase gene in breast cancer. Oncogene 28(50):4491–4500
242. Yang ZQ et al (2000) Identification of a novel gene, GASC1, within an amplicon at 9p23-24 frequently detected in esophageal cancer cell lines. Cancer Res 60(17):4735–4739
243. Italiano A et al (2006) Molecular cytogenetic characterization of a metastatic lung sarcomatoid carcinoma: 9p23 neocentromere and 9p23-p24 amplification including JAK2 and JMJD2C. Cancer Genet Cytogenet 167(2):122–130
244. Rui L et al (2010) Cooperative epigenetic modulation by cancer amplicon genes. Cancer Cell 18(6):590–605
245. Ehrbrecht A et al (2006) Comprehensive genomic analysis of desmoplastic medulloblastomas: identification of novel amplified genes and separate evaluation of the different histological components. J Pathol 208(4):554–563
246. Northcott PA et al (2009) Multiple recurrent genetic events converge on control of histone lysine methylation in medulloblastoma. Nat Genet 41(4):465–472
247. Sun LL et al (2013) Histone demethylase GASC1, a potential prognostic and predictive marker in esophageal squamous cell carcinoma. Am J Cancer Res 3(5):509–517
248. Ozaki Y et al (2015) The oncogenic role of GASC1 in chemically induced mouse skin cancer. Mamm Genome 26(11–12):591–597
249. Ishimura A et al (2009) Jmjd2c histone demethylase enhances the expression of Mdm2 oncogene. Biochem Biophys Res Commun 389(2):366–371
250. Berdel B et al (2012) Histone demethylase GASC1 – a potential prognostic and predictive marker in invasive breast cancer. BMC Cancer 12:516
251. Kim TD et al (2012) Regulation of tumor suppressor p53 and HCT116 cell physiology by histone demethylase JMJD2D/KDM4D. PLoS One 7(4):e34618
252. Hillringhaus L et al (2011) Structural and evolutionary basis for the dual substrate selectivity of human KDM4 histone demethylase family. J Biol Chem 286(48):41616–41625
253. Ng SS et al (2007) Crystal structures of histone demethylase JMJD2A reveal basis for substrate specificity. Nature 448(7149):87–91
254. Couture JF et al (2007) Specificity and mechanism of JMJD2A, a trimethyllysine-specific histone demethylase. Nat Struct Mol Biol 14(8):689–695
255. Kim J et al (2006) Tudor, MBT and chromo domains gauge the degree of lysine methylation. EMBO Rep 7(4):397–403
256. Lee J et al (2008) Distinct binding modes specify the recognition of methylated histones H3K4 and H4K20 by JMJD2A-tudor. Nat Struct Mol Biol 15(1):109–111
257. Mallette FA et al (2012) RNF8- and RNF168-dependent degradation of KDM4A/JMJD2A triggers 53BP1 recruitment to DNA damage sites. EMBO J 31(8):1865–1878
258. Pedersen MT et al (2014) The demethylase JMJD2C localizes to H3K4me3-positive transcription start sites and is dispensable for embryonic development. Mol Cell Biol 34(6):1031–1045
259. Ozboyaci M et al (2011) Molecular recognition of H3/H4 histone tails by the tudor domains of JMJD2A: a comparative molecular dynamics simulations study. PLoS One 6(3):e14765
260. Gaughan L et al (2013) KDM4B is a master regulator of the estrogen receptor signalling cascade. Nucleic Acids Res 41(14):6892–6904
261. Chen Z et al (2007) Structural basis of the recognition of a methylated histone tail by JMJD2A. Proc Natl Acad Sci U S A 104(26):10818–10823
262. Rose NR et al (2008) Inhibitor scaffolds for 2-oxoglutarate-dependent histone lysine demethylases. J Med Chem 51(22):7053–7056
263. Rose NR et al (2010) Selective inhibitors of the JMJD2 histone demethylases: combined nondenaturing mass spectrometric screening and crystallographic approaches. J Med Chem 53(4):1810–1818
264. King ON et al (2010) Quantitative high-throughput screening identifies 8-hydroxyquinolines as cell-active histone demethylase inhibitors. PLoS One 5(11):e15535

265. Chang KH et al (2011) Inhibition of histone demethylases by 4-carboxy-2,2′-bipyridyl compounds. ChemMedChem 6(5):759–764
266. Chowdhury R et al (2011) The oncometabolite 2-hydroxyglutarate inhibits histone lysine demethylases. EMBO Rep 12(5):463–469
267. Woon EC et al (2012) Linking of 2-oxoglutarate and substrate binding sites enables potent and highly selective inhibition of JmjC histone demethylases. Angew Chem Int Ed Engl 51(7):1631–1634
268. Rose NR et al (2012) Plant growth regulator daminozide is a selective inhibitor of human KDM2/7 histone demethylases. J Med Chem 55(14):6639–6643
269. Hopkinson RJ et al (2013) 5-carboxy-8-hydroxyquinoline is a broad spectrum 2-oxoglutarate oxygenase inhibitor which causes iron translocation. Chem Sci 4(8):3110–3117
270. Williams ST et al (2014) Studies on the catalytic domains of multiple JmjC oxygenases using peptide substrates. Epigenetics 9(12):1596–1603
271. Korczynska M et al (2016) Docking and linking of fragments to discover Jumonji histone demethylase inhibitors. J Med Chem 59(4):1580–1598
272. Roatsch M et al (2016) Substituted 2-(2-aminopyrimidin-4-yl)pyridine-4-carboxylates as potent inhibitors of JumonjiC domain-containing histone demethylases. Future Med Chem 8(13):1553–1571
273. Bavetsias V et al (2016) 8-Substituted pyrido[3,4-d]pyrimidin-4(3H)-one derivatives as potent, cell permeable, KDM4 (JMJD2) and KDM5 (JARID1) histone lysine demethylase inhibitors. J Med Chem 59(4):1388–1409
274. Johansson C et al (2016) Structural analysis of human KDM5B guides histone demethylase inhibitor development. Nat Chem Biol 12(7):539–545
275. Wigle TJ et al (2015) A high-throughput mass spectrometry assay coupled with redox activity testing reduces artifacts and false positives in lysine demethylase screening. J Biomol Screen 20(6):810–820
276. Krishnan S, Trievel RC (2013) Structural and functional analysis of JMJD2D reveals molecular basis for site-specific demethylation among JMJD2 demethylases. Structure 21(1):98–108
277. Westaway SM et al (2016) Cell penetrant inhibitors of the KDM4 and KDM5 families of histone lysine demethylases. 2. Pyrido[3,4-d]pyrimidin-4(3H)-one derivatives. J Med Chem 59(4):1370–1387
278. Blair LP et al (2011) Epigenetic regulation by lysine demethylase 5 (KDM5) enzymes in cancer. Cancers (Basel) 3(1):1383–1404
279. Rasmussen PB, Staller P (2014) The KDM5 family of histone demethylases as targets in oncology drug discovery. Epigenomics 6(3):277–286
280. Voigt P, Tee WW, Reinberg D (2013) A double take on bivalent promoters. Genes Dev 27(12):1318–1338
281. Bernstein BE et al (2006) A bivalent chromatin structure marks key developmental genes in embryonic stem cells. Cell 125(2):315–326
282. Horton JR et al (2016) Structural basis for KDM5A histone lysine demethylase inhibition by diverse compounds. Cell Chemical Biology 23(7):769–781
283. Vinogradova M et al (2016) An inhibitor of KDM5 demethylases reduces survival of drug-tolerant cancer cells. Nat Chem Biol 12(7):531–538
284. Yamane K et al (2007) PLU-1 is an H3K4 demethylase involved in transcriptional repression and breast cancer cell proliferation. Mol Cell 25(6):801–812
285. Hou J et al (2012) Genomic amplification and a role in drug-resistance for the KDM5A histone demethylase in breast cancer. Am J Transl Res 4(3):247–256
286. Teng YC et al (2013) Histone demethylase RBP2 promotes lung tumorigenesis and cancer metastasis. Cancer Res 73(15):4711–4721
287. Wang S et al (2013) RBP2 induces epithelial-mesenchymal transition in non-small cell lung cancer. PLoS One 8(12):e84735
288. Liang X et al (2013) Histone demethylase retinoblastoma binding protein 2 is overexpressed in hepatocellular carcinoma and negatively regulated by hsa-miR-212. PLoS One 8(7):e69784

289. Zeng J et al (2010) The histone demethylase RBP2 is overexpressed in gastric cancer and its inhibition triggers senescence of cancer cells. Gastroenterology 138(3):981–992
290. Jiping Z et al (2013) MicroRNA-212 inhibits proliferation of gastric cancer by directly repressing retinoblastoma binding protein 2. J Cell Biochem 114(12):2666–2672
291. Fattaey AR et al (1993) Characterization of the retinoblastoma binding proteins RBP1 and RBP2. Oncogene 8(11):3149–3156
292. Benevolenskaya EV et al (2005) Binding of pRB to the PHD protein RBP2 promotes cellular differentiation. Mol Cell 18(6):623–635
293. Lin W et al (2011) Loss of the retinoblastoma binding protein 2 (RBP2) histone demethylase suppresses tumorigenesis in mice lacking Rb1 or Men1. Proc Natl Acad Sci USA 108(33):13379–13386
294. Cao J et al (2014) Histone demethylase RBP2 is critical for breast cancer progression and metastasis. Cell Rep 6(5):868–877
295. Zhou D et al (2016) RBP2 induces stem-like cancer cells by promoting EMT and is a prognostic marker for renal cell carcinoma. Exp Mol Med 48:e238
296. Liang X et al (2015) Histone demethylase RBP2 promotes malignant progression of gastric cancer through TGF beta1 (p Smad3) RBP2-E-cadherin-Snail3 feedback circuit. Oncotarget 6(19):17661–17674
297. Sharma SV et al (2010) A chromatin-mediated reversible drug-tolerant state in cancer cell subpopulations. Cell 141(1):69–80
298. Banelli B et al (2015) The histone demethylase KDM5A is a key factor for the resistance to temozolomide in glioblastoma. Cell Cycle 14(21):3418–3429
299. Cancer Genome Atlas, N (2012) Comprehensive molecular portraits of human breast tumours. Nature 490(7418):61–70
300. Hayami S et al (2010) Overexpression of the JmjC histone demethylase KDM5B in human carcinogenesis: involvement in the proliferation of cancer cells through the E2F/RB pathway. Mol Cancer 9:59
301. Li X et al (2013) Connexin 26 is down-regulated by KDM5B in the progression of bladder cancer. Int J Mol Sci 14(4):7866–7879
302. Liggins AP et al (2010) A panel of cancer-testis genes exhibiting broad-spectrum expression in haematological malignancies. Cancer Immun 10:8
303. Xiang Y et al (2007) JARID1B is a histone H3 lysine 4 demethylase up-regulated in prostate cancer. Proc Natl Acad Sci U S A 104(49):19226–19231
304. Ohta K et al (2013) Depletion of JARID1B induces cellular senescence in human colorectal cancer. Int J Oncol 42(4):1212–1218
305. Dai B et al (2014) Overexpressed KDM5B is associated with the progression of glioma and promotes glioma cell growth via downregulating p21. Biochem Biophys Res Commun 454(1):221–227
306. Wang L et al (2015) Overexpression of JARID1B is associated with poor prognosis and chemotherapy resistance in epithelial ovarian cancer. Tumour Biol 36(4):2465–2472
307. Wang D et al (2016) Depletion of histone demethylase KDM5B inhibits cell proliferation of hepatocellular carcinoma by regulation of cell cycle checkpoint proteins p15 and p27. J Exp Clin Cancer Res 35:37
308. Tang B et al (2015) JARID1B promotes metastasis and epithelial-mesenchymal transition via PTEN/AKT signaling in hepatocellular carcinoma cells. Oncotarget 6(14):12723–12739
309. Scibetta AG et al (2007) Functional analysis of the transcription repressor PLU-1/JARID1B. Mol Cell Biol 27(20):7220–7235
310. Roesch A et al (2010) A temporarily distinct subpopulation of slow-cycling melanoma cells is required for continuous tumor growth. Cell 141(4):583–594
311. Roesch A et al (2013) Overcoming intrinsic multidrug resistance in melanoma by blocking the mitochondrial respiratory chain of slow-cycling JARID1B(high) cells. Cancer Cell 23(6):811–825
312. Wang Z et al (2015) KDM5B is overexpressed in gastric cancer and is required for gastric cancer cell proliferation and metastasis. Am J Cancer Res 5(1):87–100

313. Lin CS et al (2015) Silencing JARID1B suppresses oncogenicity, stemness and increases radiation sensitivity in human oral carcinoma. Cancer Lett 368(1):36–45
314. Kuo YT et al (2015) JARID1B expression plays a critical role in chemoresistance and stem cell-like phenotype of neuroblastoma cells. PLoS One 10(5):e0125343
315. Bamodu OA et al (2016) Aberrant KDM5B expression promotes aggressive breast cancer through MALAT1 overexpression and downregulation of hsa-miR-448. BMC Cancer 16:160
316. Klein BJ et al (2014) The histone-H3K4-specific demethylase KDM5B binds to its substrate and product through distinct PHD fingers. Cell Rep 6(2):325–335
317. Dalgliesh GL et al (2010) Systematic sequencing of renal carcinoma reveals inactivation of histone modifying genes. Nature 463(7279):360–363
318. Komura K et al (2016) Resistance to docetaxel in prostate cancer is associated with androgen receptor activation and loss of KDM5D expression. Proc Natl Acad Sci USA 113(22):6259–6264
319. Niu X et al (2012) The von Hippel-Lindau tumor suppressor protein regulates gene expression and tumor growth through histone demethylase JARID1C. Oncogene 31(6):776–786
320. Tu S et al (2008) The ARID domain of the H3K4 demethylase RBP2 binds to a DNA CCGCCC motif. Nat Struct Mol Biol 15(4):419–421
321. Yao W, Peng Y, Lin D (2010) The flexible loop L1 of the H3K4 demethylase JARID1B ARID domain has a crucial role in DNA-binding activity. Biochem Biophys Res Commun 396(2):323–328
322. Zhang Y et al (2014) The PHD1 finger of KDM5B recognizes unmodified H3K4 during the demethylation of histone H3K4me2/3 by KDM5B. Protein Cell 5(11):837–850
323. Torres IO et al (2015) Histone demethylase KDM5A is regulated by its reader domain through a positive-feedback mechanism. Nat Commun 6:6204
324. Chakravarty S et al (2015) Histone peptide recognition by KDM5B-PHD1: a case study. Biochemistry 54(37):5766–5780
325. Wang GG et al (2009) Haematopoietic malignancies caused by dysregulation of a chromatin-binding PHD finger. Nature 459(7248):847–851
326. Klose RJ et al (2007) The retinoblastoma binding protein RBP2 is an H3K4 demethylase. Cell 128(5):889–900
327. Sengoku T, Yokoyama S (2011) Structural basis for histone H3 Lys 27 demethylation by UTX/KDM6A. Genes Dev 25(21):2266–2277
328. van Oevelen C et al (2008) A role for mammalian Sin3 in permanent gene silencing. Mol Cell 32(3):359–370
329. Koehler C et al (2008) Backbone and sidechain 1H, 13C and 15N resonance assignments of the Bright/ARID domain from the human JARID1C (SMCX) protein. Biomol NMR Assign 2(1):9–11
330. Hong S et al (2007) Identification of JmjC domain-containing UTX and JMJD3 as histone H3 lysine 27 demethylases. Proc Natl Acad Sci U S A 104(47):18439–18444
331. Hubner MR, Spector DL (2010) Role of H3K27 demethylases Jmjd3 and UTX in transcriptional regulation. Cold Spring Harb Symp Quant Biol 75:43–49
332. Walport LJ et al (2014) Human UTY(KDM6C) is a male-specific N-methyl lysyl demethylase. J Biol Chem 289(26):18302–18313
333. Greenfield A et al (1998) The UTX gene escapes X inactivation in mice and humans. Hum Mol Genet 7(4):737–742
334. Lan F et al (2007) A histone H3 lysine 27 demethylase regulates animal posterior development. Nature 449(7163):689–694
335. Shpargel KB et al (2012) UTX and UTY demonstrate histone demethylase-independent function in mouse embryonic development. PLoS Genet 8(9):e1002964
336. Arcipowski KM, Martinez CA, Ntziachristos P (2016) Histone demethylases in physiology and cancer: a tale of two enzymes, JMJD3 and UTX. Curr Opin Genet Dev 36:59–67
337. Perrigue PM, Najbauer J, Barciszewski J (2016) Histone demethylase JMJD3 at the intersection of cellular senescence and cancer. Biochim Biophys Acta 1865(2):237–244
338. Van der Meulen J, Speleman F, Van Vlierberghe P (2014) The H3K27me3 demethylase UTX in normal development and disease. Epigenetics 9(5):658–668

339. Robinson G et al (2012) Novel mutations target distinct subgroups of medulloblastoma. Nature 488(7409):43–48
340. Gui Y et al (2011) Frequent mutations of chromatin remodeling genes in transitional cell carcinoma of the bladder. Nat Genet 43(9):875–878
341. Nickerson ML et al (2014) Concurrent alterations in TERT, KDM6A, and the BRCA pathway in bladder cancer. Clin Cancer Res 20(18):4935–4948
342. Van der Meulen J et al (2015) The H3K27me3 demethylase UTX is a gender-specific tumor suppressor in T-cell acute lymphoblastic leukemia. Blood 125(1):13–21
343. Ntziachristos P et al (2014) Contrasting roles of histone 3 lysine 27 demethylases in acute lymphoblastic leukaemia. Nature 514(7523):513–517
344. Mar BG et al (2012) Sequencing histone-modifying enzymes identifies UTX mutations in acute lymphoblastic leukemia. Leukemia 26(8):1881–1883
345. Jankowska AM et al (2011) Mutational spectrum analysis of chronic myelomonocytic leukemia includes genes associated with epigenetic regulation: UTX, EZH2, and DNMT3A. Blood 118(14):3932–3941
346. van Haaften G et al (2009) Somatic mutations of the histone H3K27 demethylase gene UTX in human cancer. Nat Genet 41(5):521–523
347. Wang JK et al (2010) The histone demethylase UTX enables RB-dependent cell fate control. Genes Dev 24(4):327–332
348. Benyoucef A et al (2016) UTX inhibition as selective epigenetic therapy against TAL1-driven T-cell acute lymphoblastic leukemia. Genes Dev 30(5):508–521
349. Kim JH et al (2014) UTX and MLL4 coordinately regulate transcriptional programs for cell proliferation and invasiveness in breast cancer cells. Cancer Res 74(6):1705–1717
350. Patani N et al (2011) Histone-modifier gene expression profiles are associated with pathological and clinical outcomes in human breast cancer. Anticancer Res 31(12):4115–4125
351. Ene CI et al (2012) Histone demethylase Jumonji D3 (JMJD3) as a tumor suppressor by regulating p53 protein nuclear stabilization. PLoS One 7(12):e51407
352. Williams K et al (2014) The histone lysine demethylase JMJD3/KDM6B is recruited to p53 bound promoters and enhancer elements in a p53 dependent manner. PLoS One 9(5):e96545
353. Agger K et al (2009) The H3K27me3 demethylase JMJD3 contributes to the activation of the INK4A-ARF locus in response to oncogene- and stress-induced senescence. Genes Dev 23(10):1171–1176
354. Barradas M et al (2009) Histone demethylase JMJD3 contributes to epigenetic control of INK4a/ARF by oncogenic RAS. Genes Dev 23(10):1177–1182
355. Tokunaga R et al (2016) The prognostic significance of histone lysine demethylase JMJD3/KDM6B in colorectal cancer. Ann Surg Oncol 23(2):678–685
356. Park WY et al (2016) H3K27 demethylase JMJD3 employs the NF-kappaB and BMP signaling pathways to modulate the tumor microenvironment and promote melanoma progression and metastasis. Cancer Res 76(1):161–170
357. Zhang Y et al (2016) JMJD3 promotes survival of diffuse large B-cell lymphoma subtypes via distinct mechanisms. Oncotarget 7(20):29387–29399
358. Kruidenier L et al (2012) A selective jumonji H3K27 demethylase inhibitor modulates the proinflammatory macrophage response. Nature 488(7411):404–408
359. Hashizume R et al (2014) Pharmacologic inhibition of histone demethylation as a therapy for pediatric brainstem glioma. Nat Med 20(12):1394–1396
360. Sakaki H et al (2015) GSKJ4, a selective Jumonji H3K27 demethylase inhibitor, effectively targets ovarian cancer stem cells. Anticancer Res 35(12):6607–6614
361. Dutta A et al (2016) Identification of an NKX3.1-G9a-UTY transcriptional regulatory network that controls prostate differentiation. Science 352(6293):1576–1580
362. Lau YF, Zhang J (2000) Expression analysis of thirty one Y chromosome genes in human prostate cancer. Mol Carcinog 27(4):308–321
363. Omichinski JG et al (1993) NMR structure of a specific DNA complex of Zn-containing DNA binding domain of GATA-1. Science 261(5120):438–446

364. Issaeva I et al (2007) Knockdown of ALR (MLL2) reveals ALR target genes and leads to alterations in cell adhesion and growth. Mol Cell Biol 27(5):1889–1903

365. Cho YW et al (2007) PTIP associates with MLL3- and MLL4-containing histone H3 lysine 4 methyltransferase complex. J Biol Chem 282(28):20395–20406

366. Burchfield JS et al (2015) JMJD3 as an epigenetic regulator in development and disease. Int J Biochem Cell Biol 67:148–157

367. Manna S et al (2015) Histone H3 lysine 27 demethylases Jmjd3 and Utx are required for T-cell differentiation. Nat Commun 6:8152

368. Park SY, Park JW, Chun YS (2016) Jumonji histone demethylases as emerging therapeutic targets. Pharmacol Res 105:146–151

369. Horton JR et al (2011) Structural basis for human PHF2 Jumonji domain interaction with metal ions. J Mol Biol 406(1):1–8

370. Baba A et al (2011) PKA-dependent regulation of the histone lysine demethylase complex PHF2-ARID5B. Nat Cell Biol 13(6):668–675

371. Hata K et al (2013) Arid5b facilitates chondrogenesis by recruiting the histone demethylase Phf2 to Sox9-regulated genes. Nat Commun 4:2850

372. Osawa T et al (2011) Increased expression of histone demethylase JHDM1D under nutrient starvation suppresses tumor growth via down-regulating angiogenesis. Proc Natl Acad Sci U S A 108(51):20725–20729

373. Ma Q et al (2015) The histone demethylase PHF8 promotes prostate cancer cell growth by activating the oncomiR miR-125b. Onco Targets Ther 8:1979–1988

374. Wang Q et al (2016) Stabilization of histone demethylase PHF8 by USP7 promotes breast carcinogenesis. J Clin Invest 126(6):2205–2220

375. Zhu G et al (2015) Elevated expression of histone demethylase PHF8 associates with adverse prognosis in patients of laryngeal and hypopharyngeal squamous cell carcinoma. Epigenomics 7(2):143–153

376. Shen Y, Pan X, Zhao H (2014) The histone demethylase PHF8 is an oncogenic protein in human non-small cell lung cancer. Biochem Biophys Res Commun 451(1):119–125

377. Sun X et al (2013) Oncogenic features of PHF8 histone demethylase in esophageal squamous cell carcinoma. PLoS One 8(10):e77353

378. Arteaga MF et al (2013) The histone demethylase PHF8 governs retinoic acid response in acute promyelocytic leukemia. Cancer Cell 23(3):376–389

379. Sun LL et al (2013) Overexpression of Jumonji AT-rich interactive domain 1B and PHD finger protein 2 is involved in the progression of esophageal squamous cell carcinoma. Acta Histochem 115(1):56–62

380. Sinha S et al (2008) Alterations in candidate genes PHF2, FANCC, PTCH1 and XPA at chromosomal 9q22.3 region: pathological significance in early- and late-onset breast carcinoma. Mol Cancer 7:84

381. Ghosh A et al (2012) Association of FANCC and PTCH1 with the development of early dysplastic lesions of the head and neck. Ann Surg Oncol 19(Suppl 3):S528–S538

382. Lee KH et al (2015) PHF2 histone demethylase acts as a tumor suppressor in association with p53 in cancer. Oncogene 34(22):2897–2909

383. Pattabiraman DR et al (2016) Activation of PKA leads to mesenchymal-to-epithelial transition and loss of tumor-initiating ability. Science 351(6277):aad3680

384. Loenarz C et al (2010) PHF8, a gene associated with cleft lip/palate and mental retardation, encodes for an Nepsilon-dimethyl lysine demethylase. Hum Mol Genet 19(2):217–222

385. Abidi F et al (2007) A novel mutation in the PHF8 gene is associated with X-linked mental retardation with cleft lip/cleft palate. Clin Genet 72(1):19–22

386. Koivisto AM et al (2007) Screening of mutations in the PHF8 gene and identification of a novel mutation in a Finnish family with XLMR and cleft lip/cleft palate. Clin Genet 72(2):145–149

387. Laumonnier F et al (2005) Mutations in PHF8 are associated with X linked mental retardation and cleft lip/cleft palate. J Med Genet 42(10):780–786

388. Yang Y et al (2010) Structural insights into a dual-specificity histone demethylase ceKDM7A from *Caenorhabditis elegans*. Cell Res 20(8):886–898

389. Feng W et al (2010) PHF8 activates transcription of rRNA genes through H3K4me3 binding and H3K9me1/2 demethylation. Nat Struct Mol Biol 17(4):445–450
390. Kleine-Kohlbrecher D et al (2010) A functional link between the histone demethylase PHF8 and the transcription factor ZNF711 in X-linked mental retardation. Mol Cell 38(2):165–178
391. Fortschegger K et al (2010) PHF8 targets histone methylation and RNA polymerase II to activate transcription. Mol Cell Biol 30(13):3286–3298
392. Liu W et al (2010) PHF8 mediates histone H4 lysine 20 demethylation events involved in cell cycle progression. Nature 466(7305):508–512
393. Qi HH et al (2010) Histone H4K20/H3K9 demethylase PHF8 regulates zebrafish brain and craniofacial development. Nature 466(7305):503–507
394. Qiu J et al (2010) The X-linked mental retardation gene PHF8 is a histone demethylase involved in neuronal differentiation. Cell Res 20(8):908–918
395. Xu W et al (2011) Oncometabolite 2-hydroxyglutarate is a competitive inhibitor of alpha-ketoglutarate-dependent dioxygenases. Cancer Cell 19(1):17–30
396. Upadhyay AK et al (2012) An analog of BIX-01294 selectively inhibits a family of histone H3 lysine 9 Jumonji demethylases. J Mol Biol 416(3):319–327
397. Yu L et al (2010) Structural insights into a novel histone demethylase PHF8. Cell Res 20(2):166–173
398. Yue WW et al (2010) Crystal structure of the PHF8 Jumonji domain, an Nepsilon-methyl lysine demethylase. FEBS Lett 584(4):825–830
399. Wen H et al (2010) Recognition of histone H3K4 trimethylation by the plant homeodomain of PHF2 modulates histone demethylation. J Biol Chem 285(13):9322–9326
400. Ahuja N, Sharma AR, Baylin SB (2016) Epigenetic therapeutics: a new weapon in the war against cancer. Annu Rev Med 67:73–89
401. Baylin SB, Ohm JE (2006) Epigenetic gene silencing in cancer - a mechanism for early oncogenic pathway addiction? Nat Rev Cancer 6(2):107–116
402. Jones PA, Baylin SB (2007) The epigenomics of cancer. Cell 128(4):683–692
403. Hoffmann I et al (2012) The role of histone demethylases in cancer therapy. Mol Oncol 6(6):683–703
404. Gale M et al (2016) Screen-identified selective inhibitor of lysine demethylase 5A blocks cancer cell growth and drug resistance. Oncotarget 7(26):39931–39944
405. Seligson DB et al (2005) Global histone modification patterns predict risk of prostate cancer recurrence. Nature 435(7046):1262–1266
406. Lohse B et al (2011) Inhibitors of histone demethylases. Bioorg Med Chem 19(12):3625–3636
407. Bradshaw JM et al (2015) Prolonged and tunable residence time using reversible covalent kinase inhibitors. Nat Chem Biol 11(7):525–531
408. Mould DP et al (2015) Reversible inhibitors of LSD1 as therapeutic agents in acute myeloid leukemia: clinical significance and progress to date. Med Res Rev 35(3):586–618
409. Hojfeldt JW, Agger K, Helin K (2013) Histone lysine demethylases as targets for anticancer therapy. Nat Rev Drug Discov 12(12):917–930
410. Khan MN, Suzuki T, Miyata N (2013) An overview of phenylcyclopropylamine derivatives: biochemical and biological significance and recent developments. Med Res Rev 33(4):873–910
411. McGrath JP et al (2016) Pharmacological inhibition of the histone lysine demethylase KDM1A suppresses the growth of multiple acute myeloid leukemia subtypes. Cancer Res 76(7):1975–1988
412. Mohammad HP, Kruger RG (2016) Antitumor activity of LSD1 inhibitors in lung cancer. Mol Cell Oncol 3(2):e1117700
413. Mohammad HP et al (2015) A DNA hypomethylation signature predicts antitumor activity of LSD1 inhibitors in SCLC. Cancer Cell 28(1):57–69
414. McAllister TE et al (2016) Recent progress in histone demethylase inhibitors. J Med Chem 59(4):1308–1329
415. Chin YW, Han SY (2015) KDM4 histone demethylase inhibitors for anti-cancer agents: a patent review. Expert Opin Ther Pat 25(2):135–144

416. Thinnes CC et al (2014) Targeting histone lysine demethylases - progress, challenges, and the future. Biochim Biophys Acta 1839(12):1416–1432
417. Shih JC, Chen K, Ridd MJ (1999) Monoamine oxidase: from genes to behavior. Annu Rev Neurosci 22:197–217
418. Lee MG et al (2006) Histone H3 lysine 4 demethylation is a target of nonselective antidepressive medications. Chem Biol 13(6):563–567
419. Schmidt DM, McCafferty DG (2007) trans-2-Phenylcyclopropylamine is a mechanism-based inactivator of the histone demethylase LSD1. Biochemistry 46(14):4408–4416
420. Ueda R et al (2009) Identification of cell-active lysine specific demethylase 1-selective inhibitors. J Am Chem Soc 131(48):17536–17537
421. Culhane JC et al (2006) A mechanism-based inactivator for histone demethylase LSD1. J Am Chem Soc 128(14):4536–4537
422. Kumarasinghe IR, Woster PM (2014) Synthesis and evaluation of novel cyclic peptide inhibitors of lysine-specific demethylase 1. ACS Med Chem Lett 5(1):29–33
423. Suzuki T, Miyata N (2011) Lysine demethylases inhibitors. J Med Chem 54(24):8236–8250
424. Maes T et al (2015) Advances in the development of histone lysine demethylase inhibitors. Curr Opin Pharmacol 23:52–60
425. Martinez ED, Gazdar AF (2016) Inhibiting the Jumonji family: a potential new clinical approach to targeting aberrant epigenetic mechanisms. Epigenomics 8(3):313–316
426. Rotili D et al (2014) Pan-histone demethylase inhibitors simultaneously targeting Jumonji C and lysine-specific demethylases display high anticancer activities. J Med Chem 57(1):42–55
427. Opocher G, Schiavi F (2011) Functional consequences of succinate dehydrogenase mutations. Endocr Pract 17(Suppl 3):64–71
428. Dang L et al (2009) Cancer-associated IDH1 mutations produce 2-hydroxyglutarate. Nature 462(7274):739–744
429. Losman JA, Kaelin WG Jr (2013) What a difference a hydroxyl makes: mutant IDH, (R)-2-hydroxyglutarate, and cancer. Genes Dev 27(8):836–852
430. Losman JA et al (2013) (R)-2-hydroxyglutarate is sufficient to promote leukemogenesis and its effects are reversible. Science 339(6127):1621–1625
431. Zhao S et al (2009) Glioma-derived mutations in IDH1 dominantly inhibit IDH1 catalytic activity and induce HIF-1alpha. Science 324(5924):261–265
432. Dang CV et al (2011) Therapeutic targeting of cancer cell metabolism. J Mol Med (Berl) 89(3):205–212
433. Choi C et al (2012) 2-hydroxyglutarate detection by magnetic resonance spectroscopy in IDH-mutated patients with gliomas. Nat Med 18(4):624–629
434. Gross S et al (2010) Cancer-associated metabolite 2-hydroxyglutarate accumulates in acute myelogenous leukemia with isocitrate dehydrogenase 1 and 2 mutations. J Exp Med 207(2):339–344
435. Lu C et al (2012) IDH mutation impairs histone demethylation and results in a block to cell differentiation. Nature 483(7390):474–478
436. Xiao M et al (2012) Inhibition of alpha-KG-dependent histone and DNA demethylases by fumarate and succinate that are accumulated in mutations of FH and SDH tumor suppressors. Genes Dev 26(12):1326–1338
437. Hamada S et al (2009) Synthesis and activity of N-oxalylglycine and its derivatives as Jumonji C-domain-containing histone lysine demethylase inhibitors. Bioorg Med Chem Lett 19(10):2852–2855
438. Heinemann B et al (2014) Inhibition of demethylases by GSK-J1/J4. Nature 514(7520):E1–E2
439. Kruidenier L et al (2014) Kruidenier et al. reply. Nature 514(7520):E2
440. Wang L et al (2013) A small molecule modulates Jumonji histone demethylase activity and selectively inhibits cancer growth. Nat Commun 4:2035
441. Nielsen AL et al (2012) Identification of catechols as histone-lysine demethylase inhibitors. FEBS Lett 586(8):1190–1194

442. Liang J et al (2016) Lead optimization of a pyrazolo[1,5-a]pyrimidin-7(4H)-one scaffold to identify potent, selective and orally bioavailable KDM5 inhibitors suitable for in vivo biological studies. Bioorg Med Chem Lett 26(16):4036–4041
443. Luo X et al (2011) A selective inhibitor and probe of the cellular functions of Jumonji C domain-containing histone demethylases. J Am Chem Soc 133(24):9451–9456
444. Wagner EK et al (2012) Identification and characterization of small molecule inhibitors of a plant homeodomain finger. Biochemistry 51(41):8293–8306
445. Merk A et al (2016) Breaking Cryo-EM resolution barriers to facilitate drug discovery. Cell 165(7):1698–1707

Misregulation of Histone Methylation Regulators in Cancer

Wen Fong Ooi*, Xiaosai Yao*, Patrick Tan, and Bin Tean Teh

Abstract Histone post-translational modifications include methylation at N-terminal of histone tails. Such modifications play important roles in many biological processes through divergent transcription activities. Recently, aberrant histone modifications have been shown to contribute significantly towards many diseases, notably cancer. Here, we summarize the known drivers leading to misregulation of DNA and histone methylation in cancer, and current therapeutic options to counter these aberrations.

Keywords Histone • Methylation • Cancer • Epigenetics

*Wen Fong Ooi and Xiaosai Yao are contributed equally to the manuscript

W.F. Ooi • X. Yao
Cancer Therapeutics and Stratified Oncology, Genome Institute of Singapore,
60 Biopolis Street, Singapore 138672, Singapore

P. Tan (✉)
Cancer Therapeutics and Stratified Oncology, Genome Institute of Singapore,
60 Biopolis Street, Singapore 138672, Singapore

Cancer and Stem Cell Biology Program, Duke–NUS Medical School,
8 College Road, Singapore 169857, Singapore

National Cancer Centre Singapore, 11 Hospital Drive, Singapore 169610, Singapore

Cancer Science Institute of Singapore, National University of Singapore,
14 Medical Drive, #12-01, Singapore 117599, Singapore

SingHealth/Duke–NUS Precision Medicine Institute, Singapore 168752, Singapore
e-mail: gmstanp@duke-nus.edu.sg

B.T. Teh (✉)
Cancer and Stem Cell Biology Program, Duke–NUS Medical School,
8 College Road, Singapore 169857, Singapore

National Cancer Centre Singapore, 11 Hospital Drive, Singapore 169610, Singapore

Cancer Science Institute of Singapore, National University of Singapore,
14 Medical Drive, #12-01, Singapore 117599, Singapore

SingHealth/Duke–NUS Precision Medicine Institute, Singapore 168752, Singapore

Institute of Molecular and Cell Biology, 61 Biopolis Drive, Singapore, Singapore, 138673
e-mail: teh.bin.tean@singhealth.com.sg

© Springer International Publishing AG 2017
A. Kaneda, Y.-i. Tsukada (eds.), *DNA and Histone Methylation as Cancer Targets*,
Cancer Drug Discovery and Development, DOI 10.1007/978-3-319-59786-7_8

1 Introduction

The advent of next-generation sequencing has substantially accelerated drug development towards targeted therapeutics. Early drug target discovery tends to focus on mutated kinases [1, 2]. For example, vemurafenib, a BRAF kinase inhibitor, is used to treat metastatic melanoma patients harboring BRAF V600E mutation [3]. Despite the profound anticancer effects of targeting activated kinase pathways, such benefit is often temporary in a subset of patients with advanced solid tumors [4]. The lack of durable response motivates the search for enzymes involved in other functional roles such as epigenetics [5] and metabolism [6] as alternative drug targets.

Epigenetic modifications occur both at DNA and histone proteins. The amino acid residues at the N-terminal histone tails are subjected to post-translational modification, such as methylation, acetylation, ubiquitination, phosphorylation and SUMOylation [7, 8]. Recent studies have shown that notably, misregulation at histone methylation leads to diseases including cancer. For example, enhancers showing gain or loss of H3 lysine 4 mono methylation (H3K4me1) can clearly distinguish between normal colon crypts and colorectal cancer [9]. Burgeoning research focusing on epigenetic alterations in cancer have identified a collection of genes involved in epigenetic programming with direct influence on chromatin structure and cell identity [10]. These findings strongly suggest that the transformation of healthy cells to cancer cells may be dependent on the underlying aberrant modifications at histone level. Therefore, identifying drivers to such aberrant transformation may provide new insights for therapeutics to treat cancer. In this chapter, we will summarize the known drivers of aberrant histone methylation in cancer, and current therapeutic strategies to counter aberrant histone methylation.

2 Regulators of Histone Methylation

Unlike the permanent DNA sequences, histone methylation is a highly dynamic process. It is constantly written and erased by histone modifying enzymes (Table 2). This dynamic process forms the basis of lineage specification during development [11], imprinting [12, 13] and disease state. The resulting histone code, containing "on" and "off" signals, is then interpreted by histone readers who can dock on the histone modifications and recruit other co-factors.

Histone can be methylated at lysine, arginine and rarely histidine. Well-characterized sites of lysine methylation include H3K4, H3K9, H3K20, H3K27, H3K36 and H3K79. Each lysine can exist as unmethylated (me0), monomethylated (me1) [14], dimethylated (me2) [15] and trimethylated (me3) [16]. Arginine residues are commonly modified at H3R2, H3R8, H3R17, and H4R3. Arginine residues exist as unmethylated (me0), monomethylated (me1) [17], symmetrically dimethylated (me2s) and asymmetrically dimethylated [18]. Symmetrically dimethylated arginines have a single methyl group on two different nitrogens whereas asymmetrically dimethylated arginines have two methyl group on a single nitrogen. It is estimated that approximately 2% of the arginine residues are methylated in total nuclear proteins of rat liver cells [19].

The different positions of lysine methylation can be associated with vastly divergent transcription activity. In general, H3K4me3 is associated with transcriptional activation. H3K4me3 is thought to be causal for transcriptional activation because TAF3, a subunit of the basal transcription factor TFIID, directly binds to the H3K4me3 [20]. TFIID mediates formation of preinitiation complex assembly for transcription [21]. In contrast, H3K27me3 is associated with transcriptional silencing [22]. The EZH2 subunit of the transcriptional repressor polycomb repressive complex (PRC) [23] catalyzes the methylation of H3K27 which in turn recruits PRC through the EED subunit and stimulates its methyltransferase activity in a positive feedback loop [24]. Similarly, H3K9me3 is also associated with transcriptional repression because it serves as the binding site for heterochromatin protein (HP1) which compacts the chromatin [25]. H3K36me3 is enriched in transcriptionally active regions as its level is sharply elevated after transcription start sites [26, 27]. However, in some other regions, such as the repressed *Snurf–Snrpn* locus, H3K36me3 is not associated with transcription activity but associated with heterochromatin [28]. H3K79 is associated with both silencing and active transcription. It regulates telomeric silencing and is thus tightly regulated during cell cycle [29]. At the same time, H3K79 methylation is associated with active transcription and correlates with euchromatin [30, 31], likely through inhibiting the nonspecific binding of the repressive Sir proteins [32].

In terms of arginine residues, activating marks are H3R8me2a, H3R17me2a and H4R3me2a [33]. H4R3me2a deposited by arginine methyltransferase 1 (PRMT1) promotes transcriptional activation by enhancing lysine acetylation by P300 [33]. Another arginine methyltransferase member, Coactivator-associated arginine methyltransferase 1 (CARM1), enhances transcriptional activation by nuclear receptors [34] and it catalyzes the methylation of H3R2, H3R17 and H3R26 [35]. Repressive marks are H4R3me2s, H3R2me2s and H3R8me2s and H3R2me2a. Lysine methylation and arginine methylation can have antagonistic roles: H3R2me2a deposited by PRMT6 exerts its repressive role by abrogating H3K4 methylation by mixed lineage leukaemia (MLL) complex [36, 37]. Conversely, H3K4me3 also prevents H3R2 methylation by PRMT6 [36, 37].

Different histone modifications mark chromatin states. H3K4me3 marks are generally associated with promoters [38]; H3K4me1 with enhancers [38] and H3K36me3 with transcribed regions [22]. Chromatin states also vary with developmental stage. Embryonic stem (ES) cells have the most permissive chromatin state, but transition to a more restrictive state by gaining H3K27me3 as ES cells differentiate into embryoid bodies, to neural progenitors and finally to differentiated neurons [39]. Large scale chromatin maps showed that chromatin states defined by combination of histone modifications can distinguish between various cell types. In particular, enhancers mark, H3K4me1, is the most tissue-specific [39–41]. Hierarchical clustering using H3K4me1 can group cell types of similar origin, for example, haemotopoietic stem cells, B cells, T cells, monocytes fall under the same module [41]. Therefore, histone modifications mark cis-regulatory regions that contain lineage-specific genes. Finally, in cancer, clusters of enhancers called superenhancers [42] or stretch enhancers [43], are located near key oncogenes, further illustrating the fact that histone modifications play integral roles to the regulation of key master regulators.

2.1 Writers

The majority of lysine methyltransferases contain the highly conserved SET domain. SET domains bind to donor S-Adenosyl-L-Methionine (SAM) and lysine substrate on opposite faces, and catalyze the transfer of methyl group through the methyltransfer pore [44]. Lysine methylation at multiple histone positions is performed by SET domain-containing histone methyltransferases. MLL family of proteins methylate H3K4 [45]. SUV39H1 [46] and G9a [47] can both methylate H3K9. EZH2 catalyzes the formation of H3K27me3 [48–50]. KMT3B/NSD1 primarily dimethylates H3K36 [51, 52] and SETD2 is responsible for forming nearly all transcription-dependent H3K36me3 [53]. Besides SET domain, another domain capable of methyltransferase activity is the DOT1 domain. DOT1L specifically mono-, di, and tri-methylates H3K79 [29], and is found at the proximal transcribed region of active genes [54].

For methylation of arginine residues, PRMTs use the same donor SAM as lysine methylation. PRMT1, a transcriptional activator, is the major enzyme catalyzing the active mark H4R3me2a which promotes subsequent histone acetylation by P300 recruitment [33, 55]. PRTM1 is a component of the MLL complex and PRTM1-MLL fusion promotes self-renewal of haematopoietic cells [56]. On the other hand, PRMT5, usually acts as a transcriptional repressor, symmetrically dimethylating H3 and H4 to produce H4R3me2s and H3R8me2s respectively [57]. Because PRMT5 can repress tumor suppressors including the RB family, it is generally considered as an oncogene [57].

2.2 Erasers

The most common domain found in histone demethylases is the JumonjiC (JmjC) domain. In the presence of co-factors Fe (II) and alpha-ketoglutarate (α-KG), JmjC domain undergoes oxidative demethylation reaction to produce hydroxylmethyl-lysine, succinate and CO_2 [58]. Because of this dependency on α-KG, mutations affecting TCA cycle enzymes *IDH1* and *IDH2* can deplete a-KG and subsequently impair histone demethylation [59]. Stable transfection of mutant *IDH* resulted in progressive accumulation of histone methylation, including H3K9. KDM5A, KDM5B and KDM5C are responsible for erasing tri-, di- and monomethylation mark of H3K4 [60–63]. UTX and JMJD3 catalyze demethylation of H3K27me3/2 [64]. JHDM1 is the first JmjC-containing enzyme that has been shown to have demethylation activity and its substrate is H3K36 [58]. JHDM2A specifically demethylates mono- and dimethyl-H3K9, and its depletion led to H3K9 demethylation and transcriptional activation [65]. No known enzyme has been found to demethylase H3K79.

Another domain capable of histone demethylation is amine oxidase, present in KDM1A/LSD1. The LSD1 can specifically demethylate H3K4me1 and H3K4me2 in a FAD (flavin adenine dinucleotide)-dependent oxidative reaction [66]. LSD1 is unable to demethylate H3K4me3 because it requires a protonated nitrogen in the substrates [66]. Because LSD1 removes methylation from H3K4, it acts as a transcriptional repressor [66]. No demethylases have been found for arginine methylation.

2.3 Readers

The most common domain found in readers of methylated lysine is the plant home-odomain (PHD domain). First discovered in ING2 tumor suppressor, the PHD domain binds with increasingly affinity to methylated H3K4, with strongest association to H3K4me3, and no association with H3K4me0/1 [67]. It is thought that PHD domain contributes to the tumor suppressive role of ING2 by stabilizing histone deacetylase, mSin3a-HDAC1, at promoters of proliferation genes [67]. At the same time, it is also found that PHD domain is present in bromodomain and PHD domain transcription factor (BPTF), the largest subunit of nucleosome remodeling factor NURF, suggesting that NURF-mediated chromatin remodeling is directly coupled to H3K4me3 [68, 69].

However, not all PHD domains have similar affinity of histone methyl lysines. Unlike the PHD domain in ING2 and BPTF, PHD domain found in BHC80 binds to unmethylated H3K4. Interestingly, BHC80 influences LSD1 binding, and its depletion leads to de-repression of LSD1 target genes [70].

PHD domains are also present in many histone writers, so there are many histone writers that read. The MLL family of histone methyltransferases all contain multiple PHD domains whose functions are not identical. For instance, the second PHD domain of KMT2A and KMT2B shows E3 ubiquitin ligase activity whereas the third PHD domain binds with the highest affinity to H3K4me3 and less to H3K4me1/2 [71]. The recognition of its own mark suggests a positive feedback system of histone methylation.

In terms of histone methylarginine, the transcriptional activator, TDRD3, reads the active marks H3R17me2a and H4R3me2a using its Tudor domain [72]. Specifically, TDRD3 can distinguish between the asymmetrical, active mark H4R3me2a from the symmetrical, repressive mark H4R3me2s [72]. TDRD3 is a transcriptional co-activator that binds to H4R3me2a and H3R17me2a located upstream of transcriptional start sites.

3 Mechanism of Misregulation

Given the multi-faceted roles of histone modifiers in gene regulation, it is no surprise that cancer hijacks them via diverse mechanisms: mutations, gene rearrangements and misregulation of gene expression. The resulting change is often genome-wide, affecting multiple gene targets and pathways.

3.1   Mutations in the Catalytic Domains

Mutations in the catalytic domains of histone methyltransferases affect methylation differently. The most common mutation residing within the SETD domain of *EZH2*, Y646 (previously Y641), is a gain of the function mutation. *EZH2* Y646 increases global H3K27me3 levels because it displays enhanced catalytic activity towards H3K27me2/3 whereas the wildtype EZH2 has the greatest affinity towards H3K27me0/1 substrate [73]. Although *EZH2* Y646F causes global increases of H3K27me3, the gain of H3K27me3 is not monotonic across the genome, as some loci exhibit a loss of H3K27me3 and increased transcription [74]. As a result, *EZH2* Y646F induces both repression and activation of polycomb target genes.

KMT2C/MLL3 is frequently inactivated in a number of different cancers by inactivating, truncating or even activating mutations [75–80]. The N4848S mutation leads to a loss of the catalytic activity of MLL3, similar to frame shifts or other inactivating mutations. In contrast, the Y4884C mutation of *MLL3* is a gain of function mutation as it adopts a higher catalytic activity towards H3K4me1 than the wildtype *MLL3*, in a manner highly analogous to *EZH2* Y646. Knockout of *MLL2/3* globally decreases H3K4me1 and H3K4me2 levels in macrophages and HCT116 colon cancer cells [81]. Since MLL3 and MLL2 co-localize with markers of enhancers including H3K4me1, P300 binding and H3K27ac [81–83], perturbation of enhancer landscape by inactivating mutations of *MLL2/3* could contribute to tumorigenesis.

Mutations can also target the catalytic domains of histone demethylases. The Jumonji-C domain-containing *KDM6A/UTX* (demethylase of H3K27me3) [11, 64] is a tumor suppressor frequently associated with inactivating mutations [84]. Ectopic expression of UTX leads to a strong decrease of H3K27me3 levels and delocalization of polycomb proteins [64, 84]. Conversely, knockdown of UTX by siRNA decreases its occupancy at promoters of polycomb target genes, *HOXA13* and *HOXC4,* and brings about a concomitant increase in the levels of H3K27me2/3 at these promoters [85]. It remains to be elucidated what is the genome-wide effect of UTX depletion on H3K27me2/3 levels. Current evidence suggests that the loss of *UTX* may be a reciprocal mechanism to *EZH2* gain, and both may lead to increasing and redistributing H3K27me3 mark, and deregulating the transcription of polycomb target genes.

Finally, chromatin readers can also be targeted by inactivating mutations that abrogate their binding to histone marks. Four mutations targeting *ING1* (C215, N216S, V218I and G221V) are either located within or near the H3K4me3 binding site of the PHD finger [86]. The hotspot C215 mutation disrupts the three-dimensional structure of the PHD finger and abolishes interaction with H3K4me3 [86]. Similarly, the other three mutations all decrease the affinity of the PHD finger with H3K4me3.

3.2 Gene Arrangement

Gene arrangement involving *MLL1* gene on chromosome band 11q23 occurs frequently in leukemia. The first form of gene rearrangement involves *MLL* gene fusions [87–89], which occur in the 8.3 kb breakpoint cluster region (BCR) of the *MLL* gene, between exons 8 and 12. The fusion forms include *MLL-AF4, MLL-AF9, MLL-AF10, MLL-AF17, MLL-AF5q31, MLL-ENL*. What is common amongst these fusion partners is that they all form stable complex with KMT4/DOT1L, a histone methyltransferase of H3K79 [90, 91]. MLL-AF9 binds to the promoters of target genes and induces H3K79me2 at the binding region. The increase in H3K79me2 induced by *MLL-AF9* causes increased expression of direct targets including HoxA [92] which are important for hematopoiesis. In addition to H3K79me2, other active marks including H3K4me3, H3K36me3 are also concomitantly elevated and the repressive mark H3K27me3 is depleted [92]. Another important histone methyltransferase targeted by *MLL-AF9* is LSD1 [93]. LSD1 sustains the leukemia stem cell potential of *MLL-AF9* cells [93]. Knockdown of LSD1 increases the level of H3K4me2 at *MLL-AF9* bound genes, suggesting that expression of *MLL-AF9* target genes is dependent upon H3K4me2 [93].

The second form of gene rearrangement involves partial tandem duplication of *MLL* from exon 5 to 11/12 (MLL PTD) in the absence of a partner gene [94], found in 5–10% of patients with acute myeloid leukemia (AML). In AML patients, *MLL* PTD also co-occurs with the loss of *MLL* in the second allele [95]. *MLL* PTD displays activation of similar target genes as *MLL* fusions such as HoxA, but through increased methylation of H3K4 [96].

Another gene fusion involves the chromatin reader, plant homeodomain (PHD) finger 23 (*PHF23*) with nucleoporin 98-KDa (*NUP98*) [97]. NUP98 fuses with either HOX or non-HOX partners. Interestingly, *NUP98-PHF23* can also achieve activation of HOX, but through binding to H3K4me3 regions spanning *HOX* genes. The binding of *NUP98-PHF23* to H3K4me3 is highly specific, occupying only 1.6% of total H3K4me3 regions, but it remains unknown how such specificity is achieved [98]. In addition to fusing with the chromatin reader *PHF23*, *NUP98* can also fuse with *NSD1*, the methyltransferase of H3K36 in AML [99]. In a manner similar to the MLL fusion and other NUP98 fusions, *NUP98–NSD1* activates HoxA and Meis proto-oncogenes by recruiting p300 (histone acetyl transferase) and suppression of EZH2 [100].

3.3 Gene Deregulation

Overexpression of EZH2 is an alternative but analogous mechanism to inactivating mutations. While mutations of *EZH2* mainly occurs in hematopoietic cancers including diffuse large B-cell lymphoma and follicular lymphoma, EZH2 overexpression can occur in a variety of solid cancers including prostate, breast, gastric, bladder, kidney, liver and ovarian [101–105]. Multiple transcription factors can stimulate EZH2 overexpression. MYC binds to *EZH2* promoter and directly activates its transcription [106]. Other transcription factors that cause EZH2 overexpression include E2F [107], EWS-FLI1 fusion [108], SOX4 [109], and HIF1α [110].

Transcriptional upregulation of MLL1 and MLL2 can be induced by gain of function (GOF) p53 mutants. R273H p53 mutant, but not wildtype p53, binds at the promoter of *MLL1* and *MLL2* [111]. GOF p53 results in slight elevation in the global levels of H3K4me3, including regions around the *hoxa* gene cluster [111]. The oncogenic role of GOF p53 mutant is dependent on MLL1 expression [111].

Another example of overexpressed histone reader is PRMT5, found in leukemia, lymphoma [57], lung, gastric cancer [112] and glioblastoma [113]. PRMT5 can be directly upregulated by MYC [114] which physically associates with PRMT5 and stimulate H4R4me2s [115]. This implies that gene misregulation of chromatin modifiers often stem from mutations in classic oncogenes or tumor suppressors.

4 How do Changes in Histone Methylation Lead to Oncogenesis?

4.1 Activation of Developmental Master Regulators

Various mutational changes and gene rearrangements converge to activate developmentally important master regulators. Often expressed in progenitor cells, these factors are essential for maintaining stemness during development but are turned off in differentiated cells. However, deregulated histone modifiers often re-activate these developmental regulators, thus contributing to tumorigenesis.

In vivo mouse model shows that Hoxa9 can collaborate with meis1a to induce AML in less than 3 months [116]. DOT1L induced by *MLL* fusion is targeted to hoxa9 [91], and the presence of DOT1L resulted in enhanced H3K79me2 at HoxA clusters and Meis1 [92]. Another translocation mentioned earlier, *NUP98-PHF23* fusion, also caused overexpression of Hoxa and Hoxb cluster. AML-derived myeloblastic cells with *NUP98-PHF23* demonstrate both enrichment of H3K4me3 and depletion of H3K27me3 across the *Hoxa*, *Hoxb* and *Meis* loci [98]. Similarly, *EZH2* Y641F causes a re-distribution of H3K27me3. Even though the global level of H3K27me3 is elevated, this repressive mark is depleted from *Hoxc* cluster and *Meis1* which are densely covered with H3K27me3 in normal B cells [74]. The liberation of the repressive H3K27me3 from developmental regulators causes their overexpression and contributes to tumorigenesis.

4.2 Suppression of Tumor Suppressors

The redistribution of histone mark can simultaneously activate oncogenes and repress tumor suppressors. The tumor suppressor *Ink4a/Arf* locus is epigenetically silenced in leukemia-initiating cells by strong enrichment of H3K27me3 [117]. *Ezh2* knockout decreases H3K27me3 at *Ink4a-Arf* locus, implying that *Ezh2* is required to maintain H3K27me3 and repression of the *Ink4a/Arf* locus [118].

Another important group of tumor suppressors inactivated by histone methylation is the retinoblastoma protein (RB family). PRMT5 recruitment to the promoters of *RB*, *RBL1* and *RBL2* is increased 3–4.7-fold, 4–9.5-fold and 3–5.2-fold respectively in transformed lymphoid cell lines compared to that of normal B cells [57]. The increase in PRMT5 recruitment results in corresponding enrichment of the repressive marks, H3R8me2s and H4R3me2s, that suppress the mRNA levels of the *RB* tumor suppressor genes [57].

An example of a histone demethylase that contributes to suppression of tumor suppressor is the H3K4 demethylase KDM5B/PLU-1. Its recruitment and resulting depletion of H3K4me3 mark represses tumor suppressors including *BRCA1*, therefore its overexpression can contribute to breast cancer cell proliferation [63].

4.3 Splicing Defects

Besides marking transcriptionally active regions, H3K36me3 also plays an important role in safeguarding splicing fidelity. H3K36me3 recruits polypyrimidine tract–binding protein (PTB) which results in exon silencing [119]. Truncating mutations of *SETD2* in ccRCC result in a global loss of H3K36me3 [120]. H3K36me3-deficient ccRCCs display a drastic increase in intron retention, affecting 95% of the transcripts [120]. Other defects in exon utilization, start and termination site usage were also observed [120]. The most affected genes include tumor suppressors, genes in the DNA repair pathway and cell cycle regulators [120].

4.4 Genomic Instability

Histone modifications may also influence genomic instability even though the exact mechanism is not completely well understood. *SETD2* loss has also been associated with genomic instability. Even though the main cause of genomic instability due to *SETD2* depletion may be a result of decreased methylation in microtubules, a non-histone substrate [121], it is also observed that chromosomal breakpoints are located away from H3K36me3 [122]. *SETD2* loss decreases nucleosomal occupancy and increases sensitivity to micrococcal nuclease, suggesting that *SETD2* plays a role in maintaining nucleosome stabilization and coordination of DNA repair [122].

Another histone modifying enzyme that safeguards genomic stability is MLL2. Tumor cells with *MLL2* knockout had higher levels of sister chromatid exchange compared with the two control cell lines [123]. Deletion of SET domain alone mimics the genomic instability seen in *MLL2* knockouts, indicating that the catalytic domain is necessary for maintaining genomic stability [123]. However intriguingly, *MLL2* deficient cells do not display differential H3K4 levels compared to *MLL2* wildtype at mutated genes since *MLL2* mutation predominantly affects H3K4 methylation at enhancers [123]. Therefore, the connection between histone methylation and genomic instability remains to be elucidated.

5 Histone Methyltransferase/Demethylase Inhibitors as Treatment in Cancer

Unlike genetic abnormalities, epigenetic alteration are reversible, enabling restoration of original function in cells showing disease phenotypes without altering the DNA sequences [124, 125]. Taken together, such findings has fueled immense interest in using chromatin-associated proteins as anticancer drug targets.

Indeed, several epigenetic inhibitors have been approved by the Food and Drug Administration (FDA). These approved drugs include azacitidine (5-azacytidine) and decitabine (5-aza-2′-deoxycytidine) as DNA methyltransferase (DNMT) inhibitors; suberoylanilide hydroxamic acid (SAHA) romidepsin (depsipeptide or FK228) as histone deacetylase (HDAC) inhibitors. On the other hand, since inhibitors of lysine methyltransferases (KMT) and demethylases (KDM) have been recently discovered, many of them are still in (pre-) clinical development (see Table 1 for a list of inhibitors and their drug development stage). Interestingly, the utility of such inhibitors in academic research demonstrated promising results in treating cancer with KMT/KDM inhibitors. Given the increasing importance of these compounds in cancer, pharmaceutical companies strive to develop more epigenetic drugs through collaborative discovery and development. Recently, Merck Sharp & Dohme (MSD) initiated collaboration with Cancer Research Technology to develop a portfolio of inhibitors of protein arginine methyltransferase 5 (PRMT5) for treatment of blood cancers. Other pharmaceutical companies developing PRMT inhibitors include Epizyme and GlaxoSmithKline [157]. Business acquisition of EpiTherapeutics by Gilead Sciences, and Quanticel Pharmaceuticals by Celgene Corporations further suggest the immense interest of pharmaceutical giants in epigenetic drugs. In essence, inhibitors targeting histone methylases/demethylases may render a previously-untapped reservoir of cancer therapeutic interventions.

Here, we highlight the clinical development of selected pharmacological inhibitors targeting histone methyltransferases and demethylases. Anti-tumour effects followed by treatment with inhibitors are also briefly discussed.

Table 1 A list of methyltransferases and demethylases, and corresponding substrates and inhibitors

Enzyme	Substrate	Inhibitor	Reference
KMT1C/EHMT2/G9a KMT1D/EHMT1/ GLP	H3K9, H1.2K187, H1.4K26	BIX-01294 UNC0642 A-366 BRD9539 UNC0224	[126] [127] [128] [129] [130]
KDM5A KDM5B/JARID1B KDM5C/JARID1C KDM5D	H3K4	EPT-103182	[131]
KDM1A/LSD1	H3K4, H3K9	Tranylcypromine ORY-1001 GSK2879552	[132] [131] [133], NCT02177812, NCT02034123
EZH2	H3K27	GSK126 GSK343 EPZ005687 EPZ-6438 EI1 UNC1999 JQEZ5	[134], NCT02082977 [135] [136] [137], NCT02601950, NCT01897571, NCT02889523 [138] [139] [140]
KDM6A/UTX	H3K27	GSK-J1	[141]
KDM6B/JMJD3	H3K27	GSK-J1 GSKJ4	[141] [142]
KMT3C/SMYD2	H3K36	AZ505	[143]
KDM4A	H3K36	C-4	[144]
DOT1L	H3K79	EPZ-5676 EPZ004777 SGC0946	[145], NCT02141828 [146] [147]
PRMT1	H4R3	AM1-1, AMI-8 allantodapsone compound 6 DCLX069, DCLX078 MHI-21 E84 Stilbamidine	[148] [149] [150] [151] [152] [153] [149]
PRMT3	RPS2, p53	14u	[154]
PRMT4/CARM1	H3R17	17b MethylGene	[155] [156]
PRMT5	H3R8	GSK3326595	NCT02783300

Inhibitors that are tested in ongoing clinical trials are indicated by the identifiers starting "NCT"

5.1 EZH2 Inhibitors

As mentioned in the previous section, EZH2 is a histone-lysine N-methyltransferase enzyme that methylates H3K27, and thus has repressive effect on gene expression. Studies have shown that EZH2 overexpression associates with cancer development and poor prognosis in human cancer, including lymphoma, breast, prostate, kidney and lung [77, 158–161]. Therefore, inhibiting EZH2 could be an important therapeutic intervention.

Recent studies have revealed an array of small molecule inhibitors targeting EZH2 (Table 2). Amongst these inhibitors, 3-Deazaneplanocin A (DZNep) was previously reported as a SAH-hydrolase inhibitor, acting as an indirect EZH2 inhibitor [188, 189]. It is also a derivative of the antibiotic neplanocin-A. Despite indirect inhibition, DZNep was shown to induce apoptosis in cancer by reactivating PRC2 target genes [188].

There are also inhibitors imposing direct inhibition on EZH2, such as GSK126 and EPZ005687 leading to global decrease of H3K27me3 and also reactivation of silenced PRC2 target genes in haematological cancers, including diffuse large B-cell lymphoma (DLBCL) [134] and non-Hodgkin's lymphoma [190]. Since activating mutations in EZH2 were reported in DLBCL and follicular lymphoma [75, 77, 191–193], inhibitors were designed to be specific to EZH2 mutants. Specifically, GSK126 (GlaxoSmithKline) effectively inhibited the proliferation of EZH2 mutant DLBCL cell lines as well as xenografts in mice [134]. EPZ005687 (Epizyme) enables apoptotic cell killing in heterozygous Y641 or A677 mutant cells with non-Hodgkin's lymphoma [136]. Treatment with UNC1999 also selectively killed DLBCL cell lines harboring the EZH2^{Y641N} mutant [139]. EI1 (Novartis) showed reduced proliferation, cell cycle arrest and apoptosis in DLBCL cells carrying the Y641 mutations.

Unlike DLBCL and NHL, EZH2 is often overexpressed but not mutated in solid tumors. Inhibition of EZH2 in solid tumors has not been studied as extensively as in haematological cancers. This raises an important problem whether existing EZH2 inhibitors are able to inhibit the expression carrying wild type EZH2. To address this concern, a previous study conducted on three-dimensional culture of epithelial ovarian cancer shows that the tumor culture is sensitive to EZH2 methyltransferase inhibition by GSK343 [135]. The inhibition results in suppression of cell growth and invasion, and induction of apoptosis. Additionally, treatment of non-small cell lung carcinoma with genetically engineered mouse models using JQEZ5 promotes regression of these tumors [140], and EPZ-6438 treatment in malignant rhabdoid tumors with mutated SMARCB1 caused apoptosis and differentiation [137]. In general, most of the EZH2 inhibitors show effect in cancer cells with mutant and wild type EZH2, but with a few exceptions. For example, EPZ005687 is effective in targeting cells carrying EZH2 mutant, but its effect on the proliferation of NHL cells with wild type EZH2 is minimal [136]. It is also worth noting that the kinetics of H3K27me3 turnover is slow, therefore prolonged EZH2 inhibition for several days is required to reduce tri-methylation of H3 lysine 27 and alter the transcriptional program in cancer cells [194].

Table 2 A list of selected histone writers, erasers and readers that are misregulated in cancer

Histone	Type	Gene	Domains	Histone mark	Misregulation in cancer	Selected cancers	Ref
Lysine							
H3K4	Writer	KMT2A/MLL	SET, PHD, bromo	H3K4me1/2/3	Translocation	Leukemia, lung cancer, endometrial cancer	[87–89, 162, 163]
	Writer	KMT2C/MLL3	SET, PHD	H3K4me1/2/3	Inactivating and activating mutations	Medulloblastoma, liver cancer, breast cancer, colon cancer, gastric cancer, transitional cell carcinoma	[76, 78–83, 164]
	Writer	KMT2D/MLL2	SET, PHD	H3K4me1/2/3	Inactivating mutations	Medulloblastoma, lymphoma, lung cancer, phyllodes tumor	[75, 76, 79, 81–83, 123, 165, 166]
	Eraser	KDM5B/JARID1B	JmjC, PHD, ARID, JmjN	H3K4me1/2/3	Overexpression, missense	Prostate cancer, breast cancer	[167, 168]
	Eraser	KDM5C/JARID1C	JmjC, PHD, ARID, JmjN	H3K4me2/3	Inactivating mutations	Renal cell carcinoma	[169, 170]
	Eraser	KDM5D	JmjC, PHD, ARID, JmjN	H3K4me2/3	Decreased expression	Castration resistant prostate cancer	[171]
	Eraser	KDM1A/LSD1	Amine oxidase, SWIRM, FAD-binding	H3K4me1/2 H3K9me1/2	Overexpression	Bladder, lung and colorectal	[66, 172]
	Reader	BPTF	PHD	H3K4	Mutations	Liver cancer	[79]
	Reader	ING1	PHD	H3K4	Mutations; decreased expression	Head and neck, neuroblastoma	[173]
	Reader	PHF8	PHD	H3K4	Overexpression	Prostate cancer	[174]

(continued)

Table 2 (continued)

Histone	Type	Gene	Domains	Histone mark	Misregulation in cancer	Selected cancers	Ref
H3K9	Writer	SUV39H1	SET, chromodomain	H3K9me2/3	Overexpression	Basal breast	[46, 175]
	Eraser	KDM4A/JMJD2A	JmjC, JmjN, Tudor	H3K9me2/3	Amplification, overexpression	Prostate, colorectal, lung, breast	[176]
	Eraser	KDM3A/JMJD1	JmjC, LXXLL	H3K9me1/2	Truncating mutation	Breast cancer	[177]
	Reader	CHD4	Chromodomain, helicase	H3K9me3	Missense and truncating mutations	Endometrial cancer	[178]
	Reader	TRIM33	PHD	H3K9me3	Reduced expression	Chronic myelomonocytic leukaemia	[179]
H3K20	Writer	KMT5B/SUV420H1	SET	H3K20me2/3	Amplification	Breast, esophageal, bladder and head and neck cancers	[180, 181]
	Eraser	PHF8	JmjC, PHD	H3K20me1	Overexpression	Prostate cancer	[174]
H3K27	Writer	EZH2	SET, CXC	H3K27me2/3	Activating mutations, overexpression	Non-Hodgkin lymphoma, myelodysplastic-myeloproliferative neoplasms, melanoma	[73, 74, 101, 104–110]
	Eraser	KDM6A UTX	JmjC	H3K27me2/3	Inactivating mutations	Multiple myeloma, transitional cell carcinoma of bladder	[80, 84, 85, 182]
	Reader	EED	WD40	H3K27me3	Overexpression; inactivating mutations	Colorectal cancer, malignant peripheral nerve sheath tumors	[24, 183, 184]

	Role	Protein	Domains	Mark	Mechanism	Cancer	Ref.
H3K36	Writer	KMT3B/NSD1	SET, AWS, PWWP	H3K36me2	Overexpression, gene silencing, translocation	AML, prostate, neuroblastoma, breast	[51, 52, 99, 100]
	Writer	SETD2	SET, AWS, WW	H3K36me3	Inactivating mutations	Renal cell carcinoma, lung adenocarcinoma, acute leukemia, glioma, phyllodes tumor	[53, 121, 122]
	Eraser	KDM4A/JMJD2A	JmjN, JmjC, JD2H, TUDOR, and PHD-type	H3K36me1/2/3	Overexpression	Prostate, colorectal, lung, breast	[176]
	Reader	PHF19	Tudor	H3K36me3	Overexpression	Colon, skin, lung, rectal, cervical, uterus, and liver cancer	[55, 185]
H3K79	Writer	DOT1L	DOT1	H3K79me1/2/3	Upregulation by MLL fusion	Leukemia	[92]
Arginine							
H3R2	Writer	PRMT5	PRMT	H3R2me2s	Overexpression due to altered expression of PRMT5-specific microRNAs	CLL	[186]
H3R8	Writer	PRMT5	PRMT	H3R8me2s	Overexpression due to altered expression of PRMT5-specific microRNAs	CLL	[186]
H4R3	Writer	PRMT1	PRMT	H4R3me2a	Overexpression	Leukemia	[55, 56]
	Writer	PRMT5	PRMT	H4R3me2s	Overexpression due to altered expression of PRMT5-specific microRNAs	CLL	[186]
	Reader	TDRD3	Tudor	H4R3me2a	Overexpression	Breast cancer	[72, 187]

5.2   DOT1L Inhibitors

As discussed in the previous section, misregulation of DOT1L, a H3K79 methyl-transferase, may serve as a potential oncogenic driver in leukaemia with MLL-fusion proteins [91]. Therefore, pharmacological inhibition of DOT1L may treat patients suffering from leukaemia.

Most DOTL1 inhibitors are SAM competitive inhibitors. Analysis of structure-activity relationships and co-crystal structures design principles using S-Adenosyl-L-Homocysteine (SAH), the demethylated form of SAM, [195] is used to identify small molecules targeting DOT1L catalytic activity. The first compound, EPZ004777, is a potent and highly selective DOT1L aminonucleoside inhibitor [146]. It competes with the universal methyl donor for binding to the DOT1L's active site. Previous studies showed that the compound exhibited cell-killing effect in murine myeloid progenitors and human AML cells harbouring MLL rearrange-ment [145–147, 196, 197]. The treatment with EPZ004777 led to dosage-dependent global depletion of H3K79 methylation [146]. However, such response to the inhib-itor was only observed in primary AML cells with both wild type MLL and IDH1/IDH2 mutations [198]. Primary AML cells with wild type MLL alone dem-onstrated limited antitumor effect [145–147, 196, 197].

EPZ-5676, an alternative DOT1L inhibitor with improved pharmacokinetics was demonstrated to activate apoptosis in MLL-translocated leukemia cell lines in a time- and dosage-dependent manner. Continuous infusion is necessary to achieve maximal efficacy. For example, complete regression of MV4-11 subcutaneous xenograft tumors in rats was observed after 21 days of continuous infusion of EPZ-5676. Similar to EPZ004777, treatment with the compound is also associated with depletion of H3K79me2 in the tumor [145]. Currently, EPZ-5676 is at phase I clini-cal trial targeting AML patients with MLL-rearrangement (http://clinicaltrials.gov).

Taken together, the results showed that the aminonucleoside DOT1L inhibitors show favorable pre-clinical outcome, including improved survival in rats (MV4-11 subcutaneous xenograft model) and treatment response. Such achievement should motivate more drug development and optimization to address some of the limita-tions including insignificant oral bioavailability [199].

5.3   PRMT Inhibitors

Protein arginine methyltransferases (PRMT) have been identified as coactivators for nuclear hormone receptors [34, 200]. Misregulation of PRMT is associated with development in multiple diseases, notably cancer. Specifically, PRMT was found to be overexpressed in a wide range of cancers, including breast, prostate, lung, blad-der and leukaemia [201]. Furthermore, aberrant activation of different PRMT iso-forms, which have distinct functional role were also implicated in cancer [202–204]. Taken together, these findings motivated drug discovery effort in identifying lead compounds targeting specifically for one particular isoform enzyme.

A series of compounds were identified as PRMT1-specific inhibitors using virtual and structure-based screening. AMI-1 and AMI-8 are among the earliest small molecule inhibitors [148], followed by allantodapsone [149]. A newer inhibitor of PRMT1, compound 6 [150], showed improvement in the selectivity profile since it is inactive to CARM1 and SET7/9. Compound 6 showed growth inhibition of breast cancer cell line MCF-7a and prostate cancer cell line LNCaP [205]. It also showed significant reduction in androgen-dependent transcription [205]. Treatment with other compounds, such as DCLX069 and DCLX078, demonstrated reduced proliferation rate by 40% in HepG2, MCF7 and leukemic monocyte cell line THP1 [151]. MHI-21 (compound 11) treatment on cervical cancer cell line HeLa caused cell arrest in the S-phase and led to cell growth inhibition [152]. Another compound E84 was tested for cellular activity in three different hemotological cancer cell lines: Meg01 (chronic myelogenous leukaemia), MOLM13 (AML) and HEL (erythroleukemia) [153]. Notably, the compound repressed cell proliferation and associated with depletion in global cellular methylation after 24 h treatment. The methylation-depleting effect is significant at 100 nM treatment for Meg01 and MOLM13 cells. Stilbamidine (compound 13) shows better activity than AMI-1 on reducing the transcription activation of an estrogen-dependent gene in MCF-7-2a cells [149]. In short, these drug treatments *in vitro* delivered promising results, but more studies are needed to bring these compounds further to clinical testing.

Overexpression of PRMT4/CARM1 was reported in hormone-dependent cancer [206, 207]. For example, CARM1 expression associates with androgen-dependent transcription in prostate carcinoma. It also promotes tumour progression in androgen-independent prostate cancer [208]. Besides prostate cancer, elevated CARM1 expression is also linked to high-grade breast cancer tumours. Interestingly, inhibition of estrogen-dependent transcription, cell cycle progression and cancer cell growth were observed in breast cancer cells with CARM1 mutant [200, 209]. Taken these findings together suggest CARM1 as a novel anti-cancer drug target. In this regard, several pharmacological inhibitors, such as compounds by Methylgene [156], 17b by Bristol-Myers Squibb [155, 210] and 7g [211] were synthesized. The compound, 7g was tested in the prostate cancer cell line LNCaP, and showed a significant reduction of the prostate-specific antigen promoter activity in a dose-dependent manner. However, such treatment did not affect cancer cell viability [211].

5.4   LSD1/2 Inhibitors

Overexpression of LSD1, histone demethylase of H3K4me1/2 and H3K9me1/2 is oncogenic in several cancers including leukaemia [93], colon [212], breast [213], prostate [214] and liver [215]. For example, high expression of LSD1 was linked to activation of epithelial-mesenchymal transition (EMT) and cancer progression in estrogen receptor-negative tumors [213]. On the contrary, depleting LSD1 expression using small interfering (si) RNAs led to the suppression of proliferation in various cancer cell lines [172]. Taken together, the LSD1 expression is important to tumorigenesis, thus making it as an attractive target for therapeutic intervention.

Tranylcypromine (TCP) is one of the firstly discovered KDM inhibitors. Interestingly, it is initially used clinically to treat depression. Mechanistically, it is an unselective compound that acts as an inhibitor of monoaminooxidase, and bonds to the cofactor of FAD at the C-terminal end of LSD1 [216]. Although the treatment with TCP showed anticancer effect in a mouse model [93], it also caused side-effects, such as dizziness, drowsiness [217, 218] and drug-induced anaemia in mice [93]. In light of these limitations, a more potent drug is desired. Treatment with ORY-1001, a potent and selective LSD1 inhibitor designed by Oryzon, demonstrated the accumulation of H3K4me2 at LSD1 target genes in a time- and dosage-dependent manner. It also activates gene expression involving in differentiation in THP-1 cells with MLL translocation (*MLL-AF9*). ORY-1001 treatment also shows reduced tumor growth in rodent MV (4;11) xenograft [219]. Its rival, GlaxoSmithKline, also reported a selective irreversible LSD1 inhibitor, GSK2879552, which is in a phase I study in AML and in small cell lung cancer. The compound promotes differentiation in AML cells. Treatment in SCLC and AML cells demonstrated a potent anti-proliferative growth effect and favourable clinical outcome in mouse models [220]. Besides the irreversible inhibitor GSK2879552, GlaxoSmithKline also developed a reversible LSD1 inhibitor, GSK690. Favorable clinical outcome after treatment could be attributed to the underlying changes in epigenomic landscape in tumors, both locally or globally. For example, a previous study showed that an elevated enrichment of H3K4me2 at gene promoters is associated with myeloid differentiation after inhibiting LSD1 in AML [132]. Another study also demonstrated a global increase of H3K4me2 and growth inhibition in breast cancer cells overexpressing LSD1 after treating with pharmacologic inhibitors targeting amine oxidases [213]. Besides targeting the enzyme directly to repress demethylation activity at H3K4, similar effect can be achieved through downregulating LSD1 expression by inhibiting Sp1 with pan-HDAC inhibitor (HDI) treatment [221].

Despite promising therapeutics effect, these preclinical studies largely focused on the treatment in haematological cancer. More studies using solid tumor samples should be conducted in future to attest the benefit of LSD1 inhibitors in a wider spectrum of cancer. Given the dual capability of LSD1 in activating and repressing different sets of gene through modification of H3K4 and H3K9, the design of therapeutic strategies for targeting LSD1 should account for its multifaceted actions.

JMJC demethylases are another class of lysine demethylase. However, unlike LSD1 inhibitors, clinical candidates targeting JMJC domain-containing demethylases are still lacking. The drug development process is hindered by two factors: (1) high structural similarity of JMJC members, thus causing poor selectivity, and (2) poor cellular permeability of the inhibitors. To address this concern, selective pharmacological intervention across the JMJ family has been achieved by designing small-molecule inhibitors [141]. For example, EPT-103182 (EpiTherapeutics) targeting KDM5B/JARID1B showed anti-proliferative growth effect in cancer lines as well as in xenograft model [131]. GlaxoSmithKline also reported another compound, GSKJ1/4 targeting KDM6 [141]. It induced cell death and caused loss of self-renewal and tumor-initiating capacity in ovarian cancer cell lines [142]. Studies to date have covered only a subset of lysine demethylases. Other lysine demethylases such H3K79 demethylase remain unknown, which might be distinct from existing classes of histone demethylase [222].

6 Application of Combined Epigenetic Therapies with Other Cancer Treatments

In the previous section, we have discussed the application of single agent alone leading to antitumor effect. However, combining epigenetic therapies with other cancer treatments has become an emerging trend. Recent reports have demonstrated that combining epigenetic therapies with other treatment exerts synergistic activity and yields significantly improved clinical outcome in AML. For example, the engraftment of primary AML cells *in vivo* in the NOD/SCID-IL-2receptor-γ-deficient (NSG) mice diminished after co-treatment with the LSD1 inhibitor tranylcypromine (TCP) and all-*trans*-retinoic acid [132]. Interestingly, a recent study using the combined therapy using a very potent LSD1 inhibitor (SP2509) and a pan-HDAC inhibitor (panobinostat) yielded synergistic lethal effect against cultured and primary AML [223]. Such co-treatment also demonstrated more superior survival outcome in mice engrafted with the human AML cells. There is also evidence that EPZ-5676, a DOT1L inhibitor shows synergistic anti-proliferative activity with standard agents (cytarabine and daunorubicin) in the treatment of patients with AML [224]. Combined therapies with all-trans retinoic acid (ATRA) differentiation therapy with KDM1A inhibition also show potent anti-leukemic effect [132]. Such combination could sensitize otherwise ATRA-insensitive cells towards differentiation. In summary, these findings highlight the importance and potential application of combined therapies with standard cancer treatments.

References

1. Vogelstein B et al (2013) Cancer genome landscapes. Science 339(6127):1546–1558
2. Torkamani A, Verkhivker G, Schork NJ (2009) Cancer driver mutations in protein kinase genes. Cancer Lett 281(2):117–127
3. Chapman PB et al (2011) Improved survival with vemurafenib in melanoma with BRAF V600E mutation. N Engl J Med 364(26):2507–2516
4. Misale S et al (2012) Emergence of KRAS mutations and acquired resistance to anti-EGFR therapy in colorectal cancer. Nature 486(7404):532–536
5. Arrowsmith CH et al (2012) Epigenetic protein families: a new frontier for drug discovery. Nat Rev Drug Discov 11(5):384–400
6. Furuhashi M, Hotamisligil GS (2008) Fatty acid-binding proteins: role in metabolic diseases and potential as drug targets. Nat Rev Drug Discov 7(6):489–503
7. Berger SL (2007) The complex language of chromatin regulation during transcription. Nature 447(7143):407–412
8. Kouzarides T (2007) Chromatin modifications and their function. Cell 128(4):693–705
9. Akhtar-Zaidi B et al (2012) Epigenomic enhancer profiling defines a signature of colon cancer. Science 336(6082):736–739
10. Wutz A (2013) Epigenetic regulation of stem cells: the role of chromatin in cell differentiation. Adv Exp Med Biol 786:307–328
11. Lan F et al (2007) A histone H3 lysine 27 demethylase regulates animal posterior development. Nature 449(7163):689–694
12. Lewis A et al (2004) Imprinting on distal chromosome 7 in the placenta involves repressive histone methylation independent of DNA methylation. Nat Genet 36(12):1291–1295

13. Umlauf D et al (2004) Imprinting along the Kcnq1 domain on mouse chromosome 7 involves repressive histone methylation and recruitment of Polycomb group complexes. Nat Genet 36(12):1296–1300
14. Murray K (1964) The occurrence of epsilon-N-methyl lysine in histones. Biochemistry 3:10–15
15. Woon Ki Paik SK (1967) Epsilon-N-dimethyllysine in histones. Biochem Biophys Res Commun 27(4):479–483
16. Hempel K, Lange HW, Birkofer L (1968) Epsilon-N-trimethyllysine, a new amino acid in histones. Naturwissenschaften 55(1):37
17. Byvoet P et al (1972) The distribution and turnover of labeled methyl groups in histone fractions of cultured mammalian cells. Arch Biochem Biophys 148(2):558–567
18. Borun TW, Pearson D, Paik WK (1972) Studies of histone methylation during the HeLa S-3 cell cycle. J Biol Chem 247(13):4288–4298
19. Boffa LC et al (1977) Distribution of NG, NG,-dimethylarginine in nuclear protein fractions. Biochem Biophys Res Commun 74(3):969–976
20. Lauberth SM et al (2013) H3K4me3 interactions with TAF3 regulate preinitiation complex assembly and selective gene activation. Cell 152(5):1021–1036
21. Buratowski S et al (1989) Five intermediate complexes in transcription initiation by RNA polymerase II. Cell 56(4):549–561
22. Mikkelsen TS et al (2007) Genome-wide maps of chromatin state in pluripotent and lineage-committed cells. Nature 448(7153):553–560
23. Boyer LA et al (2006) Polycomb complexes repress developmental regulators in murine embryonic stem cells. Nature 441(7091):349–353
24. Margueron R et al (2009) Role of the polycomb protein EED in the propagation of repressive histone marks. Nature 461(7265):762–767
25. Bannister AJ et al (2001) Selective recognition of methylated lysine 9 on histone H3 by the HP1 chromo domain. Nature 410(6824):120–124
26. Bannister AJ et al (2005) Spatial distribution of di- and tri-methyl lysine 36 of histone H3 at active genes. J Biol Chem 280(18):17732–17736
27. Barski A et al (2007) High-resolution profiling of histone methylations in the human genome. Cell 129(4):823–837
28. Chantalat S et al (2011) Histone H3 trimethylation at lysine 36 is associated with constitutive and facultative heterochromatin. Genome Res 21(9):1426–1437
29. Feng Q et al (2002) Methylation of H3-lysine 79 is mediated by a new family of HMTases without a SET domain. Curr Biol 12(12):1052–1058
30. Ng HH et al (2003) Lysine-79 of histone H3 is hypomethylated at silenced loci in yeast and mammalian cells: a potential mechanism for position-effect variegation. Proc Natl Acad Sci U S A 100(4):1820–1825
31. van Welsem T et al (2008) Synthetic lethal screens identify gene silencing processes in yeast and implicate the acetylated amino terminus of Sir3 in recognition of the nucleosome core. Mol Cell Biol 28(11):3861–3872
32. van Leeuwen F, Gafken PR, Gottschling DE (2002) Dot1p modulates silencing in yeast by methylation of the nucleosome core. Cell 109(6):745–756
33. Wang H et al (2001) Methylation of histone H4 at arginine 3 facilitating transcriptional activation by nuclear hormone receptor. Science 293(5531):853–857
34. Chen D et al (1999) Regulation of transcription by a protein methyltransferase. Science 284(5423):2174–2177
35. Schurter BT et al (2001) Methylation of histone H3 by coactivator-associated arginine methyltransferase 1. Biochemistry 40(19):5747–5756
36. Guccione E et al (2007) Methylation of histone H3R2 by PRMT6 and H3K4 by an MLL complex are mutually exclusive. Nature 449(7164):933–937
37. Kirmizis A et al (2007) Arginine methylation at histone H3R2 controls deposition of H3K4 trimethylation. Nature 449(7164):928–932
38. Heintzman ND et al (2007) Distinct and predictive chromatin signatures of transcriptional promoters and enhancers in the human genome. Nat Genet 39(3):311–318

39. Zhu J et al (2013) Genome-wide chromatin state transitions associated with developmental and environmental cues. Cell 152(3):642–654
40. Ernst J et al (2011) Mapping and analysis of chromatin state dynamics in nine human cell types. Nature 473(7345):43–49
41. Roadmap Epigenomics Consortium et al (2015) Integrative analysis of 111 reference human epigenomes. Nature 518(7539):317–330
42. Whyte WA et al (2013) Master transcription factors and mediator establish super-enhancers at key cell identity genes. Cell 153(2):307–319
43. Parker SC et al (2013) Chromatin stretch enhancer states drive cell-specific gene regulation and harbor human disease risk variants. Proc Natl Acad Sci U S A 110(44):17921–17926
44. Trievel RC et al (2002) Structure and catalytic mechanism of a SET domain protein methyltransferase. Cell 111(1):91–103
45. Milne TA et al (2002) MLL targets SET domain methyltransferase activity to Hox gene promoters. Mol Cell 10(5):1107–1117
46. Rea S et al (2000) Regulation of chromatin structure by site-specific histone H3 methyltransferases. Nature 406(6796):593–599
47. Tachibana M et al (2002) G9a histone methyltransferase plays a dominant role in euchromatic histone H3 lysine 9 methylation and is essential for early embryogenesis. Genes Dev 16(14):1779–1791
48. Kuzmichev A et al (2002) Histone methyltransferase activity associated with a human multiprotein complex containing the Enhancer of Zeste protein. Genes Dev 16(22):2893–2905
49. Czermin B et al (2002) Drosophila enhancer of Zeste/ESC complexes have a histone H3 methyltransferase activity that marks chromosomal Polycomb sites. Cell 111(2):185–196
50. Muller J et al (2002) Histone methyltransferase activity of a Drosophila Polycomb group repressor complex. Cell 111(2):197–208
51. Rayasam GV et al (2003) NSD1 is essential for early post-implantation development and has a catalytically active SET domain. EMBO J 22(12):3153–3163
52. Qiao Q et al (2011) The structure of NSD1 reveals an autoregulatory mechanism underlying histone H3K36 methylation. J Biol Chem 286(10):8361–8368
53. Edmunds JW, Mahadevan LC, Clayton AL (2008) Dynamic histone H3 methylation during gene induction: HYPB/Setd2 mediates all H3K36 trimethylation. EMBO J 27(2):406–420
54. Steger DJ et al (2008) DOT1L/KMT4 recruitment and H3K79 methylation are ubiquitously coupled with gene transcription in mammalian cells. Mol Cell Biol 28(8):2825–2839
55. Huang S, Litt M, Felsenfeld G (2005) Methylation of histone H4 by arginine methyltransferase PRMT1 is essential in vivo for many subsequent histone modifications. Genes Dev 19(16):1885–1893
56. Cheung N et al (2007) Protein arginine-methyltransferase-dependent oncogenesis. Nat Cell Biol 9(10):1208–1215
57. Wang L, Pal S, Sif S (2008) Protein arginine methyltransferase 5 suppresses the transcription of the RB family of tumor suppressors in leukemia and lymphoma cells. Mol Cell Biol 28(20):6262–6277
58. Tsukada Y et al (2006) Histone demethylation by a family of JmjC domain-containing proteins. Nature 439(7078):811–816
59. Lu C et al (2012) IDH mutation impairs histone demethylation and results in a block to cell differentiation. Nature 483(7390):474–478
60. Christensen J et al (2007) RBP2 belongs to a family of demethylases, specific for tri-and dimethylated lysine 4 on histone 3. Cell 128(6):1063–1076
61. Iwase S et al (2007) The X-linked mental retardation gene SMCX/JARID1C defines a family of histone H3 lysine 4 demethylases. Cell 128(6):1077–1088
62. Klose RJ et al (2007) The retinoblastoma binding protein RBP2 is an H3K4 demethylase. Cell 128(5):889–900
63. Yamane K et al (2007) PLU-1 is an H3K4 demethylase involved in transcriptional repression and breast cancer cell proliferation. Mol Cell 25(6):801–812
64. Agger K et al (2007) UTX and JMJD3 are histone H3K27 demethylases involved in HOX gene regulation and development. Nature 449(7163):731–734

65. Yamane K et al (2006) JHDM2A, a JmjC-containing H3K9 demethylase, facilitates transcription activation by androgen receptor. Cell 125(3):483–495
66. Shi Y et al (2004) Histone demethylation mediated by the nuclear amine oxidase homolog LSD1. Cell 119(7):941–953
67. Shi X et al (2006) ING2 PHD domain links histone H3 lysine 4 methylation to active gene repression. Nature 442(7098):96–99
68. Wysocka J et al (2006) A PHD finger of NURF couples histone H3 lysine 4 trimethylation with chromatin remodelling. Nature 442(7098):86–90
69. Li H et al (2006) Molecular basis for site-specific read-out of histone H3K4me3 by the BPTF PHD finger of NURF. Nature 442(7098):91–95
70. Lan F et al (2007) Recognition of unmethylated histone H3 lysine 4 links BHC80 to LSD1-mediated gene repression. Nature 448(7154):718–722
71. Wang Z et al (2010) Pro isomerization in MLL1 PHD3-bromo cassette connects H3K4me readout to CyP33 and HDAC-mediated repression. Cell 141(7):1183–1194
72. Yang Y et al (2010) TDRD3 is an effector molecule for arginine-methylated histone marks. Mol Cell 40(6):1016–1023
73. Sneeringer CJ et al (2010) Coordinated activities of wild-type plus mutant EZH2 drive tumor-associated hypertrimethylation of lysine 27 on histone H3 (H3K27) in human B-cell lymphomas. Proc Natl Acad Sci U S A 107(49):20980–20985
74. Souroullas GP et al (2016) An oncogenic Ezh2 mutation induces tumors through global redistribution of histone 3 lysine 27 trimethylation. Nat Med 22(6):632–640
75. Pasqualucci L et al (2011) Analysis of the coding genome of diffuse large B-cell lymphoma. Nat Genet 43(9):830–837
76. Parsons DW et al (2011) The genetic landscape of the childhood cancer medulloblastoma. Science 331(6016):435–439
77. Morin RD et al (2011) Frequent mutation of histone-modifying genes in non-Hodgkin lymphoma. Nature 476(7360):298–303
78. Zang ZJ et al (2012) Exome sequencing of gastric adenocarcinoma identifies recurrent somatic mutations in cell adhesion and chromatin remodeling genes. Nat Genet 44(5):570–574
79. Fujimoto A et al (2012) Whole-genome sequencing of liver cancers identifies etiological influences on mutation patterns and recurrent mutations in chromatin regulators. Nat Genet 44(7):760–764
80. Gui Y et al (2011) Frequent mutations of chromatin remodeling genes in transitional cell carcinoma of the bladder. Nat Genet 43(9):875–878
81. Hu D et al (2013) The MLL3/MLL4 branches of the COMPASS family function as major histone H3K4 monomethylases at enhancers. Mol Cell Biol 33(23):4745–4754
82. Lee JE et al (2013) H3K4 mono- and di-methyltransferase MLL4 is required for enhancer activation during cell differentiation. eLife 2:e01503
83. Kaikkonen MU et al (2013) Remodeling of the enhancer landscape during macrophage activation is coupled to enhancer transcription. Mol Cell 51(3):310–325
84. van Haaften G et al (2009) Somatic mutations of the histone H3K27 demethylase gene UTX in human cancer. Nat Genet 41(5):521–523
85. Lee MG et al (2007) Demethylation of H3K27 regulates polycomb recruitment and H2A ubiquitination. Science 318(5849):447–450
86. Pena PV et al (2008) Histone H3K4me3 binding is required for the DNA repair and apoptotic activities of ING1 tumor suppressor. J Mol Biol 380(2):303–312
87. Djabali M et al (1992) A trithorax-like gene is interrupted by chromosome 11q23 translocations in acute leukaemias. Nat Genet 2(2):113–118
88. Gu Y et al (1992) The t(4;11) chromosome translocation of human acute leukemias fuses the ALL-1 gene, related to Drosophila trithorax, to the AF-4 gene. Cell 71(4):701–708
89. Tkachuk DC, Kohler S, Cleary ML (1992) Involvement of a homolog of Drosophila trithorax by 11q23 chromosomal translocations in acute leukemias. Cell 71(4):691–700
90. Mohan M et al (2010) Linking H3K79 trimethylation to Wnt signaling through a novel Dot1-containing complex (DotCom). Genes Dev 24(6):574–589

91. Okada Y et al (2005) hDOT1L links histone methylation to leukemogenesis. Cell 121(2):167–178
92. Bernt KM et al (2011) MLL-rearranged leukemia is dependent on aberrant H3K79 methylation by DOT1L. Cancer Cell 20(1):66–78
93. Harris WJ et al (2012) The histone demethylase KDM1A sustains the oncogenic potential of MLL-AF9 leukemia stem cells. Cancer Cell 21(4):473–487
94. Caligiuri MA et al (1994) Molecular rearrangement of the ALL-1 gene in acute myeloid leukemia without cytogenetic evidence of 11q23 chromosomal translocations. Cancer Res 54(2):370–373
95. Whitman SP et al (2005) The MLL partial tandem duplication: evidence for recessive gain-of-function in acute myeloid leukemia identifies a novel patient subgroup for molecular-targeted therapy. Blood 106(1):345–352
96. Dorrance AM et al (2008) The Mll partial tandem duplication: differential, tissue-specific activity in the presence or absence of the wild-type allele. Blood 112(6):2508–2511
97. Reader JC et al (2007) A novel NUP98-PHF23 fusion resulting from a cryptic translocation t(11;17)(p15;p13) in acute myeloid leukemia. Leukemia 21(4):842–844
98. Gough SM et al (2014) NUP98-PHF23 is a chromatin-modifying oncoprotein that causes a wide array of leukemias sensitive to inhibition of PHD histone reader function. Cancer Discov 4(5):564–577
99. Cerveira N et al (2003) Frequency of NUP98-NSD1 fusion transcript in childhood acute myeloid leukaemia. Leukemia 17(11):2244–2247
100. Wang GG et al (2007) NUP98-NSD1 links H3K36 methylation to Hox-A gene activation and leukaemogenesis. Nat Cell Biol 9(7):804–812
101. Raman JD et al (2005) Increased expression of the polycomb group gene, EZH2, in transitional cell carcinoma of the bladder. Clin Cancer Res 11(24 Pt 1):8570–8576
102. Matsukawa Y et al (2006) Expression of the enhancer of zeste homolog 2 is correlated with poor prognosis in human gastric cancer. Cancer Sci 97(6):484–491
103. Kondo Y et al (2007) Alterations of DNA methylation and histone modifications contribute to gene silencing in hepatocellular carcinomas. Hepatol Res 37(11):974–983
104. Lee HW, Choe M (2012) Expression of EZH2 in renal cell carcinoma as a novel prognostic marker. Pathol Int 62(11):735–741
105. Rao ZY et al (2010) EZH2 supports ovarian carcinoma cell invasion and/or metastasis via regulation of TGF-beta1 and is a predictor of outcome in ovarian carcinoma patients. Carcinogenesis 31(9):1576–1583
106. Koh CM et al (2011) Myc enforces overexpression of EZH2 in early prostatic neoplasia via transcriptional and post-transcriptional mechanisms. Oncotarget 2(9):669–683
107. Bracken AP et al (2003) EZH2 is downstream of the pRB-E2F pathway, essential for proliferation and amplified in cancer. EMBO J 22(20):5323–5335
108. Richter GH et al (2009) EZH2 is a mediator of EWS/FLI1 driven tumor growth and metastasis blocking endothelial and neuro-ectodermal differentiation. Proc Natl Acad Sci U S A 106(13):5324–5329
109. Tiwari N et al (2013) Sox4 is a master regulator of epithelial-mesenchymal transition by controlling Ezh2 expression and epigenetic reprogramming. Cancer Cell 23(6):768–783
110. Mahara S et al (2016) HIFI-alpha activation underlies a functional switch in the paradoxical role of Ezh2/PRC2 in breast cancer. Proc Natl Acad Sci U S A 113(26):E3735–E3744
111. Zhu J et al (2015) Gain-of-function p53 mutants co-opt chromatin pathways to drive cancer growth. Nature 525(7568):206–211
112. Kim JM et al (2005) Identification of gastric cancer-related genes using a cDNA microarray containing novel expressed sequence tags expressed in gastric cancer cells. Clin Cancer Res 11(2 Pt 1):473–482
113. Yan F et al (2014) Genetic validation of the protein arginine methyltransferase PRMT5 as a candidate therapeutic target in glioblastoma. Cancer Res 74(6):1752–1765
114. Koh CM et al (2015) MYC regulates the core pre-mRNA splicing machinery as an essential step in lymphomagenesis. Nature 523(7558):96–100

115. Mongiardi MP et al (2015) Myc and Omomyc functionally associate with the Protein Arginine Methyltransferase 5 (PRMT5) in glioblastoma cells. Sci Rep 5:15494
116. Kroon E et al (1998) Hoxa9 transforms primary bone marrow cells through specific collaboration with Meis1a but not Pbx1b. EMBO J 17(13):3714–3725
117. Volanakis EJ, Boothby MR, Sherr CJ (2013) Epigenetic regulation of the Ink4a-Arf (Cdkn2a) tumor suppressor locus in the initiation and progression of Notch1-driven T cell acute lymphoblastic leukemia. Exp Hematol 41(4):377–386
118. Chen H et al (2009) Polycomb protein Ezh2 regulates pancreatic beta-cell Ink4a/Arf expression and regeneration in diabetes mellitus. Genes Dev 23(8):975–985
119. Zhou HL et al (2014) Regulation of alternative splicing by local histone modifications: potential roles for RNA-guided mechanisms. Nucleic Acids Res 42(2):701–713
120. Simon JM et al (2014) Variation in chromatin accessibility in human kidney cancer links H3K36 methyltransferase loss with widespread RNA processing defects. Genome Res 24(2):241–250
121. Park IY et al (2016) Dual chromatin and cytoskeletal remodeling by SETD2. Cell 166(4):950–962
122. Kanu N et al (2015) SETD2 loss-of-function promotes renal cancer branched evolution through replication stress and impaired DNA repair. Oncogene 34(46):5699–5708
123. Kantidakis T et al (2016) Mutation of cancer driver MLL2 results in transcription stress and genome instability. Genes Dev 30(4):408–420
124. Baylin SB, Jones PA (2011) A decade of exploring the cancer epigenome – biological and translational implications. Nat Rev Cancer 11(10):726–734
125. Ahuja N, Easwaran H, Baylin SB (2014) Harnessing the potential of epigenetic therapy to target solid tumors. J Clin Invest 124(1):56–63
126. Kubicek S et al (2007) Reversal of H3K9me2 by a small-molecule inhibitor for the G9a histone methyltransferase. Mol Cell 25(3):473–481
127. Liu F et al (2013) Discovery of an in vivo chemical probe of the lysine methyltransferases G9a and GLP. J Med Chem 56(21):8931–8942
128. Sweis RF et al (2014) Discovery and development of potent and selective inhibitors of histone methyltransferase g9a. ACS Med Chem Lett 5(2):205–209
129. Yuan Y et al (2012) A small-molecule probe of the histone methyltransferase G9a induces cellular senescence in pancreatic adenocarcinoma. ACS Chem Biol 7(7):1152–1157
130. Liu F et al (2009) Discovery of a 2,4-diamino-7-aminoalkoxyquinazoline as a potent and selective inhibitor of histone lysine methyltransferase G9a. J Med Chem 52(24):7950–7953
131. Maes T et al (2015) Advances in the development of histone lysine demethylase inhibitors. Curr Opin Pharmacol 23:52–60
132. Schenk T et al (2012) Inhibition of the LSD1 (KDM1A) demethylase reactivates the all-trans-retinoic acid differentiation pathway in acute myeloid leukemia. Nat Med 18(4):605–611
133. Mohammad HP, Kruger RG (2016) Antitumor activity of LSD1 inhibitors in lung cancer. Mol Cell Oncol 3(2):e1117700
134. McCabe MT et al (2012) EZH2 inhibition as a therapeutic strategy for lymphoma with EZH2-activating mutations. Nature 492(7427):108–112
135. Amatangelo MD et al (2013) Three-dimensional culture sensitizes epithelial ovarian cancer cells to EZH2 methyltransferase inhibition. Cell Cycle 12(13):2113–2119
136. Knutson SK et al (2012) A selective inhibitor of EZH2 blocks H3K27 methylation and kills mutant lymphoma cells. Nat Chem Biol 8(11):890–896
137. Knutson SK et al (2013) Durable tumor regression in genetically altered malignant rhabdoid tumors by inhibition of methyltransferase EZH2. Proc Natl Acad Sci U S A 110(19):7922–7927
138. Qi W et al (2012) Selective inhibition of Ezh2 by a small molecule inhibitor blocks tumor cells proliferation. Proc Natl Acad Sci U S A 109(52):21360–21365
139. Konze KD et al (2013) An orally bioavailable chemical probe of the Lysine Methyltransferases EZH2 and EZH1. ACS Chem Biol 8(6):1324–1334
140. Zhang H et al (2016) Oncogenic deregulation of EZH2 as an opportunity for targeted therapy in lung cancer. Cancer Discov 6(9):1006–1021

141. Kruidenier L et al (2012) A selective jumonji H3K27 demethylase inhibitor modulates the proinflammatory macrophage response. Nature 488(7411):404–408
142. Sakaki H et al (2015) GSKJ4, a selective Jumonji H3K27 demethylase inhibitor, effectively targets ovarian cancer stem cells. Anticancer Res 35(12):6607–6614
143. Ferguson AD et al (2011) Structural basis of substrate methylation and inhibition of SMYD2. Structure 19(9):1262–1273
144. Wang J et al (2016) Silencing the epigenetic silencer KDM4A for TRAIL and DR5 simultaneous induction and antitumor therapy. Cell Death Differ 23(11):1886–1896
145. Daigle SR et al (2013) Potent inhibition of DOT1L as treatment of MLL-fusion leukemia. Blood 122(6):1017–1025
146. Daigle SR et al (2011) Selective killing of mixed lineage leukemia cells by a potent small-molecule DOT1L inhibitor. Cancer Cell 20(1):53–65
147. Yu W et al (2012) Catalytic site remodelling of the DOT1L methyltransferase by selective inhibitors. Nat Commun 3:1288
148. Cheng D et al (2004) Small molecule regulators of protein arginine methyltransferases. J Biol Chem 279(23):23892–23899
149. Spannhoff A et al (2007) Target-based approach to inhibitors of histone arginine methyltransferases. J Med Chem 50(10):2319–2325
150. Hu H et al (2016) Small molecule inhibitors of protein arginine methyltransferases. Expert Opin Investig Drugs 25(3):335–358
151. Xie Y et al (2014) Virtual screening and biological evaluation of novel small molecular inhibitors against protein arginine methyltransferase 1 (PRMT1). Org Biomol Chem 12(47):9665–9673
152. Sinha SH et al (2012) Synthesis and evaluation of carbocyanine dyes as PRMT inhibitors and imaging agents. Eur J Med Chem 54:647–659
153. Hu H et al (2015) Exploration of cyanine compounds as selective inhibitors of protein arginine methyltransferases: synthesis and biological evaluation. J Med Chem 58(3):1228–1243
154. Liu F et al (2013) Exploiting an allosteric binding site of PRMT3 yields potent and selective inhibitors. J Med Chem 56(5):2110–2124
155. Wan H et al (2009) Benzo[d]imidazole inhibitors of Coactivator Associated Arginine Methyltransferase 1 (CARM1)--Hit to Lead studies. Bioorg Med Chem Lett 19(17):5063–5066
156. Allan M et al (2009) N-Benzyl-1-heteroaryl-3-(trifluoromethyl)-1H-pyrazole-5-carboxamides as inhibitors of co-activator associated arginine methyltransferase 1 (CARM1). Bioorg Med Chem Lett 19(4):1218–1223
157. Chan-Penebre E et al (2015) A selective inhibitor of PRMT5 with in vivo and in vitro potency in MCL models. Nat Chem Biol 11(6):432–437
158. Varambally S et al (2002) The polycomb group protein EZH2 is involved in progression of prostate cancer. Nature 419(6907):624–629
159. Kleer CG et al (2003) EZH2 is a marker of aggressive breast cancer and promotes neoplastic transformation of breast epithelial cells. Proc Natl Acad Sci U S A 100(20):11606–11611
160. Wagener N et al (2010) Enhancer of zeste homolog 2 (EZH2) expression is an independent prognostic factor in renal cell carcinoma. BMC Cancer 10:524
161. Takawa M et al (2011) Validation of the histone methyltransferase EZH2 as a therapeutic target for various types of human cancer and as a prognostic marker. Cancer Sci 102(7):1298–1305
162. Peifer M et al (2012) Integrative genome analyses identify key somatic driver mutations of small-cell lung cancer. Nat Genet 44(10):1104–1110
163. Cancer Genome Atlas Research Network et al (2013) Integrated genomic characterization of endometrial carcinoma. Nature 497(7447):67–73
164. Sjoblom T et al (2006) The consensus coding sequences of human breast and colorectal cancers. Science 314(5797):268–274
165. Okosun J et al (2014) Integrated genomic analysis identifies recurrent mutations and evolution patterns driving the initiation and progression of follicular lymphoma. Nat Genet 46(2):176–181
166. Tan J et al (2015) Genomic landscapes of breast fibroepithelial tumors. Nat Genet 47(11):1341–1345

167. Xiang Y et al (2007) JARID1B is a histone H3 lysine 4 demethylase up-regulated in prostate cancer. Proc Natl Acad Sci U S A 104(49):19226–19231
168. Yamamoto S et al (2014) JARID1B is a luminal lineage-driving oncogene in breast cancer. Cancer Cell 25(6):762–777
169. Dalgliesh GL et al (2010) Systematic sequencing of renal carcinoma reveals inactivation of histone modifying genes. Nature 463(7279):360–363
170. Varela I et al (2011) Exome sequencing identifies frequent mutation of the SWI/SNF complex gene PBRM1 in renal carcinoma. Nature 469(7331):539–542
171. Komura K et al (2016) Resistance to docetaxel in prostate cancer is associated with androgen receptor activation and loss of KDM5D expression. Proc Natl Acad Sci U S A 113(22):6259–6264
172. Hayami S et al (2011) Overexpression of LSD1 contributes to human carcinogenesis through chromatin regulation in various cancers. Int J Cancer 128(3):574–586
173. Gunduz M et al (2000) Genomic structure of the human ING1 gene and tumor-specific mutations detected in head and neck squamous cell carcinomas. Cancer Res 60(12):3143–3146
174. Bjorkman M et al (2012) Systematic knockdown of epigenetic enzymes identifies a novel histone demethylase PHF8 overexpressed in prostate cancer with an impact on cell proliferation, migration and invasion. Oncogene 31(29):3444–3456
175. Peters AH et al (2001) Loss of the Suv39h histone methyltransferases impairs mammalian heterochromatin and genome stability. Cell 107(3):323–337
176. Black JC et al (2013) KDM4A lysine demethylase induces site-specific copy gain and rereplication of regions amplified in tumors. Cell 154(3):541–555
177. Stephens PJ et al (2012) The landscape of cancer genes and mutational processes in breast cancer. Nature 486(7403):400–404
178. Le Gallo M et al (2012) Exome sequencing of serous endometrial tumors identifies recurrent somatic mutations in chromatin-remodeling and ubiquitin ligase complex genes. Nat Genet 44(12):1310–1315
179. Xi Q et al (2011) A poised chromatin platform for TGF-beta access to master regulators. Cell 147(7):1511–1524
180. Schotta G et al (2004) A silencing pathway to induce H3-K9 and H4-K20 trimethylation at constitutive heterochromatin. Genes Dev 18(11):1251–1262
181. Vougiouklakis T et al (2015) SUV420H1 enhances the phosphorylation and transcription of ERK1 in cancer cells. Oncotarget 6(41):43162–43171
182. Kim JH et al (2014) UTX and MLL4 coordinately regulate transcriptional programs for cell proliferation and invasiveness in breast cancer cells. Cancer Res 74(6):1705–1717
183. Liu YL et al (2015) Expression and clinicopathological significance of EED, SUZ12 and EZH2 mRNA in colorectal cancer. J Cancer Res Clin Oncol 141(4):661–669
184. Lee W et al (2014) PRC2 is recurrently inactivated through EED or SUZ12 loss in malignant peripheral nerve sheath tumors. Nat Genet 46(11):1227–1232
185. Brien GL et al (2012) Polycomb PHF19 binds H3K36me3 and recruits PRC2 and demethylase NO66 to embryonic stem cell genes during differentiation. Nat Struct Mol Biol 19(12):1273–1281
186. Zhao Q et al (2009) PRMT5-mediated methylation of histone H4R3 recruits DNMT3A, coupling histone and DNA methylation in gene silencing. Nat Struct Mol Biol 16(3):304–311
187. Nagahata T et al (2004) Expression profiling to predict postoperative prognosis for estrogen receptor-negative breast cancers by analysis of 25,344 genes on a cDNA microarray. Cancer Sci 95(3):218–225
188. Tan J et al (2007) Pharmacologic disruption of Polycomb-repressive complex 2-mediated gene repression selectively induces apoptosis in cancer cells. Genes Dev 21(9):1050–1063
189. Miranda TB et al (2009) DZNep is a global histone methylation inhibitor that reactivates developmental genes not silenced by DNA methylation. Mol Cancer Ther 8(6):1579–1588
190. Knutson SK et al (2014) Selective inhibition of EZH2 by EPZ-6438 leads to potent antitumor activity in EZH2-mutant non-Hodgkin lymphoma. Mol Cancer Ther 13(4):842–854
191. Morin RD et al (2010) Somatic mutations altering EZH2 (Tyr641) in follicular and diffuse large B-cell lymphomas of germinal-center origin. Nat Genet 42(2):181–185

192. McCabe MT et al (2012) Mutation of A677 in histone methyltransferase EZH2 in human B-cell lymphoma promotes hypertrimethylation of histone H3 on lysine 27 (H3K27). Proc Natl Acad Sci U S A 109(8):2989–2994

193. Ryan RJ et al (2011) EZH2 codon 641 mutations are common in BCL2-rearranged germinal center B cell lymphomas. PLoS One 6(12):e28585

194. Bradley WD et al (2014) EZH2 inhibitor efficacy in non-Hodgkin's lymphoma does not require suppression of H3K27 monomethylation. Chem Biol 21(11):1463–1475

195. Basavapathruni A et al (2012) Conformational adaptation drives potent, selective and durable inhibition of the human protein methyltransferase DOT1L. Chem Biol Drug Des 80(6):971–980

196. Chen L et al (2013) Abrogation of MLL-AF10 and CALM-AF10-mediated transformation through genetic inactivation or pharmacological inhibition of the H3K79 methyltransferase Dot1l. Leukemia 27(4):813–822

197. Deshpande AJ et al (2013) Leukemic transformation by the MLL-AF6 fusion oncogene requires the H3K79 methyltransferase Dot1l. Blood 121(13):2533–2541

198. Sarkaria SM et al (2014) Primary acute myeloid leukemia cells with IDH1 or IDH2 mutations respond to a DOT1L inhibitor in vitro. Leukemia 28(12):2403–2406

199. Basavapathruni A et al (2014) Nonclinical pharmacokinetics and metabolism of EPZ-5676, a novel DOT1L histone methyltransferase inhibitor. Biopharm Drug Dispos 35(4):237–252

200. Yadav N et al (2003) Specific protein methylation defects and gene expression perturbations in coactivator-associated arginine methyltransferase 1-deficient mice. Proc Natl Acad Sci U S A 100(11):6464–6468

201. Yang Y, Bedford MT (2013) Protein arginine methyltransferases and cancer. Nat Rev Cancer 13(1):37–50

202. Goulet I et al (2007) Alternative splicing yields protein arginine methyltransferase 1 isoforms with distinct activity, substrate specificity, and subcellular localization. J Biol Chem 282(45):33009–33021

203. Mathioudaki K et al (2008) The PRMT1 gene expression pattern in colon cancer. Br J Cancer 99(12):2094–2099

204. Baldwin RM et al (2012) Alternatively spliced protein arginine methyltransferase 1 isoform PRMT1v2 promotes the survival and invasiveness of breast cancer cells. Cell Cycle 11(24):4597–4612

205. Bissinger EM et al (2011) Acyl derivatives of p-aminosulfonamides and dapsone as new inhibitors of the arginine methyltransferase hPRMT1. Bioorg Med Chem 19(12):3717–3731

206. El Messaoudi S et al (2006) Coactivator-associated arginine methyltransferase 1 (CARM1) is a positive regulator of the Cyclin E1 gene. Proc Natl Acad Sci U S A 103(36):13351–13356

207. Majumder S et al (2006) Involvement of arginine methyltransferase CARM1 in androgen receptor function and prostate cancer cell viability. Prostate 66(12):1292–1301

208. Hong H et al (2004) Aberrant expression of CARM1, a transcriptional coactivator of androgen receptor, in the development of prostate carcinoma and androgen-independent status. Cancer 101(1):83–89

209. Frietze S et al (2008) CARM1 regulates estrogen-stimulated breast cancer growth through up-regulation of E2F1. Cancer Res 68(1):301–306

210. Sack JS et al (2011) Structural basis for CARM1 inhibition by indole and pyrazole inhibitors. Biochem J 436(2):331–339

211. Cheng D et al (2011) Novel 3,5-bis(bromohydroxybenzylidene)piperidin-4-ones as coactivator-associated arginine methyltransferase 1 inhibitors: enzyme selectivity and cellular activity. J Med Chem 54(13):4928–4932

212. Ding J et al (2013) LSD1-mediated epigenetic modification contributes to proliferation and metastasis of colon cancer. Br J Cancer 109(4):994–1003

213. Lim S et al (2010) Lysine-specific demethylase 1 (LSD1) is highly expressed in ER-negative breast cancers and a biomarker predicting aggressive biology. Carcinogenesis 31(3):512–520

214. Kahl P et al (2006) Androgen receptor coactivators lysine-specific histone demethylase 1 and four and a half LIM domain protein 2 predict risk of prostate cancer recurrence. Cancer Res 66(23):11341–11347

215. Zhao ZK et al (2012) Overexpression of lysine specific demethylase 1 predicts worse prognosis in primary hepatocellular carcinoma patients. World J Gastroenterol 18(45):6651–6656
216. Schmidt DM, McCafferty DG (2007) trans-2-Phenylcyclopropylamine is a mechanism-based inactivator of the histone demethylase LSD1. Biochemistry 46(14):4408–4416
217. Fiedorowicz JG, Swartz KL (2004) The role of monoamine oxidase inhibitors in current psychiatric practice. J Psychiatr Pract 10(4):239–248
218. Shulman KI et al (2009) Current prescription patterns and safety profile of irreversible monoamine oxidase inhibitors: a population-based cohort study of older adults. J Clin Psychiatry 70(12):1681–1686
219. Morera L, Lubbert M, Jung M (2016) Targeting histone methyltransferases and demethylases in clinical trials for cancer therapy. Clin Epigenetics 8:57
220. Mohammad H et al (2014) Novel anti-tumor activity of targeted LSD1 inhibition by GSK2879552. Eur J Cancer 50:72
221. Huang PH et al (2011) Histone deacetylase inhibitors stimulate histone H3 lysine 4 methylation in part via transcriptional repression of histone H3 lysine 4 demethylases. Mol Pharmacol 79(1):197–206
222. Shi YG, Tsukada Y (2013) The discovery of histone demethylases. Cold Spring Harb Perspect Biol 5(9):a017947
223. Fiskus W et al (2014) Highly effective combination of LSD1 (KDM1A) antagonist and pan-histone deacetylase inhibitor against human AML cells. Leukemia 28(11):2155–2164
224. Klaus CR et al (2014) DOT1L inhibitor EPZ-5676 displays synergistic antiproliferative activity in combination with standard of care drugs and hypomethylating agents in MLL-rearranged leukemia cells. J Pharmacol Exp Ther 350(3):646–656

Other Histone Modifications

Hiroaki Kato

Abstract There are a lot of histone modifications other than methylation, many of which are known to be dysregulated in cancer cells. This chapter briefly introduces typical histone modifications associated with cancer, and then provides an overview of the current understanding of histone acetylation. Histone acetylation, which occurs at the α amino group of the most N-terminal amino acid residue, and at the ε-amino groups of internal lysine residues in histone molecules, is catalyzed by various kinds of histone acetyltransferases. This modification causes alterations in the electrostatic property of the target residue, and thereby contributes to the dynamic regulation of the state of chromatin. N-terminal acetylation of histones is considered to occur constitutively, whereas the internal lysine acetylation is reversible, being recognized by trans-acting bromodomain-containing proteins and removed by histone deacetylases. This chapter focuses on outlining representative histone acetyltransferases and their molecular mechanisms, to provide a picture of how their substrate-specificity is ensured. Next, how bromodomains recognize their target residues is presented. Finally, the molecular mechanisms of histone deacetylation and its inhibition are briefly summarized.

Keywords Histone methylation • Histone acetylation • Histone acetyltransferase • Bromodomain • Histone deacetylase • Molecular mechanism

1 Other Histone Modifications and Cancer

There are many post-translational modifications that occur at different positions in histone molecules, some of which are shown in (Fig. 1). These modifications include histone acetylation, methylation, phosphorylation, ubiquitination and others. Histone methylation had been considered as a rather "static" modification until demethylation enzymes, which remove this modification, were identified. Additionally, various histone acetyltransferase (HAT) and deacetylase (HDAC)

H. Kato (✉)
Department of Biochemistry, Shimane University School of Medicine, Izumo, Japan
e-mail: hkato@med.shimane-u.ac.jp

© Springer International Publishing AG 2017
A. Kaneda, Y.-i. Tsukada (eds.), *DNA and Histone Methylation as Cancer Targets*, Cancer Drug Discovery and Development, DOI 10.1007/978-3-319-59786-7_9

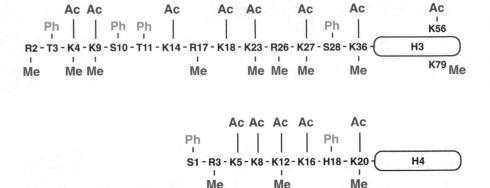

Fig. 1 Schematic representation of various posttranslational modifications of histones H3 and H4. Histone H3 and H4 amino acid residues whose side chains are targeted by posttranslational modifications are shown. *Ac* acetylation, *Ph* phosphorylation, *Me* methylation. These modifications occur in the amino terminal (N-terminal tails) of the histones, except for acetylation at Lys-56 (*K56*) and methylation at Lys-79 (*K79*) that are located in the histone-fold globular domain

enzymes were identified in rapid succession in 1995 and 1996 [1–5]. On the other hand, although the first histone methyltransferase was identified 4 years later [6], it took another 4 years for a demethylase to be identified [7]. Therefore, up until the year 2004, it remained uncertain whether histone methylation of a single histone molecule was reversible, and whether histone methylation-mediated epigenetic control was as dynamic as that mediated by acetylation. In the "pre-demethylase" period, other histone modifications such as acetylation and phosphorylation were preferentially investigated in epigenetic studies.

Patterns of several histone modifications are often altered in cancer. These include patterns of methylation as well as non-methylation modification such as acetylation, phosphorylation and ubiquitination. The discovery and analyses of those aberrant modification patterns were highly dependent on the generation of reliable antibodies that specifically recognize each modification [8–10].

A well-known hallmark of cancer cells in terms of histone modification that was reported in 2005, is the global reduction in acetylation and trimethylation of histone H4, which occurs at Lys16 (H4K16ac) and Lys20 (H4K20me3), respectively. These alterations are associated with hypomethylation of DNA repetitive sequences, which is common in tumorigenesis [11]. It was also reported in 2005 that four distinct histone modifications positively correlate with increasing grade of prostate cancer [12]: acetylation of histone H3 at Lys18 (H3K18ac) and of H4 at Lys12 (H4K12ac); and dimethylation of H3 at Lys4 (H3K4me2) and of H4 at Arg3 (H4R3me2). That study also showed that histone modification patterns can predict the risk of recurrence. Similarly, in breast tumor samples, the levels of acetylation of histone H3 at Lys9 (H3K9ac), of H3K18ac, H4K12ac, H4K16ac, H4K20me3, H4R3me2 and H3K4me2 are reduced [13].

Alteration of histone modification in cancer cells is not restricted to methylation and acetylation. Phosphorylation of histone H3 at Ser10, which occurs during the M phase of the cell cycle, often increases in proliferating cancer cells, and is indispensable for cellular transformation [14–18]. Furthermore, the immunohistochemical analyses of tissue microarrays performed by Prenzel et al. showed that a decrease in the mono-ubiquitination level of histone H2B correlates with breast cancer progression and metastasis [19].

2 Histone Acetylation

Acetylation of histone molecules can occur in two distinct ways (Fig. 2). acetylation at the α-amino group of the most N-terminal amino acid residue is termed "N α acetylation" (Fig. 3), and acetylation at the ε-amino group in the side chain of a lysine residue is termed "N-ε-acetylation" (Fig. 4). In both acetylations, a responsible HAT catalyzes the transfer of the acetyl moiety of acetyl Coenzyme A

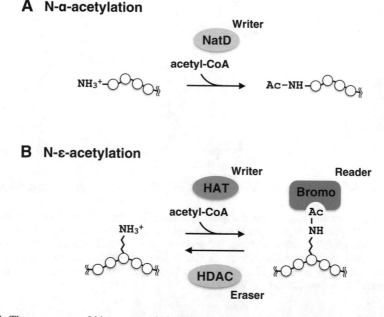

Fig. 2 The two types of histone acetylation. (**a**) In N-α-acetylation, the conserved N-terminal acetyltransferase NatD transfers the acetyl group of acetyl-CoA to the α-amino group of histones H2A and H4. This reaction is considered to occur co-translationally. No reader or eraser for this modification has been identified. (**b**) In N-ε-acetylation, the ε-amino group of the lysine side chain is acetylated by various histone acetyltransferases (HATs; "writers"). This modification can be recognized by bromodomain-containing "reader" proteins, and can be removed by "eraser" histone deacetylases (HDACs). Amino acid residues are depicted as *white* circles. Amino acid side chains, except for those of the acetylated lysine, were omitted for clarity

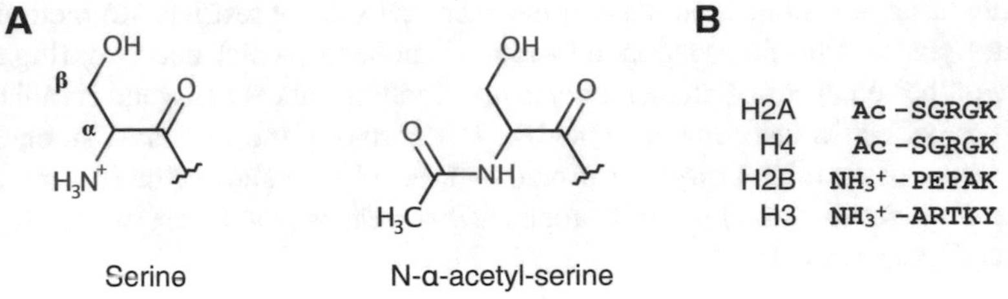

A

OH
β

α

H_3N^+

Serine

OH

O

H_3C —NH

N-α-acetyl-serine

B

H2A	Ac –SGRGK
H4	Ac –SGRGK
H2B	NH_3^+ –PEPAK
H3	NH_3^+ –ARTKY

Fig. 3 Acetylation of the N-terminal serine. (**a**) The chemical structure of an unmodified serine and an N-α-acetyl-serine at the amino terminal (N-terminal) of a peptide are shown. Subsequent residues linked through peptide bonds are omitted. The position of the carbon atoms α and β are indicated. Co-translational cleavage of the initiator methionine forms a new N-terminal α-amino group (*blue*). The positive charge of this group is neutralized by the N-terminal acetylation. (**b**) The first five amino acids in the peptide sequence of core histones, and the modification state of their N-terminal amino acids are shown. *Ac* N-α-acetylated, *NH_3^+* unmodified. The chemical structures were drawn using MarvinSketch

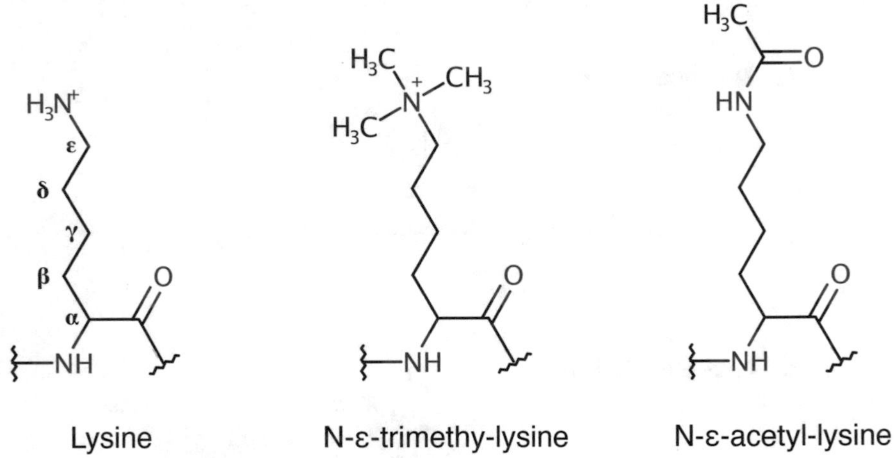

H_3N^+

ε

δ

γ

β   O

α

}—NH

Lysine

H_3C
    $\overset{+}{N}$—CH_3
H_3C

O

}—NH

N-ε-trimethy-lysine

H_3C
       =O
HN

O

}—NH

N-ε-acetyl-lysine

Fig. 4 Acetylation and methylation of a lysine side chain. The chemical structure of an unmodified lysine, N-ε-trimethyl-lysine and N-ε-acetyl-lysine residues is shown. Neighboring residues linked through peptide bonds are omitted. The positions of the α-ε carbon atoms in the lysine side chain are indicated. The ε-amino group of a lysine residue is positively charged at physiological pH, and this charge is neutralized by acetylation but not by methylation. The relatively long aliphatic part of the lysine side chain is hydrophobic

(acetyl-CoA) to the amino group. These two ways of acetylation should be distinguished with respect not only to the target amino group, but also to the catalyzing enzyme.

A variety of enzymes contribute to N-ε-acetylation, all of which belong to one of five HAT subfamilies [20–22]. Some of these enzymes are located in the cytoplasm and acetylate free full-length histones. Others act in the nucleus and often acetylate nucleosomal histones. In either case, the N-ε-acetylation occurs in a post-translational manner. In contrast to the diversity of the N-ε-acetylation enzymes, only one evolutionarily conserved enzyme, called NatD, is responsible for the N-α-acetylation of histone molecules. Since this enzyme is associated with the ribosome, N-α-acetylation of histones is considered to occur co-translationally as the target site emerges upon cleavage of the initiator methionine, which is also a co-translational event.

The enzymes that catalyze certain covalent modifications are generally referred to as "writers" (Fig. 2). Thus, HATs are writers for histone acetylation. In addition to writers, there are also specific "readers" (bromodomain-containing proteins) and "erasers" (histone deacetylases) for N-ε-acetylation. The existence of erasers allows the N-ε-acetylation of a single histone molecule to be reversed. In contrast, N-α-acetylation appears to be irreversible because no eraser for this modification has been identified so far.

N-ε-acetylation and methylation target the same ε-amino group of a lysine residue (Fig. 4). Unlike the methylation of histone molecules, acetylation results in alterations in their electrostatic properties. As shown in Fig. 4, the ε-amino group of a lysine residue is positively charged at physiological pH. This positive charge is not neutralized by methylation but is neutralized by acetylation. Similarly, N-α-acetylation also neutralizes the positive charge of the α-amino groups of histones H2A and H4 (Fig. 3). Since the positive charge on histone molecules contributes to their strong affinity for DNA, which has a negative charge on the phosphate backbone, acetylation is thought to weaken the interaction between histone molecules and DNA, and thereby allow dynamic regulation of chromatin structure.

For example, histone N-ε-acetylation increases the accessibility of DNA-binding factors to their binding sites [23, 24]. It is also known that the formation of 30 nm-like fibers of nucleosomal arrays is inhibited by acetylation of histone H4 at Lys16 (H4K16ac). H4K16ac is enriched in transcriptionally active decondensed chromatin in HeLa cells [25]. H4K16ac is also enriched in the *Drosophila* male X chromosome [26, 27], in which genes are transcribed at twice the rate as that in females, as a result of a phenomenon known as "dosage compensation".

The weakening of the interaction between histone molecules and DNA makes chromatin more relaxed and accessible to trans-acting factors. Thus, this state of chromatin is the preferred state for transcription by RNA polymerase II, the transcription machinery for protein-coding and long non-coding RNA genes. The transcription activity of this polymerase is in part regulated through chromatin structure. At the initiation step of transcription, nucleosomes must be depleted from the promoter region in order to open it up for recruitment of the polymerase and transcription factors so that the so-called pre-initiation complex can be assembled [28–30]. Furthermore, partial disruption of nucleosomes is necessary to let the polymerase pass through [31, 32]. Thus, N-ε-acetylation of histones is generally observed at actively transcribed genomic regions.

2.1 N-α-Acetylation of Histones H2A and H4

The initiator methionine residues of all four core histones are co-translationally removed from the nascent polypeptides by methionine aminopeptidase. Of the four core histones, the newly emerged N-terminal serine residue of histones H2A and H4, whose first five residues at their N-terminal amino acid sequence are identical (Fig. 3), are subsequently acetylated at their α amino groups by the evolutionarily conserved N-α-acetyltransferase NatD (also known as Naa40, Nat4 and Patt1) [33–35]. This modification is considered to occur co-translationally, on the basis that the enzyme localizes to ribosome fractions in yeast and human cells [34, 35].

The N-α-acetylation of histones H2A and H4 is considered to be irreversible and hence rather static, because no enzyme that removes such N-α-acetylation has been identified. However, as human NatD has been shown to localize not only in the cytosol but also at high levels in the nucleus [35], it is also possible that this modification occurs post-translationally after the protein has been translocated to the nucleus.

The N-α-acetylation of histone molecules appears to have important roles in epigenetic regulation. Studies of yeast NatD have shown that deletion of its encoding gene leads to sensitivity of the cell to various stresses such as amino acid depletion and microtubule dysfunction [34], suggesting that N-α-acetylation of histones contributes to the response to those stresses. Interestingly, Schiza et al. discovered that NatD-dependent N-α-acetylation of histone H4 inhibits asymmetric dimethylation of histone H4 at Arg3 (H4R3me2a), which is catalyzed by the arginine methyltransferase Hmt1. The H4R3me2a level positively correlates with calorie restriction-driven silencing of ribosomal RNA expression [36]. Consistent with that result, depletion of human NatD in colon cancer cells leads to a reduction in the expression of ribosomal RNA [37].

Mammalian NatD was first identified by Liu et al. as a Gcn5-related N-acetyltransferase (GNAT) family acetyltransferase that is highly expressed in liver and is downregulated in hepatocellular carcinoma [38]. They reported that increased expression of this enzyme in cultured hepatoma cells enhanced apoptosis [38], whereas its knockdown partially inhibited apoptosis. In contrast to their finding, knockdown of NatD was later shown to induce apoptosis in colon cancer cells [37]. Thus, the functions of NatD, and the NatD-dependent N-α-acetylation of histones, appear to be context-dependent.

In addition to the histone specific N-α-acetyltransferase NatD, there are five other N-α-acetyltransferases (NATs): NatA, NatB, NatC, NatE and NatF. These five enzymes have distinct substrate specificities, but none of them acetylate histone molecules. Similar to NatD, NatA acetylates the N-terminal α-amino group that emerges after cleavage of the initiator methionine of a protein. However, in contrast to the strict substrate specificity of NatD, NatA has a broader substrate preference; this enzyme acetylates peptide substrates whose first amino acids harbor short side chains (Ala, Cys, Gly, Ser, Thr or Val) [39, 40]. The other four NATs all acetylate the initiator methionine that has not been removed co-translationally, although they do so with different substrate specificities; for details, see the review by Varland et al. [41].

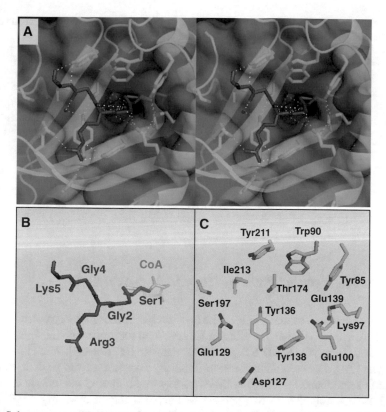

Fig. 5 Substrate recognition by NatD. (**a**) Stereo views (cross-eyed) of the binding sites of NatD with CoA and a histone H2A/H4 peptide (PDB ID: 4U9W). CoA and the histone H2A/H4 peptide are colored *orange* and *magenta*, respectively. Since the CoA is located on the opposite side of the enzyme, only the proximal part, which contains the acetyl group to be transferred to Ser1 of the H2A/H4 peptide, is visible from this point of view. NatD is shown in cartoon and transparent surface representation. The side chains of NatD involved in the contact are shown in *green*. Hydrogen bonds contributing to the substrate binding are shown as dashed *yellow* lines. Water molecules are shown as *red* spheres. Trp90 and Ile213 of NatD interact with the histone peptide via van der Waals contacts. *Blue* and *red* parts of the stick representation indicate nitrogen and oxygen atoms, respectively. (**b**) The CoA and histone H2A/H4 peptide configured as in A. (**c**) The NatD side chains configured as in A. Note that the side chain of the Lys5 in the histone peptide is not visible in this structure. The 3D structures were drawn using PyMOL

Crystal structures of human NatD with substrates indicate how this enzyme specifically recognizes its substrate [42]. In the crystal structure of NatD in a complex with coenzyme A (CoA) and a histone peptide that corresponds to the first five amino acids (Ser1-Gly2-Arg3-Gly4-Lys5) of histone H2A (or H4), the peptide is tightly packed within the structure in such a way that the α-amino group of Ser1 is located near the thiol end of CoA, from which the acetyl moiety is transferred (Fig. 5). The authors of that structural study stated that contacts between the peptide and NatD occur along the entire length of the peptide. These contacts ensure that histones H2A and H4 are the only substrates of NatD.

Table 1 Symbols of human histone acetyltransferases approved by the HUGO Gene Nomenclature Committee

Symbol	Name	Synonyms	Subfamily
HAT1	Histone acetyltransferase 1	KAT1	HAT1
KAT2A	Lysine acetyltransferase 2A	GCN5, PCAF-b	Gcn5/PCAF
KAT2B	Lysine acetyltransferase 2B	P/CAF, GCN5L	Gcn5/PCAF
CREBBP	CREB binding protein	KAT3A, CBP, RTS	p300/CBP
EP300	E1A binding protein p300	KAT3B, p300	p300/CBP
KAT5	Lysine acetyltransferase 5	TIP60, PLIP, ZC2HC5	MYST
KAT6A	Lysine acetyltransferase 6A	MOZ, ZC2HC6A	MYST
KAT6B	Lysine acetyltransferase 6B	MORF, MOZ2, ZC2HC6B	MYST
KAT7	Lysine acetyltransferase 7	HBO1, ZC2HC7	MYST
KAT8	Lysine acetyltransferase 8	MOF, hMOF, ZC2HC8	MYST

2.2   The Molecular Basis of Histone N-ε-Acetylation

The acetyltransferases that catalyze the N-ε-acetylation of histone molecules have been classified into five major subfamilies based on their primary sequence homology: Hat1, Gcn5/PCAF, MYST, p300/CBP and Rtt109 [20–22]. The Hat1, Gcn5/PCAF and MYST subfamilies are evolutionarily conserved from yeast to humans. The HAT1 and Gcn5/PCAF subfamilies belong to a higher classification called the GNAT superfamily. These two subfamilies share a region spanning ~100 amino acids that corresponds to the A, B and D regions of the GNAT family [20]. In contrast, the MYST subfamily only shares the A region which is responsible for acetyl CoA-binding [43, 44]. The proteins that belong to the p300/CBP subfamily, which is less conserved than the other subfamilies, can be divided into two subgroups; those found in metazoans, which have a bromodomain in the middle and a glutamine-rich region at the C-terminus, and those found in plants, which lack these domains [45, 46]. The p300/CBP subfamily, which has been thoroughly reviewed elsewhere [47], and the fungal-specific Rtt109 subfamily, in which the representative budding yeast protein Rtt109 acetylates histone H3 at Lys56, will not be discussed in this chapter.

The HATs that are responsible for N-ε-acetylation have generic names as well as their traditional names. For example, the human proteins hGcn5 and PCAF are also called KAT2A and KAT2B, respectively. The prefix "KAT" in these synonyms stands for lysine (denoted as K̲) a̲cetylt̲ransferase (Table 1). These generic KAT names for lysine acetyltransferases, as well as those for other chromatin-modifying enzymes (e.g. lysine methyltransferase 2A (KMT2A) and lysine demethylase 2B (KDM2B)), were proposed in 2007 to help scientists better understand their functions among different species [48]. In this regard, the budding yeast and *Tetrahymena* Gcn5 homologs should both be referred to as KAT2 since this terminology clearly shows that these enzymes are functionally related to the human homologs KAT2A and KAT2B. In this chapter, generic names will be placed at the shoulders of the traditional names in the format: yGcn5^{KAT2} or hGcn5^{KAT2} (where y and h denote yeast and human respectively).

2.2.1 The HAT1 Subfamily

Yeast and human genomes each encode one enzyme that belongs to the HAT1 subfamily. The yeast enzyme, yHat1^{KAT1}, was identified in 1995 by Kleff et al., and in 1996 by Parthun et al., as a component of a cytoplasmic HAT complex [1, 2]. Kleff et al. used a genetic approach to identify the gene encoding yHat1^{KAT1} in which they evaluated HAT activity of cell extracts from a collection of mutant strains [1]. On the other hand, Parthun et al. biochemically purified the HAT complex from a yeast cytoplasmic extract which led to identification of the non-catalytic subunit, yHat2 [2]. The human homolog of yHat1^{KAT1} is hHat1^{KAT1} and that of yHat2 is the WD40 repeat protein RbAp46, which was initially identified as the retinoblastoma tumor suppressor protein (Rb)-associated protein p46 [2, 49]. Current understanding of the function and regulation of Hat1 subfamily enzymes has been reviewed [50, 51].

The Hat1 subfamily proteins specifically acetylate Lys12 and Lys5 of newly synthesized histone H4 in the cytoplasm [1, 2, 52–55]. Both of these lysines, Lys5 and Lys12, lie within amino acid sequences that match the proposed motif (GxGKxG) for Hat1-dependent acetylation [2]. Before acetylation occurs, histone H4 forms a dimer with histone H3 with the aid of cytosolic histone chaperones [56, 57]. At least in human cells, histone H3 is mono-methylated at Lys9 by an unknown methyltransferase before dimer formation [57].

In yeast, the yHat1^{KAT1}-yHat2 complex specifically acetylates histone H4 at Lys12 but not at Lys5 [2, 58]. In this complex, yHat2 acts as an enhancer of the enzymatic activity and as a regulator of substrate specificity. Thus, although yHat1 itself, as a free molecule, can target not only Lys12 but also Lys5 to a lesser extent, incorporation of yHat2 into the complex protects Lys5 from acetylation [1, 2, 58]. In contrast, studies on this complex in other species have suggested that both Lys5 and Lys12 of H4 are the primary targets. For example, homologous enzyme complexes purified from maize, human and rat extracts apparently acetylate Lys5 as well as Lys12 of a single histone H4 molecule [52–54]. The human complex can also acetylate histone H2A at Lys5, which also lies within an amino acid sequence that matches the GxGKxG motif, yet the enzymatic activity towards histone H2A is much lower than that towards histone H4 [53]. Consistent with these data, depletion of the mouse Hat1 homolog leads to a substantial decrease in the levels of H4K5ac and H4K12ac on newly deposited nucleosomes [55]. Interestingly, a recent biochemical study on the human hHat1^{KAT1}-RbAp46 complex suggested that the second acetylation of histone H4 at Lys5 occurs after the majority of H4 substrates have been mono-acetylated at Lys12, and that the efficiency of the second acetylation at Lys5 is much lower than that of the first acetylation [59].

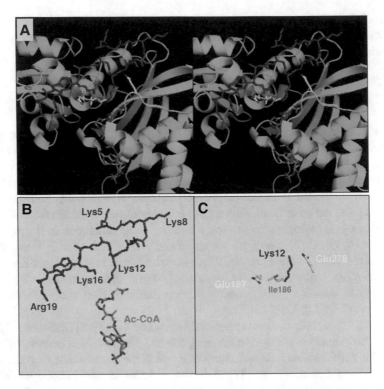

Fig. 6 Substrate recognition by Hat1. (**a**) Stereo views (cross-eyed) of the binding site of hHat-1[KAT1] with acetyl-CoA and a histone H4 peptide (PDB ID: 2P0W). The acetyl-CoA and histone H4 peptide are colored in *orange* and *magenta*, respectively. hHat1[KAT1] is shown in *green* cartoon. The side chain of Ile186, which is involved in the orientation of H4-Lys12, is shown in *light blue*. The side chains of Glu187 and Glu276, which should serve as the general base, are shown in *yellow*. *Dark blue, red* and *right orange* parts of the stick representation indicate nitrogen, oxygen and sulfur atoms, respectively. (**b**) The acetyl-CoA and histone H4 peptide configured as in A. (**c**) The side chains of Hat1 and histone H4 configured as in A

Structural studies of human and yeast Hat1 acetylation complexes indicate that Hat1 subfamily proteins specifically choose Lys12 of histone H4 as the acetylation target [58, 59]. A crystal structure of hHat1[KAT1] in complex with acetyl-CoA and a histone H4 peptide shows that the side chain of the H4 Lys12 is located deep inside a canyon in the enzyme, in close proximity to the acetyl group of acetyl-CoA (Fig. 6) [59]. Although the histone H4 peptide in this complex consisted of the first 20 amino acids, from Ser1 to Lys20, only the 15-residue region from Lys5 to Arg19 adopts a well-defined structure. In this structure, the histone H4 peptide is tightly associated with hHat1, with fourteen of the fifteen H4 residues interacting with hHat1 residues via direct and/or water-mediated ways. The conserved hydrophobic residue Ile186 of hHat1 contacts the aliphatic region of Lys12 and influences its orientation. This study suggests that the highly conserved glutamic acid residues at positions 187 and 276 of hHat1 (Glu187 and Glu276) serve as the general base for catalysis [21, 59]. These residues are within the correct distance from Lys12 of histone H4 if water molecules are considered to mediate the deprotonation of the positively charged ε-amino group [59].

A structural study of yHat1^{KAT1} in complex with yHat2, CoA and histone substrates provides insights into the substrate specificity of the yHat1-yHat2 complex (Fig. 7) [58]. This study showed that the Lys20 of histone H4, which was not observed to be involved in the human hHat1-acetyl-CoA-H4 complex [59], forms a salt bridge with Asp335 of yHat2 (see Fig. 7c). Acetylation of Lys20, which is associated with chromatin [60, 61], may compromise this interaction. Lys16 of histone H4, which is abundantly acetylated in chromatin, also contributes to complex formation by making a salt bridge contact with Glu338 of yHat2 (see Fig. 7c). In addition, the region of histone H4 between aa 29 and aa 45 in the histone fold domain forms a helix and contributes to the interaction between yHat1^{KAT1} and yHat2. The interaction between this part of histone H4 and enzyme subunits is conserved from yeast to humans [58, 62]. As a consequence, histone H4 itself partially mediates the interaction between yHat1 and yHat2. This study also showed that yHat2 can bind to the N-terminal region of histone H3 (Fig. 7). Importantly, methylation of histone H3 at Arg2 and Lys4, which is common in chromatin, inhibits the interaction between yHat2 and histone H3, while mono-methylation of Lys9 does not have such an inhibitory effect (see Fig. 7d) [58]. Therefore, the Hat1-Hat2 complex appears to choose a dimer of newly synthesized histones as a substrate, by excluding histone substrates with chromatin-associated modifications.

2.2.2   The Gcn5/PCAF Subfamily

The Gcn5/PCAF subfamily of acetyltransferases is named after two well-characterized proteins: the budding yeast general control nonderepressible 5 (yGcn5^{KAT2}) protein and one of its mammalian homologs, p300/CBP-associated factor (PCAF^{KAT2B}). The enzymes that belong to this subfamily are also referred to as Gcn5 homologs. The yeast gene encoding yGcn5^{KAT2} was cloned in 1992, as a new class of transcription regulators [63]. The HAT activity of yGcn5^{KAT2} was reported in 1996, when its _Tetrahymena_ homolog tGcn5^{KAT2} was also demonstrated to have enzymatic activity [3].

The human genome encodes two proteins that belong to the Gcn5/PCAF subfamily: hGcn5^{KAT2A} and PCAF^{KAT2B}. These proteins were both identified in 1996, as homologs of yGcn5^{KAT2} and a p300/CBP-associated factor, respectively [64, 65]. The C-terminal half of hGcn5^{KAT2A} or PCAF^{KAT2B}, which contains the evolutionarily conserved HAT and bromodomains, is highly homologous to the yeast yGcn5^{KAT2}. However, the N-terminal half is only conserved from flies to humans [66]. hGcn5^{KAT2A} and PCAF^{KAT2B} are found in evolutionarily conserved multisubunit co-activator complexes called Ada-Two-A-Containing (ATAC) and Spt-Ada-Gcn5-Acetyltransferase (SAGA) complexes [67]. The total mass of these complexes is approximately 700 kDa and 2 MDa, respectively. The complexes contain either hGcn5^{KAT2A} or PCAF^{KAT2B} as a mutually exclusive HAT subunit [68, 69]. ATAC and

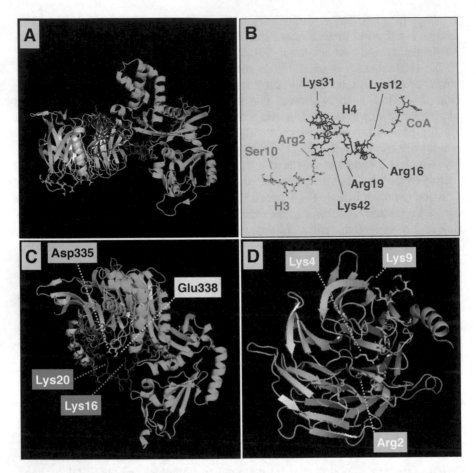

Fig. 7 Substrate recognition by the Hat1-Hat2 complex. (**a**) Overall structure of yHat1[KAT1] complexed with yHat2 and histone H3 and H4 peptides (PDB ID: 4PSX). CoA and the histone H3 and H4 peptides are colored in *orange, magenta* and *light blue*, respectively. yHat1[KAT1] and yHat2 are shown in *green* and *wheat* cartoons, respectively. Dark *blue*, *red* and *right orange* parts of the stick representation indicate nitrogen, oxygen and sulfur atoms, respectively. (**b**) The CoA and histone peptides configured as in A. (**c**) Recognition of the unmodified Lys16 and Lys20 residues of histone H4. The side chains of Glu338 and Asp335 of yHat2, which make salt bridge contacts with the histone H4 Lys16 and Lys20 residues, are shown in *yellow* and *light blue*, respectively. The structure of the histone H3 peptide, which is located at the distal side, is omitted for clarity. (**d**) Recognition of the unmodified Arg2 and Lys4 residues of histone H3 (light *blue*). The side chains of yHat2 (*wheat*) amino acid residues that make hydrogen bonds with H3-Arg2 (yHat2 Asn212 and Asp213) and with H3-Lys4 (yHat2 Glu120 and Asn162) are shown in *green* and *magenta*, respectively. Dark *blue* and *red* parts of the stick representation indicate nitrogen and oxygen atoms, respectively

SAGA share two additional subunits called hAda3 and hSgf29, respectively. These proteins are homologs of the yeast proteins yAda3 and ySgf29, respectively. In addition to a HAT subunit and these two shared subunits, the smaller ATAC complex contains nine specific subunits including hAda2a, as the complex name indicates. On the other hand, the larger SAGA complex contains 15 specific subunits including

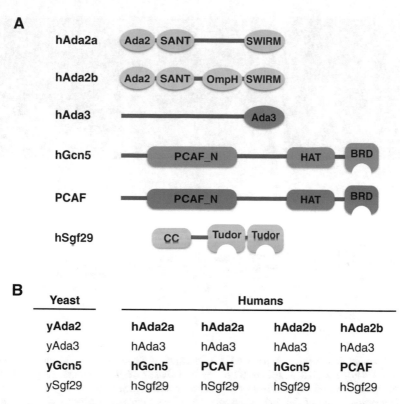

Fig. 8 Gcn5 homolog-containing HAT modules. (a) Schematic representation of the components of human Gcn5 homolog-containing histone acetyltransferase (HAT) modules. (b) Combinations of subunits for possible HAT modules. The yeast proteins yAda2, yAda3, yGcn5 and ySgf29 form the yeast HAT module. In humans, four different HAT modules with different combinations of subunits can be formed. The sole human homologs of yAda3 (hAda3) and ySgf29 (hSgf29) are incorporated into all four HAT modules. In contrast, one of the two human homologs of yAda2 (hAda2a or hAda2b) and one of the two human homologs of yGcn5[KAT2] (hGcn5[KAT2A] or PCAF[KAT2B]) are incorporated in a mutually exclusive manner

hAda2b. hAda2a and hAda2b are two distinct human homologs of the yeast protein yAda2 [66, 67].

In yeast, yAda2, yAda3, yGcn5[KAT2] and ySgf29 form a HAT module (Fig. 8) [70–74]. Similarly, in the human ATAC complex, hAda2a, hAda3, hGcn5[KAT2A] and hSgf29 act together as a HAT module, whereas hAda2a is replaced with hAda2b in the SAGA HAT module. Since PCAF[KAT2B] can replace hGcn5[KAT2A], at least four sets of Gcn5-related HAT modules are present in humans. These HAT modules have intrinsic posttranslational-modification reader domains for their proper recruitment and target selection. The Sgf29 homologs have a conserved tandem Tudor domain, which recognizes di- and tri-methylation of histone H3 at Lys4 (H3K4me2/3) [74, 75], whereas the Gcn5 homologs have a conserved bromodomain that recognizes acetylated histone tails [76–78]. A recent biochemical study

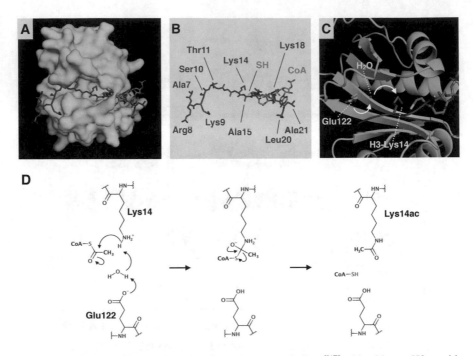

Fig. 9 Acetylation of histone H3 by Gcn5. (**a**) Structure of tGcn5^{KAT2} with a histone H3 peptide (PDB ID: 1PU9). The HAT domain of tGcn5^{KAT2} is shown as a *light blue* surface representation. CoA and the histone H3 peptide are colored in *orange* and *magenta*, respectively. Dark *blue, red* and *right orange* parts of the stick representation indicate nitrogen, oxygen and sulfur atoms, respectively. (**b**) CoA and the histone H3 peptide configured as in A. SH, the sulfhydryl group of CoA. (**c**) A magnified view of the catalytic center. The side chain of Glu122 of tGcn5^{KAT2}, which acts as the general base for the catalysis, and the target residue of histone H3 (Lys14) are shown in stick representation. *White* arrows represent proton transfer. (**d**) Mechanism of tGcn5^{KAT2} mediated catalysis of histone H3. A proton is transferred from Lys14 of histone H3 to Glu122 of tGcn5^{KAT2}, which is shuttled by the well-ordered water molecule. The activated ε-amino group makes a nucleophilic attack on the carbonyl carbon of acetyl-CoA to form a tetrahedral intermediate, which collapses to generate an acetylated lysine residue

indicated that incorporation of the human HAT modules into the ATAC or SAGA complex further increases HAT activity [79]. That study also showed that recombinant hGcn5^{KAT2A} alone and the hGcn5^{KAT2A}-containing complexes primarily acetylate histone H3 at Lys14 .

Crystal structures of the HAT domain of tGcn5^{KAT2} explain how the substrate is specifically recognized by the Gcn5 subfamily HATs and how the acetyl moiety is transferred [80, 81]. The structure shown in Fig. 9 is a ternary complex of tGcn5^{KAT2}, coenzyme A and a 19-residue histone H3 peptide that corresponds to the amino acid sequence from Gln5 to Lys23. The amino acid residues 5–6 and 22–23 are disordered. In this structure, the histone H3 peptide is buried in a long cleft in the enzyme, with the result that the ε-amino group of Lys14 is located near the sulfhydryl group (SH) of CoA. Each of the 13 residues of H3 is within H-bonding distance and/or van der Waals distance from tGcn5^{KAT2} residues [81]. Less extensive contacts are observed when tGcn5^{KAT2} forms complexes with less preferred substrates for acetylation [82, 83] Fig. 9.

A bi-bi ternary complex mechanism is proposed for the acetylation reaction catalyzed by Gcn5 homologs [21, 80, 84]. In this mechanism, binding of the two substrates is a prerequisite for the reaction to occur. The HATs in this family have a conserved glutamate residue that act as a general base for catalysis. The corresponding residue of tGcn5^{KAT2} is Glu122, whereas that of hGcn5^{KAT2A} and of PCAF^{KAT2B} is Glu575 and Glu570, respectively. In the tGcn5^{KAT2} crystal structure, there is a well-ordered water molecule that is thought to shuttle a proton from the ε-amino group of Lys14 to Glu122 (Fig. 9c, d) [80, 81, 84].

2.2.3   The MYST Subfamily

The human genome contains five genes that encode MYST (MOZ, Ybf2/Sas3, Sas2 and Tip60) subfamily proteins that each have a generic KAT name: Tip60^{KAT5} (also known as PLIP); MOZ^{KAT6A} (MYST3); MORF^{KAT6B} (MYST4); HBO1^{KAT7} (MYST2); and MOF^{KAT8} (MYST1). The HAT domain of this subfamily contains a specific C2HC zinc finger and an acetyl-CoA binding region that is homologous to that of the Hat1 and Gcn5/PCAF subfamily members [85]. In contrast to the Hat1 or Gcn5/ PCAF subfamily members, which strictly or predominantly recognize histone molecules as acetylation targets, the MYST subfamily members are known to acetylate a variety of non-histone proteins, as previously reviewed [85, 86]. This section focuses on the enzyme male-absent on the first (MOF^{KAT8}) as it has a HAT activity for H4K16Ac, which is a hallmark of cancer cells.

hMOF^{KAT8} is the human homolog of the first MOF identified, which was found in a genetic screen for genes required for dosage compensation in the fruit fly *Drosophila melanogaster* [43]. In this model organism, the genes on the X chromosome in male cells, which are heterogametic (XY), need to be transcribed at twice the rate as those in female cells, which are homogametic (XX), in order to equalize expression levels. Abrogation of this compensation system leads to the death of males as third-instar larvae or early pupae, which is referred to as the *male-specific lethal* (MSL) or *maleless* (mle) phenotype.

The hyper-active male X chromosome, but not the female X chromosomes, is cytologically associated with the characteristic chromatin mark H4K16ac, and with the MSL complex, which is responsible for this H4 acetylation [26, 27, 43]. The MSL complex contains the catalytic subunit dMOF^{KAT8}, the four protein subunits MSL1, MSL2, MSL3 and MLE, and two redundant non-coding RNAs *rna on X 1* (roX1) and roX2 [26, 27, 87, 88]. MSL1 directly binds to dMOF^{KAT8} through its PEHE domain, and to MSL3 through its most C-terminal region [89, 90]. The binding of MSL1 and MSL3 to MOF enhances its activity and restricts its action towards nucleosomal histone H4 [90, 91]. MSL3 recognition of H3K36 trimethylation through a conserved chromo-domain recruits the MSL complex to chromatin [92, 93]. The MLE subunit has an RNA helicase activity that incorporates roX1 and roX2 into the functional MSL complex, which is targeted to the X chromosome [94, 95]. Homozygous mutations in the MSL subunits lead to abrogation of the acetylation of H4K16, which is accompanied by male-specific lethality [27, 43]. In female cells, the RNA binding protein _sex-lethal_ (_sxl_) inhibits translation of the mRNA for MSL2, which ensures that the assembly of the functional MSL complex and hence the hyper-activation of chromosome X, is restricted to male cells [96, 97].

In the fruit fly, there is another complex that contains dMOF^{KAT8}, called the _non-specific lethal_ (NSL) complex [98–100]. In this complex, dMOF^{KAT8} associates with the protein subunits MBD-R2, MCRS2, NSL1, NSL2, NSL3 and WDS [98, 99]. In contrast to the male-specific role of the MSL complex in X hyper-activation, the NSL complex associates with active promoters of autosomal and X chromosomal genes in both sexes to promote transcription [99]. At the targeted promoters, which are characterized by H4K16ac as well as by H3K4me2, H3K4me3 and H3K9ac, NSL activity is required in transcription for the pre-initiation complex assembly [100]. Therefore, in contrast to the MSL complex that is specific for dosage compensation, the NSL complex appears to have general roles in transcriptional activation.

The human counterpart of dMOF^{KAT8}, hMOF^{KAT8}, is responsible for H4K16 acetylation [101–104]. As in the fruit fly, there are two distinct hMOF^{KAT8}-containing HAT complexes for H4K16 acetylation in human cells, called MSL and NSL complexes [98, 104]. The mammalian MSL complex contains homologs of the fruit fly subunits MSL1, MSL2 and MSL3, that force hMOF^{KAT8} to acetylate nucleosomal histone H4 at Lys16 [105]. In addition, MSL2 has been shown to act with MSL1 as an ubiquitin E3 ligase that ubiquitinates nucleosomal histone H2B at Lys34. [106]. Neither a non-coding RNA component nor an RNA helicase subunit has been identified for the MSL complex in human cells.

The mammalian NSL complex contains the dMBD-R2 homolog PHF20, MCRS2, NSL1, NSL2, NSL3, the WDS homolog WDR5, HCF-1 and OGT [98]. The NSL1 subunit is also referred to as MSL1v1, because it has a PEHE domain that is closely related to that in MSL1 and hence this complex is also called MOF-MSL1v1 [104]. NSL1 directly binds to hMOF^{KAT8} through the PEHE domain, and this binding is sufficient for the restriction of HAT activity to nucleosomal histone H4 [98, 105]. In contrast to the MSL complex that only acetylates nucleosomal histone H4 at Lys16, the NSL complex has a broader range of targets; it can also acetylate Lys5 and Lys8 of nucleosomal histone H4, the tumor suppressor protein p53, and the lysine-specific histone demethylase LSD1 [105, 107, 108].

Many studies have shown that mammalian MOF^{KAT8} plays important roles in transcriptional regulation, the DNA damage response and various other processes, suggesting that functional impairment of MOF^{KAT8} leads to cancer development [101, 109–117]. However, the roles of MOF^{KAT8} appear to be context dependent, and some of those previous studies did not consider which of the MOF-containing complexes act in the given context. The expression level of MOF^{KAT8} has shown to be either increased or decreased in cancer cells [112, 118–122]. Thus, the function of MOF^{KAT8} in cancer development can be said to remain poorly understood.

A recent report by Luo et al. showed that hMOF[KAT8] acts as a suppressor of epithelial-to-mesenchymal transition (EMT) and tumor metastasis [108]. According to that report, NSL1-bound hMOF[KAT8] acetylates the histone demethylase LSD1 in epithelial cells, which interferes with its demethylation of nucleosomal H3K4me2 [108]. The expression level of hMOF[KAT8] is dramatically reduced upon induction of EMT, causing LSD1 to repress epithelial gene expression via its demethylation of H3K4me2 [108, 123–125]. The study by Luo et al. indicates the importance of investigating the function of hMOF[KAT8] in terms of its subunit composition and of its target specificity in each biological context [108].

2.3 Recognition of Histone Side-Chain Acetylation

As mentioned above, acetylation of lysine residues of histones is thought to weaken the interaction between histone molecules and DNA. In addition, acetylated lysine residues of histones are themselves recognized by protein domains designed to specifically capture histone peptides including peptides with acetylated lysines (Fig. 2). Unlike the recognition of methylated lysine, where Chromo, PHD, Tudor and other domains act as readers, recognition of acetylated lysine is generally accomplished by proteins with bromodomains. Consistent with the well-known positive correlation between histone acetylation levels and transcription levels, bromodomains are often found in transcription-related proteins, including in general transcription factors, chromatin remodeling factors and HAT complexes.

The currently released human reference genome (GRCh38.p7) contains 42 genes that encode proteins with at least one bromodomain (SMART ID: SM00297) [126]. Some of these proteins are known to bind the acetylated lysine of proteins other than histones. It therefore appears that the existence of a bromodomain in a protein does not necessarily mean that the protein binds to acetylated histone.

For example, the bromodomains of BRD3 and BRD4, which belong to the Bromo and extraterminal (BET) protein family, can recognize not only acetylated histone tails but also non-histone acetylated proteins. BET family proteins each contain two bromodomains, which are referred to here as the first and second bromodomains. The first bromodomain of BRD3 binds to GATA1, which is a transcription factor that regulates the expression of erythroid and megakaryocyte-specific genes, when it is acetylated at Lys312 and Lys315 [127]. In a similar manner, the second bromodomain of BRD4 recognizes TWIST, which is a key transcription factor of epithelial-mesenchymal transition, when it is acetylated at Lys73 and Lys76 [128]. BRD4 can also bind to cycline-T1, which is a component of positive transcription elongation factor b (P-TEFb), when it is acetylated [129]. The functions and other aspects of the BET proteins have been thoroughly reviewed by Wang and Filippakopoulos [130].

Structural studies show that a bromodomain consists of a specific four-helix bundle with a left-handed twist (Fig. 10) [76, 131]. The helices are called alpha-Z, alpha-A, alpha-B and alpha-C. There is a long intervening loop named the ZA-loop

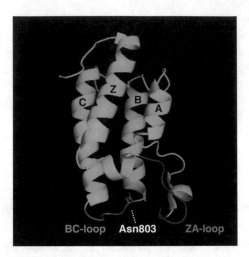

Fig. 10 Structure of a bromodomain. The structure of the bromodomain of PCAF[KAT2B] (PDB ID: 1 N72) is shown in *green* cartoon representation. The specific four alpha-helices are labeled "Z", "A", "B" and "C". The ZA- and BC-loops are colored *magenta* and *orange*, respectively. The side chain of the conserved asparagine residue Asn803 located in the BC-loop is shown in *orange* stick representation. *Dark blue* and *red* parts of the stick representation indicate nitrogen and oxygen atoms, respectively

between the alpha-Z and alpha-A helices, and another loop between the alpha-B and alpha-C helices (BC-loop). These two loops form a hydrophobic cleft that accommodates acetylated lysine residues. A good example of such binding is illustrated by the crystal structure of the bromodomain of yGcn5[KAT2] that is holding an histone H4 peptide acetylated at Lys16 (Fig. 11) [77]. The hydrophobic residues Pro351, Val361, Tyr364 and Tyr413 are present on the walls of the cleft, which contribute to hydrophobic intermolecular interactions with the neutralized acetylated lysine residue on the peptide. In this structure, as in other solved structures, the amide nitrogen of Asn-407, which is located at the beginning of the BC loop, forms a hydrogen bond with the oxygen of the acetyl carbonyl group in the acetylated lysine residue. This interaction plays a major role in orienting the N-acetyl group so that its carbonyl group fits into the hydrophobic cleft. A lysine residue that was not acetylated would be positively charged, and, as there is no compensatory negative charge within the cleft, such a lysine would be much less favorable for this interaction.

Although the overall structures of solved bromodomains are similar, each bromodomain has distinct target specificity. Some bromodomains recognize monoacetylated histone tails, whereas others recognize histone tails that are doubly acetylated, with each acetylation at a different lysine residue. The bromodomains of yGcn5[KAT2] and its homolog PCAF[KAT2B] prefer histone H4 mono acetylated at Lys8 or Lys16, and H3 acetylated at Lys9 as substrates [76–78]. In the crystal structure of the complex between yGcn5[KAT2] and an histone H4 peptide (Fig. 11), two residues (His-18 and Arg-19) of the histone H4 peptide near the acetylated Lys16 make secondary interactions with the yGcn5[KAT2] residues Phe367, Tyr406, Arg404 and

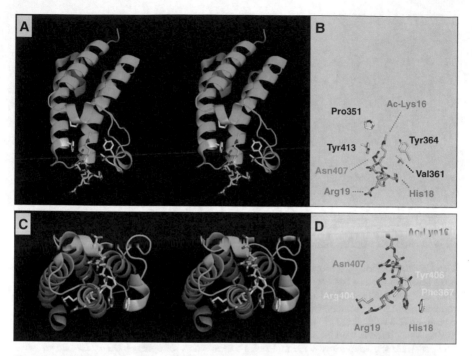

Fig. 11 Recognition of histone H4 acetylated at Lys16 by the Gcn5 bromodomain. (**a**) Stereo views (cross-eyed) of the bromodomain of yGcn5^{KAT2} associated with an histone H4 peptide acetylated at Lys16 (PDB ID: 1E6I). The histone H4 peptide is shown in light *blue* stick representation. The bromodomain is shown in *green* cartoon. The side chain of Asn407 of yGcn5^{KAT2}, which is conserved and critical for acetylated H4 recognition, is shown in *orange*. The yGcn5^{KAT2} residues Pro351, Val361, Tyr364 and Tyr413, which hydrophobically interact with the acetylated lysine residue, are shown in *gray*. *Dark blue* and *red* parts of the stick representation indicate nitrogen and oxygen atoms, respectively. (**b**) The yGcn5^{KAT2} side chains and acetylated histone H4 peptide configured as in A. (**c**) Stereo views of the complex from a different point of view. The yGcn5^{KAT2} residues Phe367, Arg404 and Tyr406, which are involved in secondary interactions, are shown in *yellow*. (**d**) The yGcn5^{KAT2} side chains and acetylated histone H4 peptide configured as in C

Asn407, raising the possibility that these four yGcn5^{KAT2} residues contribute to the specificity of its target recognition.

TAFII250, the largest subunit of the general transcription factor TFIID, contains two specific tandemly aligned bromodomains [132]. These two domains form a histone reader module that prefers a doubly acetylated histone H4 peptide (Lys5/Lys12 or Lys8/Lys16) to a mono-acetylated peptide. The distance between the two hydrophobic pockets in the solved structure of this module is 25 Å, which would require a peptide about seven amino acid residues in length to span it [132]. This required amino acid length corresponds to the distance between the acetylated lysine residues in a doubly acetylated H4 peptide (e.g., Lys5 is indeed seven amino acids away from Lys12).

It is also known that even a single bromodomain can recognize a doubly acetylated histone peptide. The first bromodomain of BRD4 provides the best example of this phenomenon (Fig. 12) [130, 133]. This domain can hold distinct but similar types of histone H4 peptides that are doubly acetylated at Lys residues in close

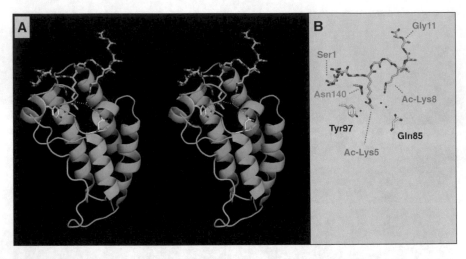

Fig. 12 Recognition by a bromodomain of a doubly acetylated histone peptide. (**a**) Stereo views (cross-eyed) of the first bromodomain of BRD4 associated with a histone H4 peptide doubly acety-lated at Lys5 and Lys8 (PDB ID: 3UVW). The histone H4 peptide is shown in *light blue* stick representation. The bromodomain is shown in *green* cartoon. The side chain of Asn140, which is conserved and critical for H4 recognition, is shown in *orange*. The BRD4 residues Gln85 and Tyr97, which interact with the acetylated lysine residues in a water-mediated manner (*dashed yellow* lines), are shown in *gray*. Water molecules are shown as red spheres. *Dark blue* and *red parts* of the stick representation indicate nitrogen and oxygen atoms, respectively. (**b**) The BRD4 side chains and histone H4 peptide configured as in A

proximity (Lys5/Lys8, Lys12/Lys16 or Lys16/Lys20). In these peptides, acetylation occurs at lysine residues that are positioned three to four amino acids away from each other. Of the two acetylated lysine residues, the most N-terminal one (e.g. Lys5) interacts with the conserved asparagine that is located at the beginning of the BC loop. This interaction plays a major role in orienting the acetylated peptide for insertion of the carbonyl group of its acetylated lysine residue into the hydrophobic cleft in a manner similar to the folding of the yGcn5^{KAT2}-histone H4 peptide complex, in which the peptide was mono-acetylated at Lys16. The second acetylated lysine residue (e.g. Lys8) participates in the formation of a water-mediated interaction network that further stabilizes the first lysine residue within the cleft.

2.4 Removal of Histone N-ε-Acetylation

The N-ε-acetylation of the lysine residues in histones and non-histone proteins is removed by histone deacetylases (HDACs), which are also referred to as protein lysine deacetylases (KDACs). Based on their primary sequences and catalytic activities, HDACs are currently classified into four groups: type I, II, III and IV [134, 135]. The type I, II and IV HDACs catalyze deacetylation in a zinc-dependent

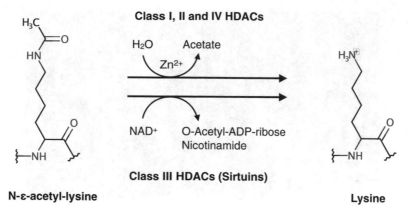

Fig. 13 Two kinds of reactions catalyzed by HDACs. Class I, II and IV HDACs catalyze lysine deacetylation in a zinc-dependent manner, whereas class III HDACs use NAD⁺ to remove the acetyl moiety from lysine residues, yielding O-acetyl-ADP-ribose and nicotinamide as reaction products

manner, whereas the type III HDACs, which are called sirtuins, utilize nicotinamide adenine dinucleotide (NAD⁺) to remove the acetyl group (Fig. 13).

Before HDAC proteins or genes were identified, the HDAC inhibitors trapoxin (TPX) and trichostatin A (TSA) were known to possess antitumorigenic activities [136, 137]. TPX is a cyclic tetrapeptide with an aliphatic epoxydecanoic acid residue that is sterically similar to acetyl lysine. This compound covalently binds to the active site of HDAC via its reactive epoxide, thereby irreversibly inhibiting HDAC activity [138]. The first HDAC, HDAC1, was identified in human Jurkat nuclear extracts following its co-precipitation with a derivative of TPX [4]. The identified protein shared homology with the yeast transcriptional regulator Rpd3, whose biochemical function was previously unknown [139]. This finding led to the subsequent identification of other HDACs.

TSA and its derivative suberoylanilide hydroxamic acid (SAHA) contain a hydroxamic acid that is important for the inhibition of HDAC. Finnin et al. reported a structural study of the manner by which these compounds bind to an HDAC [140]. They used an HDAC-like protein from the hyperthermophilic bacterium *Aquifex aeolicus* for this study. Although this bacterium does not itself express histones, this HDAC-like protein that is called histone deacetylase like protein (HDLP) can deacetylate histones in vitro, and this activity is inhibited by TSA and SAHA. They showed that HDLP has a deep narrow pocket, near the bottom of which the zinc ion that is required for catalysis is positioned. As shown in Fig. 14, the long aliphatic chain of the inhibitors is inserted into this pocket to inactivate the enzymatic activity.

Five HDAC inhibitors, Belinostat (Beleodaq), Chidamide (Epidaza), Vorinostat (SAHA), Romidepsin (Istodax) and Panobinostat (Farydak), have been approved for cancer therapy [134, 141, 142]. In addition, many other HDAC inhibitor compounds are being investigated for their effectiveness in cancer treatment. The current knowledge regarding HDAC inhibitors for cancer therapy is summarized

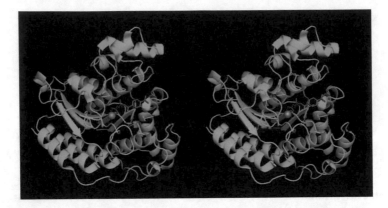

Fig. 14 Binding of a hydroxamate HDAC inhibitor to an HDAC-related protein. Stereo views (cross-eyed) of the HDAC-like protein (HDLP) from the hyperthermophilic bacterium *Aquifex aeolicus* bound to TSA (PDB ID: 1C3R). HDLP is shown in *green* cartoon representation. TSA is shown in *magenta*. The hydroxamic acid group of TSA is inserted into a pocket of HDLP, and coordinates the zinc (*orange*) at the bottom of the pocket. This zinc is required for enzymatic activity. Dark Blue and red parts of the stick representation indicate nitrogen and oxygen atoms, respectively

in excellent reviews [134, 135]. In general, HDAC inhibitors are more effective for the treatment of hematological cancers than for solid tumors, probably because of the difficulty in delivering the drug to solid tumors [134]. The exact mechanisms of action of HDAC inhibitors in cancer treatment are still unclear. Mass spectrometry studies show that more than 2000 non-histone proteins are acetylated in human cells, which could potentially be targets of HDACs [142]. Therefore, it should be taken into consideration that HDAC inhibitors will affect cellular processes that involve these non-histone proteins.

References

1. Kleff S, Andrulis ED, Anderson CW, Sternglanz R (1995) Identification of a gene encoding a yeast histone H4 acetyltransferase. J Biol Chem 270(42):24674–24677
2. Parthun MR, Widom J, Gottschling DE (1996) The major cytoplasmic histone acetyltransferase in yeast: links to chromatin replication and histone metabolism. Cell 87(1):85–94
3. Brownell JE, Zhou J, Ranalli T, Kobayashi R, Edmondson DG et al (1996) Tetrahymena histone acetyltransferase A: a homolog to yeast Gcn5p linking histone acetylation to gene activation. Cell 84(6):843–851
4. Taunton J, Hassig CA, Schreiber SL (1996) A mammalian histone deacetylase related to the yeast transcriptional regulator Rpd3p. Science 272(5260):408–411
5. Rundlett SE, Carmen AA, Kobayashi R, Bavykin S, Turner BM et al (1996) HDA1 and RPD3 are members of distinct yeast histone deacetylase complexes that regulate silencing and transcription. Proc Natl Acad Sci U S A 93(25):14503–14508
6. Rea S, Eisenhaber F, O'Carroll D, Strahl BD, Sun ZW et al (2000) Regulation of chromatin structure by site-specific histone H3 methyltransferases. Nature 406(6796):593–599

7. Shi Y, Lan F, Matson C, Mulligan P, Whetstine JR et al (2004) Histone demethylation mediated by the nuclear amine oxidase homolog LSD1. Cell 119(7):941–953
8. Suka N, Suka Y, Carmen AA, Wu J, Grunstein M (2001) Highly specific antibodies determine histone acetylation site usage in yeast heterochromatin and euchromatin. Mol Cell 8(2):473–479
9. Turner BM, Fellows G (1989) Specific antibodies reveal ordered and cell-cycle-related use of histone-H4 acetylation sites in mammalian cells. Eur J Biochem 179(1):131–139
10. Turner BM, O'Neill LP, Allan IM (1989) Histone H4 acetylation in human cells. Frequency of acetylation at different sites defined by immunolabeling with site-specific antibodies. FEBS Lett 253(1–2):141–145
11. Fraga MF, Ballestar E, Villar-Garea A, Boix-Chornet M, Espada J et al (2005) Loss of acetylation at Lys16 and trimethylation at Lys20 of histone H4 is a common hallmark of human cancer. Nat Genet 37(4):391–400
12. Seligson DB, Horvath S, Shi T, Yu H, Tze S et al (2005) Global histone modification patterns predict risk of prostate cancer recurrence. Nature 435(7046):1262–1266
13. Elsheikh SE, Green AR, Rakha FA, Powe DG, Ahmed RA et al (2009) Global histone modifications in breast cancer correlate with tumor phenotypes, prognostic factors, and patient outcome. Cancer Res 69(9):3802–3809
14. Chadee DN, Hendzel MJ, Tylipski CP, Allis CD, Bazett-Jones DP et al (1999) Increased Ser-10 phosphorylation of histone H3 in mitogen-stimulated and oncogene-transformed mouse fibroblasts. J Biol Chem 274(35):24914–24920
15. Choi HS, Choi BY, Cho YY, Mizuno H, Kang BS et al (2005) Phosphorylation of histone H3 at serine 10 is indispensable for neoplastic cell transformation. Cancer Res 65(13):5818–5827
16. Kim HG, Lee KW, Cho YY, Kang NJ, Oh SM et al (2008) Mitogen- and stress-activated kinase 1-mediated histone H3 phosphorylation is crucial for cell transformation. Cancer Res 68(7):2538–2547
17. Tange S, Ito S, Senga T, Hamaguchi M (2009) Phosphorylation of histone H3 at Ser10: its role in cell transformation by v-Src. Biochem Biophys Res Commun 386(4):588–592
18. Li B, Huang G, Zhang X, Li R, Wang J et al (2013) Increased phosphorylation of histone H3 at serine 10 is involved in Epstein-Barr virus latent membrane protein-1-induced carcinogenesis of nasopharyngeal carcinoma. BMC Cancer 13:124
19. Prenzel T, Begus-Nahrmann Y, Kramer F, Hennion M, Hsu C et al (2011) Estrogen-dependent gene transcription in human breast cancer cells relies upon proteasome-dependent monoubiquitination of histone H2B. Cancer Res 71(17):5739–5753
20. Sterner DE, Berger SL (2000) Acetylation of histones and transcription-related factors. Microbiol Mol Biol Rev 64(2):435–459
21. Yuan H, Marmorstein R (2013) Histone acetyltransferases: rising ancient counterparts to protein kinases. Biopolymers 99(2):98–111
22. McCullough CE, Marmorstein R (2016) Molecular basis for histone acetyltransferase regulation by binding partners, associated domains, and autoacetylation. ACS Chem Biol 11(3):632–642
23. Lee DY, Hayes JJ, Pruss D, Wolffe AP (1993) A positive role for histone acetylation in transcription factor access to nucleosomal DNA. Cell 72(1):73–84
24. Vettese-Dadey M, Grant PA, Hebbes TR, Crane- Robinson C, Allis CD et al (1996) Acetylation of histone H4 plays a primary role in enhancing transcription factor binding to nucleosomal DNA in vitro. EMBO J 15(10):2508–2518
25. Shogren-Knaak M, Ishii H, Sun JM, Pazin MJ, Davie JR et al (2006) Histone H4-K16 acetylation controls chromatin structure and protein interactions. Science 311(5762):844–847
26. Turner BM, Birley AJ, Lavender J (1992) Histone H4 isoforms acetylated at specific lysine residues define individual chromosomes and chromatin domains in Drosophila polytene nuclei. Cell 69(2):375–384
27. Bone JR, Lavender J, Richman R, Palmer MJ, Turner BM et al (1994) Acetylated histone H4 on the male X chromosome is associated with dosage compensation in Drosophila. Genes Dev 8(1):96–104

28. Liu X, Bushnell DA, Kornberg RD (2013) RNA polymerase II transcription: structure and mechanism. Biochim Biophys Acta 1829(1):2–8
29. Lorch Y, Kornberg RD (2015) Chromatin-remodeling and the initiation of transcription. Q Rev Biophys 48(4):465–470
30. Sainsbury S, Bernecky C, Cramer P (2015) Structural basis of transcription initiation by RNA polymerase II. Nat Rev Mol Cell Biol 16(3):129–143
31. Venkatesh S, Workman JL (2015) Histone exchange, chromatin structure and the regulation of transcription. Nat Rev Mol Cell Biol 16(3):178–189
32. Kulaeva OI, Hsieh FK, Chang HW, Luse DS, Studitsky VM (2013) Mechanism of transcription through a nucleosome by RNA polymerase II. Biochim Biophys Acta 1829(1):76–83
33. Song OK, Wang X, Waterborg JH, Sternglanz R (2003) An Nalpha-acetyltransferase responsible for acetylation of the N-terminal residues of histones H4 and H2A. J Biol Chem 278(40):38109–38112
34. Polevoda B, Hoskins J, Sherman F (2009) Properties of Nat4, an N(alpha)-acetyltransferase of *Saccharomyces cerevisiae* that modifies N termini of histones H2A and H4. Mol Cell Biol 29(11):2913–2924
35. Hole K, Van Damme P, Dalva M, Aksnes H, Glomnes N et al (2011) The human N-alpha-acetyltransferase 40 (hNaa40p/hNatD) is conserved from yeast and N-terminally acetylates histones H2A and H4. PLoS One 6(9):e24713
36. Schiza V, Molina-Serrano D, Kyriakou D, Hadjiantoniou A, Kirmizis A (2013) N-alpha-terminal acetylation of histone H4 regulates arginine methylation and ribosomal DNA silencing. PLoS Genet 9(9):e1003805
37. Pavlou D, Kirmizis A (2016) Depletion of histone N-terminal-acetyltransferase Naa40 induces p53-independent apoptosis in colorectal cancer cells via the mitochondrial pathway. Apoptosis 21(3):298–311
38. Liu Z, Liu Y, Wang H, Ge X, Jin Q et al (2009) Patt1, a novel protein acetyltransferase that is highly expressed in liver and downregulated in hepatocellular carcinoma, enhances apoptosis of hepatoma cells. Int J Biochem Cell Biol 41(12):2528–2537
39. Polevoda B, Norbeck J, Takakura H, Blomberg A, Sherman F (1999) Identification and specificities of N-terminal acetyltransferases from *Saccharomyces cerevisiae*. EMBO J 18(21):6155–6168
40. Arnesen T, Van Damme P, Polevoda B, Helsens K, Evjenth R et al (2009) Proteomics analyses reveal the evolutionary conservation and divergence of N-terminal acetyltransferases from yeast and humans. Proc Natl Acad Sci U S A 106(20):8157–8162
41. Varland S, Osberg C, Arnesen T (2015) N-terminal modifications of cellular proteins: the enzymes involved, their substrate specificities and biological effects. Proteomics 15(14):2385–2401
42. Magin RS, Liszczak GP, Marmorstein R (2015) The molecular basis for histone H4- and H2A-specific amino-terminal acetylation by NatD. Structure 23(2):332–341
43. Hilfiker A, Hilfiker-Kleiner D, Pannuti A, Lucchesi JC (1997) mof, a putative acetyl transferase gene related to the Tip60 and MOZ human genes and to the SAS genes of yeast, is required for dosage compensation in Drosophila. EMBO J 16(8):2054–2060
44. Kuo MH, Allis CD (1998) Roles of histone acetyltransferases and deacetylases in gene regulation. BioEssays 20(8):615–626
45. Bordoli L, Netsch M, Luthi U, Lutz W, Eckner R (2001) Plant orthologs of p300/CBP: conservation of a core domain in metazoan p300/CBP acetyltransferase-related proteins. Nucleic Acids Res 29(3):589–597
46. Pandey R, Muller A, Napoli CA, Selinger DA, Pikaard CS et al (2002) Analysis of histone acetyltransferase and histone deacetylase families of *Arabidopsis thaliana* suggests functional diversification of chromatin modification among multicellular eukaryotes. Nucleic Acids Res 30(23):5036–5055
47. Dancy BM, Cole PA (2015) Protein lysine acetylation by p300/CBP. Chem Rev 115(6):2419–2452

48. Allis CD, Berger SL, Cote J, Dent S, Jenuwien T et al (2007) New nomenclature for chromatin-modifying enzymes. Cell 131(4):633–636
49. Huang S, Lee WH, Lee EY (1991) A cellular protein that competes with SV40 T antigen for binding to the retinoblastoma gene product. Nature 350(6314):160–162
50. Parthun MR (2012) Histone acetyltransferase 1: more than just an enzyme? Biochim Biophys Acta 1819(3–4):256–263
51. Keck KM, Pemberton LF (2013) Histone chaperones link histone nuclear import and chromatin assembly. Biochim Biophys Acta 1819(3–4):277–289
52. Eberharter A, Lechner T, Goralik-Schramel M, Loidl P (1996) Purification and characterization of the cytoplasmic histone acetyltransferase B of maize embryos. FEBS Lett 386(1):75–81
53. Verreault A, Kaufman PD, Kobayashi R, Stillman B (1998) Nucleosomal DNA regulates the core-histone-binding subunit of the human Hat1 acetyltransferase. Curr Biol 8(2):96–108
54. Kolle D, Sarg B, Lindner H, Loidl P (1998) Substrate and sequential site specificity of cytoplasmic histone acetyltransferases of maize and rat liver. FEBS Lett 421(2):109–114
55. Nagarajan P, Ge Z, Sirbu B, Doughty C, Agudelo Garcia PA et al (2013) Histone acetyl transferase 1 is essential for mammalian development, genome stability, and the processing of newly synthesized histones H3 and H4. PLoS Genet 9(6):e1003518
56. Poveda A, Pamblanco M, Tafrov S, Tordera V, Sternglanz R et al (2004) Hif1 is a component of yeast histone acetyltransferase B, a complex mainly localized in the nucleus. J Biol Chem 279(16):16033–16043
57. Campos EI, Fillingham J, Li G, Zheng H, Voigt P et al (2010) The program for processing newly synthesized histones H3.1 and H4. Nat Struct Mol Biol 17(11):1343–1351
58. Li Y, Zhang L, Liu T, Chai C, Fang Q et al (2014) Hat2p recognizes the histone H3 tail to specify the acetylation of the newly synthesized H3/H4 heterodimer by the Hat1p/Hat2p complex. Genes Dev 28(11):1217–1227
59. Wu H, Moshkina N, Min J, Zeng H, Joshua J et al (2012) Structural basis for substrate specificity and catalysis of human histone acetyltransferase 1. Proc Natl Acad Sci U S A 109(23):8925–8930
60. Zheng Y, Thomas PM, Kelleher NL (2013) Measurement of acetylation turnover at distinct lysines in human histones identifies long-lived acetylation sites. Nat Commun 4:2203
61. Kaimori JY, Maehara K, Hayashi-Takanaka Y, Harada A, Fukuda M et al (2016) Histone H4 lysine 20 acetylation is associated with gene repression in human cells. Sci Rep 6:24318
62. Murzina NV, Pei XY, Zhang W, Sparkes M, Vicente-Garcia J et al (2008) Structural basis for the recognition of histone H4 by the histone-chaperone RbAp46. Structure 16(7):1077–1085
63. Georgakopoulos T, Thireos G (1992) Two distinct yeast transcriptional activators require the function of the GCN5 protein to promote normal levels of transcription. EMBO J 11(11):4145–4152
64. Candau R, Moore PA, Wang L, Barlev N, Ying CY et al (1996) Identification of human proteins functionally conserved with the yeast putative adaptors ADA2 and GCN5. Mol Cell Biol 16(2):593–602
65. Yang XJ, Ogryzko VV, Nishikawa J, Howard BH, Nakatani Y (1996) A p300/CBP-associated factor that competes with the adenoviral oncoprotein E1A. Nature 382(6589):319–324
66. Nagy Z, Tora L (2007) Distinct GCN5/PCAF-containing complexes function as co-activators and are involved in transcription factor and global histone acetylation. Oncogene 26(37):5341–5357
67. Spedale G, Timmers HT, Pijnappel WW (2012) ATAC-king the complexity of SAGA during evolution. Genes Dev 26(6):527–541
68. Krebs AR, Demmers J, Karmodiya K, Chang NC, Chang AC et al (2010) ATAC and Mediator coactivators form a stable complex and regulate a set of non-coding RNA genes. EMBO Rep 11(7):541–547
69. Nagy Z, Riss A, Fujiyama S, Krebs A, Orpinell M et al (2010) The metazoan ATAC and SAGA coactivator HAT complexes regulate different sets of inducible target genes. Cell Mol Life Sci 67(4):611–628

70. Marcus GA, Silverman N, Berger SL, Horiuchi J, Guarente L (1994) Functional similarity and physical association between GCN5 and ADA2: putative transcriptional adaptors. EMBO J 13(20):4807–4815
71. Horiuchi J, Silverman N, Marcus GA, Guarente L (1995) ADA3, a putative transcriptional adaptor, consists of two separable domains and interacts with ADA2 and GCN5 in a trimeric complex. Mol Cell Biol 15(3):1203–1209
72. Pollard KJ, Peterson CL (1997) Role for ADA/GCN5 products in antagonizing chromatin-mediated transcriptional repression. Mol Cell Biol 17(11):6212–6222
73. Lee KK, Sardiu ME, Swanson SK, Gilmore JM, Torok M et al (2011) Combinatorial depletion analysis to assemble the network architecture of the SAGA and ADA chromatin remodeling complexes. Mol Syst Biol 7:503
74. Bian C, Xu C, Ruan J, Lee KK, Burke TL et al (2011) Sgf29 binds histone H3K4me2/3 and is required for SAGA complex recruitment and histone H3 acetylation. EMBO J 30(14):2829–2842
75. Vermeulen M, Eberl HC, Matarese F, Marks H, Denissov S et al (2010) Quantitative interaction proteomics and genome-wide profiling of epigenetic histone marks and their readers. Cell 142(6):967–980
76. Dhalluin C, Carlson JE, Zeng L, He C, Aggarwal AK et al (1999) Structure and ligand of a histone acetyltransferase bromodomain. Nature 399(6735):491–496
77. Owen DJ, Ornaghi P, Yang JC, Lowe N, Evans PR et al (2000) The structural basis for the recognition of acetylated histone H4 by the bromodomain of histone acetyltransferase gcn5p. EMBO J 19(22):6141–6149
78. Hassan AH, Prochasson P, Neely KE, Galasinski SC, Chandy M et al (2002) Function and selectivity of bromodomains in anchoring chromatin-modifying complexes to promoter nucleosomes. Cell 111(3):369–379
79. Riss A, Scheer E, Joint M, Trowitzsch S, Berger I et al (2015) Subunits of ADA-two-A-containing (ATAC) or Spt-Ada-Gcn5-acetyltrasferase (SAGA) Coactivator complexes enhance the Acetyltransferase activity of GCN5. J Biol Chem 290(48):28997–29009
80. Rojas JR, Trievel RC, Zhou J, Mo Y, Li X et al (1999) Structure of Tetrahymena GCN5 bound to coenzyme A and a histone H3 peptide. Nature 401(6748):93–98
81. Clements A, Poux AN, Lo WS, Pillus L, Berger SL et al (2003) Structural basis for histone and phosphohistone binding by the GCN5 histone acetyltransferase. Mol Cell 12(2):461–473
82. Trievel RC, Li FY, Marmorstein R (2000) Application of a fluorescent histone acetyltransferase assay to probe the substrate specificity of the human p300/CBP-associated factor. Anal Biochem 287(2):319–328
83. Poux AN, Marmorstein R (2003) Molecular basis for Gcn5/PCAF histone acetyltransferase selectivity for histone and nonhistone substrates. Biochemistry 42(49):14366–14374
84. Clements A, Marmorstein R (2003) Insights into structure and function of GCN5/PCAF and yEsa 1 histone acetyltransferase domains. Methods Enzymol 371:545–564
85. Sapountzi V, Cote J (2011) MYST-family histone acetyltransferases: beyond chromatin. Cell Mol Life Sci 68(7):1147–1156
86. Su J, Wang F, Cai Y, Jin J (2016) The functional analysis of histone acetyltransferase MOF in tumorigenesis. Int J Mol Sci 17(1):E99
87. Meller VH, Rattner BP (2002) The roX genes encode redundant male-specific lethal transcripts required for targeting of the MSL complex. EMBO J 21(5):1084–1091
88. Deng X, Meller VH (2006) roX RNAs are required for increased expression of X-linked genes in *Drosophila melanogaster* males. Genetics 174(4):1859–1866
89. Marin I (2003) Evolution of chromatin-remodeling complexes: comparative genomics reveals the ancient origin of "novel" compensasome genes. J Mol Evol 56(5):527–539
90. Morales V, Straub T, Neumann MF, Mengus G, Akhtar A et al (2004) Functional integration of the histone acetyltransferase MOF into the dosage compensation complex. EMBO J 23(11):2258–2268
91. Morales V, Regnard C, Izzo A, Vetter I, Becker PB (2005) The MRG domain mediates the functional integration of MSL3 into the dosage compensation complex. Mol Cell Biol 25(14):5947–5954

92. Larschan E, Alekseyenko AA, Gortchakov AA, Peng S, Li B et al (2007) MSL complex is attracted to genes marked by H3K36 trimethylation using a sequence-independent mechanism. Mol Cell 28(1):121–133

93. Sural TH, Peng S, Li B, Workman JL, Park PJ et al (2008) The MSL3 chromodomain directs a key targeting step for dosage compensation of the Drosophila melanogaster X chromosome. Nat Struct Mol Biol 15(12):1318–1325

94. Ilik IA, Quinn JJ, Georgiev P, Tavares-Cadete F, Maticzka D et al (2013) Tandem stem-loops in roX RNAs act together to mediate X chromosome dosage compensation in Drosophila. Mol Cell 51(2):156–173

95. Maenner S, Muller M, Frohlich J, Langer D, Becker PB (2013) ATP-dependent roX RNA remodeling by the helicase maleless enables specific association of MSL proteins. Mol Cell 51(2):174–184

96. Kelley RL, Wang J, Bell L, Kuroda MI (1997) Sex lethal controls dosage compensation in Drosophila by a non-splicing mechanism. Nature 387(6629):195–199

97. Beckmann K, Grskovic M, Gebauer F, Hentze MW (2005) A dual inhibitory mechanism restricts msl-2 mRNA translation for dosage compensation in Drosophila. Cell 122(4):529–540

98. Mendjan S, Taipale M, Kind J, Holz H, Gebhardt P et al (2006) Nuclear pore components are involved in the transcriptional regulation of dosage compensation in Drosophila. Mol Cell 21(6):811–823

99. Raja SJ, Charapitsa I, Conrad T, Vaquerizas JM, Gebhardt P et al (2010) The nonspecific lethal complex is a transcriptional regulator in Drosophila. Mol Cell 38(6):827–841

100. Lam KC, Muhlpfordt F, Vaquerizas JM, Raja SJ, Holz H et al (2012) The NSL complex regulates housekeeping genes in Drosophila. PLoS Genet 8(6):e1002736

101. Gupta A, Sharma GG, Young CS, Agarwal M, Smith ER et al (2005) Involvement of human MOF in ATM function. Mol Cell Biol 25(12):5292–5305

102. Dou Y, Milne TA, Tackett AJ, Smith ER, Fukuda A et al (2005) Physical association and coordinate function of the H3 K4 methyltransferase MLL1 and the H4 K16 acetyltransferase MOF. Cell 121(6):873–885

103. Taipale M, Rea S, Richter K, Vilar A, Lichter P et al (2005) hMOF histone acetyltransferase is required for histone H4 lysine 16 acetylation in mammalian cells. Mol Cell Biol 25(15):6798–6810

104. Smith ER, Cayrou C, Huang R, Lane WS, Cote J et al (2005) A human protein complex homologous to the Drosophila MSL complex is responsible for the majority of histone H4 acetylation at lysine 16. Mol Cell Biol 25(21):9175–9188

105. Li X, Wu L, Corsa CA, Kunkel S, Dou Y (2009) Two mammalian MOF complexes regulate transcription activation by distinct mechanisms. Mol Cell 36(2):290–301

106. Wu L, Zee BM, Wang Y, Garcia BA, Dou Y (2011) The RING finger protein MSL2 in the MOF complex is an E3 ubiquitin ligase for H2B K34 and is involved in crosstalk with H3 K4 and K79 methylation. Mol Cell 43(1):132–144

107. Cai Y, Jin J, Swanson SK, Cole MD, Choi SH et al (2010) Subunit composition and substrate specificity of a MOF-containing histone acetyltransferase distinct from the male-specific lethal (MSL) complex. J Biol Chem 285(7):4268–4272

108. Luo H, Shenoy AK, Li X, Jin Y, Jin L et al (2016) MOF acetylates the histone demethylase LSD1 to suppress epithelial-to-mesenchymal transition. Cell Rep 15(12):2665–2678

109. Gupta A, Hunt CR, Hegde ML, Chakraborty S, Chakraborty S et al (2014) MOF phosphorylation by ATM regulates 53BP1-mediated double-strand break repair pathway choice. Cell Rep 8(1):177–189

110. Li X, Corsa CA, Pan PW, Wu L, Ferguson D et al (2010) MOF and H4 K16 acetylation play important roles in DNA damage repair by modulating recruitment of DNA damage repair protein Mdc1. Mol Cell Biol 30(22):5335–5347

111. Sharma GG, So S, Gupta A, Kumar R, Cayrou C et al (2010) MOF and histone H4 acetylation at lysine 16 are critical for DNA damage response and double-strand break repair. Mol Cell Biol 30(14):3582–3595

112. Gupta A, Guerin-Peyrou TG, Sharma GG, Park C, Agarwal M et al (2008) The mammalian ortholog of Drosophila MOF that acetylates histone H4 lysine 16 is essential for embryogenesis and oncogenesis. Mol Cell Biol 28(1):397–409

113. Thomas T, Dixon MP, Kueh AJ, Voss AK (2008) Mof (MYST1 or KAT8) is essential for progression of embryonic development past the blastocyst stage and required for normal chromatin architecture. Mol Cell Biol 28(16):5093–5105

114. Kumar R, Hunt CR, Gupta A, Nannepaga S, Pandita RK et al (2011) Purkinje cell-specific males absent on the first (mMof) gene deletion results in an ataxia-telangiectasia-like neurological phenotype and backward walking in mice. Proc Natl Acad Sci U S A 108(9):3636–3641

115. Gupta A, Hunt CR, Pandita RK, Pae J, Komal K et al (2013) T-cell-specific deletion of Mof blocks their differentiation and results in genomic instability in mice. Mutagenesis 28(3):263–270

116. Horikoshi N, Hunt CR, Pandita TK (2016) More complex transcriptional regulation and stress response by MOF. Oncogene 35(21):2681–2683

117. Sheikh BN, Bechtel-Walz W, Lucci J, Karpiuk O, Hild I et al (2016) MOF maintains transcriptional programs regulating cellular stress response. Oncogene 35(21):2698–2710

118. Cao L, Zhu L, Yang J, Su J, Ni J et al (2014) Correlation of low expression of hMOF with clinicopathological features of colorectal carcinoma, gastric cancer and renal cell carcinoma. Int J Oncol 44(4):1207–1214

119. Liu N, Zhang R, Zhao X, Su J, Bian X et al (2013) A potential diagnostic marker for ovarian cancer: involvement of the histone acetyltransferase, human males absent on the first. Oncol Lett 6(2):393–400

120. Pfister S, Rea S, Taipale M, Mendrzyk F, Straub B et al (2008) The histone acetyltransferase hMOF is frequently downregulated in primary breast carcinoma and medulloblastoma and constitutes a biomarker for clinical outcome in medulloblastoma. Int J Cancer 122(6):1207–1213

121. Zhang J, Liu H, Pan H, Yang Y, Huang G et al (2014) The histone acetyltransferase hMOF suppresses hepatocellular carcinoma growth. Biochem Biophys Res Commun 452(3):575–580

122. Zhao L, Wang DL, Liu Y, Chen S, Sun FL (2013) Histone acetyltransferase hMOF promotes S phase entry and tumorigenesis in lung cancer. Cell Signal 25(8):1689–1698

123. Lin T, Ponn A, Hu X, Law BK, Lu J (2010) Requirement of the histone demethylase LSD1 in Snail-mediated transcriptional repression during epithelial-mesenchymal transition. Oncogene 29(35):4896–4904

124. Tang M, Shen H, Jin Y, Lin T, Cai Q et al (2013) The malignant brain tumor (MBT) domain protein SFMBT1 is an integral histone reader subunit of the LSD1 demethylase complex for chromatin association and epithelial-to-mesenchymal transition. J Biol Chem 288(38):27680–27691

125. Lin Y, Wu Y, Li J, Dong C, Ye X et al (2010) The SNAG domain of Snail1 functions as a molecular hook for recruiting lysine-specific demethylase 1. EMBO J 29(11):1803–1816

126. Herrero J, Muffato M, Beal K, Fitzgerald S, Gordon L et al (2016) Ensembl comparative genomics resources. Database (Oxford) 2016:bav096

127. Gamsjaeger R, Webb SR, Lamonica JM, Billin A, Blobel GA et al (2011) Structural basis and specificity of acetylated transcription factor GATA1 recognition by BET family bromodomain protein Brd3. Mol Cell Biol 31(13):2632–2640

128. Shi J, Wang Y, Zeng L, Wu Y, Deng J et al (2014) Disrupting the interaction of BRD4 with diacetylated twist suppresses tumorigenesis in basal-like breast cancer. Cancer Cell 25(2):210–225

129. Schroder S, Cho S, Zeng L, Zhang Q, Kaehlcke K et al (2012) Two-pronged binding with bromodomain-containing protein 4 liberates positive transcription elongation factor b from inactive ribonucleoprotein complexes. J Biol Chem 287(2):1090–1099

130. Wang CY, Filippakopoulos P (2015) Beating the odds: BETs in disease. Trends Biochem Sci 40(8):468–479

131. Smith SG, Zhou MM (2016) The Bromodomain: a new target in emerging epigenetic medicine. ACS Chem Biol 11(3):598–608
132. Jacobson RH, Ladurner AG, King DS, Tjian R (2000) Structure and function of a human TAFII250 double bromodomain module. Science 288(5470):1422–1425
133. Filippakopoulos P, Picaud S, Mangos M, Keates T, Lambert JP et al (2012) Histone recognition and large-scale structural analysis of the human bromodomain family. Cell 149(1):214–231
134. Mottamal M, Zheng S, Huang TL, Wang G (2015) Histone deacetylase inhibitors in clinical studies as templates for new anticancer agents. Molecules 20(3):3898–3941
135. Benedetti R, Conte M, Altucci L (2015) Targeting histone deacetylases in diseases: where are we? Antioxid Redox Signal 23(1):99–126
136. Yoshida M, Beppu T (1988) Reversible arrest of proliferation of rat 3Y1 fibroblasts in both the G1 and G2 phases by trichostatin A. Exp Cell Res 177(1):122–131
137. Yoshida H, Sugita K (1992) A novel tetracyclic peptide, trapoxin, induces phenotypic change from transformed to normal in sis-oncogene-transformed NIH3T3 cells. Jpn J Cancer Res 83(4):324–328
138. Kijima M, Yoshida M, Sugita K, Horinouchi S, Beppu T (1993) Trapoxin, an antitumor cyclic tetrapeptide, is an irreversible inhibitor of mammalian histone deacetylase. J Biol Chem 268(30):22429–22435
139. Vidal M, Gaber RF (1991) RPD3 encodes a second factor required to achieve maximum positive and negative transcriptional states in Saccharomyces cerevisiae. Mol Cell Biol 11(12):6317–6327
140. Finnin MS, Donigian JR, Cohen A, Richon VM, Rifkind RA et al (1999) Structures of a histone deacetylase homologue bound to the TSA and SAHA inhibitors. Nature 401(6749):188–193
141. Simon RP, Robaa D, Alhalabi Z, Sippl W, Jung M (2016) KATching-up on small molecule modulators of lysine acetyltransferases. J Med Chem 59(4):1249–1270
142. Gil J, Ramirez-Torres A, Encarnacion-Guevara S (2017) Lysine acetylation and cancer: a proteomics perspective. J Proteome 150:297–309

Part III
DNA and Histone Methylation-Related Events Underlying Cancer

DNA Methylation and Dysregulation of miRNA in Cancer

Feedback Loop Between Dysregulated miRNAs and Epigenetic Pathways in Cancer

Akira Kurozumi, Yusuke Goto, Atsushi Okato, and Naohiko Seki

Abstract The discovery of microRNAs (miRNAs) has resulted in major advancements in cancer research. miRNAs are small noncoding RNAs that function to fine tune the expression of protein coding/noncoding RNAs by repressing translation or cleaving RNA transcripts in a sequence-depending manner. The unique characteristic function of miRNAs is to regulate RNA transcripts in human cells. Therefore, dysregulated expression of miRNAs can disrupt tightly regulated RNA networks in cancer cells. miRNAs play critical roles in various biological processes, and their dysregulation has been observed in several human diseases, including cancers.

Recent studies of cancer epigenome analysis have demonstrated that epigenetic mechanisms, including DNA methylation and histone modification, regulate the expression of a number of miRNAs, and conversely, these miRNAs control the expression of various epigenetic modulators, including DNA methyltransferases (DNMTs), histone deacetylases (HDACs), and polycomb group genes. When this complicated feedback loop between miRNAs and epigenetics is dysregulated by aberrant expression of miRNAs, normal physiological functions are disrupted, and as a result, several diseases occur, including cancer. That is, dysregulation of miRNAs can affect epigenetic alterations in cancer. The present review focuses on some tumor-suppressive miRNAs that have been shown to regulate epigenetic modulators in cancer; the functional roles of these miRNAs in epigenetics are described. Elucidation of the relationship between miRNA dysregulation and epigenetic alterations will lead to the discovery of new therapeutic strategies for cancer.

Keywords microRNA • Epigenetics • DNA methylation • Histone modification • Cancer

A. Kurozumi • Y. Goto • A. Okato • N. Seki (✉)
Department of Functional Genomics, Chiba University Graduate School of Medicine,
1-8-1 Inohana Chuo-ku, Chiba 260-8670, Japan
e-mail: naoseki@faculty.chiba-u.jp

© Springer International Publishing AG 2017
A. Kaneda, Y.-i. Tsukada (eds.), *DNA and Histone Methylation as Cancer Targets*,
Cancer Drug Discovery and Development, DOI 10.1007/978-3-319-59786-7_10

1   Introduction

MicroRNAs (miRNAs) are endogenous, short, noncoding, single-stranded RNAs (18–23 nucleotides in length) that post-transcriptionally regulate protein/nonprotein-coding gene expression by repressing mRNA translation or cleaving mRNA transcripts through binding to the 3'-untranslated region (UTR) of mRNAs [1]. Lee et al. identified the first miRNAs in *Caenorhabditis elegans* in 1993 [2]. Currently, 2588 human miRNAs are registered in the miRBase (Release 21, June 2014). A number of studies have indicated that miRNAs play critical roles in various cellular processes, including cell proliferation, differentiation, and apoptosis [1, 3]. Furthermore, aberrantly expressed miRNAs disrupt normal RNA regulatory networks, promoting the development of various human diseases, including cancers. miRNAs can behave as oncogenes or tumor suppressors depending on the functions of target genes. In general, downregulated miRNAs in cancer tissues appear to act as tumor-suppressor genes, and conversely, upregulated miRNAs in cancer tissues appear to act as oncogenes [4]. Recent studies have identified a number of aberrantly expressed miRNAs in human cancer. However, the underlying molecular mechanisms of miRNA dysregulation in cancer have still not been fully elucidated.

Recently, the expression of miRNAs has been shown to be regulated by genetic and epigenetic mechanisms [5, 6]. Many miRNAs are located in cancer-associated genomic regions, and their promoter regions are epigenetically regulated by DNA methylation and histone modification. Furthermore, these miRNAs, called epi-miRNAs, can affect the expression of epigenetic modulators, including DNA methyltransferases (DNMTs) and histone deacetylases (HDACs) [7]. This complicated feedback loop between dysregulated miRNAs and epigenetic pathways has become increasingly recognized as an important factor contributing to cancer development [8].

In the present review, we focused on some epi-miRNAs in several cancers and described current knowledge regarding the roles of these miRNAs in targeting epigenetic modulators in cancer. Although the network of miRNAs and epigenetics is highly complicated, increasing our understanding of this feedback loop will provide insights into the discovery of new cancer treatment strategies.

2   miRNA Biogenesis

miRNA genes are transcribed by RNA polymerase II or RNA polymerase III (mainly RNA polymerase II) and form primary miRNAs (pri-miRNAs) measuring approximately 200 to several thousand nucleotides in length. Pri-miRNAs are single-stranded RNAs that contain loop sequences. The 5'-ends of pri-miRNAs are cleaved by the ribonuclease III enzyme Drosha and its binding partner DiGeorge syndrome chromosomal region 8 (DGCR8) [9]. The products form small hairpin-shaped RNAs called precursor miRNAs (pre-miRNAs). Pre-miRNAs are 70–100 nucleotides in length and are transported from the nucleus to the cytoplasm via exportin-5 with Ran-GTP as a cofactor. The terminal ends of the pre-miRNAs are then cleaved by another RNase, Dicer, generating duplex guide-passenger duplex miRNAs (miRNA/miRNA* complex). Duplex miRNAs are about 22 nucleotides in length and can be arranged in two directions; the resulting miRNAs are called guide strand or passenger strand miRNAs (miRNA or miRNA*) or can be labeled according to their direction (*miRNA-5p* or *miRNA-3p*). The mature miRNA strands are incorporated into the RNA-induced silencing complex (RISC), which contains Argonaut (AGO) protein. AGO protein plays central roles in the RISC and consists of N, PAZ, MID, and PIWI domains. miRNAs assemble with AGO protein family members. miRNAs are loaded onto AGO proteins by chaperones (e.g., heat-shock cognate protein [Hsc70]/heat-shock protein 90 [Hsp90]), and one end of the duplex is opened by AGO proteins, followed by release of the passenger strand [10]. In the RISC, the 5′-end of miRNAs, which is called the seed sequence, binds to the 3′-untranlsated region (UTR) of the target mRNA in a sequence-specific manner and consequently represses mRNA translation or cleaves mRNA. Previous study suggested that the miRNA passenger strand (miRNA*) was degraded, and only the miRNA guide strand (miRNA) exerted its functions. However, recent analyses revealed that both strands have functions and are incorporated into the RISC. The precise mechanisms of the miRNA-RISC complex are unclear.

These are canonical biogenesis pathways for miRNAs; however, recent research had indicated alternative pathways for miRNA biogenesis. Through this alternative pathway, miRNAs called miRtrons are generated [11]. miRtrons are produced from short introns with hairpin potential. After splicing, these introns debranch and fold to form miRNA hairpins and then enter the canonical miRNA biogenesis pathway before transportation into the cytoplasm. This pathway bypasses Drosha cleavage. miRtron pathways were originally reported in flies and worms and were subsequently confirmed in other species, including humans.

3 Epigenetically Dysregulated miRNAs in Cancer

As described the previous section, miRNA biogenesis has been well-studied. However, the mechanisms regulating miRNAs are still not fully understood. In addition to protein-coding genes, miRNAs appear to be regulated by both genetic and epigenetic mechanisms. In general, the expression of miRNAs is epigenetically regulated by DNA methylation and histone modifications.

DNA methylation is the most common epigenetic regulation mechanism and involves addition of a methyl group at the carbon 5 position of cytosine in CpG islands by three DNMTs (*DNMT1*, *DNMT3A*, and *DNMT3B*). *DNMT3A* and

DNMT3B have de novo methylation activity, and *DNMT1* maintains methylated DNA replication. In cancer, DNA hypermethylation of CpG islands within the promoter region leads to the silencing of several tumor-suppressive miRNAs, and conversely, DNA hypomethylation activates several oncogenic miRNAs.

Histone modification is also the most important epigenetic mechanism; this pathway involves the activities of HDACs and histone acetyltransferases (HATs). HDACs condense chromatin by removing acetyl groups from lysine residues of histones, leading to transcriptional repression [12]. Recent studies have shown that HDAC silences tumor-suppressive miRNAs in cancer. Furthermore, HDAC inhibition leads to the increase of active histone marks at the promoters of the miRNAs, thereby upregulating miRNAs.

4 miRNAs Targeting Epigenetic Pathway-Related Genes

Many studies have indicated that a single miRNA can regulate multiple genes; conversely, a single gene can be regulated by several different miRNAs. Table 1 lists several epi-miRNAs and the targeted epigenetic pathway-related genes in various human cancers. Additionally, Table 2 shows some typical epigenetic effectors regulated by different miRNAs. In this review, we focus on some miRNAs that function as tumor suppressors by targeting epigenetic pathway-related genes and describe them in detail.

4.1 miR-7

Zhang et al. indicated that *miR-7* suppresses colorectal cancer tumorigenesis by targeting the oncogenic *Yin Yang 1* (*YY1*) gene directly [13]. *YY1* is a transcription factor of the polycomb group protein family and exerts its oncogenic functions by inhibiting the transcription factor *p53* and promoting Wnt-dependent signaling pathways [13, 14]. *YY1* expression has been shown to be positively associated with poor survival in patients with colorectal cancer.

4.2 miR-25

miR-25 inhibits the proliferation of thyroid carcinoma cells by targeting *EZH2* [15]. EZH2 is a member of the polycomb group proteins and functions as the conserved catalytic subunit within the polycomb repressive complex 2 (PRC2). EZH2 regulates histone (H3) trimethylation at lysine 27 (H3K27me3) [16]. EZH2 is a master regulator of epigenetic modifications.

Table 1 miRNAs and targeting epigenetic pathway-related genes in several cancers

miRNAs	Target genes	Cancer type	Citation
miR-7	YY1	Colorectal cancer	[13]
miR-25	EZH2	Thyroid carcinoma	[15]
miR-26a	EZH2	Nasopharyngeal carcinoma	[21]
miR-29 s	DNMT3A, DNMT3B	Lung cancer, Glioblastoma	[22, 23]
miR-30d	EZH2	Thyroid carcinoma	[15]
miR-34a	YY1	Esophageal squamous cell carcinoma, Gastric cancer	[26]
miR-34b	DNMT1, DNMT3B, HDAC1, HDAC2, HDAC4	Prostate cancer	[25]
	YY1	Gastric cancer	[26]
miR-34c	YY1	Gastric cancer	[26]
miR-101	UHRF1, EZH2	Renal cell carcinoma	[27]
	EZH2	Hepatocellular carcinoma	[28]
	DNMT3A	Lung cancer	[29]
miR-125a	HDAC4	Breast cancer	[30]
miR-138	EZH2	Osteosarcoma	[31]
miR-140	HDAC4	Osteosarcoma	[33]
miR-143	DNMT3A	Colorectal cancer	[39]
miR-145	DNMT3B	Prostate cancer	[40]
	UHRF1	Bladder cancer	[41]
miR-148a	DNMT1	Cholangiocarcinoma	[43, 44]
miR-152	DNMT1	Cholangiocarcinoma, Hepatocellular carcinoma	[43, 44]
miR-181	YY1	Cervical cancer	[46]
miR-182	DNMT3A	Cervical cancer	[48]
miR-185	DNMT1	Glioma	[49]
miR-200b	BMI1	Hepatocellular carcinoma	[51]
miR-212	MeCP2	Gastric cancer	[52]
miR-338	BMI1	Gastric cancer	[54]
miR-340	EZH2	Laryngeal squamous cell carcinoma	[58]
miR-342	DNMT1	Colorectal cancer	[60]
miR-376c	BMI1	Cervical cancer	[63]
miR-449a	HDAC1	Prostate caner, Lung cancer	[65, 66]
miR-449b	HDAC1	Lung cancer	[66]
miR-452	BMI1	Lung cancer	[68]
miR-506	EZH2	Colon cancer	[72]

4.3 miR-26a

miR-26a has been shown to have a tumor-suppressive role in various type of cancers, such as prostate cancer, renal cell carcinoma, oral squamous cell carcinoma, and head and neck squamous cell carcinoma [17–20]. Lu et al. reported that miR-26a exhibits tumor-suppressive effects in nasopharyngeal carcinoma by repressing EZH2 [21].

Table 2 Epigenetic pathway-related genes regulated by miRNA

Target genes	miRNAs	Citation
DNMT3A	miR-29s, miR-101, miR-143, miR-182	[22, 23, 29, 39, 48]
DNMT3B	miR-29s,miR-34b, miR-145, miR-148, miR-221	[22, 23, 25, 40, 42]
DNMT1	miR-34b, miR-148, miR-152, miR-185, miR-342	[25, 43, 44, 49, 60]
HDAC1	miR-34b, miR-449a, miR-449b, miR-874	[25, 65, 66, 78]
HDAC2	miR-34b	[25]
HDAC4	miR-34b, miR-125a-5p, miR-140	[25, 30, 33]
EZH2	miR-25, miR-26a, miR-30d, miR-101, miR-138, miR-340, miR-506	[15, 21, 27, 31, 58, 72, 76]
UHRF1	miR-101, miR-145	[27, 28, 41]
BMI1	miR-200b, miR-141/200c, miR-338-5p, miR-376c, miR-452	[50, 51, 54, 63, 68]
YY1	miR-7, miR-34, miR-181	[13, 26, 46]
MeCP2	miR-212	[52]

4.4   The miR-29 Family

The *miR-29* family (*miR-29a*, *miR-29b*, and *miR-29c*) targets *DNMT3A* and *DNMT3B* directly in lung cancer and glioblastoma and targets *DNMT1* indirectly in acute myeloid leukemia [22, 23].

4.5   miR-30d

miR-30d has been reported to be downregulated in non-small cell lung cancer and thyroid carcinoma [15, 24]. Moreover, ectopic expression of *miR-30d* suppresses the proliferation of thyroid carcinoma cells by regulating *EZH2* [15].

4.6   The miR-34 Family

Majid et al. reported that *miR-34b* is silenced by CpG hypermethylation in prostate cancer and that ectopic expression of *miR-34b* reduces the expression of both DNMTs (*DNMT1* and *DNMT3B*) and HDACs (*HDAC1*, *HDAC2*, and *HDAC4*) [25]. Additionally, *YY1* is directly targeted by the *miR-34* family (*miR-34a*, *miR-34b*, and *miR-34c*) in gastric cancer [26].

4.7   miR-101

The tumor-suppressive roles of *miR-101* have been reported in several cancers, including renal cell carcinoma, lung cancer, hepatocellular carcinoma, gastric cancer, and breast cancer [27]. In particular, we showed that *UHRF1* and *EZH2* are directly suppressed by *miR-101* in RCC cells [27]. In addition to EZH2, UHRF1 is a master regulator of epigenetic modifications and is required for DNMT1 function through direct binding to DNMT1 and activation of DNMT1 function for maintenance of DNA methylation. Furthermore, genomic loss of *miR-101* in cancer leads to overexpression of *EZH2*, resulting in cancer progression [28]. *miR-101* also suppresses lung tumorigenesis by targeting *DNMT3A* [29].

4.8   miR-125a

Low circulating *miR-125a-5p* has been shown to be an independent prognostic biomarker associated with poor survival rates in breast cancer, and *miR-125a-5p* directly targets *HDAC4* mRNA [30].

4.9   miR-138

miR-138 acts as a tumor suppressor in gallbladder carcinoma, non-small cell lung cancer, and osteosarcoma. Some miRNAs play pivotal roles in cancer chemoresistance. *miR-138* was shown to have a tumor-suppressive function by targeting *EZH2* and enhancing cisplatin-induced apoptosis in osteosarcoma [31].

4.10   miR-140

miR-140 has been reported to have tumor-suppressive functions in non-small cell lung cancer, osteosarcoma, and esophageal cancer [32–34]. Additionally, ectopic expression of *miR-140* inhibits osteosarcoma cell proliferation by targeting *HDAC4* [33].

4.11   miR-143/145

miR-143 forms a cluster with *miR-145* on chromosome 5q32-q33, and these cluster miRNAs have been shown to be downregulated in several types of human cancer, such as prostate cancer, bladder cancer, renal cell carcinoma, and colorectal cancer [35–38]. In colorectal cancer, *miR-143* targets *DNMT3A* [39]. Furthermore, crosstalk occurs between *miR-145* and *DNMT3B* via a double-negative feedback loop in prostate cancer [40]. Our recent report indicated that dual-strand *miR-145* (*miR-145-5p* and *miR-145-3p*) inhibits bladder cancer cell aggressiveness by targeting *UHRF1* [41].

4.12   miR-148

miR-148 has been shown to target *DNMT3B* directly by binding a recognition site located in the coding region [42]. Braconi et al. demonstrated that *miR-148a* and *miR-152* directly regulate *DNMT1* in human cholangiocarcinoma [43, 44]. Downregulation of *DNMT1* restores the expression of the methylation-sensitive tumor-suppressor genes *Rassf1a* and *p16INK4a*.

4.13   miR-152

Braconi et al. reported that *DNMT1* is directly regulated by *miR-152* in human cholangiocarcinoma [43]. Additionally, Huang et al. reported that *miR-152* is downregulated in tissues from patients with hepatitis B virus-related hepatocellular carcinoma and is inversely correlated with *DNMT1* expression [44].

4.14   miR-181

miR-181 has been shown to act as a tumor suppressor by suppressing the epithelial-mesenchymal transition (EMT) pathway in glioblastoma [45]. Furthermore, *miR-181* inhibits cervical cancer progression by targeting *YY1* [46].

4.15   miR-182

miR-182 is silenced by HDACs in acute myelogenous leukemia (AML), and inhibition of HDACs induces *miR-182*, leading to sensitization of AML cells to DNA-damaging agents [47]. Additionally, Sun et al. showed that *miR-182* inhibits DNMT3a and induces cervical cancer cell apoptosis [48].

4.16   miR-185

Zhang et al. reported that *miR-185* is downregulated in glioma cells and targets *DNMT1* [49]. In glioma, the *miR-185* locus on chromosome 22q11.2 has been reported to exhibit loss of heterozygosity (LOH), and ectopic expression of *miR-185* inhibits global DNA methylation and induces the expression of promoter-hypermethylated genes.

4.17   miR-200 *Family*

The miR-*200* family is classified into two groups (*miR-141/200c* and *miR-200a/200b/429*). *miR-141* and *miR-200c* are located on chromosome 12p13.31, whereas *miR-200a*, *miR-200b*, and *miR-429* are located on chromosome 1p36.33. *miR-141 and miR-200c* have been reported to function as tumor suppressors by targeting B cell-specific Moloney murine leukemia virus integration site 1 (*BMI1*) [50]. BMI1 is a member of the polycomb repressive complex 1 (PRC1) and functions as a transcriptional repressor. Furthermore, Wu et al. reported that *miR-200b* had tumor-suppressive functions by targeting *BMI1* in hepatocellular carcinoma [51].

4.18   *miR-212*

miR-212 is downregulated in gastric cancer and targets methyl-CpG-binding protein (*MeCP2*) [52]. MeCP2 is a nuclear protein containing a methyl-CpG-binding domain (MBD) [53]. MBDs are able to bind to methylated DNA specifically. MeCP2 is a global transcriptional repressor and has a role in mediating epigenetic signaling and tumor progression.

4.19   *miR-338-5p*

miR-338-5p has been shown to suppress gastric cancer cell growth by targeting *BMI1* directly; this anti-proliferative effect can be suppressed by *MeCP2* [54].

4.20   *miR-340*

miR-340 has a tumor-suppressive role in various types of cancers, such as breast cancer, hepatocellular carcinoma, colorectal cancer, and laryngeal squamous cell carcinoma [55–58]. Moreover, *miR-340* inhibits laryngeal squamous cell carcinoma progression by targeting *EZH2* [58].

4.21   *miR-342*

miR-342 has been reported to be frequently silenced epigenetically in colorectal cancer [59]. Wang et al. reported that *miR-342* is downregulated in colorectal cancer cells and directly targets *DNMT1* [60].

4.22 miR-376c

miR-376c has been reported to be downregulated in various types of cancers, such as osteosarcoma, non-small-cell lung cancer, cervical cancer, and melanoma [61–64]. Deng et al. reported that *miR-376c* targets *BMI1* and inhibits cervical cancer cell invasion [63].

4.23 miR-449 Family

miR-449a regulates *HDAC1* directly in prostate cancer and lung cancer [65, 66]. In lung cancer, the *miR-449* family (*miR-449a* and *miR-449b*) has been shown to regulate *HDAC1*.

4.24 miR-452

The tumor-suppressive function of *miR-452* has been demonstrated in glioma, non-small cell lung cancer, and prostate cancer [67–69]. *miR-452* suppresses non-small cell lung cancer metastasis by targeting *BMI1* directly [68].

4.25 miR-506

miR-506 has a tumor-suppressive role in ovarian cancer and cervical cancer [70, 71]. Zhang et al. showed that *miR-506* suppresses colon cancer metastasis by targeting *EZH2* directly [72].

4.26 miR-874

miR-874 acts as a tumor suppressor in various types of cancers, such as gastric cancer, colorectal cancer, osteosarcoma, maxillary sinus squamous cell carcinoma, and head and neck squamous cell carcinoma [73–78]. Nohata et al. reported that *miR-874* acts as a tumor suppressor by directly targeting *HDAC1* in head and neck squamous cell carcinoma [78] (Fig. 1).

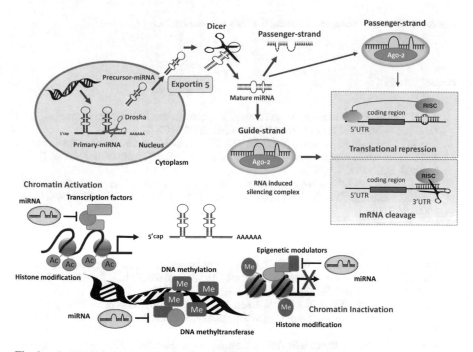

Fig. 1 pri-miRNAs are transcribed in the nucleus, and the 5'-ends of them are cleaved by Drosha. The products, called pre-miRNAs, are transported from the nucleus to the cytoplasm via exportin-5. The terminal ends of the pre-miRNAs are cleaved by Dicer, generating mature miRNAs. They can be arranged in two directions, guide strand or passenger strand miRNAs. Both of them are incorporated into the RISC, and have function by repressing mRNA translation or cleaving mRNA. DNA methylation and histone modification are the most common epigenetic regulation mechanisms. DNA methylation inactivates the transcription of CpG in the promoter regions of tumor suppressor genes and leads to gene silencing. DNA methyltransferases (DNMTs) is involved in the process of methylation, and the expression of them is regulated by several miRNAs. Histone modification plays a critical role in the regulation of chromatin, and the major roles are histone methylation and histone acetylation. Histone methylation condenses chromatin, and is involved in the regulation of chromatin inactivation (heterochromatin). Several epigenetic modulators are involved in the process of histone methylation, and the expression of them is regulated by several miRNAs. Histone acetylation reduces affinity between DNA and histones, leading to the chromatin activation (euchromatin). Several transcription factors are involved in the process of histone acetylation, and the expression of them is regulated by several miRNAs

5   Conclusions

In this review, we focused on some tumor-suppressive miRNAs and described their regulatory epigenetic mechanisms in cancer. Epigenetic alterations lead to aberrant miRNA expression, and miRNA dysregulation leads to epigenetic abnormalities in cancer. Additional studies of the relationship between miRNAs and epigenetics will facilitate the discovery of new therapeutic strategies in the treatment of human cancers.

A. Kurozumi et al.

Conflict of Interest The authors declare that they have no conflicts of interest.

References

1. Bartel DP (2004) MicroRNAs: genomics, biogenesis, mechanism, and function. Cell 116(2):281–297. PubMed PMID: 14744438, Epub 2004/01/28. eng.
2. Lee RC, Feinbaum RL, Ambros V (1993) The *C. elegans* heterochronic gene lin-4 encodes small RNAs with antisense complementarity to lin-14. Cell 75(5):843–854. PubMed PMID: 8252621. Epub 1993/12/03. Eng
3. Bartel DP (2009) MicroRNAs: target recognition and regulatory functions. Cell 136(2): 215–233. PubMed PMID: 19167326. Pubmed Central PMCID: PMC3794896. Epub 2009/01/27. Eng
4. Goto Y, Kurozumi A, Enokida H, Ichikawa T, Seki N (2015) Functional significance of aberrantly expressed microRNAs in prostate cancer. Int J Urol 22(3):242–252. PubMed PMID: 25599923. Epub 2015/01/21. eng
5. Lopez-Serra P, Esteller M (2012) DNA methylation-associated silencing of tumor-suppressor microRNAs in cancer. Oncogene 31(13):1609–1622. PubMed PMID: 21860412. Pubmed Central PMCID: PMC3325426. Epub 2011/08/24. Eng
6. Loginov VI, Rykov SV, Fridman MV, Braga EA (2015) Methylation of miRNA genes and oncogenesis. Biochemistry (Biokhimiia) 80(2):145–162. PubMed PMID: 25756530. Epub 2015/03/11. Eng
7. Iorio MV, Piovan C, Croce CM (2010) Interplay between microRNAs and the epigenetic machinery: an intricate network. Biochim Biophys Acta 1799(10–12):694–701. PubMed PMID: 20493980. Epub 2010/05/25. Eng
8. Sato F, Tsuchiya S, Meltzer SJ, Shimizu K (2011) MicroRNAs and epigenetics. FEBS J 278(10):1598–1609. PubMed PMID: 21395977. Epub 2011/03/15. Eng
9. Iorio MV, Croce CM (2012) MicroRNA dysregulation in cancer: diagnostics, monitoring and therapeutics. A comprehensive review. EMBO Mol Med 4(3):143–159. PubMed PMID: 22351564. Pubmed Central PMCID: PMC3376845. Epub 2012/02/22. Eng
10. Kobayashi H, Tomari Y (2016) RISC assembly: coordination between small RNAs and Argonaute proteins. Biochim Biophys Acta 1859(1):71–81. PubMed PMID: 26303205. Epub 2015/08/26. Eng
11. Curtis HJ, Sibley CR, Wood MJ (2012) Mirtrons, an emerging class of atypical miRNA. Wiley Interdiscip Rev RNA 3(5):617–632. PubMed PMID: 22733569. Epub 2012/06/27. Eng
12. Marks PA (2010) The clinical development of histone deacetylase inhibitors as targeted anticancer drugs. Expert Opin Investig Drugs 19(9):1049–1066. PubMed PMID: 20687783. Pubmed Central PMCID: PMC4077324. Epub 2010/08/07. Eng
13. Zhang N, Li X, Wu CW et al (2013) microRNA-7 is a novel inhibitor of YY1 contributing to colorectal tumorigenesis. Oncogene 32(42):5078–5088. PubMed PMID: 23208495. Epub 2012/12/05. eng
14. Gronroos E, Terentiev AA, Punga T, Ericsson J (2004) YY1 inhibits the activation of the p53 tumor suppressor in response to genotoxic stress. Proc Natl Acad Sci U S A 101(33):12165–12170. PubMed PMID: 15295102. Pubmed Central PMCID: PMC514451. Epub 2004/08/06. Eng
15. Esposito F, Tornincasa M, Pallante P et al (2012) Down-regulation of the miR-25 and miR-30d contributes to the development of anaplastic thyroid carcinoma targeting the polycomb protein EZH2. J Clin Endocrinol Metab 97(5):E710–E718. PubMed PMID: 22399519. Epub 2012/03/09. Eng
16. Volkel P, Dupret B, Le Bourhis X, Angrand PO (2015) Diverse involvement of EZH2 in cancer epigenetics. Am J Transl Res 7(2):175–193. PubMed PMID: 25901190. Pubmed Central PMCID: PMC4399085. Epub 2015/04/23. Eng

17. Kato M, Goto Y, Matsushita R et al (2015) MicroRNA-26a/b directly regulate La-related protein 1 and inhibit cancer cell invasion in prostate cancer. Int J Oncol 47(2):710–718. PubMed PMID: 26063484. Epub 2015/06/13. eng
18. Kurozumi A, Kato M, Goto Y et al (2016) Regulation of the collagen cross-linking enzymes LOXL2 and PLOD2 by tumor-suppressive microRNA-26a/b in renal cell carcinoma. Int J Oncol 48(5):1837–1846. PubMed PMID: 26983694. Pubmed Central PMCID: PMC4809659. Epub 2016/03/18. eng
19. Fukumoto I, Hanazawa T, Kinoshita T et al (2015) MicroRNA expression signature of oral squamous cell carcinoma: functional role of microRNA-26a/b in the modulation of novel cancer pathways. Br J Cancer 112(5):891–900. PubMed PMID: 25668004. Pubmed Central PMCID: PMC4453953. Epub 2015/02/11. eng
20. Fukumoto I, Kikkawa N, Matsushita R et al (2016) Tumor-suppressive microRNAs (miR-26a/b, miR-29a/b/c and miR-218) concertedly suppressed metastasis-promoting LOXL2 in head and neck squamous cell carcinoma. J Hum Genet 61(2):109–118. PubMed PMID: 26490187. Epub 2015/10/23. Eng
21. Lu J, He ML, Wang L et al (2011) MiR-26a inhibits cell growth and tumorigenesis of nasopharyngeal carcinoma through repression of EZH2. Cancer Res 71(1):225–233. PubMed PMID: 21199804. Epub 2011/01/05. eng
22. Fabbri M, Garzon R, Cimmino A et al (2007) MicroRNA-29 family reverts aberrant methylation in lung cancer by targeting DNA methyltransferases 3A and 3B. Proc Natl Acad Sci U S A 104(40):15805–15810. PubMed PMID: 17890317. Pubmed Central PMCID: PMC2000384. Epub 2007/09/25. eng
23. Xu H, Sun J, Shi C et al (2015) miR-29s inhibit the malignant behavior of U87MG glioblastoma cell line by targeting DNMT3A and 3B. Neurosci Lett 590:40–46. PubMed PMID: 25625222. Epub 2015/01/28. eng
24. Chen D, Guo W, Qiu Z et al (2015) MicroRNA-30d-5p inhibits tumour cell proliferation and motility by directly targeting CCNE2 in non-small cell lung cancer. Cancer Lett 362(2):208–217. PubMed PMID: 25843294. Epub 2015/04/07. Eng
25. Majid S, Dar AA, Saini S et al (2013) miRNA-34b inhibits prostate cancer through demethylation, active chromatin modifications, and AKT pathways. Clin Cancer Res 19(1):73–84. PubMed PMID: 23147995. Pubmed Central PMCID: PMC3910324. Epub 2012/11/14. Eng
26. Wang AM, Huang TT, Hsu KW et al (2014) Yin Yang 1 is a target of microRNA-34 family and contributes to gastric carcinogenesis. Oncotarget 5(13):5002–5016. PubMed PMID: 24970812. Pubmed Central PMCID: PMC4148117. Epub 2014/06/28. eng
27. Goto Y, Kurozumi A, Nohata N et al (2016) The microRNA signature of patients with sunitinib failure: regulation of UHRF1 pathways by microRNA-101 in renal cell carcinoma. Oncotarget 7(37):59070–59086. PubMed PMID: 27487138. Epub 2016/08/04. Eng
28. Varambally S, Cao Q, Mani RS et al (2008) Genomic loss of microRNA-101 leads to overexpression of histone methyltransferase EZH2 in cancer. Science (New York, NY) 12;322(5908):1695–1699. PubMed PMID: 19008416. Pubmed Central PMCID: PMC2684823. Epub 2008/11/15. Eng
29. Yan F, Shen N, Pang J et al (2014) Restoration of miR-101 suppresses lung tumorigenesis through inhibition of DNMT3a-dependent DNA methylation. Cell Death Dis 5:e1413. PubMed PMID: 25210796. Pubmed Central PMCID: PMC4540207. Epub 2014/09/12. eng
30. Hsieh TH, Hsu CY, Tsai CF et al (2015) miR-125a-5p is a prognostic biomarker that targets HDAC4 to suppress breast tumorigenesis. Oncotarget 6(1):494–509. PubMed PMID: 25504437. Pubmed Central PMCID: PMC4381610. Epub 2014/12/17. eng
31. Zhu Z, Tang J, Wang J, Duan G, Zhou L, Zhou X (2016) MiR-138 acts as a tumor suppressor by targeting EZH2 and enhances cisplatin-induced apoptosis in osteosarcoma cells. PLoS One 11(3):e0150026. PubMed PMID: 27019355. Pubmed Central PMCID: PMC4809565. Epub 2016/03/29. eng
32. Li W, Jiang G, Zhou J et al (2014) Down-regulation of miR-140 induces EMT and promotes invasion by targeting slug in esophageal cancer. Cell Physiol Biochem 34(5):1466–1476. PubMed PMID: 23147995. Pubmed Central PMCID: PMC3910324. Epub 2012/11/14. Eng

33. Xiao Q, Huang L, Zhang Z et al (2017) Overexpression of miR-140 inhibits proliferation of osteosarcoma cells via suppression of histone deacetylase 4. Oncol Res 25(2):267–275. PubMed PMID: 27624383. Epub 2016/09/15. Eng

34. Yuan Y, Shen Y, Xue L, Fan H (2013) miR-140 suppresses tumor growth and metastasis of non-small cell lung cancer by targeting insulin-like growth factor 1 receptor. PLoS One 8(9):e73604. PubMed PMID: 23147995. Pubmed Central PMCID: PMC3910324. Epub 2012/11/14. Eng

35. Kojima S, Enokida H, Yoshino H et al (2014) The tumor-suppressive microRNA-143/145 cluster inhibits cell migration and invasion by targeting GOLM1 in prostate cancer. J Hum Genet 59(2):78–87. PubMed PMID: 24284362. Epub 2013/11/29. eng

36. Kurozumi A, Goto Y, Okato A, Ichikawa T, Seki N (2017) Aberrantly expressed microR-NAs in bladder cancer and renal cell carcinoma. J Hum Genet 62(1):49–56. PubMed PMID: 27357429. Epub 2016/07/01. Eng

37. Yoshino H, Enokida H, Itesako T et al (2013) Tumor-suppressive microRNA-143/145 cluster targets hexokinase-2 in renal cell carcinoma. Cancer Sci 104(12):1567–1574. PubMed PMID: 24033605. Epub 2013/09/17. eng

38. Su J, Liang H, Yao W et al (2014) MiR-143 and MiR-145 regulate IGF1R to suppress cell proliferation in colorectal cancer. PLoS One 9(12):e114420. PubMed PMID: 25474488. Pubmed Central PMCID: PMC4256231. Epub 2014/12/05. Eng

39. Ng EK, Tsang WP, Ng SS et al (2009) MicroRNA-143 targets DNA methyltransferases 3A in colorectal cancer. Br J Cancer 101(4):699–706. PubMed PMID: 19638978. Pubmed Central PMCID: PMC2736825. Epub 2009/07/30. eng

40. Xue G, Ren Z, Chen Y et al (2015) A feedback regulation between miR-145 and DNA methyltransferase 3b in prostate cancer cell and their responses to irradiation. Cancer Lett 361(1):121–127. PubMed PMID: 25749421. Epub 2015/03/10. eng

41. Matsushita R, Yoshino H, Enokida H et al (2016) Regulation of UHRF1 by dual-strand tumor-suppressor microRNA-145 (miR-145-5p and miR-145-3p): inhibition of bladder cancer cell aggressiveness. Oncotarget 7(19):28460–28487. PubMed PMID: 27072587. Epub 2016/04/14. Eng

42. Duursma AM, Kedde M, Schrier M, le Sage C, Agami R (2008) miR-148 targets human DNMT3b protein coding region. RNA (New York, NY) 14(5):872–877. PubMed PMID: 18367714. Pubmed Central PMCID: PMC2327368. Epub 2008/03/28. Eng

43. Braconi C, Huang N, Patel T (2010) MicroRNA-dependent regulation of DNA methyltransferase-1 and tumor suppressor gene expression by interleukin-6 in human malignant cholangiocytes. Hepatology (Baltimore, MD) 51(3):881–890. PubMed PMID: 20146264. Pubmed Central PMCID: PMC3902044. Epub 2010/02/11. Eng

44. Huang J, Wang Y, Guo Y, Sun S (2010) Down-regulated microRNA-152 induces aberrant DNA methylation in hepatitis B virus-related hepatocellular carcinoma by targeting DNA methyltransferase 1. Hepatology (Baltimore, MD) 52(1):60–70. PubMed PMID: 20578129. Epub 2010/06/26. Eng

45. Wang H, Tao T, Yan W et al (2015) Upregulation of miR-181s reverses mesenchymal transition by targeting KPNA4 in glioblastoma. Sci Rep 5:13072. PubMed PMID: 26283154. Pubmed Central PMCID: PMC4539550. Epub 2015/08/19. Eng

46. Zhou WY, Chen JC, Jiao TT, Hui N, Qi X (2015) MicroRNA-181 targets Yin Yang 1 expression and inhibits cervical cancer progression. Mol Med Rep 11(6):4541–4546. PubMed PMID: 25672374. Epub 2015/02/13. eng

47. Lai TH, Ewald B, Zecevic A et al (2016) HDAC inhibition induces microRNA-182, which targets RAD51 and impairs HR repair to sensitize cells to sapacitabine in acute myelogenous leukemia. Clin Cancer Res 22(14):3537–3549. PubMed PMID: 26858310. Pubmed Central PMCID: PMC4947457. Epub 2016/02/10. Eng

48. Sun J, Ji J, Huo G, Song Q, Zhang X (2015) miR-182 induces cervical cancer cell apoptosis through inhibiting the expression of DNMT3a. Int J Clin Exp Pathol 8(5):4755–4763. PubMed PMID: 26191165. Pubmed Central PMCID: PMC4503037. Epub 2015/07/21. Eng

49. Zhang Z, Tang H, Wang Z et al (2011) MiR-185 targets the DNA methyltransferases 1 and regulates global DNA methylation in human glioma. Mol Cancer 10:124. PubMed PMID: 23147995. Pubmed Central PMCID: PMC3910324. Epub 2012/11/14. Eng

50. Dimri M, Kang M, Dimri GP (2016) A miR-200c/141-BMI1 autoregulatory loop regulates oncogenic activity of BMI1 in cancer cells. Oncotarget 7(24):36220–36234. PubMed PMID: 27105531. Epub 2016/04/23. Eng

51. Wu WR, Sun H, Zhang R et al (2016) Methylation-associated silencing of miR-200b facilitates human hepatocellular carcinoma progression by directly targeting BMI1. Oncotarget 7(14):18684–18693. PubMed PMID: 26919246. Pubmed Central PMCID: PMC4951320. Epub 2016/02/27. Eng

52. Wada R, Akiyama Y, Hashimoto Y, Fukamachi H, Yuasa Y (2010) miR-212 is downregulated and suppresses methyl-CpG-binding protein MeCP2 in human gastric cancer. Int J Cancer 127(5):1106–1114. PubMed PMID: 20020497. Epub 2009/12/19. eng

53. Nan X, Campoy FJ, Bird A (1997) MeCP2 is a transcriptional repressor with abundant binding sites in genomic chromatin. Cell 88(4):471–481. PubMed PMID: 9038338. Epub 1997/02/21. Eng

54. Tong D, Zhao L, He K et al (2016) MECP2 promotes the growth of gastric cancer cells by suppressing miR- 338-mediated antiproliferative effect. Oncotarget 7(23):34845–34859. PubMed PMID: 27166996. Epub 2016/05/12. Eng

55. Wu ZS, Wu Q, Wang CQ et al (2011) miR-340 inhibition of breast cancer cell migration and invasion through targeting of oncoprotein c-Met. Cancer 117(13):2842–2852. PubMed PMID: 21692045. Epub 2011/06/22. Eng

56. Shi L, Chen ZG, Wu LL et al (2014) miR-340 reverses cisplatin resistance of hepatocellular carcinoma cell lines by targeting Nrf2-dependent antioxidant pathway. Asian Pac J Cancer Prev 15(23):10439–10444. PubMed PMID: 25556489. Epub 2015/01/06. Eng

57. Sun Y, Zhao X, Zhou Y, Hu Y (2012) miR-124, miR-137 and miR-340 regulate colorectal cancer growth via inhibition of the Warburg effect. Oncol Rep 28(4):1346–1352. PubMed PMID: 22895557. Epub 2012/08/17. Eng

58. Yu W, Zhang G, Lu B et al (2016) MiR-340 impedes the progression of laryngeal squamous cell carcinoma by targeting EZH2. Gene 577(2):193–201. PubMed PMID: 26656176. Epub 2015/12/15. eng

59. Grady WM, Parkin RK, Mitchell PS et al (2008) Epigenetic silencing of the intronic microRNA hsa-miR-342 and its host gene EVL in colorectal cancer. Oncogene 27(27):3880–3888. PubMed PMID: 18264139. Epub 2008/02/12. Eng

60. Wang H, Wu J, Meng X et al (2011) MicroRNA-342 inhibits colorectal cancer cell proliferation and invasion by directly targeting DNA methyltransferase 1. Carcinogenesis 32(7): 1033–1042. PubMed PMID: 21565830. Epub 2011/05/14. Eng

61. Jin Y, Peng D, Shen Y et al (2013) MicroRNA-376c inhibits cell proliferation and invasion in osteosarcoma by targeting to transforming growth factor-alpha. DNA Cell Biol 32(6): 302–309. PubMed PMID: 23631646. Epub 2013/05/02. Eng

62. Jiang W, Tian Y, Jiang S, Liu S, Zhao X, Tian D (2016) MicroRNA-376c suppresses non-small-cell lung cancer cell growth and invasion by targeting LRH-1-mediated Wnt signaling pathway. Biochem Biophys Res Commun 473(4):980–986. PubMed PMID: 27049310. Epub 2016/04/07. Eng

63. Deng Y, Xiong Y, Liu Y (2016) miR-376c inhibits cervical cancer cell proliferation and invasion by targeting BMI1. Int J Exp Pathol 97(3):257–265. PubMed PMID: 27345009. Pubmed Central PMCID: PMC4960580. Epub 2016/06/28. eng

64. Zehavi L, Avraham R, Barzilai A et al (2012) Silencing of a large microRNA cluster on human chromosome 14q32 in melanoma: biological effects of mir-376a and mir-376c on insulin growth factor 1 receptor. Mol Cancer 11:44. PubMed PMID: 22747855. Pubmed Central PMCID: PMC3444916. Epub 2012/07/04. Eng

65. Noonan EJ, Place RF, Pookot D et al (2009) miR-449a targets HDAC-1 and induces growth arrest in prostate cancer. Oncogene 28(14):1714–1724. PubMed PMID: 19252524. Epub 2009/03/03. eng

66. Jeon HS, Lee SY, Lee EJ et al (2012) Combining microRNA-449a/b with a HDAC inhibitor has a synergistic effect on growth arrest in lung cancer. Lung Cancer (Amsterdam, Netherlands) 76(2):171–176. PubMed PMID: 22078727. Epub 2011/11/15. Eng

67. Liu L, Chen K, Wu J et al (2013) Downregulation of miR-452 promotes stem-like traits and tumorigenicity of gliomas. Clin Cancer Res 19(13):3429–3438. PubMed PMID: 23695168. Pubmed Central PMCID: PMC3725315. Epub 2013/05/23. Eng

68. He Z, Xia Y, Pan C et al (2015) Up-regulation of MiR-452 inhibits metastasis of non-small cell lung cancer by regulating BMI1. Cell Physiol Biochem 37(1):387–398. PubMed PMID: 26316085. Epub 2015/09/01. eng

69. Goto Y, Kojima S, Kurozumi A et al (2016) Regulation of E3 ubiquitin ligase-1 (WWP1) by microRNA-452 inhibits cancer cell migration and invasion in prostate cancer. Br J Cancer 114(10):1135–1144. PubMed PMID: 27070713. Pubmed Central PMCID: PMC4865980. Epub 2016/04/14. eng

70. Sun Y, Hu L, Zheng H et al (2015) MiR-506 inhibits multiple targets in the epithelial-to-mesenchymal transition network and is associated with good prognosis in epithelial ovarian cancer. J Pathol 235(1):25–36. PubMed PMID: 25230372. Pubmed Central PMCID: PMC4268369. Epub 2014/09/18. Eng

71. Wen SY, Lin Y, Yu YQ et al (2015) miR-506 acts as a tumor suppressor by directly targeting the hedgehog pathway transcription factor Gli3 in human cervical cancer. Oncogene 34(6):717–725. PubMed PMID: 24608427. Epub 2014/03/13. Eng

72. Zhang Y, Lin C, Liao G et al (2015) MicroRNA-506 suppresses tumor proliferation and metastasis in colon cancer by directly targeting the oncogene EZH2. Oncotarget 6(32):32586–32601. PubMed PMID: 26452129. Pubmed Central PMCID: PMC4741714. Epub 2015/10/10. eng

73. Jiang B, Li Z, Zhang W et al (2014) miR-874 Inhibits cell proliferation, migration and invasion through targeting aquaporin-3 in gastric cancer. J Gastroenterol 49(6):1011–1025. PubMed PMID: 23800944. Epub 2013/06/27. Eng

74. Zhang X, Tang J, Zhi X et al (2015) miR-874 functions as a tumor suppressor by inhibiting angiogenesis through STAT3/VEGF-A pathway in gastric cancer. Oncotarget 6(3):1605–1617. PubMed PMID: 25596740. Pubmed Central PMCID: PMC4359318. Epub 2015/01/19. Eng

75. Han J, Liu Z, Wang N, Pan W (2016) MicroRNA-874 inhibits growth, induces apoptosis and reverses chemoresistance in colorectal cancer by targeting X-linked inhibitor of apoptosis protein. Oncol Rep 36(1):542–550. PubMed PMID: 27221209. Epub 2016/05/26. Eng

76. Zhang LQ, Sun SL, Li WY et al (2015) Decreased expression of tumor suppressive miR-874 and its clinical significance in human osteosarcoma. Genet Mol Res 14(4):18315–18324. PubMed PMID: 26782479. Epub 2016/01/20. Eng

77. Nohata N, Hanazawa T, Kikkawa N et al (2011) Tumour suppressive microRNA-874 regulates novel cancer networks in maxillary sinus squamous cell carcinoma. Br J Cancer 105(6):833–841. PubMed PMID: 21847129. Pubmed Central PMCID: PMC3171017. Epub 2011/08/19. Eng

78. Nohata N, Hanazawa T, Kinoshita T et al (2013) Tumour-suppressive microRNA-874 contributes to cell proliferation through targeting of histone deacetylase 1 in head and neck squamous cell carcinoma. Br J Cancer 108(8):1648–1658. PubMed PMID: 23558898. Pubmed Central PMCID: PMC3668462. Epub 2013/04/06. eng

Genomic Imprinting Syndromes and Cancer

Ken Higashimoto, Keiichiro Joh, and Hidenobu Soejima

Abstract Genomic imprinting is an epigenetic phenomenon that leads to parent-specific differential expression of a subset of mammalian genes. Some imprinted genes are expressed from the maternal allele and repressed on the paternal allele, whereas others are expressed from the paternal and not the maternal allele. Because most imprinted genes play important roles in growth and development, and metabolism, the aberrant expression of imprinted genes due to epigenetic or genetic alterations often causes human disorders. These include genomic imprinting syndromes and tumors. Since loss of imprinting (LOI) of *IGF2* (which means biallelic expression of *IGF2*) was first reported in Wilms tumor in 1993, aberrant methylation of differentially methylated regions (DMRs), which regulate expression of imprinted genes and/or aberrant expression of imprinted genes, have been reported in various tumors. In this section, general imprinting mechanisms, representative clinical features and causative molecular alterations of eight imprinting syndromes are described. In addition, representative molecular alterations of imprinted DMRs or imprinted genes associated with tumors are also described.

Keywords Genomic imprinting • Imprinting syndromes • Imprinted genes • Differentially methylated regions (DMRs) • Imprinting control regions (ICRs)

1 Genomic Imprinting

1.1 Genomic Imprinting and Human Disorders

Genomic imprinting is an epigenetic phenomenon that leads to parent-specific differential expression of a subset of mammalian genes. Some imprinted genes are expressed from the maternal allele and repressed on the paternal allele, whereas others are expressed from the paternal not maternal allele. Because most imprinted

K. Higashimoto • K. Joh • H. Soejima (✉)
Division of Molecular Genetics & Epigenetics, Department of Biomolecular Sciences, Saga University, 5-1-1 Nabeshima, Saga 849-8501, Japan
e-mail: soejimah@cc.saga-u.ac.jp

© Springer International Publishing AG 2017
A. Kaneda, Y.-i. Tsukada (eds.), *DNA and Histone Methylation as Cancer Targets*, Cancer Drug Discovery and Development, DOI 10.1007/978-3-319-59786-7_11

genes play important roles in the growth and development of embryos, placental formation, and metabolism, the aberrant expression of imprinted genes due to epigenetic or genetic alterations often cause human disorders, such as genomic imprinting syndromes and tumors [2, 220]. In addition, recent studies show that imprinted genes are involved in wide biological phenomena, such as feeding, maintenance of body temperature, neurological and behavioral processes, sleep, and stem cell maintenance and renewal. These indicate that altered expression of imprinted genes may influence the development of a wide-range of human disorders [181].

Genomic imprinting in mammals was identified by pronuclear transplantation experiments in the early 1980s [150, 214]. Such experiments indicated that maternal and paternal contributions to the mouse embryonic genome are not equivalent. It is noteworthy that ovarian teratoma developed by parthenogenesis and complete hydatidiform mole developed by androgenesis both also indicate separate contributions of the two parental genomes in humans. In 1991, three imprinted genes were firstly identified in mice. These include: insulin-like growth factor 2 (*Igf2*), insulin-like growth factor 2 receptor (*Igf2r*), and *H19*, a non-coding RNA. In humans, uniparental disomy was described as a new genetic concept in 1980 [50]. This was defined as the inheritance of two copies of a chromosome or part of a chromosome from one parent and no copies from the other parent. In addition, Prader-Willi syndrome (PWS) was identified as the first imprinting disorder in 1989 [170]. Thus far, eight genomic imprinting syndromes are known. These are: Beckwith-Wiedemann syndrome (BWS), Silver-Russell syndrome (SRS), Prader-Willi syndrome (PWS), Angelman syndromes (AS), Kagami-Ogata syndrome (KOS), Temple syndrome (TS), pseudohypoparathyroidism (PHP), and transient neonatal diabetes mellitus type 1 (TNDM1).

1.2   The Control of DNA Methylation Imprints

To date, approximately 150 imprinted genes have been identified in the mouse with approximately 70% conserved in humans. Many imprinted genes form clusters, or imprinting domains. The expression of imprinted genes within these domains is regulated by imprinting control regions (ICRs) [181, 209]. ICRs show differential methylation between the two parental alleles, forming so-called differentially methylated regions (DMRs). DMRs are classified into maternally and paternally methylated DMRs, as well as into gametic and somatic DMRs. Maternally methylated DMRs are methylated maternal alleles only, and not paternal alleles, and vice versa for paternally methylated DMRs. Gametic DMRs acquire DNA methylation in the maternal and paternal germ cells and most gametic DMRs are identical to ICRs. In contrast, methylations of somatic DMRs are established after fertilization in response to nearby gametic DMRs (ICRs) [55, 209].

To date, there are 28 known gametic DMRs (ICRs) in the mouse and 38 in humans [153]. DNA methylation of the genome, including DMRs, is erased in primordial germ cells (PGCs). After this, sex-specific methylation marks at DMRs

(ICRs) are acquired and established in developing germ cells. The establishment of methylation marks requires *de novo* DNA methyltransferase Dnmt3a and its regulatory factor Dnmt3l [18, 96]. In mouse developing oocytes, the Dnmt3a-Dnmt3l complex shows low affinity to H3K4me3, but interacts with unmethylated H3K4. This suggests that demethylation of H3K4 is a prerequisite for *de novo* DNA methylation at some ICRs [30, 176]. Transcription through the ICR regions would thus be critical for methylation acquisition in developing oocytes because transcription may make the chromatin more accessible via the Dnmt3a-Dnmt3l complex [29, 55].

After fertilization, zygotes undergo global demethylation until implantation. The paternal genome is rapidly demethylated, indicating an active mechanism associated with Tet3-mediated oxidation of 5 mC converting to 5 hmC [66]. The maternal genome is gradually demethylated due to a passive replication-dependent dilution mechanism. During the global demethylation, methylation of ICRs must be maintained. Dppa3 (also known as Pgc7 or Stella) is a factor protecting methylation of the maternal genome, including ICRs. Dppa3 recognizes and binds to H3K9me2 on the methylated ICRs and prevents them from Tet3-mediated demethylation [166, 236]. Dppa3 also protects paternally methylated ICRs, such as *H19*-DMR and *Rasgrf1*, in the mouse [166].

Zfp57 is another factor, which protects imprinted methylation. This KRAB zinc-finger protein binds to a methylated sequence, such as TGCCGC, and interacts with Trim28 (also known as Kap1) to recruit Dnmt1 and H3K9 methyltransferase Setdb1. This results in protection of methylated ICRs [125, 186]. In humans, homozygous recessive mutations of *ZFP57* have been found in TNDM1 patients. Such patients show loss of DNA methylation (LOM) at several ICRs other than *ZAC*-DMR, which is an ICR responsible for TNDM1 [138].

After implantation, the global DNA methylation level increases. Dnmt3b is a responsible *de novo* methyltransferase for this increase [153]. At this stage, it is important to protect unmethylated DMRs against *de novo* methylation. CTCF binds to unmethylated maternal *H19*-DMR and protects it from *de novo* methylation [51, 205]. Rex1/Zfp42 also protects *Peg3* and *Gnas* DMRs [131]. In addition, most unmethylated ICRs overlap promoter CpG islands with active transcription enriched with H3K4me3. Since H3K4me3 prevents binding of DNMT3L, which leads to impairment in *de novo* methylation, those ICRs may be protected [176]. Furthermore, formation of R-loops (double-stranded RNA-DNA structures forming on the transcribed DNA strand) on the unmethylated transcriptional active ICRs protects the unmethylated status against *de novo* DNA methylation by Dnmt3b in the early embryo [63].

1.3 Regulation of Imprinted Gene Expression by ICRs

Imprinting domains contain both maternally and paternally expressed genes, as well as genes that encode proteins and those that encode non-coding RNAs. Gene expression within the domains is also regulated by ICRs, as previously mentioned [181].

Maternally methylated ICRs are found at promoters of protein-coding genes or non-coding RNA genes, whereas paternally methylated ICRs are found in intergenic regions [55]. ICRs act in *cis* to express genes within the domains monoallelically. Although the precise mechanisms differ among loci, there are two principal models—the long non-coding RNA (lncRNA) model and the insulator model [181].

The lncRNA model is thought to implicate four imprinting domains: *Igf2r*, *Kcnq1ot1*, *Snrpn*, and *Gnas* [55, 181]. Maternally methylated ICRs at promoters repress lncRNAs, but unmethylated ICRs on the paternal alleles are active in transcription and repression of neighboring protein-coding genes in *cis*. The best characterized locus for the insulator model is *H19*-DMR. When CTCF binds to unmethylated *H19*-DMR on the maternal allele, it insulates the *Igf2* promoter from downstream enhancers, resulting in silencing of *Igf2* [14, 71].

2 Genomic Imprinting Syndromes

2.1 Beckwith-Wiedemann Syndrome

Beckwith-Wiedemann syndrome (BWS; OMIM 130650) is a model of imprinting disorder, which shows prenatal and postnatal macrosomia, macroglossia, abdominal wall defects, a predisposition to tumorigenesis, and other variable features. Incidence is approximately one in 13,700 live births [208]. The chromosomal locus for BWS is 11p15.5, which consists of two imprinting domains: *IGF2/H19* and *CDKN1C/KCNQ1OT1*. *H19*-DMR and *Kv*DMR1 are the ICRs for the *IGF2/ H19* and *CDKN1C/KCNQ1OT1* domains, respectively (Fig. 1a). The important genes in the *IGF2/H19* domain are insulin-like growth factor 2 (*IGF2*) and lncRNA, *H19*. *IGF2* is expressed from the paternal allele and *H19* is expressed from the maternal allele. For the *CDKN1C/KCNQ1OT1* domain, the important genes are *CDKN1C* and *KCNQ1OT1*. *CDKN1C* encodes cyclin-dependent kinase (CDK) inhibitor and shows preferential maternal expression. *KCNQ1OT1* is a paternally expressed gene encoding lncRNA.

So far, several causative alterations have been identified. These are gain of methylation (GOM) at *H19*-DMR (~5% of patients), loss of methylation (LOM) at *Kv*DMR1 (~50% of patients), paternal uniparental disomy (pUPD) encompassing 11p15.5 (~20% of patients), loss of function mutation of *CDKN1C* (~5% of patients), and chromosomal rearrangement involving 11p15.5 (<1% of patients). However, no alteration of 11p15.5 can be found for ~20% of BWS patients [209]. *H19*-DMR-GOM leads to biallelic expression, or *IGF2* LOI and reduced expression of *H19*. *Kv*DMR1-LOM leads to expression of *KCNQ1OT1* RNA, which in turn results in repression of *CDKN1C* expression on the maternal chromosome. In Sects. 3.1 and 3.2 the detailed molecular mechanisms of the domains are described. The minimal region of pUPD is 2.7 Mb from the 11p telomere, which includes both *H19*-DMR and *Kv*DMR1-LOM, leading to both *IGF2* LOI and silencing of *CDKN1C* [175].

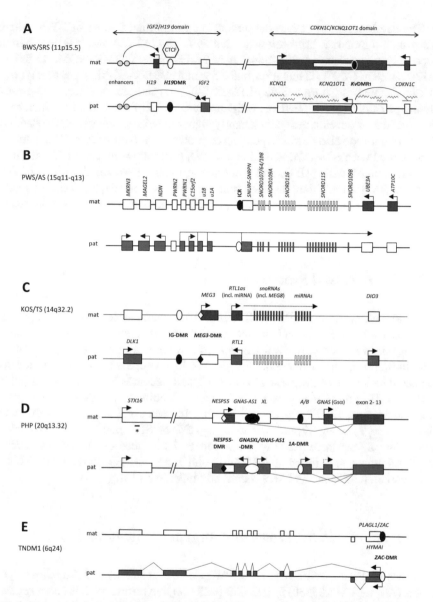

Fig. 1 Human imprinting domains and representative imprinted genes associated with imprinting syndromes. (**a**) Beckwith-Wiedemann syndrome (*BWS*)/Silver-Russell syndrome (*SRS*) locus at 11p15.5. The *IGF2/H19* domain is the best characterized domain for the insulator model. The *CDKN1C/KCNQ1OT1* domain is one of the representatives of the lncRNA model. Yellow circles: enhancers; wavy line: non-coding RNA transcribed from the paternal *KCNQ1OT1* gene. Blue: paternally expressed genes; red: maternally expressed genes; filled ovals: methylated gametic DMRs; open ovals: unmethylated gametic DMRs; filled diamonds: methylated somatic DMRs; open diamonds: unmethylated somatic DMRs. (**b**) Prader-Willi syndrome (*PWS*)/Angelman syndrome (*AS*) locus at 15q11-q13. (**c**) Kagami-Ogata syndrome (*KOS*)/Temple syndrome (*TS*) locus at 14q32.2. (**d**) Pseudohypoparathyroidism (*PHP*) locus at 20q13.32. *: a deleted region in familial PHP1b, suggesting the existence of a *cis* regulatory element for *A/B*-DMR methylation status. (**e**) Transient neonatal diabetes mellitus type 1 (TNDM1) locus at 6q24

The development of embryonal tumors is an important feature of BWS, where the overall tumor risk has been estimated at 7.4% [163]. Tumor risk is different depending on molecular alterations. It is 22.8% in *H19*-DMR-GOM, 13.8% in pUPD, 8.6% in *CDKN1C* mutation, and 2.5% in *Kv*DMR1-LOM. A specific type of pUPD, denoted as genome-wide pUPD (GWpUPD) mosaic, has been recognized among patients of pUPD. Patients with mosaic GWpUPD showed a high incidence (81%) of tumor development, significantly higher than in segmental pUPD patients [175]. Tumor type also differs depending on molecular alteration, e.g. Wilms tumor is associated with *H19*-DMR-GOM and pUPD, hepatoblastoma and adrenal carcinoma associated with pUPD, and neuroblastic tumors associated with *CDKN1C* mutation [163]. In addition, there are reports of altered gene expressions and methylation status of DMRs in many tumors (Table 1). These alterations are described in detail in Sects. 3.1 and 3.2.

2.2   Silver-Russell Syndrome

Silver-Russell syndrome (SRS; OMIM 180860) is characterized by clinical phenotypes opposite to BWS, such as intrauterine growth restriction, poor postnatal growth, relative macrocephaly, triangular face, asymmetry, and feeding difficulties [46]. Incidence is one in 100,000. SRS patients do not appear to have a significantly increased incidence of neoplasia [197]. *H19*-DMR becomes hypomethylated (*H19*-DMR-LOM) in more than 45% of SRS patients, leading to increased *H19* expression and decreased *IGF2* expression [46] (Fig. 1a). Maternal uniparental disomy of chromosome 7, or upd(7)mat, is found in 4.5% of SRS patients. The disturbed expression of imprinted genes on chromosome 7 has been estimated and several imprinted genes were found at 7p11.2-p13 and 7q31-qter. However, the molecular link between upd(7)mat and SRS is currently unknown [46].

2.3   Prader-Willi Syndrome and Angelman Syndrome

Incidence of Prader-Willi syndrome (PWS; OMIM 176270) and Angelman syndrome (AS; OMIM 105830) is 1:15,000–1:25,000 live births. PWS is characterized by severe hypotonia and feeding difficulties in early infancy, followed in later infancy or early childhood by excessive eating and gradual development of morbid obesity [23]. The evaluation of the cancer risk using the PWS registry in the US showed an increased risk of myeloid leukemia, but not other cancers [39]. AS is characterized by microcephaly, gait ataxia, severe mental retardation, and absent or severely limited speech [23]. Tumor development in AS has been rarely reported.

These two distinct disorders develop as a result of imprinting disruption of 15q11-q13 (Fig. 1b). ICR is maternally methylated and regulates expression of the genes within this region [23]. Approximately 70% of patients with PWS show

Table 1 Aberrantly methylated DMRs in tumors

Chromosomal location	Imprinted locus	DMR	Normally methylated allele	Aberrant methylation	Tumor	Refs
1p31.3	DIRAS3 (ARHI)	DIRAS3-DMRs	Mat	Hyper	Breast cancer	[12, 53, 248]
					Follicular thyroid carcinoma	[233]
					Hepatocellular carcinoma	[80]
					Oligodendroglioma	[190]
				Hypo	Ovarian cancer	[54]
					Breast cancer	[12, 248]
2q33.3	ZDBF2	ZDBF2-DMR	Pat	Hypo	Hepatoblastoma	[196]
4q22.1	NAP1L5	NAP1L5-DMR	Mat	Hyper	Hepatoblastoma	[196]
5q31	nc886	nc886	Mat	Hyper	Hepatoblastoma	[196]
					Bladder cancer	[195]
					Breast cancer	[195]
					Colon cancer	[195]
					Lung cancer	[195]
				Hypo	Bladder cancer	[195]
					Breast cancer	[195]
					Colon cancer	[195]
					Lung cancer	[195]
6q24	ZAC/PLAGL1	ZAC-DMR	Mat	Hyper	Ovarian cancer	[91]
				Hypo	Diffuse large B-cell lymphoma	[224]
					Diffuse large B-cell lymphoma	[224]
6p25.2	FAM50B	FSM50B-DMR	Mat	Hypo	Testicular germ cell tumor	[249]
6q25.3	IGF2R	IGF2R-DMR (Region2)	Mat	Hypo	Osteosarcoma	[202]

(continued)

Table 1 (continued)

Chromosomal location	Imprinted locus	DMR	Normally methylated allele	Aberrant methylation	Tumor	Refs
7p12.1	GRB10	GRB10-DMR	Mat	Hypo	Ovarian cancer	[83]
				Hyper	Breast cancer	[12]
				Hypo	Breast cancer	[12]
7q32.2	MEST	MEST-DMR	Mat	Hyper	Breast cancer	[12]
					Dermoid cyst	[191]
					Glioblastoma multiforme	[146]
				Hypo	Breast cancer	[12]
					Testicular type I teratoma	[191]
					Seminoma	[191]
7q21.3	PEG10	PEG10-DMR	Mat	Hypo	Hepatoblastoma	[196]
10q26.1	INPP5F	INPP5Fv2-DMR	Mat	Hyper	Hepatoblastoma	[196]
11p13	WT1	WT1-AS-DMR		Hyper	Hepatoblastoma	[196]
11p15.5	CDKN1C/KCNQ1OT1	KvDMR1	Mat	Hyper	Breast cancer	[194]
					Colorectal cancer	[167]
					Ovalian teratoma	[4]
					Yolk sac tumor	[4]
				Hypo	Breast cancer	[12, 194, 204]
					Cervical carcinoma	[204]
					Colorectal cancer	[167]
					Esophageal cancer	[210]
					Extragonadal teratoma	[4]
					Gastric carcinoma	[204]
					Germ cell tumor	[4]

					Cancer	Ref
11p15.5	IGF2/H19	CDKN1C promoter		Hyper	Hepatoblastoma	[196]
					Hepatocarcinoma	[204]
					Teratoma	[4]
					Vulva carcinoma	[204]
					Wilms tumor	[201, 204]
					Acute lymphocytic leukemia	[207]
					Acute myeloid leukemia	[103]
					Breast cancer	[107]
					Diffuse large B-cell lymphoma (DLBCL)	[69, 118, 130]
					Follicular lymphoma	[130]
					Gastric cancer	[103]
					Hepatocellular cancer	[103]
					Leukemia	[111]
					Lung cancer	[107]
					Malignant mesothelioma	[107]
					Pancreatic cancer	[103]
		PHLDA2 promoter		Hypo	B cell lymphoma	[184]
				Hypo	Osteosarcoma	[128]
		H19-DMR	Pat	Hyper	Osteosarcoma	[127]
				Hyper	Adrenal tumor	[171]
					Breast cancer	[12]
					Choriocarcinoma	[9]
					Colo-rectal cancer	[165]
					Germ cell tumor	[84, 60, 191]
					Head-and-neck squamouse cell carcinoma	[40]

(continued)

Table 1 (continued)

Chromosomal location	Imprinted locus	DMR	Normally methylated allele	Aberrant methylation	Tumor	Refs
					Hepatoblastoma	(Li 1998; Honda 2008; Rumbajan 2013)
					Hepatocellular carcinoma	[237]
					Osteosarcoma	[223]
					Ovarian carcinoma	[38]
					Prostate hyperplasia	[179]
					Wilms tumor	[16, 25, 34, 61, 162, 164, 201, 247]
				Hypo	Bladder cancer	[12, 160, 215]
					Cervical carcinoma	[44]
					Colorectal cancer	[28, 35]
					Dermoid cyst	[191]
					Germ cell tumor	[4, 60, 84, 100]
					Hepatocellular carcinoma	[237]
					Lung cancer	[109]
					Malignant mixed Müllerian tumor	[72]
					Osteosarcoma	[128, 223]
					Rhabdmyosarcoma	[137]
					Synovial sarcoma	[213]

Region	Parental origin	Methylation	Cancer type	References
H19 promoter	Pat	Hyper	Teratoma	[4, 191]
		Hypo	Hepatoblastoma	[196]
IGF2-DMR0	Pat	Hyper	Hepatocellular carcinoma	[114]
			Lung cancer	[109]
			Adrenal tumor	[171]
			Breast cancer	[86, 87]
			Leukemia	[86]
			Lung cancer	[86]
			Esophageal cancer	[239]
		Hypo	Bladder cancer	[24]
			Breast cancer	[12, 86, 87]
			Colorectal cancer	[11, 28, 35, 86, 87]
			Esophageal squamous cell carcinoma	[157]
			Gastrinoma	[42]
			Hepatoblastoma	[52, 126, 185, 196]
			Non-functioning pancreatic endocrine tumor (PET)	[42]
			Osteosarcoma	[129]
			Ovarian cancer	[38, 158]
			Wilms tumor	[162, 212]
IGF2-DMR2	Pat	Hyper	Breast cancer	[86]
			Colorectal cancer	[86]
			Hepatoblastoma	[196]

(continued)

Table 1 (continued)

Chromosomal location	Imprinted locus	DMR	Normally methylated allele	Aberrant methylation	Tumor	Refs
					Leukemia	[86]
					Lung cancer	[86]
					Insulinoma	[42]
				Hypo	Adrenal tumor	[171]
					Breast cancer	[12]
					Hepatoblastoma	[196]
		IGF2-DMR[a]	Pat	Hypo	Teratoma	[4]
				Hypo	Germ cell tumor	[4]
13q14.2	RB1	CpG85	Mat	Hyper	Hepatoblastoma	[196]
					Hepatocellular carcinoma	[7]
					Retinoblastoma	[49]
				Hypo	Hepatocellular carcinoma	[7]
14q32.2	DLK1/DIO3	IG-DMR	Pat	Hyper	Cholangiocarcinoma	[5]
					Giant Cell Tumor of bone	[119]
					Hepatoblastoma	[196]
					Hepatocellular carcinoma	[6, 81]
					Meningioma	[250]
					Neuroblastoma	[10]
					Phaeochromocytoma	[10]
					Pituitary tumor	[62]
					Renal cell carcinoma	[99]
					Wilms tumor	[10]
				Hypo	Hepatocellular carcinoma	[6]

Location	Gene	DMR	Parent	Methylation	Tumor	Reference
		MEG3-DMR	Pat	Hyper	Colorectal adenoma	[151]
					Hepatoblastoma	[196]
					Hepatocellular carcinoma	[6]
					Meningioma	[250]
					Neuroblastoma	[10]
					Pheochromocytoma	[10]
					Pituitary tumor	[252]
					Wilms tumor	[10]
15q11.2	SNRPN/SNURF	SNRPN-DMR	Mat	Hypo	Hepatocellular carcinoma	[6]
				Hyper	Acute myeloid leukemia	[15]
					Germ cell tumor	[84, 60]
					Ovarian teratoma	[4]
				Hypo	Biparental complete hydatidifrom mole	[48]
					Breast cancer	[12]
					Extragonadal teratoma	[4]
					Germ cell tumor	[4, 60, 84, 117, 191]
					Hepatocellular carcinoma	[114]
					Ovarian teratoma	[4]
15q26.3	IRAIN	IRAIN promoter	Unknown	Hypo	Breast cancer	[97]
17q13.1	(pri-miR)-497/195	(pri-miR)-497/195 promoter	Unknown	Hyper	Hepatocellular carcinoma	[114]

(continued)

Table 1 (continued)

Chromosomal location	Imprinted locus	DMR	Normally methylated allele	Aberrant methylation	Tumor	Refs
19q13.4	PEG3	PEG3-DMR	Mat	Hyper	Breast cancer	[12]
					Glioma	[140, 177]
					Ovarian cancer	[45, 54, 64]
					Ovarian teratoma	[4]
					Yolk sac tumor	[4]
				Hypo	Biparental complete hydatidifrom mole	[48]
					Breast cancer	[12]
					Extragonadal teratoma	[4]
					Germinoma	[4]
20q11.21	MCTS2P	MCTS2P-DMR	Mat	Hypo	Hepatoblastoma	[196]
20q11.23	NNAT	NNAT-DMR	Mat	Hyper	Acute myeloid leukaemia	[112]
					Pituitary adenoma	[189]
20q13.12	L3MBTL	L3MBTL-DMR	Mat	Hyper	Myeloid malignancy	[121]
				Hypo	Myeloid malignancy	[121]
20q13.32	GNAS	NESP55-DMR	Pat	Hyper	Biparental complete hydatidifrom mole	[48]
				Hypo	Hepatoblastoma	[196]
		GNAS-AS1-DMR	Mat	Hyper	Colorectal adenoma	[151]
				Hypo	Colorectal adenoma	[151]
		XLαs-DMR	Mat	Hyper	Hepatoblastoma	[196]
		A/B-DMR	Mat	Hypo	Hepatoblastoma	[196]

aThe precise location of this DMR is not described in the reference

5–7 Mb *de novo* interstitial deletion of paternal 15q11-q13. In addition, PWS develops as a result of maternal uniparental disomy 15 (upd(15)mat) (20–30%) and GOM at the ICR (1–3%). These alterations lose or reduce the expression of paternal genes, including *SNORD116*, which is a probable major gene contributing to the PWS phenotype [41, 198]. As for AS, maternal deletion of 15q11-q13 (70%), paternal uniparental disomy (15upd(15)pat) (3–7%), LOM at the ICR (2–4%), and mutation in the *UBE3A* (10%) are found. A causative gene, *UBE3A*, which is expressed from the maternal allele in the brain, is inactivated by the alterations [23, 106].

2.4 Kagami-Ogata Syndrome and Temple Syndrome

Since chromosome 14q32.2 harbors an imprinting domain, paternal uniparental disomy 14 (upd(14)pat) results in Kagami–Ogata syndrome (KOS, OMIM 608149) and maternal uniparental disomy 14 (upd(14)mat) results in Temple syndrome (TS, OMIM 616222). This domain contains three paternally expressed protein-coding genes and numerous maternally expressed genes that encode noncoding RNAs (Fig. 1c). The IG-DMR and the *MEG3*-DMR are paternally methylated and function as ICRs for the domain [173].

The two disorders are very rare with approximately 50 reported patients for each syndrome [85, 173].

KOS shows unique phenotypic features, which include increased coat-hanger angle to the ribs and decreased ratio of the mid to widest thorax diameter, abdominal wall defects, prenatal overgrowth/overweight, and developmental delay. The ribs and thorax abnormalities are detectable by chest roentgenogram. KOS is developed as a result of upd(14)pat (65%), deletion of maternal 14q32.2 (19%), and GOM at the IG-DMR and the *MEG3*-DMR (19%). These alterations induce the excessive *RTL1* expression and reduced expression of maternally expressed genes, which are the primary underlying factors for phenotypic development [173]. Hepatoblastoma has been identified in three infantile patients with KOS, which invariably occurred before 4 years of age [173]. Aberrant methylations of DMRs within this imprinted region were reported in several tumors (Table 1), which are described in Sect. 3.3.

The cardinal features of TS are low birth weight, hypotonia and motor delay, feeding problems early in life, early puberty onset, and significantly reduced final height. Many of the clinical features are nonspecific, making diagnosis difficult [85]. Tumor development has been rarely reported in TS. TS is developed by upd(14)mat (70–80%), microdeletion of paternal 14q32.2 (~12%), and LOM at the IG-DMR and the *MEG3*-DMR (~12%). Such alterations decrease *DLK1* and *RTL1* expression, which both play a major role in the development of TS phenotypes [85, 90].

2.5 Pseudohypoparathyroidism

Pseudohypoparathyroidism (PHP) is an endocrine disorder characterized by resistance to the parathyroid hormone. The GNAS locus at 20q13.32, a disease locus for PHP, is imprinted and contains three protein coding transcripts. These are: the *GNAS* gene encoding α–subunit of heterotrimeric guanine nucleotide-binding protein (Gsα), extra large Gsα (XL*αs*), neuroendocrine secretory protein 55 (NESP55). And two noncoding RNAs, including the *A/B* transcript and an antisense *GNAS* transcript (*GNAS-AS1*) are also contained in this locus (Fig. 1d). The imprinted expressions are regulated by multiple DMRs (see Sect. 3.4). *GNAS* is a tissue-specific imprinted gene showing maternal expression in renal proximal tubules, thyroid, gonads, hypothalamus, and pituitary. There are several disorders associated with *GNAS* mutations or defective imprinting. These are pseudohypoparathyroidism type 1A (PHP1a, OMIM 103580), PHP1b (OMIM 603233), pseudo-PHP (PPHP, OMIM 612463), progressive osseous heteroplasia (POH; OMIM 166350), and McCune-Albright syndrome (MAS; OMIM 174800) [101, 144]. Of these, PHP1a and PHP1b are related to genomic imprinting. PHP1a is caused by maternally transmitted inactivating mutations of *GNAS*, resulting in loss of function in imprinted tissues. Sporadic PHP1b is caused by LOM at *A/B*-DMR, which is normally methylated on the maternal allele. The LOM induces expression of *A/B* transcript, resulting in suppression of *GNAS*. Familial PHP1b shows a microdeletion within the maternal *STX16* gene, which is located approximately 220 Kb upstream of *A/B*-DMR (Fig. 1d). The deletion induces LOM at *A/B*-DMR, which also results in suppression of *GNAS*. PPHP and POH are caused by paternally transmitted inactivating mutations of *GNAS*, and results in haploinsufficiency in non-imprinted tissues. MAS is caused by activating mutations of *GNAS*. Several cancers including bone, thyroid, testicular, and breast have been reported in MAS [19]. Aberrant methylations of DMRs within the *GNAS* locus were reported in several tumors (Table 1), which are described in Sect. 3.4.

2.6 Transient Neonatal Diabetes Mellitus Type 1

Transient neonatal diabetes mellitus type 1 (TNDM1; OMIM #601410) is a subtype of neonatal diabetes. It presents as hyperglycemia that begins in the neonatal period and resolves by age 18 months, as well as dehydration, absence of ketoacidosis, and intrauterine growth retardation [139]. Approximately 50% of TNDM1 patients relapse diabetes in adolescence or early adulthood. Its incidence was estimated at 1:215,000 to 1:400,000 births [216]. TNDM1 is caused by overexpression of the imprinted genes *PLAGL1/ZAC*, which encode a transcription factor and *HYMAI*, a non-coding RNA, on chromosome 6q24. It is due to paternal uniparental disomy of chromosome 6 (40%), duplication of the imprinted region at 6q24 (32%), and maternal hypomethylation of the ZAC-DMR (28%), which is normally methylated on the maternal allele (Fig. 1e). Tumor development in TNDM1 has not been reported, however, *PLAGL1* is downregulated in cancers, including breast, ovarian and cervical cancer, hepatocellular carcinoma (HCC), and squamous cell carcinoma of the head and neck [1].

3 Imprinted Genes and Cancer

As previously mentioned, imprinted genes play an important role in growth and development. Disruption of imprinting due to aberrant methylation of DMRs and/or aberrant expression of imprinted genes is associated with tumor growth. Indeed, global loss of imprinting is associated with increased tumorigenesis in mice [77]. In humans, loss of imprinting (LOI) of *IGF2*, which is the same as biallelic expression of *IGF2*, was first reported in Wilms tumor in 1993 [174, 187]. *IGF2* LOI in Wilms tumor has been associated with hypermethylation of *H19*-DMR [155, 211]. *IGF2* LOI is also reported in many adult tumors [31]. To date, aberrant methylation of DMRs and/or aberrant expression of imprinted genes occurs in various tumors from individuals lacking imprinting disorders [181]. Aberrant methylation of DMRs involved in tumors is summarized in Table 1. In this section, representative imprinted domains or DMRs associated with tumors are described.

3.1 IGF2/H19

3.1.1 The Regulation of the Imprinted *IGF2/ H19* Domain

The *IGF2/H19* domain is one of the firstly identified imprinted domains. The ICR of this domain is *H19*-DMR, located upstream of *H19*, and is DNA methylated on paternal but not maternal allele. For unmethylated maternal *H19*-DMR, the CTCF insulator protein can successfully bind as a result of methylation sensitive binding to *H19*-DMR. In maternal allele, the existence of CTCF at *H19*-DMR blocks access of enhancers downstream of *H19* to the *IGF2* promoters. This instead activates the *H19* promoter, resulting in maternal *H19* expression. Conversely, in paternal allele, *IGF2* is activated by allowing the promoters to access the enhancers due to the unbound of CTCF on methylated *H19*-DMR, resulting in paternal *IGF2* expression [74] (Fig. 1a).

The CTCF also involves the formation of chromatin looping in addition to insulator function. Studies of chromosome conformation capture (3C) show that, depending on the methylation status of *H19*-DMR, *H19*-DMR alters interaction regions, such as *Igf2*-DMR1, DMR2, or *Igf2* promoters, and *Igf2/H19* domain forms allele specific chromatin-looping that regulates the expression of *Igf2* and *H19* [113, 161, 243]. Furthermore, interaction between CTCF bound maternal *H19*-DMR and *Igf2* promoters forms chromatin-loop and polycomb repressive complex 2 (PRC2)

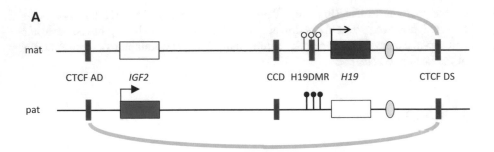

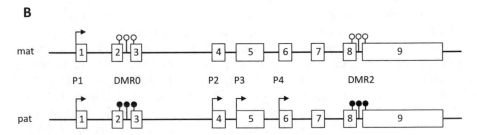

Fig. 2 (**a**) Simplified model of CTCF/cohesin complex mediated interactions in the human *IGF2/H19* domain. The CTCF/cohesin binding region and enhancer are indicated by purple rectangles and yellow ovals, respectively. Methylated and unmethylated CpG dinucleotides regions are shown by black and open lollipops, respectively. On the maternal allele, unmethylated *H19*-DMR interacts with CTCF DS, resulting in maternal *H19* expression. Conversely, on the paternal allele, CTCF DS interacts with CTCF AD because methylated *H19*-DMR prevents CTCF binding, resulting in paternal *IGF2* expression. The allele specific chromatin-loops, formed by these interactions, regulate imprinted expression in this domain by bringing enhancers into the proximity of the promoters. The interaction between CTCF AD and CCD on both alleles is omitted. (**b**) Structure characteristics of the human *IGF2* gene. The nine exons of the *IGF2* gene are indicated by the numbered boxes and the promoters (P1–P4) are indicated by *arrows*. The transcripts from P2, P3, and P4 promoters are expressed from the paternal allele, whereas transcripts from P1 are expressed from both parental alleles. *IGF2*-DMR0 and DMR2 are methylated on the paternal allele

is recruited through the CTCF. This results in maternal specific histone H3 lysine 27 methylation (H3K27me) and represses maternal *Igf2* promoters [123]. Subsequently, genome-wide analyses of CTCF and cohesin, a ring-like protein complex, reveal that both proteins were largely co-localized [235]. Cohesin is required to stabilize CTCF-mediated chromatin-loop in the *IGF2/H19* domain [169].

Most of the above studies have been performed using mice. In human cells, novel CTCF/cohesin-binding sites, were identified at the upstream site of the *IGF2* gene (CTCF AD), upstream site of *H19*-DMR (CCD), and at the downstream site of the enhancer (CTCF DS) (Fig. 2a). CTCF/cohesin bound to all these sites on both alleles because they were unmethylated. 3C studies show that unmethylated *H19*-DMR interacted with CTCF DS on the maternal allele, while CTCF DS interacts with CTCF AD on the paternal allele. The allele specific chromatin-loop formed by these interactions regulates imprinted expression in this domain by bringing enhancers into the proximity of the promoters [168].

3.1.2 The Role of IGF2 in Cancer

IGF2 is a potent mitogenic growth factor, which is particularly important for embryonic and placental growth during embryogenesis [21]. IGF2 signals occur via the IGF1 receptor (IGF1R), insulin receptor isoform A (IR-A), and the IGF1R/ IR-A hybrid receptor. The binding of IGF2 to IGF1R activates the tyrosine kinase receptor. Tyrosine kinase phosphorylates two main substrates: the insulin receptor substrates (IRSs) and Src homologous and collagen (Shc). Phosphorylated IRSs recruit the phosphatidylinositol 3-kinase (PI3K) and activates the PI3K/AKT pathway. The PI3K/AKT pathway exerts a variety of functions, such as releasing the anti-apoptotic protein Bcl-2 from BAD, activating protein synthesis via mTOR and promoting glucose metabolism by inhibiting GSK-3β, which is implicated in preventing cell death [43]. Conversely, activating Shc by IGF1R stimulates the Ras/mitogen-activated protein (MAP) kinase pathway, resulting in increased cellular proliferation [43].

The upregulation of *IGF2*, observed in various tumors, is associated with promoting tumor development, tumor angiogenesis, drug resistance, and prognosis [21]. One cause of this upregulation is *IGF2* LOI, which occurs in childhood tumors (*e.g.*, Wilms tumor, rhabdomyosarcoma, and hepatoblastoma) and a majority of adult tumors (*e.g.*, prostate, breast, lung, colon, and liver cancer) [31]. Theoretically, the *IGF2* LOI leads to a 2-fold increase in *IGF2* expression. In fact, Wilms tumors with *IGF2* LOI showed a 2.2-fold increase in *IGF2* expression compared with normal imprinting of *IGF2* [188]. The relationship between LOI and intestinal tumorigenesis was investigated using a mouse model of *Igf2* LOI in the *APCmin* background. Compared with LOI negative *APCmin* mice, LOI positive *APCmin* mice develop about twice the adenomas in both the small intestine and colon. LOI positive *APCmin* also show a shift toward a less differentiated normal intestinal epithelium. The same phenomenon is seen in the normal colonic mucosa with LOI in humans [199]. In addition, *Igf2* LOI *per se* led to increased expression of proliferation-related genes in intestinal crypts and enhancement of sensitivity to IGF2 signaling in *Igf2* LOI mice [95].

Endothelial progenitor cells (EPCs) contribute to tumor angiogenesis, which plays a critical role in tumor growth and progression. Both recruiting and incorporating EPCs to ischemic sites are involved in IGF2-IGF2R-PLCβ2 axis [141]. IGF2 also promotes embryonic stem cell differentiation into endothelial cells through IGF1R [183]. Thus, IGF2 may contribute to tumor angiogenesis.

The development of drug-resistant tumors is an obstacle to effective treatment. The ovarian cancer cell lines resistant to Taxol and other microtubule-stabilizing drugs increase *IGF2* expression compared with their drug sensitive cell lines of origin. Inhibition of IGF2 signaling in the Taxol-resistant ovarian tumor cell lines by IGF1R/IR inhibitor NVP-AEW541 or *IGF2* RNAi restores Taxol sensitivity

[79]. High *IGF2* mRNA expression is also significantly associated with clinically evident drug resistance and poor prognosis in ovarian tumor patients [22, 79].

Increased *IGF2* expression is associated with a poor prognosis in various tumors, including: ovarian, breast, esophageal tumor, and chronic myeloid leukemia [132]. Meanwhile, *IGF2* LOI can occur in normal colonic mucosa and peripheral blood of patients with LOI in cancer tissues and, less frequently, in normal individuals [33]. These results suggest the possibility that LOI may be an effective marker of colorectal cancer risk. In a pilot study, the adjusted odds ratio for LOI in lymphocytes was 5.15 for patients with a positive family history, 3.46 for those with adenomas, and 21.7 for those with colorectal cancer. This supports that LOI in lymphocytes may be able to predict colorectal cancer risk [32].

3.1.3 The Mechanisms of *IGF2* LOI

The mechanisms of *IGF2* LOI can be caused by alteration in *IGF2* promoter usage, *H19*-DMR hypermethylation, and the aberrant methylation of *IGF2*-DMRs. There are, however, many unsolved and controversial issues (Table 1).

3.1.3.1 Alterations in *IGF2* Promoter Usage

IGF2 mRNA is transcribed from separate promoters (P1-P4), which are activated in a developmental stage, in a tissue-specific manner. The transcripts from P2, P3, and P4 promoters are imprinted and activated during fetal development. Conversely, the transcripts from P1 are expressed from both parental alleles in the liver and chondrocytes (Fig. 2b). P1 promoter activity is very weak in the fetal, but increases in the adult liver [47, 124, 229]. This suggests that *IGF2* LOI may occur by promoter switching from imprinted promoters P2–P4 to non-imprinted promoter P1. This assumption has been tested in several types of tumor. However, it was recognized only in cervical carcinoma [105]. Many other tumors, such as laryngeal squamous cell carcinoma and Wilms tumor, did not show the promoter switch [65, 228].

3.1.3.2 *H19*-DMR Hypermethylation

Given regulation of the imprinted *IGF2/H19* domain, gain of methylation of unmethylated maternal *H19*-DMR (*H19*-DMR hypermethylation) leads to *IGF2* LOI and *H19* repression because the maternal *H19*-DMR changes to paternal mode. *IGF2* LOI and *H19* repression by *H19*-DMR hypermethylation has been identified in Wilms tumor and hepatoblastoma [16, 78, 201]. Conversely, some Wilms tumors with *H19*-DMR hypermethylation show normal *IGF2* imprinting. This indicates that hypermethylation is necessary, but not sufficient for *IGF2* LOI in Wilms tumor [34]. Of note, *IGF2* LOI and *H19* LOI (biallelic expression of *H19*) are accompanied by *H19*-DMR hypermethylation and hypomethylation, respectively, in osteosarcoma [223].

3.1.3.3 Aberrant Methylation of *IGF2*-DMRs

The human *IGF2* gene contains two DMRs, DMR0 and DMR2. The aberrant methylation of these DMRs is reported in various tumors. *IGF2*-DMR0, which is paternally methylated, is located between exons 2 and 3 of *IGF2* (Fig. 2b). *IGF2* LOI is tightly connected with *IGF2*-DMR0 hypomethylation, but not *H19*-DMR methylation status, in colorectal tumors and matched normal mucosae [35]. This suggests that *IGF2*-DMR0 hypomethylation is a different mechanism for LOI from *H19*-DMR aberrant methylation [35]. However, *IGF2*-DMR0 hypomethylation was not always associated with LOI because some tumors with *IGF2*-DMR0 hypomethylation showed normal *IGF2* monoallelic expression in colorectal tumors [87]. Further, there was no association between DMR0 hypomethylation and LOI in osteosarcoma, bladder, and ovarian tumors [24, 158, 223]. These results suggest that *IGF2*-DMR0 hypomethylation does not directly induce LOI. Furthermore, since it appears unlikely that paternally methylated *IGF2*-DMR0 contributes to *IGF2* repression from maternal allele in *trans*, no association is plausible. Determining the function of *IGF2*-DMR0 could resolve the above controversy. Meanwhile, *IGF2*-DMR0 hypomethylation is associated with poor prognosis in colorectal tumor and esophageal squamous cell carcinoma, suggesting its potential role as a prognostic marker [11, 157].

IGF2-DMR2, which is paternally methylated, is located between exons 8 and 9 of *IGF2* (Fig. 2b). The function of *IGF2*-DMR2 is unknown. In pancreatic endocrine tumors (PETs), *IGF2*-DMR2 hypermethylation occurs specifically in insulinomas, but not in any of other tumor types, namely gastrinomas or non-functioning PETs. DMR2 hypermethylation in insulinomas is also correlated with *IGF2* LOI and overexpression. Gastrinomas and non-functioning PETs also show significant DMR0 hypomethylation and some degree of DMR2 hypomethylation while exhibiting less *IGF2* expression than normal pancreatic tissue. In addition, decreased levels of methylation in DMRs is associated well with worse malignancy according to the World Health Organization (WHO) classification of PETs, except insulinomas, which suggests it has a potential role as a methylation-based biomarker for classification and staging [42].

3.1.4 The Role of *H19* in Cancer

H19 is the first imprinted ncRNA identified. It is highly expressed during embryonic development, but decreases significantly in most tissues after birth [93]. *H19* has been identified as a tumor suppressor candidate due to its inactivation in Wilms tumors [155, 211]. The growth inhibition by exogenous expression in embryonal tumor cell lines and the tumorigenesis in murine models lacking *H19* indicate the tumor suppressor activity [70, 244].

Conversely, exogenous expression of *H19* in choriocarcinoma cell lines and its expression pattern in the testicular germ cell tumors of adolescents and adults suggests *H19* shows oncogenic activity [135, 225]. Indeed, overexpression of *H19* is observed in several tumors [147] and the molecular evidence for oncogenic *H19* functions has been demonstrated recently. For example, tumor suppressor p53 was partially inactivated via the association between p53 and *H19* in a gastric cancer cell line [241]. *H19* is also associated with EZH2, which is known to methylate H3K27. This association results in inhibition of E-cadherin, associated with invasion and metastasis of tumor cells through Wnt/β-catenin activation in bladder cancer [133]. Furthermore, *H19* acts as a molecular sponge for *let-7* tumor suppressor miRNA. *H19* trapping of *let-7* promotes tumor metastasis [240]. *H19* is also a primary miRNA precursor of *miR-675*. Although *miR-675* is expressed exclusively in the placenta under normal physiological conditions, aberrant expression of *miR-675* can directly suppress the tumor suppressor *RB1* in colorectal cancer [102, 221]. The above results underline the oncogenic functions of *H19*. Thus, this gene may play contrary roles in tumorigenesis and may differ between embryonal and adult tumors in the human and mouse.

3.1.5 *H19* LOI and its Mechanism

H19 LOI (biallelic expression of *H19)* is observed in several tumor types and can result in its overexpression [147]. Indeed, previous work shows *H19* LOI is associated with its overexpression in lung and esophageal cancers [75, 109]. Hypomethylation of *H19*-DMR and *H19* promoter has also been correlated with *H19* LOI in osteosarcoma and lung cancer, respectively [109, 223] (Table 1). However, due to a lack of comprehensive research into the association between LOI, DNA methylation, and/or histone modifications in *H19*-DMR and *H19* promoter in various tumors, the mechanism behind LOI has not been fully elucidated.

3.2   KCNQ1OT1/CDKN1C

3.2.1   The Regulation of the Imprinted *KCNQ1OT1/CDKN1C* Domain

The ICR of this domain is *Kv*DMR1, located in intron 10 of *KCNQ1*, and is methylated on the maternal but not paternal allele. It also contains the promoter of *KCNQ1OT1*, a long non-coding RNA. The paternal *KCNQ1OT1* is expressed from unmethylated paternal *Kv*DMR1 in the antisense direction to *KCNQ1*, resulting in *cis*-repression of neighboring genes [143]. On the maternal allele, neighboring genes, such as *CDKN1C*, *KCNQ1*, *SLC22A18*, and *PHLDA2* are expressed due to lack of *KCNQ1OT1* expression (Fig. 1a). The regulatory mechanisms have been studied in genetically engineered mice and *in vitro* systems, *e.g.* episomal vector system in detail. In mice, when deletion of *Kv*DMR1 or the *Kcnq1ot1* promoter within *Kv*DMR1 is paternally transmitted, the paternal *Kcnq1ot1* transcript is eliminated and leads to LOI in maternal expressed genes within the domain [57, 143].

However, in the above results, it is difficult to distinguish which is important for imprinting regulation: the act of *Kcnq1ot1* transcription or *Kcnq1ot1* RNA itself. It was documented conclusively that *Kcnq1ot1* RNA was necessary for imprinting by truncating *Kcnq1ot1* in an episomal vector system and in mice, in which transcription was preserved, and by flanking the destabilizing sequences from the c-*fos* 3'UTR to the *Kcnq1ot1* in an episomal vector system [143, 178, 219]. Furthermore, *Kcnq1ot1* RNA interacts with H3K9 methyltransferase G9a and the H3K27 methyltransferase complex PRC2. It does so by recruiting these proteins in *cis* to neighboring gene promoters to deposit repressive chromatin marks, such as H3K9me3 and H3K27me3 in mouse placenta, but not in the liver [178, 217, 230]. In the mouse liver, *Kcnq1ot1* RNA interacts with Dnmt1 and contribute to maintaining somatic DMRs of *Cdkn1c* and *Slc22a18* [152]. In normal human fibroblast cell lines, accumulation of *KCNQ1OT1* RNA has been recognized at *CDKN1C* and *SLC22A18* [156]. Together, these findings indicate that paternal *KCNQ1OT1* RNA is pivotal in imprinting, although the imprinting regulation of this domain shows lineage-specific differences.

Conversely, *Kv*DMR1 itself can function as a regulatory element, such as a silencer or an insulator in enhancer-blocking assays [94, 142, 218]. The insulator protein CTCF binding sites conserved between mouse and human have also been identified, whereby CTCF binds to *Kv*DMR1 *in vivo* in a methylation-sensitive manner [56]. Currently, it is unclear whether *Kv*DMR1 represses paternal *Cdkn1c* expression by a *Kcnq1ot1* RNA-independent mechanism. However, given that imprinting regulation differs between extra-embryonic tissues and the embryo proper [120, 152], this suggests that the mechanistic differences of imprinting regulation may exist among various embryonic lineages.

3.2.2   The Role of CDKN1C in Cancer

CDKN1C is a type of cyclin-dependent kinase inhibitor (CKI) belonging to the Cip/Kip family and the first imprinted cell-cycle regulator. CDKN1C binds to cyclin-CDK complexes and inhibits cell cycle progression [116, 148]. In addition, CDKN1C regulates tumor differentiation, apoptosis, cell invasion and metastasis, and angiogenesis [98]. For example, *CDKN1C*-overexpressed LNCaP prostate cancer cells reduce invasive ability *in vitro* and, when transplanted to a nude mouse, can form well-differentiated squamous lesions [89]. Induction of *CDKN1C* expression in HeLa cells enhances sensitivity to apoptotic agents through the mitochondrial apoptotic cell death pathway [227]. The interaction between CDKN1C and the actin cytoskeleton modifying enzyme, LIM-kinase 1 (LIMK-1), can enhance the kinase activity of LIMK-1 and thereby stabilize actin filaments. This results in inhibited cell migration [226]. In placenta of mice lacking *Cdkn1c*, the expression of vascular endothelial growth factor (VEGF), a potent angiogenic factor, increased compared with wild type mice [149]. The aforementioned studies combined with reports of decreased *CDKN1C* expression in various tumors [17] suggest that *CDKN1C* is a multifunctional tumor suppressor gene [98].

3.2.3 The Mechanism of CDKN1C Inactivation

CDKN1C inactivation occurs in various tumors but mutation is infrequent. Abnormal expression of CDKN1C is caused by multiple mechanisms at transcriptional and posttranscriptional levels, as well as by posttranslational modification. Here, we focus on the mechanisms of epigenetic transcriptional silencing in *CDKN1C*.

3.2.3.1 *CDKN1C* Promoter Silencing by DNA Methylation

Aberrant DNA methylation in the promoter region is often invoked as a mechanism, which causes transcriptional inactivation of tumor suppressor genes. Aberrant DNA methylation at *CDKN1C* promoter is also a strong mechanism, which attenuates CDKN1C expression in many tumors. These include gastric, hepatocellular, pancreatic, and breast cancers, and acute myeloid leukemia [17, 103, 107] (Table 1). The clinical significance of the *CDKN1C* methylation status was reported in hematological malignancies. In acute lymphocytic leukemia (ALL), the methylation status in *p73*, *p15*, and *CDKN1C* composing a cell-cycle regulatory pathway was investigated. Philadelphia chromosome-negative patients with two or three methylated genes of this pathway showed significantly worse overall survival compared with those with zero or one methylated genes. Although, *CDKN1C* methylation status alone had no relevance to any clinical parameters [207]. In diffuse large B-cell lymphoma (DLBCL), *CDKN1C* promoter methylation occurs frequently [130]. Thus is may be applied as a biomarker for detecting minimal residual disease in DLBCL [69]. However, *CDKN1C* methylation was proposed as a favorable prognostic marker for a low-risk DLBCL group based on the International Prognostic Index. This is because patients with rather than without methylation show longer overall survival despite the unknown mechanism behind this favorable prognosis [118].

3.2.3.2 *CDKN1C* Promoter Silencing by Histone Modifications

The chromatin structure is regulated by histone modifications, such as acetylation, methylation, phosphorylation, and ubiquitination, as well as DNA methylation [110]. The chromatin structure in gene regulatory elements such as promoter and enhancer could influence the accessibility of transcriptional factors. In rhabdoid tumor cell lines lacking SMARCB1, a subunit of the SWI/SNF ATP-dependent chromatin-remodeling complex, induction of SMARCB1 upregulates *CDKN1C* expression by increasing permissive modifications, H3 and H4 acetylation at the *CDKN1C* promoter. In addition, the histone deacetylase (HDAC) inhibitor can restore *CDKN1C* expression in these cell lines [3]. In breast cancer cell lines, *CDKN1C* is repressed by repressive modification, H3K27me3 by histone methyltransferase EZH2 [242]. These results highlight the important role of histone modifications in *CDKN1C* repression.

3.2.3.3 *CDKN1C* Repression by DNA Hypomethylation at *Kv*DMR1

DNA hypomethylation of maternal *Kv*DMR1, leading to aberrant maternal *KCNQ1OT1* expression, is consequently associated with *CDKN1C* repression. Such methylation abnormalities have previously been described in various tumors, such as liver, breast, cervical, gastric, vulva, Wilms tumors, and colorectal cancer cell lines [167, 201, 204] (Table 1). However, *CDKN1C* expression is not associated with *Kv*DMR1 methylation status in colorectal cancer cell lines and Wilms tumors [167, 201]. Conversely, in esophageal cancer cell lines, diminished *CDKN1C* expression is statistically correlated with *Kv*DMR1 hypomethylation, but not methylation of the *CDKN1C* promoter itself [210]. Thus, the *CDKN1C* silencing mechanism associated with *Kv*DMR1 may depend on cancer type. In addition, it is difficult to explain the mechanisms of *CDKN1C* repression in only the epigenetic status of *CDKN1C* promoter and *Kv*DMR1, as the expression is also regulated by microRNAs and signaling pathways [67].

3.2.4 PHLDA2 in Cancer

PHLDA2, a homologue of mouse *TDAG51*, is the first apoptosis-related imprinted gene. *PHLDA2* is related to growth inhibition and apoptosis induction via the mitochondrial apoptosis pathway, and enhanced chemosensitivity, as well as stemness decrease in osteosarcoma [37, 82]. Furthermore, it is regulated by EGFR/ErbB2 signaling and inhibits cell proliferation through repressing AKT activation in lung cancers in a negative feedback loop [232]. Thus, PHLDA2 plays a potent role in tumor suppression.

The loss of *PHLDA2* expression has been reported in Wilms tumors, complete hydatidiform moles, and osteosarcomas [37, 203, 206]. Previous work has shown that DNA methylation or EZH2-associated H3K27me3 of the promoter in osteosarcoma cell lines mediates transcriptional repression of *PHLDA2* (Table 1), although its molecular mechanisms in primary tumors have not been well investigated [127, 136].

3.3 DLK1/MEG3

The human *DLK1-MEG3* locus spans about 840 kb at 14q32.2. This imprinted domain contains three paternally expressed protein-coding genes and numerous maternally expressed genes that encode noncoding RNAs, such as lncRNAs, miRNAs, and small nucleolar RNAs (snoRNAs) (Fig. 1c) [36, 173]. Parental allele-specific expression of the imprinted genes is controlled by two paternally methylated DMRs: IG-DMR and *MEG3*-DMR. The methylation of IG-DMR is established in germ cells and *MEG3*-DMR methylation is established after fertilization. The *MEG3* gene (referred to as *Gtl2* in mice) encodes an lncRNA and is expressed in many normal human tissues, but repressed in various types of human cancers and cancer cell lines. Ectopic gene expression shows various tumor suppressor functions, such as inhibited cellular proliferation, induced apoptosis, and induced p53 activity in many types of cancer and normal cell lines [20, 231, 250, 251]. *RTL1* is a paternally expressed protein-coding gene in this locus. In mice, hepatic expression of this gene can promote cell growth *in vitro* and drive carcinogenesis of HCC *in vivo*. 30% (10/33) of human HCC also shows *RTL1* expression, while normal livers show no significant expression of this gene [192].

Silencing or reduced *MEG3* expression is observed in many types of tumors, such as pituitary tumors [252], neuroblastoma [10], meningioma and meningioma cell lines [250], HCC and HCC cell lines [20], and glioma [231]. In addition to reduced expression, hypermethylation at the *MEG3*-DMR occurs in these tumors and cell lines. *MEG3*-DMR hypermethylation also occurs in a small fraction of pheochromocytomas and Wilms' tumors [10]. Further, treatment with 5-aza-dC can reactivate *MEG3* in neuroblastoma, meningioma, and HCC cell lines [10, 20, 250]. In addition to reactivation by 5-aza-dC, overexpression of *miR-29*, which modulates the expression of DNMT1 and DNMT3B, can also reactivate *MEG3* expression in HCC cell lines [20]. Furthermore, HCC tissues show frequently reduced *miR-29* expression [238]. These results indicate that *MEG3* is inactivated by hypermethylation of maternal *MEG3*-DMR in many types of cancers.

miR-370, maternally expressed from the genomic region between *RTL1* and *MEG8* in the locus, is downregulated in cholangiocarcinoma [5]. Cancers with reduced *miR-370* expression harbor hypermethylation at IG-DMR. Further, *miR-370* expression levels show negative correlations with methylation levels of the DMR. Among the possible targets of *miR-370* is *WNT10B*, whose role is not clear, but enhances cellular proliferation. *miR-127-3p*, *miR-154*, and *miR-495*, are expressed from the *anti-RTL1* region, the proximal miRNA cluster, and the snoRNA region in *DLK1-MEG3* locus, respectively. Hypermethylation at *MEG3*-DMR is found in majority of colorectal adenomas [151]. Two of the three miRNAs: *miR-127-3p* and *miR-154*, show lower expression in adenomas with hypermethylation than in adenomas with normal methylation. Conversely, *miR-495* is expressed in similar or slightly higher levels in adenomas with hypermethylation. These four miRNAs inhibit cellular proliferation when overexpressed in cancer cell lines [26, 27, 58]. In contrast to the downregulation in adenomas, expression of *miR-379* from the snoRNA region and *miR-154* is elevated in prostate cancer cell lines and primary cancer tissues [68]. Expression levels are correlated with cancer malignancy and overexpression of these miRNAs induces epithelial to mesenchymal transition in prostate cancer cells. DNA methylation was not analyzed in these cancer tissues and cell lines. Some miRNAs expressed from this imprinting locus, may have oncogenic or tumor suppressing functions. Further investigation is needed to elucidate how such miRNAs are involved in carcinogenesis of various types of cancer.

3.4 GNAS *Locus*

The *GNAS* complex locus occurs on the long arm of human chromosome 20 (20q13.32) and is a complex imprinted domain, which contains multiple imprinted genes and DMRs [13, 222] (Fig. 1d). As mentioned in Sect. 2.5, this locus expresses multiple transcripts that encode Gsα (*GNAS* gene), XLαs, and NESP55. The transcripts initiate from unique first exons: *GNAS*, *XL*, and *NESP55*, and are spliced onto a common set of exons 2-13.

Gsα is involved in a signaling pathway that mediates the actions of various hormones by elevating intracellular cyclic AMP levels. The roles of the proteins, XLαs and NESP55, are not yet well understood. Two noncoding RNAs: *A/B* and *GNAS-AS1*, are expressed from the locus in addition to the protein-coding transcripts. Transcript *A/B* is transcribed from exon A/B and is spliced onto the common exons 2-13 (Fig. 1d). *GNAS-AS1* initiates from exon AS1 and is transcribed in an antisense orientation to other transcripts.

The transcripts, *XLαs, GNAS-AS1*, and *A/B* are expressed only from the paternal allele, while *NESP55* is expressed only from the maternal allele. *GNAS* is expressed biallelically in most human tissues, but shows maternal expression in some tissues, such as renal proximal tubules, thyroid, gonads, hypothalamus, and pituitary. The imprinted expressions are regulated by multiple DMRs. The *GNAS-AS1*, *XL*, and *A/B* promoters are DMRs that are methylated on the maternal allele, while the *NESP55* promoter is a DMR methylated on the paternal allele. The promoter of *GNAS* is not methylated on both alleles. The *A/B* transcript and/or *A/B*-DMR is involved in the tissue-specific imprinting of *GNAS*.

Constitutively activating *GNAS* mutations have been reported in endocrine tumors. Further, elevated activity of the Gsα signaling pathway may contribute to the pathogenesis of endocrine tumors. The mutations are always of maternal origin in growth hormone-secreting pituitary adenoma, consistent with the imprinted maternal expression of *GNAS* in the pituitary [115, 145]. De-repression of the *GNAS* paternal allele was found in somatotroph pituitary adenomas [73, 182]. However, the loss of imprinting did not result in the increase of total *GNAS* mRNA levels because decrease of the maternal expression was concomitant with increased paternal expression [182]. This result suggests that imprinting relaxation is not involved in tumorigenesis, but is a secondary phenomenon that is part of the tumorigenic process.

Recently, human miRNAs: *miR-296* and *miR-298*, were found to lie within the *GNAS-AS1* transcription unit and show paternal allele-specific expression as members of the *GNAS* imprinting locus [193]. Prostate cancer cell lines and cancer tissues express *miR-296* at low levels and *HMGA1*, a high-mobility group AT-hook gene, at high levels. The expression of *miR-296* inversely correlates with the expression of *HMGA1* mRNA and the HMGA1 protein. *HMGA1* is an oncogene involved in carcinogenesis of prostate cancer and one of the target genes of *miR-296* [234]. Reduced expression of the miRNA was also observed in pancreatic intraepithelial tumors and pancreatic ductal adenocarcinomas [245]. The more progressed pancreatic

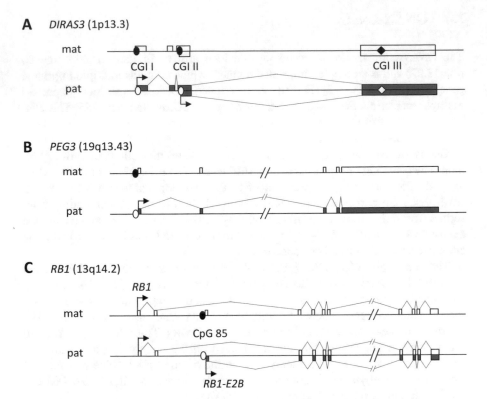

Fig. 3 Representative human imprinting loci associated with tumors. (**a**) *DIRAS3* locus at 1p13.3. (**b**) *PEG3* locus at 19q13.43. (**c**) *RB1* locus at 13q14.2. Blue: paternally expressed genes; filled ovals: methylated gametic DMRs; open ovals: unmethylated gametic DMRs; filled diamond: methylated somatic DMR; open diamond: unmethylated somatic DMR

tumors expressed the lower *miR-296*. Methylation analysis at *GNAS-AS1*-DMR was not performed in these tumors, but colorectal adenoma showed reduced expression of *miR-296* along with aberrant methylation at *GNAS-AS1*-DMR [151]. Frequent hypermethylation (ca. 50%) and some hypomethylation were found in 50 colorectal adenomas. Expression of *miR-296* in adenomas with hypermethylation is lower than those in adenomas with normal methylation [151].

3.5   DIRAS3/ARHI

The *DIRAS3* gene at 1p13.3, also known as *ARHI*, encodes small 26 kDa GTP binding GTPase belonging to the Ras/Rap superfamily. This is a maternally imprinted tumor suppressor gene that is expressed exclusively from the paternal allele in many adult human tissues. The gene contains two start exons and three CpG islands designated as CGI I, CGI II, and CGI III (Fig. 3a). The CGI I and the CGI II identify the first and second start exons, respectively, and are gametic DMRs with maternal methylation. The CGI III lies within the last exon and its methylation level varies from hypermethylation to intermediate levels among different tissues, so is presumably a tissue-specific somatic DMR [134, 172, 248] (UCSC browser, chr1:68,045,962-68,051,631, hg38, http://genome.ucsc.edu/).

DIRAS3 is silenced in most ovarian and breast cancer cell lines [246] and can inhibit growth of breast and ovarian cancer cell lines when the expression constructs are introduced in the cancer cells. This growth inhibition is accomplished by down-regulation of cyclin D1 and up-regulation of p21$^{WAF1/CIP1}$. In a study of ovarian cancer, cancer cell lines showed DIRAS3 silencing and CGI I hypermethylation with frequencies of 80% (8/10) and 60% (6/10), respectively [54]. Analysis of cancer tissues showed 88% (35/40) of the cancers expressed lower levels of DIRAS3 than normal ovarian tissues. CGI I and CGI II were hypermethylated in 31% (13/42) and 12% (5/42) of cancers, respectively. All cancers with hypermethylation showed reduced expression of the gene. Frequent LOH (41%, 9/22) occurred in these cancers, which led to loss of the active paternal allele. In spite of the frequent LOH, there were many cancers that retained heterozygosity and thus the gene was also silenced by aberrant hypermethylation at the CGIs.

CGI methylation status of the DIRAS3 gene has also been reported in breast cancer cell lines, in which DIRAS3 was silenced. CGIs I and III were frequently hypermethylated and CGI II showed either hypermethylation or hypomethylation in the cell lines [248]. Aberrant methylation at the DIRAS3-CGIs was also observed in breast cancer tissues [53, 248]. However, no characteristic feature was seen in the aberrant methylation, such as hypermethylation or hypomethylation, and frequencies at each of the CGIs. Because DIRAS3 expression and chromosomal abnormality were not analyzed in either of these studies on breast cancer tissues, it is not clear whether the observed aberrant methylation alters DIRAS3 expression and whether aberrant methylation is due to changes in DNA methylation or loss of methylated or unmethylated alleles. On the other hand, some studies suggest that histone modifications are also involved in inactivation of the DIRAS3 gene. A histone deacetylase inhibitor, trichostatin A, could reactivate gene expression in breast cancer cells, in which DIRAS3 is repressed without hypermethylation at CGI II [59]. Breast cancer tissues highly express JMJD2A, a histone demethylase, which acts on tri- and di-methylated H3K9 and H3K36. Expression of this enzyme is positively correlated with progression of cancers and negatively correlated with DIRAS3 expression. JMJD2A binds the DIRAS3 promoter together with HDAC1 and HDAC3 and represses gene expression [122].

Many other types of cancer, such as follicular thyroid carcinoma, oligodendroglioma, and HCC, have downregulated DIRAS3 and shown aberrant methylation of DIRAS3 CGIs. LOH of the DIRAS3 locus was found in 64% (9/14) of follicular thyroid carcinoma [233] and 53% (20/38) of oligodendrogliomas [190]. A LOH case of follicular thyroid carcinoma showed hypermethylation at all DIRAS3 CGIs and most LOH cases of oligodendroglioma showed hypermethylation of at least one of three CGIs. These indicate deletion of the paternal allele. Furthermore, among oligodendroglioma cases with ROH, several cases showed hypermethylation of the CGIs, resulting in reduced expression of the gene. In contrast to the above two types of tumors, LOH of the *DIRAS3* locus was a very rare event in HCC, which showed frequent reduction of *DIRAS3* expression [80]. Downregulation of the gene was observed in 79% (33/42) of HCCs; however, only one HCC showed LOH of the locus. Methylation analysis of the CGIs detected hypermethylation only at CGI II with a 47% (8/17) frequency. No aberrant methylation was observed at CGIs I and III. These results strongly suggest that hypermethylation at the promoter of *DIRAS3* occurred in HCCs and such hypermethylation caused downregulation of the gene.

3.6   PEG3

The *PEG3* gene on chromosome 19q13.43 encodes a Krüppel-C2H2 type zinc finger protein and is expressed in a wide variety of human tissues. The gene is imprinted and is expressed from the paternal allele the same as its mouse homologue, *Peg3* [76, 140, 159]. Exon 1 of the gene lies within a CpG island, which is a maternally methylated gametic DMR (*PEG3*-DMR) (Fig. 3b) [140, 159]. *PEG3* shows tumor suppressor activity in human glioma cell lines upon its overexpression [108].

This gene is silenced or downregulated with hypermethylation of *PEG3*-DMR in glioma cell lines [108, 140]. Treatment with 5-aza-dC can reactivate the silenced *PEG3* [140]. Primary glioma tissues also show aberrant hypo- or hypermethylation at *PEG3*-DMR together with changes in *PEG3* expression [177]. Hypermethylation at *PEG3*-DMR and downregulation of the gene are more frequent in grade IV glioblastoma than lower-grade gliomas, such as astrocytoma, oligodendroglioma, and ependymoma. Further, hypomethylation is observed only in lower-grade gliomas. In contrast to glioma cell lines, methylation levels at *PEG3*-DMR correlate weakly with *PEG3* expression in glioma tissues and some tumors with normal methylation also show reduced *PEG3* expression [177]. These results suggest that *PEG3* is downregulated by various mechanisms, including hypermethylation at *PEG3*-DMR in glioma.

Further work shows *PEG3* is downregulated and *PEG3*-DMR is hypermethylated in ovarian cancer cell lines and cancer tissues. Gene expression is also shown to be negatively correlated with DMR methylation level [45, 54, 64]. Treatment with 5-aza-dC and/or a histone deacetylase inhibitor, trichostatin A, can reactivate the gene in silenced cell lines [45, 54]. Overexpression of *PEG3* also inhibits proliferation of ovarian cancer cells [54]. *PEG3* silencing and *PEG3*-DMR hypermethylation are also found in two other gynecologic cancer cell lines, endometrial cancer and cervical cancer [45].

Pediatric germ cell tumors show aberrant methylation at *PEG3*-DMR with patterns characteristic of histologic tumor subtypes. Hypermethylation has been observed in ovarian teratoma and yolk sac tumors, and hypomethylation in female germinoma [4]. Aberrant methylation, mainly hypermethylation, at *PEG3*-DMR also occurs in invasive breast cancers [12].

3.7 RB1

RB1 was the first identified tumor suppressor gene and is frequently inactivated in several cancers. This gene is expressed biallelically; however, a variant transcript, *RB1-E2B*, was found to be imprinted and expressed only from the paternal allele in lower levels than the main *RB1* transcript (Fig. 3c) [92]. The variant transcript initiates from a novel first exon, called *E2B*, which lies in intron 2, and is spliced onto exon 3 of the *RB1* gene. The *RB1-E2B* transcript harbors a coding sequence in the same reading frame as one of the *RB1* mRNAs, which encodes a shortened version of pRb.

The function, if any, of the presumptive protein is not well understood yet. The exon *E2B* lies in a CpG island called CpG85 that is a maternally methylated DMR. The *RB1-E2B* transcription interferes with expression of the main *RB1* mRNA. This results in an allelic imbalance of the *RB1* expression in favor of the maternal allele. Frequent aberrant methylation, hyper- or hypomethylation, at CpG85 has been found in HCC [7]. Some HCCs with hyper- or hypomethylation retains both alleles, suggesting that aberrant methylation occurs on the methylated or unmethylated allele. Further work suggests hypermethylation at CpG85 causes reduced *RB1-E2B* expression, which results in increased primary *RB1* expression [7, 92]. Hypermethylation at CpG85 is also associated with reduced overall survival of HCC patients. These results are contradictory to the tumor suppressor activity of pRB1 [7]. Eloy *et al.* also reported frequent hypermethylation (93%, 42/45) at CpG85 in retinoblastoma, although no expression analysis was performed [49].

3.8 Multilocus Methylation Defects at Imprinted DMRs in Cancers

Complete hydatidiform mole (CHM) is an abnormal form of pregnancy carrying diploid genomes with the risk of developing into choriocarcinoma. Most CHMs are sporadic and carry only paternal genomes (androgenetic CHM). A fraction of CHMs can be recurrent and familial. These CHMs have biparental genomes (biparental CHM). Biallelic mutations of *NLRP7* and *KHDC3L* genes occur in patients with familial biparental CHM [154, 180]. Multilocus methylation defects at imprinted loci have been reported in androgenetic CHM and familial biparental CHM from mothers with *NLRP7* mutations [200]. Hypomethylation occurs in the majority of more than 30 maternal gametic DMR analyzed in androgenetic and biparental CHM. *H19*-DMR is the only analyzed DMR of paternal gametic imprinting and is hypermethylated in androgenetic CHM, but normally (ca. 50%) methylated in biparental CHM. Multilocus methylation analysis has not yet been reported in biparental CHM with *KHDC3L* mutation. It is highly possible that *NLRP7* and *KHDC3L* involves establishment and/or maintenance of maternal imprints and that mutations in these genes may cause methylation defects at maternally methylated imprinted loci. Multilocus aberrant methylation at imprinted loci could result in abnormal proliferation of trophoblastic tissue to form CHM, and may result in tumors, such as choriocarcinoma.

These days, DNA methylation analysis of cancer genomes is performed in a more comprehensive or genome-wide manner. Recent work has analyzed 33 imprinted DMRs for aberrant methylation in hepatoblastoma tissues by quantitative methylation analysis with MALDI-TOF MS [196]. Such research has found frequent hypermethylation at *INPP5Fv2*-DMR, CpG85 (*RB1*-DMR), and *GNASXL*-DMR. *IGF2*-DMR0 and *Kv*DMR1 showed frequent hypomethylation. Bisulfite-pyrosequencing at *IGF2*-DMR2, *IGF2*-DMR0, *DIRAS3*-DMR, *GRB10*-DMR, *PEG3*-DMR, *MEST*-DMR, *H19*-DMR, *Kv*DMR1, and *SNRPN*-DMR has also revealed aberrant DNA methylation in breast cancer tissues [12].

DNA methylation microarray analyses can identify aberrant methylation of genes, including imprinted genes in cancers. DNA methylome analyses were performed in three subtypes of pediatric germ cell tumors, including germinoma, teratoma, and yolk sac tumor. Hyper- or hypomethylation were found at several imprinted genes, such as *H19*-DMR, *IGF2*, *Kv*DMR1, *SNRPN*, and *PEG3* [4]. Similarly, 22 out of 56 imprinted genes analyzed were aberrantly methylated in prostate tumors. This work also found that hypermethylation was more frequent than hypomethylation [88]. In contrast, in HCC, hypomethylation was observed more frequently than hypermethylation [8, 114]. Aberrant methylation, mainly hypomethylation, was observed in 27 genes out of 59 imprinted genes [114]. These results suggest that paternally expressed imprinted genes are more susceptible to epigenetic disruption. Hypomethylation at imprinted loci correlates with global loss of DNA methylation, mutation in *CTNNB1* gene encoding β-catenin, and shortened overall survival of HCC patients [8].

Kim *et al.* analyzed data sets from TCGA (The Cancer Genome Atlas) to identify aberrant expression and epigenetic change at promoters and/or ICRs of imprinted genes in multiple human cancers [104]. They found some abnormal characteristics of imprinted genes in cancer. The number of cancers showing aberrant expression of imprinted genes is greater than those showing aberrant methylation at imprinted loci. DNA methylation instability among the imprinted genes is relatively higher than those among total genes. The number of imprinted genes with hypermethylation is much greater than those with hypomethylation. Some imprinted genes, such as *PEG3*, *DLK1*, *MEST*, and *GNAS*, are more susceptible to epigenetic change than others.

References

1. Abdollahi A (2007) LOT1 (ZAC1/PLAGL1) and its family members: mechanisms and functions. J Cell Physiol 210(1):16–25. doi:10.1002/jcp.20835
2. Abramowitz LK, Bartolomei MS (2012) Genomic imprinting: recognition and marking of imprinted loci. Curr Opin Genet Dev 22(2):72–78. doi:10.1016/j.gde.2011.12.001

3. Algar EM, Muscat A, Dagar V, Rickert C, Chow CW, Biegel JA, Ekert PG, Saffery R, Craig J, Johnstone RW, Ashley DM (2009) Imprinted CDKN1C is a tumor suppressor in rhabdoid tumor and activated by restoration of SMARCB1 and histone deacetylase inhibitors. PLoS One 4(2):e4482. doi:10.1371/journal.pone.0004482

4. Amatruda JF, Ross JA, Christensen B, Fustino NJ, Chen KS, Hooten AJ, Nelson H, Kuriger JK, Rakheja D, Frazier AL, Poynter JN (2013) DNA methylation analysis reveals distinct methylation signatures in pediatric germ cell tumors. BMC Cancer 13:313. doi:10.1186/1471-2407-13-313

5. An F, Yamanaka S, Allen S, Roberts LR, Gores GJ, Pawlik TM, Xie Q, Ishida M, Mezey E, Ferguson-Smith AC, Mori Y, Selaru FM (2012) Silencing of miR-370 in human cholangio-carcinoma by allelic loss and interleukin-6 induced maternal to paternal epigenotype switch. PLoS One 7(10):e45606. doi:10.1371/journal.pone.0045606

6. Anwar SL, Krech T, Hasemeier B, Schipper E, Schweitzer N, Vogel A, Kreipe H, Lehmann U (2012) Loss of imprinting and allelic switching at the DLK1-MEG3 locus in human hepa-tocellular carcinoma. PLoS One 7(11):e49462. doi:10.1371/journal.pone.0049462

7. Anwar SL, Krech T, Hasemeier B, Schipper E, Schweitzer N, Vogel A, Kreipe H, Lehmann U (2014) Deregulation of RB1 expression by loss of imprinting in human hepatocellular carcinoma. J Pathol 233(4):392–401. doi:10.1002/path.4376

8. Anwar SL, Krech T, Hasemeier B, Schipper E, Schweitzer N, Vogel A, Kreipe H, Lehmann U (2015) Loss of DNA methylation at imprinted loci is a frequent event in hepatocellular car-cinoma and identifies patients with shortened survival. Clin Epigenetics 7:110. doi:10.1186/s13148-015-0145-6

9. Arima T, Matsuda T, Takagi N, Wake N (1997) Association of IGF2 and H19 imprinting with choriocarcinoma development. Cancer Genet Cytogenet 93(1):39–47

10. Astuti D, Latif F, Wagner K, Gentle D, Cooper WN, Catchpoole D, Grundy R, Ferguson-Smith AC, Maher ER (2005) Epigenetic alteration at the DLK1-GTL2 imprinted domain in human neoplasia: analysis of neuroblastoma, phaeochromocytoma and Wilms' tumour. Br J Cancer 92(8):1574–1580. doi:10.1038/sj.bjc.6602478

11. Baba Y, Nosho K, Shima K, Huttenhower C, Tanaka N, Hazra A, Giovannucci EL, Fuchs CS, Ogino S (2010) Hypomethylation of the IGF2 DMR in colorectal tumors, detected by bisul-fite pyrosequencing, is associated with poor prognosis. Gastroenterology 139(6):1855–1864. doi:10.1053/j.gastro.2010.07.050

12. Barrow TM, Barault L, Ellsworth RE, Harris HR, Binder AM, Valente AL, Shriver CD, Michels KB (2015) Aberrant methylation of imprinted genes is associated with negative hor-mone receptor status in invasive breast cancer. Int J Cancer 137(3):537–547. doi:10.1002/ijc.29419

13. Bastepe M (2007) The GNAS Locus: Quintessential Complex Gene Encoding Gsalpha, XLalphas, and other Imprinted Transcripts. Curr Genomics 8(6):398–414. doi:10.2174/138920207783406488

14. Bell AC, Felsenfeld G (2000) Methylation of a CTCF-dependent boundary controls imprinted expression of the Igf2 gene. Nature 405(6785):482–485. doi:10.1038/35013100

15. Benetatos L, Hatzimichael E, Dasoula A, Dranitsaris G, Tsiara S, Syrrou M, Georgiou I, Bourantas KL (2010) CpG methylation analysis of the MEG3 and SNRPN imprinted genes in acute myeloid leukemia and myelodysplastic syndromes. Leuk Res 34(2):148–153. doi:10.1016/j.leukres.2009.06.019

16. Bjornsson HT, Brown LJ, Fallin MD, Rongione MA, Bibikova M, Wickham E, Fan JB, Feinberg AP (2007) Epigenetic specificity of loss of imprinting of the IGF2 gene in Wilms tumors. J Natl Cancer Inst 99(16):1270–1273. doi:10.1093/jnci/djm069

17. Borriello A, Caldarelli I, Bencivenga D, Criscuolo M, Cucciolla V, Tramontano A, Oliva A, Perrotta S, Della Ragione F (2011) p57(Kip2) and cancer: time for a critical appraisal. Mol Cancer Res 9(10):1269–1284. doi:10.1158/1541-7786.MCR-11-0220

18. Bourc'his D, Xu GL, Lin CS, Bollman B, Bestor TH (2001) Dnmt3L and the establishment of maternal genomic imprints. Science 294(5551):2536–2539. doi:10.1126/science.1065848

19. Boyce AM, Collins MT (1993) Fibrous dysplasia/McCune-Albright syndrome. In: Pagon RA, Adam MP, Ardinger HH et al (eds) GeneReviews®. University of Washington, Seattle, WA

20. Braconi C, Kogure T, Valeri N, Huang N, Nuovo G, Costinean S, Negrini M, Miotto E, Croce CM, Patel T (2011) microRNA-29 can regulate expression of the long non-coding RNA gene MEG3 in hepatocellular cancer. Oncogene 30(47):4750–4756. doi:10.1038/onc.2011.193

21. Brouwer-Visser J, Huang GS (2015) IGF2 signaling and regulation in cancer. Cytokine Growth Factor Rev 26(3):371–377. doi:10.1016/j.cytogfr.2015.01.002

22. Brouwer-Visser J, Lee J, McCullagh K, Cossio MJ, Wang Y, Huang GS (2014) Insulin-like growth factor 2 silencing restores taxol sensitivity in drug resistant ovarian cancer. PLoS One 9(6):e100165. doi:10.1371/journal.pone.0100165

23. Buiting K (2010) Prader-Willi syndrome and Angelman syndrome. Am J Med Genet C Semin Med Genet 154C(3):365–376. doi:10.1002/ajmg.c.30273

24. Byun HM, Wong HL, Birnstein EA, Wolff EM, Liang G, Yang AS (2007) Examination of IGF2 and H19 loss of imprinting in bladder cancer. Cancer Res 67(22):10753–10758. doi:10.1158/0008-5472.CAN-07-0329

25. Charlton J, Williams RD, Sebire NJ, Popov S, Vujanic G, Chagtai T, Alcaide-German M, Morris T, Butcher LM, Guilhamon P, Beck S, Pritchard-Jones K (2015) Comparative methylome analysis identifies new tumour subtypes and biomarkers for transformation of nephrogenic rests into Wilms tumour. Genome Med 7(1):11. doi:10.1186/s13073-015-0136-4

26. Chen J, Wang M, Guo M, Xie Y, Cong YS (2013) miR-127 regulates cell proliferation and senescence by targeting BCL6. PLoS One 8(11):e80266. doi:10.1371/journal.pone.0080266

27. Chen XP, Chen YG, Lan JY, Shen ZJ (2014) MicroRNA-370 suppresses proliferation and promotes endometrioid ovarian cancer chemosensitivity to cDDP by negatively regulating ENG. Cancer Lett 353(2):201–210. doi:10.1016/j.canlet.2014.07.026

28. Cheng YW, Idrees K, Shattock R, Khan SA, Zeng Z, Brennan CW, Paty P, Barany F (2010) Loss of imprinting and marked gene elevation are 2 forms of aberrant IGF2 expression in colorectal cancer. Int J Cancer 127(3):568–577. doi:10.1002/ijc.25086

29. Chotalia M, Smallwood SA, Ruf N, Dawson C, Lucifero D, Frontera M, James K, Dean W, Kelsey G (2009) Transcription is required for establishment of germline methylation marks at imprinted genes. Genes Dev 23(1):105–117. doi:10.1101/gad.495809

30. Ciccone DN, Su H, Hevi S, Gay F, Lei H, Bajko J, Xu G, Li E, Chen T (2009) KDM1B is a histone H3K4 demethylase required to establish maternal genomic imprints. Nature 461(7262):415–418. doi:10.1038/nature08315

31. Cui H (2007) Loss of imprinting of IGF2 as an epigenetic marker for the risk of human cancer. Dis Markers 23(1-2):105–112

32. Cui H, Cruz-Correa M, Giardiello FM, Hutcheon DF, Kafonek DR, Brandenburg S, Wu Y, He X, Powe NR, Feinberg AP (2003) Loss of IGF2 imprinting: a potential marker of colorectal cancer risk. Science 299(5613):1753–1755. doi:10.1126/science.1080902

33. Cui H, Horon IL, Ohlsson R, Hamilton SR, Feinberg AP (1998) Loss of imprinting in normal tissue of colorectal cancer patients with microsatellite instability. Nat Med 4(11):1276–1280. doi:10.1038/3260

34. Cui H, Niemitz EL, Ravenel JD, Onyango P, Brandenburg SA, Lobanenkov VV, Feinberg AP (2001) Loss of imprinting of insulin-like growth factor-II in Wilms' tumor commonly involves altered methylation but not mutations of CTCF or its binding site. Cancer Res 61(13):4947–4950

35. Cui H, Onyango P, Brandenburg S, Wu Y, Hsieh CL, Feinberg AP (2002) Loss of imprinting in colorectal cancer linked to hypomethylation of H19 and IGF2. Cancer Res 62(22):6442–6446

36. da Rocha ST, Edwards CA, Ito M, Ogata T, Ferguson-Smith AC (2008) Genomic imprinting at the mammalian Dlk1-Dio3 domain. Trends Genet 24(6):306–316. doi:10.1016/j.tig.2008.03.011

37. Dai H, Huang Y, Li Y, Meng G, Wang Y, Guo QN (2012) TSSC3 overexpression associates with growth inhibition, apoptosis induction and enhances chemotherapeutic effects in human osteosarcoma. Carcinogenesis 33(1):30–40. doi:10.1093/carcin/bgr232

38. Dammann RH, Kirsch S, Schagdarsurengin U, Dansranjavin T, Gradhand E, Schmitt WD, Hauptmann S (2010) Frequent aberrant methylation of the imprinted IGF2/H19 locus and LINE1 hypomethylation in ovarian carcinoma. Int J Oncol 36(1):171–179

39. Davies HD, Leusink GL, McConnell A, Deyell M, Cassidy SB, Fick GH, Coppes MJ (2003) Myeloid leukemia in Prader-Willi syndrome. J Pediatr 142(2):174–178. doi:10.1067/mpd.2003.81

40. De Castro Valente Esteves LI, De Karla CN, Do Carmo Javaroni A, Magrin J, Kowalski LP, Rainho CA, Rogatto SR (2006) H19-DMR allele-specific methylation analysis reveals epigenetic heterogeneity of CTCF binding site 6 but not of site 5 in head-and-neck carcinomas: a pilot case-control analysis. Int J Mol Med 17(2):397–404

41. de Smith AJ, Purmann C, Walters RG, Ellis RJ, Holder SE, Van Haelst MM, Brady AF, Fairbrother UL, Dattani M, Keogh JM, Henning E, Yeo GS, O'Rahilly S, Froguel P, Farooqi IS, Blakemore AI (2009) A deletion of the HBII-85 class of small nucleolar RNAs (snoRNAs) is associated with hyperphagia, obesity and hypogonadism. Hum Mol Genet 18(17):3257–3265. doi:10.1093/hmg/ddp263

42. Dejeux E, Olaso R, Dousset B, Audebourg A, Gut IG, Terris B, Tost J (2009) Hypermethylation of the IGF2 differentially methylated region 2 is a specific event in insulinomas leading to loss-of-imprinting and overexpression. Endocr Relat Cancer 16(3):939–952. doi:10.1677/ERC-08-0331

43. Denduluri SK, Idowu O, Wang Z, Liao Z, Yan Z, Mohammed MK, Ye J, Wei Q, Wang J, Zhao L, Luu HH (2015) Insulin-like growth factor (IGF) signaling in tumorigenesis and the development of cancer drug resistance. Genes Dis 2(1):13–25. doi:10.1016/j.gendis.2014.10.004

44. Douc-Rasy S, Barrois M, Fogel S, Ahomadegbe JC, Stéhelin D, Coll J, Riou G (1996) High incidence of loss of heterozygosity and abnormal imprinting of H19 and IGF2 genes in invasive cervical carcinomas. Uncoupling of H19 and IGF2 expression and biallelic hypomethylation of H19. Oncogene 12(2):423–430

45. Dowdy SC, Gostout BS, Shridhar V, Wu X, Smith DI, Podratz KC, Jiang SW (2005) Biallelic methylation and silencing of paternally expressed gene 3 (PEG3) in gynecologic cancer cell lines. Gynecol Oncol 99(1):126–134. doi:10.1016/j.ygyno.2005.05.036

46. Eggermann T (2010) Russell-Silver syndrome. Am J Med Genet C Semin Med Genet 154C(3):355–364. doi:10.1002/ajmg.c.30274

47. Ekstrom TJ, Cui H, Li X, Ohlsson R (1995) Promoter-specific IGF2 imprinting status and its plasticity during human liver development. Development 121(2):309–316

48. El-Maarri O, Seoud M, Coullin P, Herbiniaux U, Oldenburg J, Rouleau G, Slim R (2003) Maternal alleles acquiring paternal methylation patterns in biparental complete hydatidiform moles. Hum Mol Genet 12(12):1405–1413

49. Eloy P, Dehainault C, Sefta M, Aerts I, Doz F, Cassoux N, Lumbroso le Rouic L, Stoppa-Lyonnet D, Radvanyi F, Millot GA, Gauthier-Villars M, Houdayer C (2016) A Parent-of-Origin Effect Impacts the Phenotype in Low Penetrance Retinoblastoma Families Segregating the c.1981C>T/p.Arg661Trp Mutation of RB1. PLoS Genet 12(2):e1005888. doi:10.1371/journal.pgen.1005888

50. Engel E (1980) A new genetic concept: uniparental disomy and its potential effect, isodisomy. Am J Med Genet 6(2):137–143. doi:10.1002/ajmg.1320060207

51. Engel N, Thorvaldsen JL, Bartolomei MS (2006) CTCF binding sites promote transcription initiation and prevent DNA methylation on the maternal allele at the imprinted H19/Igf2 locus. Hum Mol Genet 15(19):2945–2954. doi:10.1093/hmg/ddl237

52. Eriksson T, Frisk T, Gray SG, von Schweinitz D, Pietsch T, Larsson C, Sandstedt B, Ekström TJ (2001) Methylation changes in the human IGF2 p3 promoter parallel IGF2 expression in the primary tumor, established cell line, and xenograft of a human hepatoblastoma. Exp Cell Res 270(1):88–95. doi:10.1006/excr.2001.5336

53. Feng W, Lu Z, Luo RZ, Zhang X, Seto E, Liao WS, Yu Y (2007) Multiple histone deacetylases repress tumor suppressor gene ARHI in breast cancer. Int J Cancer 120(8):1664–1668. doi:10.1002/ijc.22474

54. Feng W, Marquez RT, Lu Z, Liu J, Lu KH, Issa JP, Fishman DM, Yu Y, Bast RC (2008) Imprinted tumor suppressor genes ARHI and PEG3 are the most frequently down-regulated in human ovarian cancers by loss of heterozygosity and promoter methylation. Cancer 112(7):1489–1502. doi:10.1002/cncr.23323
55. Ferguson-Smith AC (2011) Genomic imprinting: the emergence of an epigenetic paradigm. Nat Rev Genet 12(8):565–575. doi:10.1038/nrg3032
56. Fitzpatrick GV, Pugacheva EM, Shin JY, Abdullaev Z, Yang Y, Khatod K, Lobanenkov VV, Higgins MJ (2007) Allele-specific binding of CTCF to the multipartite imprinting control region KvDMR1. Mol Cell Biol 27(7):2636–2647. doi:10.1128/MCB.02036-06
57. Fitzpatrick GV, Soloway PD, Higgins MJ (2002) Regional loss of imprinting and growth deficiency in mice with a targeted deletion of KvDMR1. Nat Genet 32(3):426–431. doi:10.1038/ng988
58. Formosa A, Markert EK, Lena AM, Italiano D, Finazzi-Agro' E, Levine AJ, Bernardini S, Garabadgiu AV, Melino G, Candi E (2014) MicroRNAs, miR-154, miR-299-5p, miR-376a, miR-376c, miR-377, miR-381, miR-487b, miR-485-3p, miR-495 and miR-654-3p, mapped to the 14q32.31 locus, regulate proliferation, apoptosis, migration and invasion in metastatic prostate cancer cells. Oncogene 33(44):5173–5182. doi:10.1038/onc.2013.451
59. Fujii S, Luo RZ, Yuan J, Kadota M, Oshimura M, Dent SR, Kondo Y, Issa JP, Bast RC, Yu Y (2003) Reactivation of the silenced and imprinted alleles of ARHI is associated with increased histone H3 acetylation and decreased histone H3 lysine 9 methylation. Hum Mol Genet 12(15):1791–1800
60. Furukawa S, Haruta M, Arai Y, Honda S, Ohshima J, Sugawara W, Kageyama Y, Higashi Y, Nishida K, Tsunematsu Y, Nakadate H, Ishii M, Kaneko Y (2009) Yolk sac tumor but not seminoma or teratoma is associated with abnormal epigenetic reprogramming pathway and shows frequent hypermethylation of various tumor suppressor genes. Cancer Sci 100(4):698–708. doi:10.1111/j.1349-7006.2009.01102.x
61. Gadd S, Huff V, Huang CC, Ruteshouser EC, Dome JS, Grundy PE, Breslow N, Jennings L, Green DM, Beckwith JB, Perlman EJ (2012) Clinically relevant subsets identified by gene expression patterns support a revised ontogenic model of Wilms tumor: a Children's Oncology Group Study. Neoplasia 14(8):742–756
62. Gejman R, Batista DL, Zhong Y, Zhou Y, Zhang X, Swearingen B, Stratakis CA, Hedley-Whyte ET, Klibanski A (2008) Selective loss of MEG3 expression and intergenic differentially methylated region hypermethylation in the MEG3/DLK1 locus in human clinically nonfunctioning pituitary adenomas. J Clin Endocrinol Metab 93(10):4119–4125. doi:10.1210/jc.2007-2633
63. Ginno PA, Lott PL, Christensen HC, Korf I, Chédin F (2012) R-loop formation is a distinctive characteristic of unmethylated human CpG island promoters. Mol Cell 45(6):814–825. doi:10.1016/j.molcel.2012.01.017
64. Gloss BS, Patterson KI, Barton CA, Gonzalez M, Scurry JP, Hacker NF, Sutherland RL, O'Brien PM, Clark SJ (2012) Integrative genome-wide expression and promoter DNA methylation profiling identifies a potential novel panel of ovarian cancer epigenetic biomarkers. Cancer Lett 318(1):76–85. doi:10.1016/j.canlet.2011.12.003
65. Grbesa I, Ivkic M, Pegan B, Gall-Troselj K (2006) Loss of imprinting and promoter usage of the IGF2 in laryngeal squamous cell carcinoma. Cancer Lett 238(2):224–229. doi:10.1016/j.canlet.2005.07.003
66. Gu TP, Guo F, Yang H, Wu HP, Xu GF, Liu W, Xie ZG, Shi L, He X, Jin SG, Iqbal K, Shi YG, Deng Z, Szabo PE, Pfeifer GP, Li J, Xu GL (2011) The role of Tet3 DNA dioxygenase in epigenetic reprogramming by oocytes. Nature 477(7366):606–610. doi:10.1038/nature10443
67. Guo H, Tian T, Nan K, Wang W (2010) p57: A multifunctional protein in cancer (Review). Int J Oncol 36(6):1321–1329
68. Gururajan M, Josson S, Chu GC, Lu CL, Lu YT, Haga CL, Zhau HE, Liu C, Lichterman J, Duan P, Posadas EM, Chung LW (2014) miR-154* and miR-379 in the DLK1-DIO3

microRNA mega-cluster regulate epithelial to mesenchymal transition and bone metastasis of prostate cancer. Clin Cancer Res 20(24):6559–6569. doi:10.1158/1078-0432.ccr-14-1784

69. Hagiwara K, Li Y, Kinoshita T, Kunishma S, Ohashi H, Hotta T, Nagai H (2010) Aberrant DNA methylation of the p57KIP2 gene is a sensitive biomarker for detecting minimal residual disease in diffuse large B cell lymphoma. Leuk Res 34(1):50–54. doi:10.1016/j.leukres.2009.06.028

70. Hao Y, Crenshaw T, Moulton T, Newcomb E, Tycko B (1993) Tumour-suppressor activity of H19 RNA. Nature 365(6448):764–767. doi:10.1038/365764a0

71. Hark AT, Schoenherr CJ, Katz DJ, Ingram RS, Levorse JM, Tilghman SM (2000) CTCF mediates methylation-sensitive enhancer-blocking activity at the H19/Igf2 locus. Nature 405(6785):486–489. doi:10.1038/35013106

72. Hashimoto K, Azuma C, Tokugawa Y, Nobunaga T, Aki TA, Matsui Y, Yanagida T, Izumi H, Saji F, Murata Y (1997) Loss of H19 imprinting and up-regulation of H19 and SNRPN in a case with malignant mixed Müllerian tumor of the uterus. Hum Pathol 28(7):862–865

73. Hayward BE, Barlier A, Korbonits M, Grossman AB, Jacquet P, Enjalbert A, Bonthron DT (2001) Imprinting of the G(s)alpha gene GNAS1 in the pathogenesis of acromegaly. J Clin Invest 107(6):R31–R36. doi:10.1172/jci11887

74. Herold M, Bartkuhn M, Renkawitz R (2012) CTCF: insights into insulator function during development. Development 139(6):1045–1057. doi:10.1242/dev.065268

75. Hibi K, Nakamura H, Hirai A, Fujikake Y, Kasai Y, Akiyama S, Ito K, Takagi H (1996) Loss of H19 imprinting in esophageal cancer. Cancer Res 56(3):480–482

76. Hiby SE, Lough M, Keverne EB, Surani MA, Loke YW, King A (2001) Paternal monoallelic expression of PEG3 in the human placenta. Hum Mol Genet 10(10):1093–1100

77. Holm TM, Jackson-Grusby L, Brambrink T, Yamada Y, Rideout WM 3rd, Jaenisch R (2005) Global loss of imprinting leads to widespread tumorigenesis in adult mice. Cancer Cell 8(4):275–285. doi:10.1016/j.ccr.2005.09.007

78. Honda S, Arai Y, Haruta M, Sasaki F, Ohira M, Yamaoka H, Horie H, Nakagawara A, Hiyama E, Todo S, Kaneko Y (2008) Loss of imprinting of IGF2 correlates with hypermethylation of the H19 differentially methylated region in hepatoblastoma. Br J Cancer 99(11):1891–1899. doi:10.1038/sj.bjc.6604754. Epub 2008 Oct 28

79. Huang GS, Brouwer-Visser J, Ramirez MJ, Kim CH, Hebert TM, Lin J, Arias-Pulido H, Qualls CR, Prossnitz ER, Goldberg GL, Smith HO, Horwitz SB (2010) Insulin-like growth factor 2 expression modulates Taxol resistance and is a candidate biomarker for reduced disease-free survival in ovarian cancer. Clin Cancer Res 16(11):2999–3010. doi:10.1158/1078-0432.CCR-09-3233

80. Huang J, Lin Y, Li L, Qing D, Teng XM, Zhang YL, Hu X, Hu Y, Yang P, Han ZG (2009) ARHI, as a novel suppressor of cell growth and downregulated in human hepatocellular carcinoma, could contribute to hepatocarcinogenesis. Mol Carcinog 48(2):130–140. doi:10.1002/mc.20461

81. Huang J, Zhang X, Zhang M, Zhu JD, Zhang YL, Lin Y, Wang KS, Qi XF, Zhang Q, Liu GZ, Yu J, Cui Y, Yang PY, Wang ZQ, Han ZG (2007) Up-regulation of DLK1 as an imprinted gene could contribute to human hepatocellular carcinoma. Carcinogenesis 28(5):1094–1103. doi:10.1093/carcin/bgl215

82. Huang Y, Dai H, Guo QN (2012) TSSC3 overexpression reduces stemness and induces apoptosis of osteosarcoma tumor-initiating cells. Apoptosis 17(8):749–761. doi:10.1007/s10495-012-0734-1

83. Huang Z, Wen Y, Shandilya R, Marks JR, Berchuck A, Murphy SK (2006) High throughput detection of M6P/IGF2R intronic hypermethylation and LOH in ovarian cancer. Nucleic Acids Res 34(2):555–563. doi:10.1093/nar/gkj468

84. Ichikawa M, Arai Y, Haruta M, Furukawa S, Ariga T, Kajii T, Kaneko Y (2013) Meiosis error and subsequent genetic and epigenetic alterations invoke the malignant transformation of germ cell tumor. Genes Chromosomes Cancer 52(3):274–286. doi:10.1002/gcc.22027

85. Ioannides Y, Lokulo-Sodipe K, Mackay DJ, Davies JH, Temple IK (2014) Temple syndrome: improving the recognition of an underdiagnosed chromosome 14 imprinting disorder: an analysis of 51 published cases. J Med Genet 51(8):495–501. doi:10.1136/jmedgenet-2014-102396

86. Issa JP, Vertino PM, Boehm CD, Newsham IF, Baylin SB (1996) Switch from monoallelic to biallelic human IGF2 promoter methylation during aging and carcinogenesis. Proc Natl Acad Sci U S A 93(21):11757–11762

87. Ito Y, Koessler T, Ibrahim AE, Rai S, Vowler SL, Abu-Amero S, Silva AL, Maia AT, Huddleston JE, Uribe-Lewis S, Woodfine K, Jagodic M, Nativio R, Dunning A, Moore G, Klenova E, Bingham S, Pharoah PD, Brenton JD, Beck S, Sandhu MS, Murrell A (2008) Somatically acquired hypomethylation of IGF2 in breast and colorectal cancer. Hum Mol Genet 17(17):2633–2643. doi:10.1093/hmg/ddn163

88. Jacobs DI, Mao Y, Fu A, Kelly WK, Zhu Y (2013) Dysregulated methylation at imprinted genes in prostate tumor tissue detected by methylation microarray. BMC Urol 13:37. doi:10.1186/1471-2490-13-37

89. Jin RJ, Lho Y, Wang Y, Ao M, Revelo MP, Hayward SW, Wills ML, Logan SK, Zhang P, Matusik RJ (2008) Down-regulation of p57Kip2 induces prostate cancer in the mouse. Cancer Res 68(10):3601–3608. doi:10.1158/0008-5472.CAN-08-0073

90. Kagami M, Sekita Y, Nishimura G, Irie M, Kato F, Okada M, Yamamori S, Kishimoto H, Nakayama M, Tanaka Y, Matsuoka K, Takahashi T, Noguchi M, Tanaka Y, Masumoto K, Utsunomiya T, Kouzan H, Komatsu Y, Ohashi H, Kurosawa K, Kosaki K, Ferguson-Smith AC, Ishino F, Ogata T (2008) Deletions and epimutations affecting the human 14q32.2 imprinted region in individuals with paternal and maternal upd(14)-like phenotypes. Nat Genet 40(2):237–242. doi:10.1038/ng.2007.56

91. Kamikihara T, Arima T, Kato K, Matsuda T, Kato H, Douchi T, Nagata Y, Nakao M, Wake N (2005) Epigenetic silencing of the imprinted gene ZAC by DNA methylation is an early event in the progression of human ovarian cancer. Int J Cancer 115(5):690–700. doi:10.1002/ijc.20971

92. Kanber D, Berulava T, Ammerpohl O, Mitter D, Richter J, Siebert R, Horsthemke B, Lohmann D, Buiting K (2009) The human retinoblastoma gene is imprinted. PLoS Genet 5(12):e1000790. doi:10.1371/journal.pgen.1000790

93. Kanduri C (2016) Long noncoding RNAs: Lessons from genomic imprinting. Biochim Biophys Acta 1859(1):102–111. doi:10.1016/j.bbagrm.2015.05.006

94. Kanduri C, Fitzpatrick G, Mukhopadhyay R, Kanduri M, Lobanenkov V, Higgins M, Ohlsson R (2002) A differentially methylated imprinting control region within the Kcnq1 locus harbors a methylation-sensitive chromatin insulator. J Biol Chem 277(20):18106–18110. doi:10.1074/jbc.M200031200

95. Kaneda A, Wang CJ, Cheong R, Timp W, Onyango P, Wen B, Iacobuzio-Donahue CA, Ohlsson R, Andraos R, Pearson MA, Sharov AA, Longo DL, Ko MS, Levchenko A, Feinberg AP (2007) Enhanced sensitivity to IGF-II signaling links loss of imprinting of IGF2 to increased cell proliferation and tumor risk. Proc Natl Acad Sci U S A 104(52):20926–20931. doi:10.1073/pnas.0710359105

96. Kaneda M, Okano M, Hata K, Sado T, Tsujimoto N, Li E, Sasaki H (2004) Essential role for de novo DNA methyltransferase Dnmt3a in paternal and maternal imprinting. Nature 429(6994):900–903. doi:10.1038/nature02633

97. Kang L, Sun J, Wen X, Cui J, Wang G, Hoffman AR, Hu JF, Li W (2015) Aberrant allele-switch imprinting of a novel IGF1R intragenic antisense non-coding RNA in breast cancers. Eur J Cancer 51(2):260–270. doi:10.1016/j.ejca.2014.10.031

98. Kavanagh E, Joseph B (2011) The hallmarks of CDKN1C (p57, KIP2) in cancer. Biochim Biophys Acta 1816(1):50–56. doi:10.1016/j.bbcan.2011.03.002

99. Kawakami T, Chano T, Minami K, Okabe H, Okada Y, Okamoto K (2006a) Imprinted DLK1 is a putative tumor suppressor gene and inactivated by epimutation at the region upstream of GTL2 in human renal cell carcinoma. Hum Mol Genet 15(6):821–830. doi:10.1093/hmg/ddl001

100. Kawakami T, Zhang C, Okada Y, Okamoto K (2006b) Erasure of methylation imprint at the promoter and CTCF-binding site upstream of H19 in human testicular germ cell tumors of adolescents indicate their fetal germ cell origin. Oncogene 25(23):3225–3236. doi:10.1038/sj.onc.1209362

101. Kelsey G (2010) Imprinting on chromosome 20: tissue-specific imprinting and imprinting mutations in the GNAS locus. Am J Med Genet C Semin Med Genet 154C(3):377–386. doi:10.1002/ajmg.c.30271

102. Keniry A, Oxley D, Monnier P, Kyba M, Dandolo L, Smits G, Reik W (2012) The H19 lin-cRNA is a developmental reservoir of miR-675 that suppresses growth and Igf1r. Nat Cell Biol 14(7):659–665. doi:10.1038/ncb2521

103. Kikuchi T, Toyota M, Itoh F, Suzuki H, Obata T, Yamamoto H, Kakiuchi H, Kusano M, Issa JP, Tokino T, Imai K (2002) Inactivation of p57KIP2 by regional promoter hypermethylation and histone deacetylation in human tumors. Oncogene 21(17):2741–2749. doi:10.1038/sj.onc.1205376

104. Kim J, Bretz CL, Lee S (2015) Epigenetic instability of imprinted genes in human cancers. Nucleic Acids Res 43(22):10689–10699. doi:10.1093/nar/gkv867

105. Kim SJ, Park SE, Lee C, Lee SY, Jo JH, Kim JM, Oh YK (2002) Alterations in promoter usage and expression levels of insulin-like growth factor-II and H19 genes in cervical carcinoma exhibiting biallelic expression of IGF-II. Biochim Biophys Acta 1586(3):307–315

106. Kishino T, Lalande M, Wagstaff J (1997) UBE3A/E6-AP mutations cause Angelman syndrome. Nat Genet 15(1):70–73. doi:10.1038/ng0197-70

107. Kobatake T, Yano M, Toyooka S, Tsukuda K, Dote H, Kikuchi T, Toyota M, Ouchida M, Aoe M, Date H, Pass HI, Doihara H, Shimizu N (2004) Aberrant methylation of p57KIP2 gene in lung and breast cancers and malignant mesotheliomas. Oncology reports 12(5):1087–1092

108. Kohda T, Asai A, Kuroiwa Y, Kobayashi S, Aisaka K, Nagashima G, Yoshida MC, Kondo Y, Kagiyama N, Kirino T, Kaneko-Ishino T, Ishino F (2001) Tumour suppressor activity of human imprinted gene PEG3 in a glioma cell line. Genes Cells 6(3):237–247

109. Kondo M, Suzuki H, Ueda R, Osada H, Takagi K, Takahashi T, Takahashi T (1995) Frequent loss of imprinting of the H19 gene is often associated with its overexpression in human lung cancers. Oncogene 10(6):1193–1198

110. Kouzarides T (2007) Chromatin modifications and their function. Cell 128(4):693–705. doi:10.1016/j.cell.2007.02.005

111. Kuang SQ, Ling X, Sanchez-Gonzalez B, Yang H, Andreeff M, Garcia-Manero G (2007) Differential tumor suppressor properties and transforming growth factor-beta responsiveness of p57KIP2 in leukemia cells with aberrant p57KIP2 promoter DNA methylation. Oncogene 26(10):1439–1448. doi:10.1038/sj.onc.1209907

112. Kuerbitz SJ, Pahys J, Wilson A, Compitello N, Gray TA (2002) Hypermethylation of the imprinted NNAT locus occurs frequently in pediatric acute leukemia. Carcinogenesis 23(4):559–564

113. Kurukuti S, Tiwari VK, Tavoosidana G, Pugacheva E, Murrell A, Zhao Z, Lobanenkov V, Reik W, Ohlsson R (2006) CTCF binding at the H19 imprinting control region mediates maternally inherited higher-order chromatin conformation to restrict enhancer access to Igf2. Proc Natl Acad Sci U S A 103(28):10684–10689. doi:10.1073/pnas.0600326103

114. Lambert MP, Ancey PB, Esposti DD, Cros MP, Sklias A, Scoazec JY, Durantel D, Hernandez-Vargas H, Herceg Z (2015) Aberrant DNA methylation of imprinted loci in hepatocellular carcinoma and after in vitro exposure to common risk factors. Clin Epigenetics 7(1):15. doi:10.1186/s13148-015-0053-9

115. Landis CA, Masters SB, Spada A, Pace AM, Bourne HR, Vallar L (1989) GTPase inhibiting mutations activate the alpha chain of Gs and stimulate adenylyl cyclase in human pituitary tumours. Nature 340(6236):692–696. doi:10.1038/340692a0

116. Lee MH, Reynisdottir I, Massague J (1995) Cloning of p57KIP2, a cyclin-dependent kinase inhibitor with unique domain structure and tissue distribution. Genes Dev 9(6):639–649

117. Lee SH, Appleby V, Jeyapalan JN, Palmer RD, Nicholson JC, Sottile V, Gao E, Coleman N, Scotting PJ (2011) Variable methylation of the imprinted gene, SNRPN, supports a relationship between intracranial germ cell tumours and neural stem cells. J Neurooncol 101(3):419–428. doi:10.1007/s11060-010-0275-9

118. Lee SM, Lee EJ, Ko YH, Lee SH, Maeng L, Kim KM (2009) Prognostic significance of O6-methylguanine DNA methyltransferase and p57 methylation in patients with diffuse large B-cell lymphomas. APMIS 117(2):87–94. doi:10.1111/j.1600-0463.2008.00017.x

119. Lehner B, Kunz P, Saehr H, Fellenberg J (2014) Epigenetic silencing of genes and microRNAs within the imprinted Dlk1-Dio3 region at human chromosome 14.32 in giant cell tumor of bone. BMC Cancer 14:495. doi:10.1186/1471-2407-14-495

120. Lewis A, Mitsuya K, Umlauf D, Smith P, Dean W, Walter J, Higgins M, Feil R, Reik W (2004) Imprinting on distal chromosome 7 in the placenta involves repressive histone methylation independent of DNA methylation. Nat Genet 36(12):1291–1295. doi:10.1038/ng1468

121. Li J, Bench AJ, Vassiliou GS, Fourouclas N, Ferguson-Smith AC, Green AR (2004) Imprinting of the human L3MBTL gene, a polycomb family member located in a region of chromosome 20 deleted in human myeloid malignancies. Proc Natl Acad Sci U S A 101(19):7341–7346. doi:10.1073/pnas.0308195101

122. Li LL, Xue AM, Li BX, Shen YW, Li YH, Luo CL, Zhang MC, Jiang JQ, Xu ZD, Xie JH, Zhao ZQ (2014a) JMJD2A contributes to breast cancer progression through transcriptional repression of the tumor suppressor ARHI. Breast Cancer Res 16(3):R56. doi:10.1186/bcr3667

123. Li T, Hu JF, Qiu X, Ling J, Chen H, Wang S, Hou A, Vu TH, Hoffman AR (2008a) CTCF regulates allelic expression of Igf2 by orchestrating a promoter-polycomb repressive complex 2 intrachromosomal loop. Mol Cell Biol 28(20):6473–6482. doi:10.1128/MCB.00204-08

124. Li X, Cui H, Sandstedt B, Nordlinder H, Larsson E, Ekstrom TJ (1996) Expression levels of the insulin-like growth factor-II gene (IGF2) in the human liver: developmental relationships of the four promoters. J Endocrinol 149(1):117–124

125. Li X, Ito M, Zhou F, Youngson N, Zuo X, Leder P, Ferguson-Smith AC (2008b) A maternal-zygotic effect gene, Zfp57, maintains both maternal and paternal imprints. Dev Cell 15(4):547–557. doi:10.1016/j.devcel.2008.08.014

126. Li X, Kogner P, Sandstedt B, Haas OA, Ekström TJ (1998) Promoter-specific methylation and expression alterations of Igf2 and H19 are involved in human hepatoblastoma. Int J Cancer 75(2):176–180

127. Li Y, Huang Y, Lv Y, Meng G, Guo QN (2014b) Epigenetic regulation of the pro-apoptosis gene TSSC3 in human osteosarcoma cells. Biomed Pharmacother 68(1):45–50. doi:10.1016/j.biopha.2013.10.006

128. Li Y, Meng G, Guo QN (2008c) Changes in genomic imprinting and gene expression associated with transformation in a model of human osteosarcoma. Exp Mol Pathol 84(3):234–239. doi:10.1016/j.yexmp.2008.03.013

129. Li Y, Meng G, Huang L, Guo QN (2009) Hypomethylation of the P3 promoter is associated with up-regulation of IGF2 expression in human osteosarcoma. Hum Pathol 40(10):1441–1447. doi:10.1016/j.humpath.2009.03.003

130. Li Y, Nagai H, Ohno T, Yuge M, Hatano S, Ito E, Mori N, Saito H, Kinoshita T (2002) Aberrant DNA methylation of p57(KIP2) gene in the promoter region in lymphoid malignancies of B-cell phenotype. Blood 100(7):2572–2577. doi:10.1182/blood-2001-11-0026

131. Kim JD, Kim H, Ekram MB, Yu S, Faulk C, Kim J (2011) Rex1/Zfp42 as an epigenetic regulator for genomic imprinting. Hum Mol Genet 20(7):1353–1362. doi:10.1093/hmg/ddr017

132. Livingstone C (2013) IGF2 and cancer. Endocr Relat Cancer 20(6):R321–R339. doi:10.1530/ERC-13-0231

133. Luo M, Li Z, Wang W, Zeng Y, Liu Z, Qiu J (2013) Long non-coding RNA H19 increases bladder cancer metastasis by associating with EZH2 and inhibiting E-cadherin expression. Cancer Lett 333(2):213–221. doi:10.1016/j.canlet.2013.01.033

134. Luo RZ, Peng H, Xu F, Bao J, Pang Y, Pershad R, Issa JP, Liao WS, Bast RC, Yu Y (2001) Genomic structure and promoter characterization of an imprinted tumor suppressor gene ARHI. Biochim Biophys Acta 1519(3):216–222
135. Lustig-Yariv O, Schulze E, Komitowski D, Erdmann V, Schneider T, de Groot N, Hochberg A (1997) The expression of the imprinted genes H19 and IGF-2 in choriocarcinoma cell lines. Is H19 a tumor suppressor gene? Oncogene 15(2):169–177. doi:10.1038/sj.onc.1201175
136. Lv YF, Yan GN, Meng G, Zhang X, Guo QN (2015) Enhancer of zeste homolog 2 silencing inhibits tumor growth and lung metastasis in osteosarcoma. Sci Rep 5:12999. doi:10.1038/srep12999
137. Lynch CA, Tycko B, Bestor TH, Walsh CP (2002) Reactivation of a silenced H19 gene in human rhabdomyosarcoma by demethylation of DNA but not by histone hyperacetylation. Mol Cancer 1:2
138. Mackay DJ, Callaway JL, Marks SM, White HE, Acerini CL, Boonen SE, Dayanikli P, Firth HV, Goodship JA, Haemers AP, Hahnemann JM, Kordonouri O, Masoud AF, Oestergaard E, Storr J, Ellard S, Hattersley AT, Robinson DO, Temple IK (2008) Hypomethylation of multiple imprinted loci in individuals with transient neonatal diabetes is associated with mutations in ZFP57. Nat Genet 40(8):949–951. doi:10.1038/ng.187
139. Mackay DJ, Temple IK (2010) Transient neonatal diabetes mellitus type 1. Am J Med Genet C Semin Med Genet 154C(3):335–342. doi:10.1002/ajmg.c.30272
140. Maegawa S, Yoshioka H, Itaba N, Kubota N, Nishihara S, Shirayoshi Y, Nanba E, Oshimura M (2001) Epigenetic silencing of PEG3 gene expression in human glioma cell lines. Mol Carcinog 31(1):1–9
141. Maeng YS, Choi HJ, Kwon JY, Park YW, Choi KS, Min JK, Kim YH, Suh PG, Kang KS, Won MH, Kim YM, Kwon YG (2009) Endothelial progenitor cell homing: prominent role of the IGF2-IGF2R-PLCbeta2 axis. Blood 113(1):233–243. doi:10.1182/blood-2008-06-162891
142. Mancini-DiNardo D (2003) A differentially methylated region within the gene Kcnq1 functions as an imprinted promoter and silencer. Human Molecular Genetics 12(3):283–294. doi:10.1093/hmg/ddg024
143. Mancini-Dinardo D, Steele SJ, Levorse JM, Ingram RS, Tilghman SM (2006) Elongation of the Kcnq1ot1 transcript is required for genomic imprinting of neighboring genes. Genes Dev 20(10):1268–1282. doi:10.1101/gad.1416906
144. Mantovani G (2011) Clinical review: Pseudohypoparathyroidism: diagnosis and treatment. J Clin Endocrinol Metab 96(10):3020–3030. doi:10.1210/jc.2011-1048
145. Mantovani G, Bondioni S, Lania AG, Corbetta S, de Sanctis L, Cappa M, Di Battista E, Chanson P, Beck-Peccoz P, Spada A (2004) Parental origin of Gsalpha mutations in the McCune-Albright syndrome and in isolated endocrine tumors. J Clin Endocrinol Metab 89(6):3007–3009. doi:10.1210/jc.2004-0194
146. Martinez R, Martin-Subero JI, Rohde V, Kirsch M, Alaminos M, Fernandez AF, Ropero S, Schackert G, Esteller M (2009) A microarray-based DNA methylation study of glioblastoma multiforme. Epigenetics 4(4):255–264
147. Matouk IJ, DeGroot N, Mezan S, Ayesh S, Abu-lail R, Hochberg A, Galun E (2007) The H19 non-coding RNA is essential for human tumor growth. PLoS One 2(9):e845. doi:10.1371/journal.pone.0000845
148. Matsuoka S, Edwards MC, Bai C, Parker S, Zhang P, Baldini A, Harper JW, Elledge SJ (1995) p57KIP2, a structurally distinct member of the p21CIP1 Cdk inhibitor family, is a candidate tumor suppressor gene. Genes Dev 9(6):650–662
149. Matsuura T, Takahashi K, Nakayama K, Kobayashi T, Choi-Miura NH, Tomita M, Kanayama N (2002) Increased expression of vascular endothelial growth factor in placentas of p57(Kip2) null embryos. FEBS Lett 532(3):283–288
150. McGrath J, Solter D (1984) Completion of mouse embryogenesis requires both the maternal and paternal genomes. Cell 37(1):179–183
151. Menigatti M, Staiano T, Manser CN, Bauerfeind P, Komljenovic A, Robinson M, Jiricny J, Buffoli F, Marra G (2013) Epigenetic silencing of monoallelically methylated miRNA loci in precancerous colorectal lesions. Oncogenesis 2:e56. doi:10.1038/oncsis.2013.21

152. Mohammad F, Mondal T, Guseva N, Pandey GK, Kanduri C (2010) Kcnq1ot1 noncoding RNA mediates transcriptional gene silencing by interacting with Dnmt1. Development 137(15):2493–2499. doi:10.1242/dev.048181

153. Monk D (2015) Germline-derived DNA methylation and early embryo epigenetic reprogramming: The selected survival of imprints. Int J Biochem Cell Biol 67:128–138. doi:10.1016/j.biocel.2015.04.014

154. Ito Y, Maehara K, Kaneki E, Matsuoka K, Sugahara N, Miyata T, Kamura H, Yamaguchi Y, Kono A, Nakabayashi K, Migita O, Higashimoto K, Soejima H, Okamoto A, Nakamura H, Kimura T, Wake N, Taniguchi T, Hata K (2016) Novel Nonsense Mutation in the NLRP7 Gene Associated with Recurrent Hydatidiform Mole. Gynecol Obstet Invest 81(4):353–358. doi:10.1159/000441780

155. Moulton T, Crenshaw T, Hao Y, Moosikasuwan J, Lin N, Dembitzer F, Hensle T, Weiss L, McMorrow L, Loew T et al (1994) Epigenetic lesions at the H19 locus in Wilms' tumour patients. Nat Genet 7(3):440–447. doi:10.1038/ng0794-440

156. Murakami K, Oshimura M, Kugoh H (2007) Suggestive evidence for chromosomal localization of non-coding RNA from imprinted LIT1. J Hum Genet 52(11):926–933. doi:10.1007/s10038-007-0196-4

157. Murata A, Baba Y, Watanabe M, Shigaki H, Miyake K, Ishimoto T, Iwatsuki M, Iwagami S, Yoshida N, Oki E, Morita M, Nakao M, Baba H (2014) IGF2 DMR0 methylation, loss of imprinting, and patient prognosis in esophageal squamous cell carcinoma. Ann Surg Oncol 21(4):1166–1174. doi:10.1245/s10434-013-3414-7

158. Murphy SK, Huang Z, Wen Y, Spillman MA, Whitaker RS, Simel LR, Nichols TD, Marks JR, Berchuck A (2006) Frequent IGF2/H19 domain epigenetic alterations and elevated IGF2 expression in epithelial ovarian cancer. Mol Cancer Res 4(4):283–292. doi:10.1158/1541-7786.MCR-05-0138

159. Murphy SK, Wylie AA, Jirtle RL (2001) Imprinting of PEG3, the human homologue of a mouse gene involved in nurturing behavior. Genomics 71(1):110–117. doi:10.1006/geno.2000.6419

160. Murrell A (2006) Genomic imprinting and cancer: from primordial germ cells to somatic cells. ScientificWorldJournal 6:1888–1910. doi:10.1100/tsw.2006.318

161. Murrell A, Heeson S, Reik W (2004) Interaction between differentially methylated regions partitions the imprinted genes Igf2 and H19 into parent-specific chromatin loops. Nat Genet 36(8):889–893. doi:10.1038/ng1402

162. Murrell A, Ito Y, Verde G, Huddleston J, Woodfine K, Silengo MC, Spreafico F, Perotti D, De Crescenzo A, Sparago A, Cerrato F, Riccio A (2008) Distinct methylation changes at the IGF2-H19 locus in congenital growth disorders and cancer. PLoS One 3(3):e1849. doi:10.1371/journal.pone.0001849

163. Mussa A, Molinatto C, Baldassarre G, Riberi E, Russo S, Larizza L, Riccio A, Ferrero GB (2016a) Cancer Risk in Beckwith-Wiedemann Syndrome: A Systematic Review and Meta-Analysis Outlining a Novel (Epi)Genotype Specific Histotype Targeted Screening Protocol. J Pediatr. 176:142–149.e1. doi:10.1016/j.jpeds.2016.05.038

164. Mussa A, Russo S, De Crescenzo A, Freschi A, Calzari L, Maitz S, Macchiaiolo M, Molinatto C, Baldassarre G, Mariani M, Tarani L, Bedeschi MF, Milani D, Melis D, Bartuli A, Cubellis MV, Selicorni A, Cirillo Silengo M, Larizza L, Riccio A, Ferrero GB (2016b) (Epi)genotype-phenotype correlations in Beckwith-Wiedemann syndrome. Eur J Hum Genet 24(2):183–190. doi:10.1038/ejhg.2015.88

165. Nakagawa H, Chadwick RB, Peltomaki P, Plass C, Nakamura Y, de La Chapelle A (2001) Loss of imprinting of the insulin-like growth factor II gene occurs by biallelic methylation in a core region of H19-associated CTCF-binding sites in colorectal cancer. Proc Natl Acad Sci U S A 98(2):591–596. doi:10.1073/pnas.011528698

166. Nakamura T, Liu YJ, Nakashima H, Umehara H, Inoue K, Matoba S, Tachibana M, Ogura A, Shinkai Y, Nakano T (2012) PGC7 binds histone H3K9me2 to protect against conversion of 5mC to 5hmC in early embryos. Nature 486(7403):415–419. doi:10.1038/nature11093

167. Nakano S, Murakami K, Meguro M, Soejima H, Higashimoto K, Urano T, Kugoh H, Mukai T, Ikeguchi M, Oshimura M (2006) Expression profile of LIT1/KCNQ1OT1 and epigenetic status at the KvDMR1 in colorectal cancers. Cancer Sci 97(11):1147–1154. doi:10.1111/j.1349-7006.2006.00305.x

168. Nativio R, Sparago A, Ito Y, Weksberg R, Riccio A, Murrell A (2011) Disruption of genomic neighbourhood at the imprinted IGF2-H19 locus in Beckwith-Wiedemann syndrome and Silver-Russell syndrome. Hum Mol Genet 20(7):1363–1374. doi:10.1093/hmg/ddr018

169. Nativio R, Wendt KS, Ito Y, Huddleston JE, Uribe-Lewis S, Woodfine K, Krueger C, Reik W, Peters JM, Murrell A (2009) Cohesin is required for higher-order chromatin conformation at the imprinted IGF2-H19 locus. PLoS Genet 5(11):e1000739. doi:10.1371/journal.pgen.1000739

170. Nicholls RD, Knoll JH, Butler MG, Karam S, Lalande M (1989) Genetic imprinting suggested by maternal heterodisomy in nondeletion Prader-Willi syndrome. Nature 342(6247):281–285. doi:10.1038/342281a0

171. Nielsen HM, How-Kit A, Guerin C, Castinetti F, Vollan HK, De Micco C, Daunay A, Taieb D, Van Loo P, Besse C, Kristensen VN, Hansen LL, Barlier A, Sebag F, Tost J (2015) Copy number variations alter methylation and parallel IGF2 overexpression in adrenal tumors. Endocr Relat Cancer 22(6):953–967. doi:10.1530/erc-15-0086

172. Niemczyk M, Ito Y, Huddleston J, Git A, Abu-Amero S, Caldas C, Moore GE, Stojic L, Murrell A (2013) Imprinted chromatin around DIRAS3 regulates alternative splicing of GNG12-AS1, a long noncoding RNA. Am J Hum Genet 93(2):224–235. doi:10.1016/j.ajhg.2013.06.010

173. Ogata T, Kagami M (2016) Kagami-Ogata syndrome: a clinically recognizable upd(14) pat and related disorder affecting the chromosome 14q32.2 imprinted region. J Hum Genet 61(2):87–94. doi:10.1038/jhg.2015.113

174. Ogawa O, Eccles MR, Szeto J, McNoe LA, Yun K, Maw MA, Smith PJ, Reeve AE (1993) Relaxation of insulin-like growth factor II gene imprinting implicated in Wilms' tumour. Nature 362(6422):749–751. doi:10.1038/362749a0

175. Ohtsuka Y, Higashimoto K, Oka T, Yatsuki H, Jozaki K, Maeda T, Kawahara K, Hamasaki Y, Matsuo M, Nishioka K, Joh K, Mukai T, Soejima H (2016) Identification of consensus motifs associated with mitotic recombination and clinical characteristics in patients with paternal uniparental isodisomy of chromosome 11. Hum Mol Genet 25(7):1406–1419. doi:10.1093/hmg/ddw023

176. Ooi SK, Qiu C, Bernstein E, Li K, Jia D, Yang Z, Erdjument-Bromage H, Tempst P, Lin SP, Allis CD, Cheng X, Bestor TH (2007) DNMT3L connects unmethylated lysine 4 of histone H3 to de novo methylation of DNA. Nature 448(7154):714–717. doi:10.1038/nature05987

177. Otsuka S, Maegawa S, Takamura A, Kamitani H, Watanabe T, Oshimura M, Nanba E (2009) Aberrant promoter methylation and expression of the imprinted PEG3 gene in glioma. Proc Jpn Acad Ser B Phys Biol Sci 85(4):157–165

178. Pandey RR, Mondal T, Mohammad F, Enroth S, Redrup L, Komorowski J, Nagano T, Mancini-Dinardo D, Kanduri C (2008) Kcnq1ot1 antisense noncoding RNA mediates lineage-specific transcriptional silencing through chromatin-level regulation. Mol Cell 32(2):232–246. doi:10.1016/j.molcel.2008.08.022

179. Paradowska A, Fenic I, Konrad L, Sturm K, Wagenlehner F, Weidner W, Steger K (2009) Aberrant epigenetic modifications in the CTCF binding domain of the IGF2/H19 gene in prostate cancer compared with benign prostate hyperplasia. Int J Oncol 35(1):87–96

180. Parry DA, Logan CV, Hayward BE, Shires M, Landolsi H, Diggle C, Carr I, Rittore C, Touitou I, Philibert L, Fisher RA, Fallahian M, Huntriss JD, Picton HM, Malik S, Taylor GR, Johnson CA, Bonthron DT, Sheridan EG (2011) Mutations causing familial biparental hydatidiform mole implicate c6orf221 as a possible regulator of genomic imprinting in the human oocyte. Am J Hum Genet 89(3):451–458. doi:10.1016/j.ajhg.2011.08.002

181. Peters J (2014) The role of genomic imprinting in biology and disease: an expanding view. Nat Rev Genet 15(8):517–530. doi:10.1038/nrg3766

182. Picard C, Silvy M, Gerard C, Buffat C, Lavaque E, Figarella-Branger D, Dufour H, Gabert J, Beckers A, Brue T, Enjalbert A, Barlier A (2007) Gs alpha overexpression and loss of Gs alpha imprinting in human somatotroph adenomas: association with tumor size and response to pharmacologic treatment. Int J Cancer 121(6):1245–1252. doi:10.1002/ijc.22816

183. Piecewicz SM, Pandey A, Roy B, Xiang SH, Zetter BR, Sengupta S (2012) Insulin-like growth factors promote vasculogenesis in embryonic stem cells. PLoS One 7(2):e32191. doi:10.1371/journal.pone.0032191

184. Pike BL, Greiner TC, Wang X, Weisenburger DD, Hsu YH, Renaud G, Wolfsberg TG, Kim M, Weisenberger DJ, Siegmund KD, Ye W, Groshen S, Mehrian-Shai R, Delabie J, Chan WC, Laird PW, Hacia JG (2008) DNA methylation profiles in diffuse large B cell lymphoma and their relationship to gene expression status. Leukemia 22(5):1035–1043. doi:10.1038/leu.2008.18

185. Poirier K, Chalas C, Tissier F, Couvert P, Mallet V, Carrié A, Marchio A, Sarli D, Gicquel C, Chaussade S, Beljord C, Chelly J, Kerjean A, Terris B (2003) Loss of parental-specific methylation at the IGF2 locus in human hepatocellular carcinoma. J Pathol 201(3):473–479. doi:10.1002/path.1477

186. Quenneville S, Verde G, Corsinotti A, Kapopoulou A, Jakobsson J, Offner S, Baglivo I, Pedone PV, Grimaldi G, Riccio A, Trono D (2011) In embryonic stem cells, ZFP57/KAP1 recognize a methylated hexanucleotide to affect chromatin and DNA methylation of imprinting control regions. Mol Cell 44(3):361–372. doi:10.1016/j.molcel.2011.08.032

187. Rainier S, Johnson LA, Dobry CJ, Ping AJ, Grundy PE, Feinberg AP (1993) Relaxation of imprinted genes in human cancer. Nature 362(6422):747–749. doi:10.1038/362747a0

188. Ravenel JD, Broman KW, Perlman EJ, Niemitz EL, Jayawardena TM, Bell DW, Haber DA, Uejima H, Feinberg AP (2001) Loss of imprinting of insulin-like growth factor-II (IGF2) gene in distinguishing specific biologic subtypes of Wilms tumor. J Natl Cancer Inst 93(22):1698–1703

189. Revill K, Dudley KJ, Clayton RN, McNicol AM, Farrell WE (2009) Loss of neuronatin expression is associated with promoter hypermethylation in pituitary adenoma. Endocr Relat Cancer 16(2):537–548. doi:10.1677/erc-09-0008

190. Riemenschneider MJ, Reifenberger J, Reifenberger G (2008) Frequent biallelic inactivation and transcriptional silencing of the DIRAS3 gene at 1p31 in oligodendroglial tumors with 1p loss. Int J Cancer 122(11):2503–2510. doi:10.1002/ijc.23409

191. Rijlaarsdam MA, Tax DM, Gillis AJ, Dorssers LC, Koestler DC, de Ridder J, Looijenga LH (2015) Genome wide DNA methylation profiles provide clues to the origin and pathogenesis of germ cell tumors. PLoS One 10(4):e0122146. doi:10.1371/journal.pone.0122146

192. Riordan JD, Keng VW, Tschida BR, Scheetz TE, Bell JB, Podetz-Pedersen KM, Moser CD, Copeland NG, Jenkins NA, Roberts LR, Largaespada DA, Dupuy AJ (2013) Identification of rtl1, a retrotransposon-derived imprinted gene, as a novel driver of hepatocarcinogenesis. PLoS Genet 9(4):e1003441. doi:10.1371/journal.pgen.1003441

193. Robson JE, Eaton SA, Underhill P, Williams D, Peters J (2012) MicroRNAs 296 and 298 are imprinted and part of the GNAS/Gnas cluster and miR-296 targets IKBKE and Tmed9. RNA 18(1):135–144. doi:10.1261/rna.029561.111

194. Rodriguez BA, Weng YI, Liu TM, Zuo T, Hsu PY, Lin CH, Cheng AL, Cui H, Yan PS, Huang TH (2011) Estrogen-mediated epigenetic repression of the imprinted gene cyclin-dependent kinase inhibitor 1C in breast cancer cells. Carcinogenesis 32(6):812–821. doi:10.1093/carcin/bgr017

195. Romanelli V, Nakabayashi K, Vizoso M, Moran S, Iglesias-Platas I, Sugahara N, Simón C, Hata K, Esteller M, Court F, Monk D (2014) Variable maternal methylation overlapping the nc886/vtRNA2-1 locus is locked between hypermethylated repeats and is frequently altered in cancer. Epigenetics 9(5):783–790. doi:10.4161/epi.28323

196. Rumbajan JM, Maeda T, Souzaki R, Mitsui K, Higashimoto K, Nakabayashi K, Yatsuki H, Nishioka K, Harada R, Aoki S, Kohashi K, Oda Y, Hata K, Saji T, Taguchi T, Tajiri T, Soejima H, Joh K (2013) Comprehensive analyses of imprinted differentially methylated

regions reveal epigenetic and genetic characteristics in hepatoblastoma. BMC Cancer 13:608. doi:10.1186/1471-2407-13-608

197. Saal HM (1993) Russell-Silver syndrome. In: Pagon RA, Adam MP, Ardinger HH et al (eds) GeneReviews®. University of Washington, Seattle, WA

198. Sahoo T, del Gaudio D, German JR, Shinawi M, Peters SU, Person RE, Garnica A, Cheung SW, Beaudet AL (2008) Prader-Willi phenotype caused by paternal deficiency for the HBII-85 C/D box small nucleolar RNA cluster. Nat Genet 40(6):719–721. doi:10.1038/ng.158

199. Sakatani T, Kaneda A, Iacobuzio-Donahue CA, Carter MG, de Boom WS, Okano H, Ko MS, Ohlsson R, Longo DL, Feinberg AP (2005) Loss of imprinting of Igf2 alters intestinal maturation and tumorigenesis in mice. Science 307(5717):1976–1978. doi:10.1126/science.1108080

200. Sanchez-Delgado M, Martin-Trujillo A, Tayama C, Vidal E, Esteller M, Iglesias-Platas I, Deo N, Barney O, Maclean K, Hata K, Nakabayashi K, Fisher R, Monk D (2015) Absence of Maternal Methylation in Biparental Hydatidiform Moles from Women with NLRP7 Maternal-Effect Mutations Reveals Widespread Placenta-Specific Imprinting. PLoS Genet 11(11):e1005644. doi:10.1371/journal.pgen.1005644

201. Satoh Y, Nakadate H, Nakagawachi T, Higashimoto K, Joh K, Masaki Z, Uozumi J, Kaneko Y, Mukai T, Soejima H (2006) Genetic and epigenetic alterations on the short arm of chromosome 11 are involved in a majority of sporadic Wilms' tumours. Br J Cancer 95(4):541–547. doi:10.1038/sj.bjc.6603302

202. Savage SA, Woodson K, Walk E, Modi W, Liao J, Douglass C, Hoover RN, Chanock SJ, Group NOES (2007) Analysis of genes critical for growth regulation identifies Insulin-like Growth Factor 2 Receptor variations with possible functional significance as risk factors for osteosarcoma. Cancer Epidemiol Biomarkers Prev 16(8):1667–1674. doi:10.1158/1055-9965.epi-07-0214

203. Saxena A (2003) The Product of the Imprinted Gene IPL Marks Human Villous Cytotrophoblast and is Lost in Complete Hydatidiform Mole. Placenta 24(8-9):835–842. doi:10.1016/s0143-4004(03)00130-9

204. Scelfo RA, Schwienbacher C, Veronese A, Gramantieri L, Bolondi L, Querzoli P, Nenci I, Calin GA, Angioni A, Barbanti-Brodano G, Negrini M (2002) Loss of methylation at chromosome 11p15.5 is common in human adult tumors. Oncogene 21(16):2564–2572. doi:10.1038/sj.onc.1205336

205. Schoenherr CJ, Levorse JM, Tilghman SM (2003) CTCF maintains differential methylation at the Igf2/H19 locus. Nat Genet 33(1):66–69. doi:10.1038/ng1057

206. Schwienbacher C, Angioni A, Scelfo R, Veronese A, Calin GA, Massazza G, Hatada I, Barbanti-Brodano G, Negrini M (2000) Abnormal RNA expression of 11p15 imprinted genes and kidney developmental genes in Wilms' tumor. Cancer Res 60(6):1521–1525

207. Shen L, Toyota M, Kondo Y, Obata T, Daniel S, Pierce S, Imai K, Kantarjian HM, Issa JP, Garcia-Manero G (2003) Aberrant DNA methylation of p57KIP2 identifies a cell-cycle regulatory pathway with prognostic impact in adult acute lymphocytic leukemia. Blood 101(10):4131–4136. doi:10.1182/blood-2002-08-2466

208. Shuman C, Beckwith JB, Smith AC, Weksberg R (1993) Beckwith-Wiedemann syndrome. In: Pagon RA, Adam MP, Ardinger HH et al (eds) GeneReviews®. University of Washington, Seattle, WA

209. Soejima H, Higashimoto K (2013) Epigenetic and genetic alterations of the imprinting disorder Beckwith-Wiedemann syndrome and related disorders. J Hum Genet 58(7):402–409. doi:10.1038/jhg.2013.51

210. Soejima H, Nakagawachi T, Zhao W, Higashimoto K, Urano T, Matsukura S, Kitajima Y, Takeuchi M, Nakayama M, Oshimura M, Miyazaki K, Joh K, Mukai T (2004) Silencing of imprinted CDKN1C gene expression is associated with loss of CpG and histone H3 lysine 9 methylation at DMR-LIT1 in esophageal cancer. Oncogene 23(25):4380–4388. doi:10.1038/sj.onc.1207576

211. Steenman MJ, Rainier S, Dobry CJ, Grundy P, Horon IL, Feinberg AP (1994) Loss of imprinting of IGF2 is linked to reduced expression and abnormal methylation of H19 in Wilms' tumour. Nat Genet 7(3):433–439. doi:10.1038/ng0794-433

212. Sullivan MJ, Taniguchi T, Jhee A, Kerr N, Reeve AE (1999) Relaxation of IGF2 imprinting in Wilms tumours associated with specific changes in IGF2 methylation. Oncogene 18(52):7527–7534. doi:10.1038/sj.onc.1203096

213. Sun Y, Gao D, Liu Y, Huang J, Lessnick S, Tanaka S (2006) IGF2 is critical for tumorigenesis by synovial sarcoma oncoprotein SYT-SSX1. Oncogene 25(7):1042–1052. doi:10.1038/sj.onc.1209143

214. Surani MA, Barton SC, Norris ML (1984) Development of reconstituted mouse eggs suggests imprinting of the genome during gametogenesis. Nature 308(5959):548–550

215. Takai D, Gonzales FA, Tsai YC, Thayer MJ, Jones PA (2001) Large scale mapping of methylcytosines in CTCF-binding sites in the human H19 promoter and aberrant hypomethylation in human bladder cancer. Hum Mol Genet 10(23):2619–2626

216. Temple IK, Mackay DJG, Docherty LE (1993) Diabetes mellitus, 6q24-related transient neonatal. In: Pagon RA, Adam MP, Ardinger HH et al (eds) GeneReviews®. University of Washington, Seattle, WA

217. Terranova R, Yokobayashi S, Stadler MB, Otte AP, van Lohuizen M, Orkin SH, Peters AH (2008) Polycomb group proteins Ezh2 and Rnf2 direct genomic contraction and imprinted repression in early mouse embryos. Dev Cell 15(5):668–679. doi:10.1016/j.devcel.2008.08.015

218. Thakur N, Kanduri M, Holmgren C, Mukhopadhyay R, Kanduri C (2003) Bidirectional silencing and DNA methylation-sensitive methylation-spreading properties of the Kcnq1 imprinting control region map to the same regions. J Biol Chem 278(11):9514–9519. doi:10.1074/jbc.M212203200

219. Thakur N, Tiwari VK, Thomassin H, Pandey RR, Kanduri M, Gondor A, Grange T, Ohlsson R, Kanduri C (2004) An antisense RNA regulates the bidirectional silencing property of the Kcnq1 imprinting control region. Mol Cell Biol 24(18):7855–7862. doi:10.1128/MCB.24.18.7855-7862.2004

220. Tomizawa S, Sasaki H (2012) Genomic imprinting and its relevance to congenital disease, infertility, molar pregnancy and induced pluripotent stem cell. J Hum Genet 57(2):84–91. doi:10.1038/jhg.2011.151

221. Tsang WP, Ng EK, Ng SS, Jin H, Yu J, Sung JJ, Kwok TT (2010) Oncofetal H19-derived miR-675 regulates tumor suppressor RB in human colorectal cancer. Carcinogenesis 31(3):350–358. doi:10.1093/carcin/bgp181

222. Turan S, Bastepe M (2015) GNAS Spectrum of Disorders. Curr Osteoporos Rep 13(3):146–158. doi:10.1007/s11914-015-0268-x

223. Ulaner GA, Vu TH, Li T, Hu JF, Yao XM, Yang Y, Gorlick R, Meyers P, Healey J, Ladanyi M, Hoffman AR (2003) Loss of imprinting of IGF2 and H19 in osteosarcoma is accompanied by reciprocal methylation changes of a CTCF-binding site. Hum Mol Genet 12(5):535–549

224. Valleley EM, Cordery SF, Carr IM, MacLennan KA, Bonthron DT (2010) Loss of expression of ZAC/PLAGL1 in diffuse large B-cell lymphoma is independent of promoter hypermethylation. Genes Chromosomes Cancer 49(5):480–486. doi:10.1002/gcc.20758

225. Verkerk AJ, Ariel I, Dekker MC, Schneider T, van Gurp RJ, de Groot N, Gillis AJ, Oosterhuis JW, Hochberg AA, Looijenga LH (1997) Unique expression patterns of H19 in human testicular cancers of different etiology. Oncogene 14(1):95–107. doi:10.1038/sj.onc.1200802

226. Vlachos P, Joseph B (2009) The Cdk inhibitor p57(Kip2) controls LIM-kinase 1 activity and regulates actin cytoskeleton dynamics. Oncogene 28(47):4175–4188. doi:10.1038/onc.2009.269

227. Vlachos P, Nyman U, Hajji N, Joseph B (2007) The cell cycle inhibitor p57(Kip2) promotes cell death via the mitochondrial apoptotic pathway. Cell Death Differ 14(8):1497–1507. doi:10.1038/sj.cdd.4402158

228. Vu TH, Hoffman A (1996) Alterations in the promoter-specific imprinting of the insulin-like growth factor-II gene in Wilms' tumor. J Biol Chem 271(15):9014–9023

229. Vu TH, Hoffman AR (1994) Promoter-specific imprinting of the human insulin-like growth factor-II gene. Nature 371(6499):714–717. doi:10.1038/371714a0

230. Wagschal A, Sutherland HG, Woodfine K, Henckel A, Chebli K, Schulz R, Oakey RJ, Bickmore WA, Feil R (2008) G9a histone methyltransferase contributes to imprinting in the mouse placenta. Mol Cell Biol 28(3):1104–1113. doi:10.1128/MCB.01111-07

231. Wang P, Ren Z, Sun P (2012) Overexpression of the long non-coding RNA MEG3 impairs in vitro glioma cell proliferation. J Cell Biochem 113(6):1868–1874. doi:10.1002/jcb.24055

232. Wang X, Li G, Koul S, Ohki R, Maurer M, Borczuk A, Halmos B (2015) PHLDA2 is a key oncogene-induced negative feedback inhibitor of EGFR/ErbB2 signaling via interference with AKT signaling. Oncotarget. doi:10.18632/oncotarget.3674

233. Weber F, Aldred MA, Morrison CD, Plass C, Frilling A, Broelsch CE, Waite KA, Eng C (2005) Silencing of the maternally imprinted tumor suppressor ARHI contributes to follicular thyroid carcinogenesis. J Clin Endocrinol Metab 90(2):1149–1155. doi:10.1210/jc.2004-1447

234. Wei JJ, Wu X, Peng Y, Shi G, Basturk O, Olca B, Yang X, Daniels G, Osman I, Ouyang J, Hernando E, Pellicer A, Rhim JS, Melamed J, Lee P (2011) Regulation of HMGA1 expression by microRNA-296 affects prostate cancer growth and invasion. Clin Cancer Res 17(6):1297–1305. doi:10.1158/1070-0432.ccr-10-0993

235. Wendt KS, Yoshida K, Itoh T, Bando M, Koch B, Schirghuber E, Tsutsumi S, Nagae G, Ishihara K, Mishiro T, Yahata K, Imamoto F, Aburatani H, Nakao M, Imamoto N, Maeshima K, Shirahige K, Peters JM (2008) Cohesin mediates transcriptional insulation by CCCTC-binding factor. Nature 451(7180):796–801. doi:10.1038/nature06634

236. Wossidlo M, Nakamura T, Lepikhov K, Marques CJ, Zakhartchenko V, Boiani M, Arand J, Nakano T, Reik W, Walter J (2011) 5-Hydroxymethylcytosine in the mammalian zygote is linked with epigenetic reprogramming. Nat Commun 2:241. doi:10.1038/ncomms1240

237. Wu J, Qin Y, Li B, He WZ, Sun ZL (2008) Hypomethylated and hypermethylated profiles of H19DMR are associated with the aberrant imprinting of IGF2 and H19 in human hepatocellular carcinoma. Genomics 91(5):443–450. doi:10.1016/j.ygeno.2008.01.007

238. Xiong Y, Fang JH, Yun JP, Yang J, Zhang Y, Jia WH, Zhuang SM (2010) Effects of microRNA-29 on apoptosis, tumorigenicity, and prognosis of hepatocellular carcinoma. Hepatology 51(3):836–845. doi:10.1002/hep.23380

239. Xu W, Fan H, He X, Zhang J, Xie W (2006) LOI of IGF2 is associated with esophageal cancer and linked to methylation status of IGF2 DMR. J Exp Clin Cancer Res 25(4):543–547

240. Yan L, Zhou J, Gao Y, Ghazal S, Lu L, Bellone S, Yang Y, Liu N, Zhao X, Santin AD, Taylor H, Huang Y (2015) Regulation of tumor cell migration and invasion by the H19/let-7 axis is antagonized by metformin-induced DNA methylation. Oncogene 34(23):3076–3084. doi:10.1038/onc.2014.236

241. Yang F, Bi J, Xue X, Zheng L, Zhi K, Hua J, Fang G (2012) Up-regulated long non-coding RNA H19 contributes to proliferation of gastric cancer cells. FEBS J 279(17):3159–3165. doi:10.1111/j.1742-4658.2012.08694.x

242. Yang X, Karuturi RK, Sun F, Aau M, Yu K, Shao R, Miller LD, Tan PB, Yu Q (2009) CDKN1C (p57) is a direct target of EZH2 and suppressed by multiple epigenetic mechanisms in breast cancer cells. PLoS One 4(4):e5011. doi:10.1371/journal.pone.0005011

243. Yoon YS, Jeong S, Rong Q, Park KY, Chung JH, Pfeifer K (2007) Analysis of the H19ICR insulator. Mol Cell Biol 27(9):3499–3510. doi:10.1128/MCB.02170-06

244. Yoshimizu T, Miroglio A, Ripoche MA, Gabory A, Vernucci M, Riccio A, Colnot S, Godard C, Terris B, Jammes H, Dandolo L (2008) The H19 locus acts in vivo as a tumor suppressor. Proc Natl Acad Sci U S A 105(34):12417–12422. doi:10.1073/pnas.0801540105

245. Yu J, Li A, Hong SM, Hruban RH, Goggins M (2012) MicroRNA alterations of pancreatic intraepithelial neoplasias. Clin Cancer Res 18(4):981–992. doi:10.1158/1078-0432.ccr-11-2347

246. Yu Y, Xu F, Peng H, Fang X, Zhao S, Li Y, Cuevas B, Kuo WL, Gray JW, Siciliano M, Mills GB, Bast RC (1999) NOEY2 (ARHI), an imprinted putative tumor suppressor gene in ovarian and breast carcinomas. Proc Natl Acad Sci U S A 96(1):214–219

247. Yuan E, Li CM, Yamashiro DJ, Kandel J, Thaker H, Murty VV, Tycko B (2005) Genomic profiling maps loss of heterozygosity and defines the timing and stage dependence of epigenetic and genetic events in Wilms' tumors. Mol Cancer Res 3(9):493–502. doi:10.1158/1541-7786. mcr-05-0082

248. Yuan J, Luo RZ, Fujii S, Wang L, Hu W, Andreeff M, Pan Y, Kadota M, Oshimura M, Sahin AA, Issa JP, Bast RC, Yu Y (2003) Aberrant methylation and silencing of ARHI, an imprinted tumor suppressor gene in which the function is lost in breast cancers. Cancer Res 63(14):4174–4180

249. Zhang A, Skaar DA, Li Y, Huang D, Price TM, Murphy SK, Jirtle RL (2011) Novel retrotransposed imprinted locus identified at human 6p25. Nucleic Acids Res 39(13):5388–5400. doi:10.1093/nar/gkr108

250. Zhang X, Gejman R, Mahta A, Zhong Y, Rice KA, Zhou Y, Cheunsuchon P, Louis DN, Klibanski A (2010) Maternally expressed gene 3, an imprinted noncoding RNA gene, is associated with meningioma pathogenesis and progression. Cancer Res 70(6):2350–2358. doi:10.1158/0008-5472.CAN-09-3885

251. Zhang X, Zhou Y, Mehta KR, Danila DC, Scolavino S, Johnson SR, Klibanski A (2003) A pituitary-derived MEG3 isoform functions as a growth suppressor in tumor cells. J Clin Endocrinol Metab 88(11):5119–5126. doi:10.1210/jc.2003-030222

252. Zhao J, Dahle D, Zhou Y, Zhang X, Klibanski A (2005) Hypermethylation of the promoter region is associated with the loss of MEG3 gene expression in human pituitary tumors. J Clin Endocrinol Metab 90(4):2179–2186. doi:10.1210/jc.2004-1848

Part IV
DNA and Histone Methylation in Particular Types of Cancer

DNA and Histone Methylation in Brain Cancer

Sung-Hun Lee and Young Zoon Kim

Abstract Brain tumors are not rare solid cancer. Among them, gliomas are the most frequently occurring primary brain tumors in adults. Although they exist in different malignant stages, including histologically benign forms and highly aggressive states, most gliomas are clinically challenging for neuro-oncologists because of their infiltrative growth patterns and inherent relapse tendency with increased malignancy and dismal prognosis. Extensive genetic analyses of glioma have revealed a variety of deregulated genetic pathways involved in DNA repair, apoptosis, cell migration/adhesion, and cell cycle. Recently, it has become evident that epigenetic alterations may also be an important factor for glioma genesis. Epigenetic events can be defined as mitotically heritable changes in gene expression that are not due to changes in the primary DNA sequence. Epigenetic mechanisms, including those involving enzymatic modifications to DNA or histone proteins, thereby regulating gene expression, are increasingly recognized as a source of phenotypic variability in biology. Of epigenetic marks, DNA and histone methylation is a key mark that regulates gene expression and thus modulates a wide range of oncogenic processes. In this review, I discuss the neuro-oncological significance of DNA and histone methylation in patients with brain cancer while briefly overviewing the biological roles of histone modifications.

Keywords Epigenome • Histone • Methylation • Glioma • Glioblastoma • Neuro-oncology

S.-H. Lee
Department of Molecular and Cellular Oncology, The University of Texas MD Anderson Cancer Center, Houston, TX, USA

Y.Z. Kim, MD, PhD (✉)
Division of Neurooncology and Department of Neurosurgery, Samsung Changwon Hospital, Samsung Medical Center, Sungkyunkwan University School of Medicine, 158 Paryong-ro, Masanhoewon-gu, Changwon, Gyeongnam 51353, South Korea
e-mail: yzkim@skku.edu

© Springer International Publishing AG 2017
A. Kaneda, Y.-i. Tsukada (eds.), *DNA and Histone Methylation as Cancer Targets*, Cancer Drug Discovery and Development, DOI 10.1007/978-3-319-59786-7_12

347

1 Introduction

Epigenetics can be defined as mitotically heritable changes in gene expression that are not due to changes in the primary DNA sequence. Epigenetic mechanisms, including those involving enzymatic modifications to DNA or histone proteins, thereby regulating gene expression, are increasingly recognized as a source of phenotypic variability in biology. The discovery of altered epigenetic profiles in human neoplasia has been a major factor in constructing a new paradigm, in which epigenetic variability contributes significantly to human disease. Because of their reversible nature and their role in gene expression and DNA structure, epigenetic alterations, especially those related to changes in histone acetylation, are a current focus for therapeutic drug targeting in clinical trials.

Covalent modifications of DNA and amino acids on histones are two major mechanisms of epigenetic gene regulation (Fig. 1). First, DNA methylation results from the addition of a methyl group to cytosine thereby creating 5-methylcytosine. In mammals, this almost always occurs at the 5'-CpG-3' dinucleotide, though occasionally methylation is also observed at CpNpGs [10]. DNA methylation is controlled by DNA methyltransferases (DNMT) that create (DNMT3A, DNMT3B) or maintain (DNMT1) patterns of methylation [53]. DNA methylation is required to silence genes on the inactive X chromosome [26] or for the allele-specific expression of some imprinted loci [37]. Methylation is also required to silence transposable elements, to maintain genomic stability [17] and is a critical regulator of genes that contribute to cell pluripotency [20].

Another major epigenetic mechanism is the post-translational modification of the N-terminal tails of histone proteins by acetylation, methylation, phosphorylation, ubiquitylation, sumoylation, ADP ribosylation, biotinylation and other potential modifications [80]. Several families of enzymes catalyze post-translational modifications of histones, including acetyltransferases and deacetylases, methyltransferases and demethylases. Additionally, multiple types of modifications can take place on a single histone molecule, increasing combinatorial complexity. In addition, each amino acid residues can be modified in different states, such as mono-, di-, or tri-methylation at lysine residues.

In addition to DNA methylation and histone modifications, there are other potential epigenetic mechanisms that include specific deposition of histone variants, noncoding RNAs, chromatin remodeling, or nuclear organization of DNA. The interplay between histone modifications and other chromatin modifications leads to the dynamic regulation of chromatin structure and thereby affects several relevant cellular processes including transcription, DNA replication, DNA repair, and genomic stability [66]. Together, these add additional layers to the regulation of gene expression in both normal and diseased states.

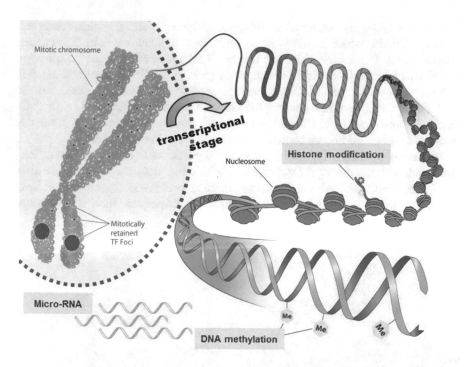

Fig. 1 Three major mechanisms of inheritable epigenetics. Mammalian gene expression is tightly controlled by genetic as well as epigenetic mechanisms. Epigenetics modifies the phenotype without altering the genotype of a cell. Shown here are some well-defined epigenetic mechanisms that include histone modifications, DNA methylation, and the noncoding RNA-mediated modulation of gene expression. Some of these mechanisms are inheritable through successive cell divisions and contribute to the maintenance of cellular phenotype. Recent studies show that the association of components of transcriptional regulatory machinery with target genes on mitotic chromosomes is a novel epigenetic mechanism that poises genes involved in key cellular processes, such as growth, proliferation, and lineage commitment, for expression in progeny cells (Adapted by Zaidi et al. [92] and modified by authors) [93]

2 Histone Modifications

Chromatin is the condensed combination of DNA and histones within the nucleus of a cell. The structural and functional unit of chromatin is the nucleosome, which consists of a disc-shaped octamer composed of two copies of each histone protein (H2A, H2B, H3, and H4), around which 147 base-pairs of DNA are wrapped twice (Fig. 2a) [34]. Electron microscopy studies have revealed that organization of nucleosomal arrays structurally resembles a series of "beads on a string", with the "beads" being the individual nucleosomes and the "string" being the linker DNA [26]. Linker histones, such as histone H1, and other non-histone proteins interact with the nucleosomal arrays to further package the nucleosomes into higher-order chromatin structures [66].

Histones are highly conserved across species. These proteins contain a conserved globular domain, which mediates histone-histone interactions within the octamer (Fig. 2a) [34]. In addition, there are two small tails protruding from the globular domain: an amino(N)-terminal domain, constituted by 20–35 residues that are rich in basic amino acids, and a short, protease accessible carboxy(C)-terminal domain [34]. Histone H2A is unique among the histones due to its possession of an additional 37 amino acids in the carboxy-terminal domain that protrudes from the nucleosome [34]. Additional histone variants have been identified [56].

In particular, their tails can be subject to a remarkable number of modifications, although examples of modifications within the globular domain have also been identified. Histone modifications include acetylation, methylation and phosphorylation, but also some less-studied modifications such as ubiquity-

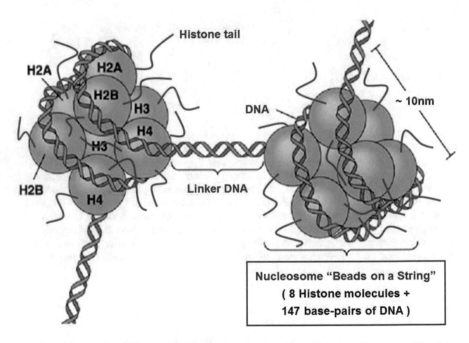

Fig. 2 Schematic representation of the nucleosome and mammalian core histone modifications. (**a**) Histones provide the basis for the nucleosome, the basic unit of chromatin structure, as seen as "beads-on-a-string" structures on electron micrographs. The nucleosome core is comprised of a histone octamer [(H2A-H2B)X2, (H3-H4)X2]. The DNA double helix is wrapped around (~1.7 times) the histone octamer. With nuclease digestion, 146 bps of DNA are tightly associated with the nucleosome but ~200 bps of DNA in total are associated with the nucleosome (modified image which was obtained at the website of http://www.mun.ca/biology/desmid/brian/BIOL2060/ BIOL2060-18/18_21.jpg). (**b**) N- and C-terminal histone tails extend from the globular domains of histones H2A, H2B, H3, and H4. DNA is wrapped around the nucleosome octamer made up of two H2A-H2B dimers and an H3-H4 tetramer. Post-translational covalent modifications include acetylation, methylation, phosphorylation, and ubiquitination. Human histone tail amino acid sequences are shown. Lysine positions 56 and 79 on histone H3 are located within the globular domain of the histone (Adapted by Mercurio et al. [43] and modified by authors)

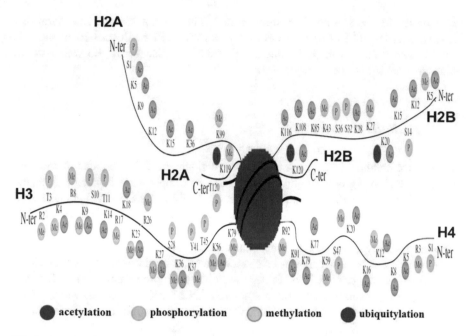

Fig. 2 (continued)

Table 1 Different classes of histone modifications and its regulated biological functions

Chromatin modification	Residues modified	Function regulated
Acetylation	Lysine	Transcription, DNA repair, replication and condensation
Methylation (lysine)	Lysine me1, me2, me3	Transcription, DNA repair
Methylation (arginine)	Arginine-me1, Arginine-me2a, Arginine-me2s	Transcription
Phosphorylation	Serine, threonine, tyrosine	Transcription, DNA repair and condensation
Ubiquitination	Lysine	Transcription, DNA repair
Sumoylation	Lysine	Transcription
ADP ribosylation	Glutamic	Transcription
Deimination	Arginine	Transcription
Proline isomerization	P-cis, P-trans	Transcription

lation, sumoylation, ADP ribosylation, deamination and proline somerization (Fig. 2b) [28, 34, 36]. Each of these histone modifications directly or indirectly affect chromatin structure, thereby leading to alterations in DNA repair, replication and gene transcription (Table 1). The effect of histone modifications on gene transcription can broadly be categorized into active versus passive marks. Moreover, numerous studies have reported the presence of site-specific combinations and interdependence of different histone modifications, which may be interpreted as the so-called "histone code". The role of histone modifications and their crosstalk in different cellular processes will be described in the following two sections. In particular, I will focus on discussing the well-studied histone marks: histone methylation.

2.1 Histone Methylation

Protein methylation is a covalent post-translational modification that commonly occurs on carboxyl groups of glutamate, leucine, and isoprenylated cysteine, or on the side-chain nitrogen atoms of lysine, arginine, and histidine residues [51]. As described in 1964, histones have long been known to be substrates for methylation [11]. For histones, methylation occurs on the side chain nitrogen atoms of lysines and arginines. The most heavily methylated histone is histone H3, followed by histone H4.

Arginine can be either mono- or di-methylated, with the latter in symmetric or asymmetric configuration [49]. Protein arginine methyltransferases (PRMTs) are the enzymes that catalyze arginine methylation. PRMTs share a conserved catalytic core but are very different on the N- and C- terminal regions, which likely determine substrate specificity [21]. There are two types of PRMTs: type I enzymes catalyze mono and asymmetric di-methylation of arginine and type II enzymes catalyze mono- and symmetric di-methylation of arginine [88]. Several studies have suggested that certain arginine methyltransferases, such as PRMT5, may repress the expression of genes involved in tumor suppression [88].

Similar to arginine methylation, lysine methylation can occur in mono-, di-, and tri-methylated forms. Some of the lysine residues methylated in histones H3 and H4 are also found to be substrates for acetylation. The enzymes that catalyze methylation on lysine residues have been grouped into two classes: lysine-specific, SET domain-containing histone methyltransferases (HMTs) share a strong homology with a 140-amino acid catalytic domain known as the SET (Su(var), Enhancer of Zeste, and Trithorax) domain, and non-SET containing HMTs. It is important to note that not all SET domain-containing proteins are HMTs nor are all HMT activities mediated by SET domains [54].

The consequences of lysine methylation are extremely diverse. Depending upon a particular lysine, methylation may serve as a marker of transcriptionally active euchromatin or transcriptionally repressed heterochromatin [19]. For instance, methylation of histones H3K9, H3K27, and H4K20 are mainly involved in formation of heterochromatin (closed chromatin conformation). On the other hand, methylation of H3K4, H3K36, and H3K79 are correlated with euchromatin (open chromatin conformation) (Table 2). Moreover, it seems that H3 clipping, a mechanism involving the cleavage of 21 amino acids of histone tails following the induction of gene transcription and histone eviction, occurs on histone tails that carry repressive histone marks [72].

Until very recently, the dogma was that methylation was an irreversible process. With the identification of the first lysine demethylase, lysine-specific demethylase 1 (LSD1) in 2004, the view of histone methylation regulation became much more dynamic, opening the way for identification of many more histone

Table 2 Major modifications of histone and their genetic regulations

Modification of histone	Mono-methylation	Di-methylation	Tri-methylation	Acetylation
H2AK5				Activation
H2AK7				Activation
H2AK9				Activation
H2AK13				Activation
H2BK5				Activation
H2BK12				Activation
H2BK15				Activation
H2BK20				Activation
H2BK120				Activation
H3R2	Activation			
H3K4	Activation	Activation	Activation	
H3K9	Activation/repression	Repression	Activation/repression	
H3K11				Activation
H3R17	Activation			
H3K18				Activation
H3K23				Activation
H3R26	Activation			
H3K27	Activation	Repression	Repression	Activation
H3K36		Activation	Activation	
H3K56				Activation
H3K79	Activation	Repression	Repression	
H3K115				Activation
H4R3		Activation		
H4K5				Activation
H4K8				Activation
H4K12				Activation
H4K16				Activation
H4K20	Activation/repression	Repression	Repression	Activation
H4K59	Repression			
H4K91				Activation

demethylases [60]. LSD1 demethylates both mono- and di-methylated K4 on H3 [60]. In 2006, the protein JHDM1A was identified as the first jumonji-domain-containing histone demethylase that removes methyl groups from mono- and di-methyl H3K36 [68]. The jumonji (JmjC)-domain-containing proteins belong to the deoxygenase superfamily and use a demethylation mechanism distinct from that of LSD1/KDM1 [79]. These enzymes can demethylate tri-methylated lysine residues. The JMJD2/KDM4 demethylases are tri-methyl demethylase families that were reported soon after the first JHDM1A was discovered [1]. Over the past few years, a series of studies have identified additional jumonji-domain-containing families that have methylated substrates K4, K9, K27 and K36. Despite the tremendous and exciting progress in the last few years, the field of histone demethylases is still in its early days and our knowledge of the biological role of these enzymes is still rather limited.

2.2 Protein Lysine Methylation

Protein lysine methylation has gained tremendous attention since the discovery of SUV39H1 as the first histone lysine methyltransferase in 2000 [58]. Following the discovery, numerous proteins have been found to possess methyltransferase activity, such as G9a/GLP [76, 77], MLLs [47], EZH2 [8], SET2 [73], SET7/9 [87], DOT1 [19, 84] and PR-SET7 (also known as SETD8) [50]. These enzymes catalyze the transfer of methyl group from the co factor S-adenosyl-L-methionine (SAM) to the lysine residues of histones. More recently, many non-histone proteins have been identified as substrates for these enzymes, hence the name protein lysine (K)

Table 3 Genetic alterations in the cancers associated with the protein methylases and demethylases

Target	Genetic alterations	Cancer type
Methylase		
EZH2	1. Heterozygous activating mutations occurring at Y641, A677 & A687 that result in hypermethylation of H3K27me3 2. Deletion of miR-101 leads to EZH2 overexpression 3. Deletion of SNF5 leads to EZH2 dependency	1. Lymphoma 2. Prostate cancer 3. Malignant rhabdoid tumor
DOT1L	1. 11q23 chromosomal translocations fusing MLL1 (without its catalytic SET domain) to DOT1L binding partners such as AF4, AF9, AF-10 and ENL leading to aberrant H3K79 methylation 2. CALM-AF10 and SET-NUP214 fusions are known to mis-target DOT1L	Leukemia
NSD1	t(5;11)(q35;p15.5) translocation create NSD1-NUP98 fusions	Acute myeloid leukemia
WHSC1	t(4;14)(p16;q32) chromosomal translocations that places WHSC1 gene under the control of the IGH promoter and results in the overexpression of WHSC1	Multiple myeloma
WHSC1L1	1. t(8;11)(p11.2;p15) chromosomal translocations fuses WHSC1L1 to NUP98 2. 8p11–12 focal amplifications	1. Acute myeloid leukemia breast cancer 2. Squamous cell lung cancer
SETDB1	1q21 amplifications	Melanoma
SMYD2	1q32 amplifications	Esophageal squamous cell carcinoma
Demethylase		
JMJD2C	1. 9p23–24 amplifications 2. t(9;14)(9p24.1q32) translocations creating fusions to IGH	1. Esophageal squamous cell carcinoma Squamous cell lung cancer 2. Medulloblastoma basal breast cancer
LSD2	6p22 amplifications	Urothelial carcinomas
UTX	Inactivating mutations of UTX lead to pro-oncogenic hypermethylation of H3K27me3 and dependence on EZH2	Multiple blood and solid cancers

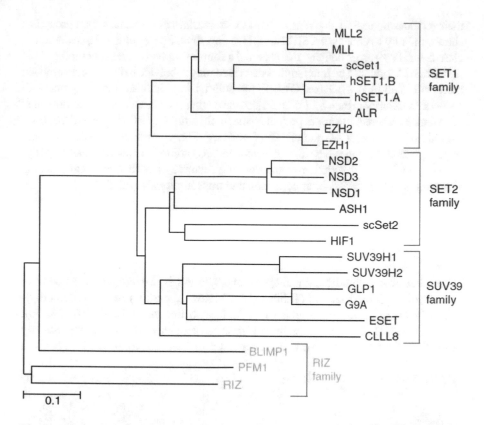

Fig. 3 A dendogram showing the relationship between some of the more characterized human SET-domain proteins. The comparison is based on the homology within the SET-domain. The Clustal W program was used to generate the figure. On the *right* are the four families defined by the homologues (Adapted from Kouzarides [35])

methyltransferases (PKMTs) (Table 3). It is worth pointing out that PKMTs play important roles in other biological processes including developmental biology and stem cell differentiation. However, here we will focus on the implications of PKMTs in cancers, especially.

Methylation of lysines residues is known to occur usually on histone H3 (K4, K9 and K27) and H4 (K20). As mentioned above, the SUV39 protein was the first histone methyltransferase to be discovered [58]. The methyltransferase activity of SUV39 is directed against lysine 9 of histone H3 and its catalytic domain resides within a highly conserved structure, the SET domain. The sequences within the SET domain are not however sufficient for enzymatic activity. Methylation is only seen when two flanking cystein-rich sequences (PRE-SET and POST-SET) are fused to the SET domain. Use of the simple modular architectural research tool (SMART) indicates that there are 73 entries in the human database which possess a SET domain. In contrast, there are 6 SET domain proteins in *Saccharomyces cerevisiae*, 11 in Schizosaccharomyces pombe, 41 in Drosophila and 37 in *Caenorhabditis elegans*. Previously characterized human proteins possess a SET domain showing that they can be grouped into four classes (Fig. 3). The classification is based on the similarity between the human SET domains as primary and their relationship to SET domains in yeast (*S. cerevisiae*) as secondary. Two groupings show similarity to either yeast SET1 or SET2, thus defining two of the classes. Another class has SUV39 as its defining member and a fourth family represents homologues of the RIZ SET domain. The four families described may subdivide to further classes when more information is available. Overall, the subdivisions indicate that enzymes with sequence similarity in their SET domain also have other structural features (i.e. domains) in common. Figure 4 illustrates protein lysine methylation/demethylation and their biological roles in terms of transcriptional activity, Fig. 5 summaries methylase and demethylase at the major 6 lysines of histone tail according to genetic regulatory activity. Next topic is a description of the defining features of each family emphasizing wherever possible, their links to chromatin and transcriptional regulation.

2.3 Protein Lysine Demethylation

Like other protein modifications, lysine methylation is also subject to its counter modification, demethylation (Table 4). For histones, the first reported demethylase is lysine-specific demethylase 1 (LSD1, also known as BHC110) [24, 70]. However, LSD1 can only demethylate mono- or di-methylated lysines. Shortly after the discovery of LSD1, a second family of enzymes, Jmj C-domain

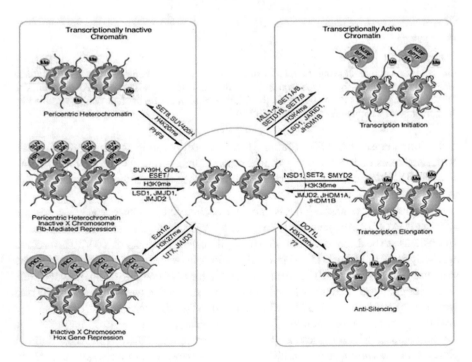

Fig. 4 Summaries of protein lysine methylation/demethylation and their biological roles in terms of transcriptional activity

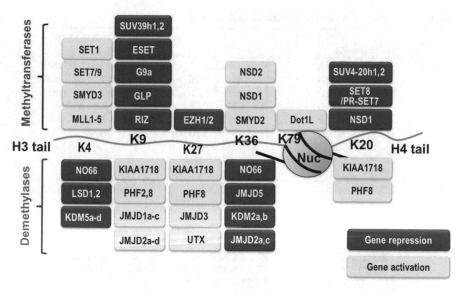

Fig. 5 Illustration of the methylase and demethylase at the six major lysines of histone tail according to genetic regulatory activity

containing proteins, was found to have demethylation activity for tri-methylated, as well as mono- and di-methylated lysines [79]. These enzymes are referred to as protein lysine demethylases (PKDMs). The roles for PKDMs in human diseases, including cancer and neurological disorders, are beginning to be delineated [63, 67]. The clinical relevance of demethylase inhibitors has not been demonstrated using a small molecule; however, a few interesting inhibitors have been disclosed. Demethylases of the LSD1/KDM1 family share some sequence and structural similarities to amine oxidases [91] and monoamine oxidase. Inhibitors, such as tranylcypromine, have been shown to inhibit LSD 1 by forming a covalent adducts between the flavin cofactor and the inhibitor [81]. The Jmj C-domain containing demethylase (JHDM) family conforms to a different catalytic mechanism, relying on an active site iron and a 2-oxoglutarate cofactor. Analogs of the 2-oxoglutarate cofactor have been shown to be inhibitors of recombinant enzyme and to increase methylation in cell systems [25].

2.4 Protein Arginine Methylation

Apart from lysine methylation, arginine (R) methylation has been also known to play certain roles in cancer. The history of arginine methylation was recently surveyed [30]. Several arginine residues are also modified by methylation. These include, R2, R8, R17, and R26 of histone H3, and R3 of histone H4. Arginine residues may undergo mono-methylation, symmetric di-methylation, or asymmetric di-methylation. There

Table 4 Summary of histone lysine methyltransferases and demethylases

Mark	Methylation	Demethylation	Catalytic specificity of the demethylase
H3K4	MLL1/KMT2A MLL2/KMT2B MLL3/KMT2C MLL4/KMT2D MLL5/KMT2E hSET1A/KMT2F hSET1B/KMT2G ASH1/KMT2H SET7–9/KMT7	LSD1/KDM1 JARID1A/RBP2/ KDM5A JARID1B/ PLU-1/KDM5B JARID1C/SMCX/ KDM5C JARID1D/ SMCY/KDM5D NDY1/JHDM1B/ FBXL10/KDM2B	me2/me1 → me0 me3/ me2/me1 → me0 me3/ me2/me1 → me0 me3/ me2 → me1 me3/ me2 → me1 me3 → me2
H3K9	SUV39H1/KMT1A SUV39H2/KMT1B G9a/KMT1C EuHMTase/GLP/ KMT1D ESET/SETDB1/ KMT1E CLL8/KMT1F RIZ1/KMT8	LSD1/KDM1 JHDM2A/JMJD1A/ KDM3A JHDM2B/5qNCA/ KDM3B JHDM2C/ TRIP8/KDM3C JMJD2A/JHDM3/ KDM4A JMJD2B/ KDM4B JMJD2C/ GASC1/KDM4C JMJD2D/KDM4D	me2/me1 → me0 me2/ me1 → me0 me2 me3/me2 → me1 me3/ me2 → me1 me3/ me2 → me1 me3/me2/ me1 → me0
H3K27	KMT6/EZH2	UTX/KDM6A JMJD3/KDM6B UTY	me3/me2 → me1 me3/ me2 → me1
H3K36	SET2/KMT3A NSD1/KMT3B SMYD2/KMT3C	NDY2/JHDM1A/ FBXL11/KDM2A NDY1/JHDM1B/ FBXL10/KDM2B JMJD2A/JHDM3/ KDM4A JMJD2B/KDM4B JMJD2C/GASC1/ KDM4C	me2/me1 → me0 me2/ me1 → me0 me3/ me2 → me1 me3
H3K79	DOT1L/KMT4		
H4K20	PR-SET7–8/KMT5A SUV4–20H1/KMT5B SUV4–20H2/KMT5C		

Adapted from Kampranis et al. [33]

are five known arginine methyltransferases that have a highly conserved catalytic domain. PRMT1, PRMT3 and PRMT4/CARM1 are classified as Class I enzymes as they can catalyze the formation of asymmetric di-methylated arginine whereas PRMT5/JBP1 is classified as a class II enzyme as it catalyzes symmetric di-methylation. The PRMT2 protein has not yet been established as an enzyme [42]. H3R2 is asymmetrically di-methylated by CARM1/PRMT4 [64] and PRMT6 [23]. H3R8 is methylated by PRMT5 [12], while H3R17 and H3R26 are asymmetrically di-methylated by CARM1/PRMT4, which also methylates H3R2 [64]. Finally, H4R3 is mono-methylated by PRMT1 and di-methylated, both symmetrically and asymmetrically by PRMT5 [2]. The methylation of specific arginine residues contributes to the regulation of cell fate. For example, ectopic expression of CARM1 in mouse blastomers increases the levels of arginine methylation and promotes the dramatic upregulation of the pluripotency genes NANOG and SOX2. This, in turn, promotes the cycling of pluripotent cells and the expansion of the inner cell mass of the blastocyst [78].

The molecular mechanisms by which arginine methylation contributes to chromatin structure and transcriptional regulation are not yet clear. However, it has been shown that arginine methylation may regulate the modification or recognition of neighboring histone residues. Thus, it has been shown that methylation of H3R2 prevents the tri-methylation of H3K4 and vice versa [76]. Furthermore, it has been shown that asymmetric methylation of H3R2 inhibits the association of the TFIID subunit TAF3 with H3K4me3 [85].

2.5   Histone Code

Over the past few years, the field of epigenetics has provided a great deal of evidence arguing that histone modifications act in a combinatorial and consistent manner, leading to the concept of the "histone code" (Table 5) [90]. Different histone modifications present on histone tails generate a "code", which can be read by different cellular machineries thereby dictating different cellular outcomes, such as activation or repression of transcription, DNA replication, and DNA repair (Fig. 6) [90]. The histone code hypothesizes that the transcription of genetic information encoded in DNA is in part regulated by chemical modifications to histone proteins, primarily on their unstructured ends. Along with similar modifications such as DNA methylation, it is part of the epigenetic code. Many of the histone tail modifications are associated with chromatin structure, and both histone modification state and chromatin structure are correlated with gene expression levels. The histone code hypothesis is that histone modifications serve to recruit other proteins by specific recognition of the modified histone via specialized protein domains, rather than through simply stabilizing or destabilizing the interaction between a histone and the underlying DNA. These recruited proteins then act to actively alter chromatin structure or to promote transcription. The combinatorial nature of different histone marks therefore adds a layer of complexity in recruiting epigenetic modifiers and regulating cellular processes. For instance, Msk1/2-mediated H3S10 phosphorylation enhances binding of GCN5, which leads to acetylation of H3K14, methylation of H3K4, and inhibition of H3K9 methylation, the sequence of which results in open chromatin conformation [31]. Moreover, phosphorylation of H3S10 favors H3K9 acetylation since Aurora-B kinase can only bind unmodified or acetylated histone H3K9, thus preventing SUV39H1 binding and histone H3K9 methylation [58]. On the other hand, histone H3K9 methylation inhibits H3S10 phosphorylation and represses gene transcription [31]. Recently, phosphorylation of histone H3T6 by protein kinase C beta I was shown to be a major event in preventing LSD1 from demethylating histone H3K4 during androgen receptor-dependent gene activation [29].

Table 5 Two major histone modifications driving histone code hypothesis

Modification	Histone	Residue	Enzyme	Possible role
Acetylation	H2A	K4	Esa1	TA
		K5	Tip60, Hat1, P300/CBP	TA, RA
		K7	Hat1, Esa1	TA
	H2B	K5	ATF2	TA
		K11	Gcn5	TA
		K12	ATF2, P300/CBP	TA
		K15	ATF2, P300/CBP	TA
		K16	Gcn5, Esa1	TA
		K20	P300	TA
	H3	K4	Esa1, Hpa2	TA
		K9	Gcn5, SRC-1	TA, RA
		K14	Gcn5, PCAF, Tip60, SRC-1, hTFIIIC90, TAF1, p300/ Gcn5, Esa1, Elp3, Hpa2, TAF1, Sas2, Sas3	TA, RA, RE
		K18	P300, CBP/Gcn5 (SAGA)	TA, RA
		K23	P300, CBP/Gcn5 (SAGA), Sas3	TA, RA
		K27	Gcn5	TA, RA
	H4	K5	Hat1, Tip60, ATF2, p300/Hat1, Esa1, Hpa2	TA, RA, RE
		K8	Gcn5, PCAF, Tip60, ATF2, p300/Esa1, Elp3	TA, RA, RE
		K12	Hat1, Tip60/Hat1, Esa1, Hpa2	TA, RA, RE
		K16	MOF, Gcn5, Tip60, ATF2/Gcn5, Esa1, Sas2	TA, RA
Methylation	H1	K26	EZH2	TR
	H3	R2	CARM1	TA
		K4	MLL4, SET1, MLL1, SET7/9, MYD3/ Set1	TA
		R8	PMRT5	TR
		K9	SUV39h1, SUV39h2, ESET, G9A, EZH2, Eu-HMTase1/Clr4, S.p. Clr4	TA, TR
		R17	CARM1	TA
		R26	CARM1	TA
		K27	EZH2, G9A	TA, TR
		K36	HYPB, NSD1/Set2, S.c.	TA
		K79	DOT1L/S.c. Dot-1	TA, TR, RA
	H4	R3	PRMT1, PRMT5	TA
		K20	PR-SET7, SUV4-20/SET9	TA, TR, RA

TA transcriptional activation, *TR* transcriptional repression, *RA* DNA repair, *RE* DNA replication

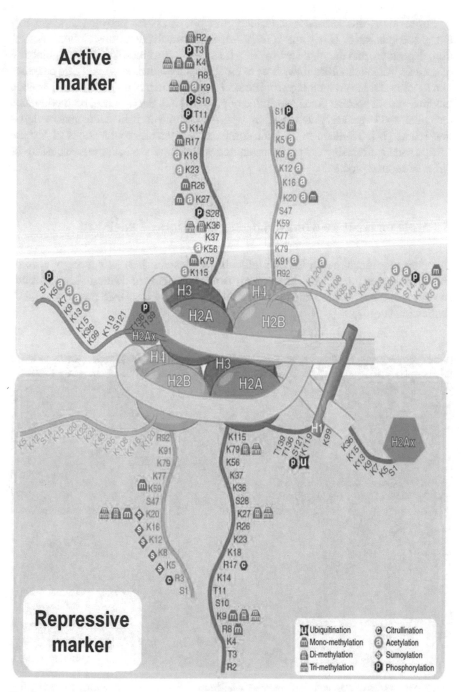

Fig. 6 Illustration of histone code according to active and repressive markers. DNA is wrapped around histone octamer of the four core histones H2A, H2B, H3, and H4. Histone H1, the linker protein, is bound to DNA between nucleosomes. Different amino acids constituting histone tails are represented along with the different covalent modification specific of each residue. Active marks are represented in the upper part of the figure and repressive marks are represented in the lower part of the figure. *K* lysine, *R* arginine, *S* serine, *T* threonine (Adapted by Sawan et al. [61] and modified by authors)

Furthermore, this histone modification crosstalk can occur between different histones. Methylation of H3K4 and H3K79, which are involved in transcriptional activation, depend on, and are regulated by, H2BK123 ubiquitination [45]. The combination of specific histone modifications is due to the specificity of histone-modifying enzymes to a specific residue on their target substrate. Epigenetic marks on histone tails provide binding sites for specific domains of effector proteins [90]. For instance, bromodomains recognize and target acetylated residues, whereas chromo domains recognize methylation marks [74]. Together, the combinatorial and sequential modifications of histone tails provide a promising field of research that will allow for a better understanding of different cellular processes.

3   Role of Histone Modifications in Cellular Processes

Covalent modifications on histone tails are now established as key regulators of chromatin-based processes. This section discusses the role of different histone modifications in the regulation and coordination of transcription, DNA repair, and DNA replication (Fig. 7).

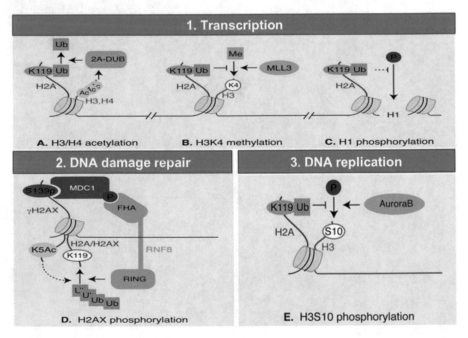

Fig. 7 Summaries of cellular role of histone modification. Functional implications in transcription regulation (**a–c**), DNA damage response (**d**) and DNA replication (**e**) are illustrated. The labels "Ub", "Ac", "Me" and "P" refer to mono-ubiquitination, acetylation, di- and trimethylation, and phosphorylation respectively (Adapted by Vissers et al. [86] and modified by authors)

3.1 Transcription

In response to different stimuli, the regulation of gene expression in eukaryotes requires certain chromatin modifiers and specific histone modifications that allow for an "open", permissive chromatin (Fig. 8). These epigenetic modifiers facilitate and open the way for transcription factors to bind the DNA and activate a cascade of events resulting in gene transcription. On the contrary, other histone modifications and modifiers can result in transcriptional repression by inducing a condensed chromatin state and closing DNA accessibility to transcription factors. Thus, histone modifications dictate whether the chromatin state is transcriptionally permissive or not (Fig. 8).

As mentioned earlier, histone methylation plays two different roles in gene transcription. COMPASS-catalyzed histone H3K4 methylation is associated with RNA polymerase II in its initiating form. Methylated histone H3K36 is found at

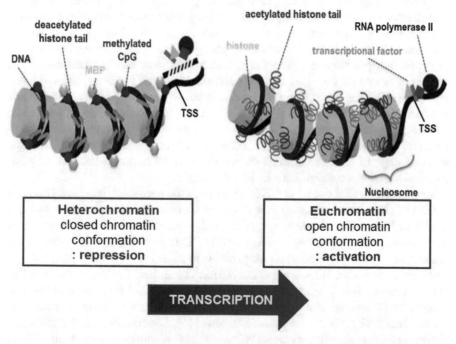

Fig. 8 Schematic diagram illustrating euchromatin and heterochromatin. Heterochromatin on the left is characterized by DNA methylation and deacetylated histones, is condensed and inaccessible to transcription factors (closed chromatin conformation), which is repressive regulation of transcription. On the contrary, euchromatin on the right is in a loose form and transcriptionally active; DNA is unmethylated and histone tails acetylated (open chromatin conformation), which is active regulation of transcription (Adapted by Benetatos et al. [3] and modified by authors)

the 3′ end of active genes in combination with the elongating form of RNA polymerase II [69]. Similar to the above mechanisms, methylated histone H3K4 may provide docking sites for downstream effectors that are involved with transcriptional activation, thus affecting gene expression [71]. Conversely, the methyltransferase for H3K9, H4K20, and H3K27 leads to a repressive effect on gene transcription. Chromatin modifiers that mediate these methylation marks function by inducing a repressive chromatin state and recruiting repressive complexes to transcription sites [71]. Lysine demethylation usually antagonizes the effect of methylation at the specific sites [44].

3.2 DNA Repair

Eukaryotic cells continuously face numerous endogenous and exogenous genotoxic stresses that can cause deleterious DNA lesions, including DNA double-strand breaks (DSBs). To combat these threats, cells have evolved mechanisms of DNA damage repair to maintain genomic stability and prevent oncogenic transformation or development of disease [46]. Compacted chromatin can be a major obstacle in the orchestration of DNA repair and other chromatin-based processes. After the induction of DNA damage, chromatin must first be relaxed to give repair proteins access to the site of breaks. Biochemical and molecular studies have revealed the link between different histone modifications and DNA repair highlighting the major role of chromatin-remodeling enzymes in repair mechanisms [83]. For efficient repair, chromatin structure needs to be altered and access to the break sites must be available; both of which require post-translational histone modifications, ATP-dependent nucleosome mobilization, and exchange of histone variants. In this section, we focus on the role of post-translational histone modifications in DNA repair.

One of the earliest events in DSB signaling is the phosphorylation of H2AX, a variant of H2A. This phosphorylation is carried out by the phosphatase inositol-3 family of kinase (PI3K) and is spread over kilo-bases (in yeast) and mega-bases (in mammal cells) from the break site [70]. This modification is required for retention and accumulation of repair proteins to damaged sites [15]. Moreover, it has been shown that H2AX phosphorylation is required for the recruitment of HATs to break sites. The recruitment of HATs is mediated by Arp4 and leads to acetylation of the chromatin surrounding the breaks, thereby relaxing the chromatin and facilitating access for repair proteins [55]. Binding of NuA4 HAT complexes and the subsequent acetylation of H4 is concomitant with H2AX phosphorylation [14]. Moreover, defects in H3 acetylation results in sensitivity to DNA damaging agents, which is consistent with its importance in DNA repair [41]. Related to the important role of histone acetylation in DNA repair, a recent study provided evidence that TRRAP/TIP60 is essential for the recruitment and loading of repair proteins to the site of breaks [48].

The role of histone methylation in DNA repair has recently received considerable attention. Methylation of histone H4K20 in fission yeast was shown to be essential for the recruitment of Crb2, a checkpoint adaptor protein with homology to 53BP1, to sites of DNA breaks to insure proper checkpoint activation in response to DNA damage [5]. In human cells, BP1 may function in a very similar manner [58, 59]. Interestingly, TIP60 binds to the heterochromatic histone mark H3K9me3 [63], triggering acetylation and activation of DNA DSB repair. Although H3K9me3 is not required for the recruitment of TIP60 to sites of DNA damage, the interaction of TIP60/ATM with the MRN complex is sufficient for chromatin localization. However, the interaction with H3K9me3 is essential for TIP60 HAT stimulation and the initiation of downstream repair events [75].

3.3 DNA Replication

DNA replication occurs during the S phase of the cell cycle and it is initiated at discrete sites on the chromosome called origins of replication. DNA replication is a delicate process for cells since it requires a high fidelity during the duplication of DNA sequences and maintenance and propagation of chromatin states. This cellular process involves several critical steps: access to DNA for the replication machinery, disruption of the parental nucleosomes ahead of the replication fork, nucleosome assembly on the daughter duplex of DNA, and propagation of the epigenetic state. All of these events are regulated by a network of histone-modifying complexes that control access to DNA and nucleosomal organization. Although the role of chromatin modifications in DNA replication remains poorly understood, several studies have provided evidence that histone post-translational modifications can control the efficiency and timing of replication origin activities [93]. As compacted chromatin can limit and prevent access for replication machinery to the DNA, it can be hypothesized that histone modifications play a critical role in setting the chromatin status for both early and late origins of DNA replication. Related to this idea, it has been shown in yeast that histone acetylation in the vicinity of the origin of replication affects replication timing. Indeed, higher levels of histone acetylation coincide with earlier induction of replication at an origin [93]. In humans, acetylation of histone tails has also been demonstrated to correlate with replication timing [9]. Consistent with the idea that acetylation opens the way for DNA replication machinery; several studies have shown that HAT HBO1 is associated with both replication factor, MCM2 and the origin recognition complex 1 subunit of the human initiator protein. These findings suggest that the targeting of histone acetylation to the origin of replication establishes a chromatin structure that is favorable for DNA replication [6]. Interestingly, ING5-containing HBO1 HAT complex associates with MCM2-7 helicase and appears to be essential for DNA replication in humans, which is consistent with the finding that depletion of either ING5 or HBO1 impairs S phase progression

[16]. Recent studies in *S. cerevisiae* showed a dynamic regulation of acetylation of H3 and H4 around an origin of replication [82]. Further studies are needed to examine the exact mechanisms and implications of other histone modifications such as methylation, phosphorylation, and ubiquination. It is likely that histone phosphorylation, similar to acetylation, could also play roles in making DNA accessible to DNA replication machinery and in restoring chromatin to a compact configuration after DNA replication is completed.

4   Epigenetic Role of Histone Methylations in Glioma

According to the nationwide, hospital-based cancer registry, as reported by the Korean Ministry of Health and Welfare in 2010, there were 10,004 newly diagnosed brain tumors in a population of 49.9 million in 2010 [32]. Among them, most of the neuroectodermal tumors were gliomas (91.7%), which accounted for 15.1% of all primary brain tumors. Glioblastoma accounted for 5.2% of all primary tumors and 34.4% of all gliomas. Among histologically confirmed cases, glioblastoma accounted for 40.6% of all gliomas [32]. Despite recent advances in surgery, radiotherapy, and chemotherapy, survival of glioma patients remains poor. The 5-year survival rate of patients with low-grade gliomas is 30–70% depending on histology, and the median survival time is only 12–15 months for the most frequent malignant glioma, glioblastoma multiforme (GBM) [89, 90].

Besides genetic alterations, epigenetic modifications are critical to the development and progression of cancer. The best-known epigenetic marker in gliomas is DNA methylation. Hypermethylation of the CpG island promoter can induce silencing of genes affecting the cell cycle, DNA repair, metabolism of carcinogens, cell-to-cell interaction, apoptosis, and angiogenesis, all of which may occur at different stages in glioma development and interact with genetic lesions [18]. In addition to DNA promoter hypermethylation, epigenetic alterations of histone modification patterns have the potential to affect the structure and integrity of the genome and disrupt normal patterns of gene expression, which may also contribute to carcinogenesis [18]. These modifications occur in different histone proteins, histone variants, and histone residues, involve different chemical groups, and have different degrees of methylation.

4.1   Alterations of Histone Modifications in Glioma Genesis

Mounted evidence from recent data shows that alterations at the histone level may also play a role in glioma genesis. These alterations encompass a globally deregulated expression of genes involved in histone modifications as well as changes in the histone modification pattern of individual genes (Table 6). Global aberrations at the histone

Table 6 Major epigenetic alteration of histone modification in human gliomas

Mutation	
Histone deacetylase	HDAC2, HDAC9
Histone demethylase	JMJD1A, JMJD1B
Histone methyltransferase	SET7, SETD7, MLL, MLL3, MLL4
Altered expression level	
Histone deacetylase	HDAC1, HDAC2, HDAC2
Modification of individual genes	
RPR22	Repression expression
P21	Repression expression
HOXA9	Enhanced expression

level result from mutations in regulatory genes, as detected in a large-scale genomic analysis of GBM samples, including HDACs (HDAC2 and HDAC9), histone demethylases (JMJD1A and JMJD1B), and histone methyltransferases (SET7, SETD7, MLL3 and MLL4) [55]. Furthermore, altered expression levels of HDACs, due to reasons that have yet to be defined, have been linked to tumor recurrence and progression (HDAC1, HDAC2, and HDAC3) [7]. Histone modifications regulating individual genes have been reported in several studies. For example, a repressed expression of the tumor suppressor RRP22 and the cell cycle regulator p21, combined with an enhanced expression of the pro-proliferative transcription factor HOXA9 have been linked to alterations in histone modification patterns [62]. However, the actual functional roles of histone modifications in gliomas, and their potential to serve as biomarkers and/or therapeutic targets, still remain to be fully elucidated. Additionally, in order to determine the exact incidence and characteristic patterns of these alterations of histone modification in human gliomas, there is a necessity of further study and more analysis.

4.2 Alterations of Histone Modifications in GBM

As previously mentioned, epigenetically silenced loci, in addition to being hypermethylated DNA, are characterized by aberrant patterns of histone modifications. Silenced CpG island promoters are characterized by increased histone H3K9 methylation and loss of H3K9 acetylation. In embryonic stem (ES) cells, the dual presence of deactivating H3K27 methylation and activation-associated H3K4 methylation, called bivalent domains, is thought to create a "poised" chromatin state for developmentally regulated genes, allowing for silencing in ES cells and subsequent transcriptional activation or repression in differentiated cells [4]. Bivalent domains, along with additional repressive marks (dimethylated H3K9 and trimethylated H3K9), are found in embryonic carcinoma cells in genes that are frequently silenced by DNA hypermethylation in adult human cancer cells. These histone modifications are hypothesized to predispose tumor suppressor genes to DNA hypermethylation and heritable gene silencing [52].

There are many instances of genetic alterations and/or deregulated expression levels of genes encoding for histone-modifying enzymes. In acute leukemias for example, it is common to observe translocations involving the mixed lineage leukemia (*MLL*) gene, encoding for H3K4 methyltransferase [13]. These translocations result in MLL fusion proteins that have lost H3K4 methyltransferase activity. Mutations resulting in altered histone HAT activity also occur in cancer related diseases: *CREB*-binding protein (CBP) mutations, abolishing HAT activity, cause Rubenstein-Taybi syndrome, a developmental disorder that is associated with a higher risk of cancer [57]. In GBM, there is also some preliminary evidence for the deregulation of genes controlling histone modifications. The gene encoding BMI-1, a member of the polycomb group complex that regulates histone H3K27 methylation, is frequently subjected to copy number alterations in both low- and high-grade gliomas, and *BMI-1* deletions are associated with poor prognosis in patients [27]. It has also been reported that expression levels of some HDAC proteins are altered in GBM. Class II and class IV HDACs displayed decreased mRNA expression in GBMs compared to low-grade astrocytomas and normal brain samples, and overall, histone H3 was more acetylated in GBMs [40]. Large-scale sequencing of protein-coding genes in GBMs uncovered mutations in many genes involved in epigenetic regulation, including histone deacetylases *HDAC2* and *HDAC9*, histone demethylases *JMJD1A* and *JMJD1B*, histone methyltransferases *SET7*, *SETD7*, *MLL3*, *MLL4* and methyl-CpG binding domain protein 1 (*MBD1*) [55]. Screening of a large cohort of gliomas of various grades and histologies (n = 784) showed H3F3A mutations to be specific to GBM and highly prevalent in children and young adults [65]. Furthermore, the presence of H3F3A/ATRX-DAXX/TP53 mutations was strongly associated with alternative lengthening of telomeres and specific gene expression profiles in GBM, which results explained the recurrent mutations in a regulatory histone [65]. These intriguing initial studies suggest that alterations in epigenetic mechanisms could be a major defect in GBM.

4.3   Global Histone Modification Patterns as Prognostic Marker in Glioma Patients

Liu et al. reported the relationship between multiple histone modifications and patient prognosis, which was analyzed by a recursive partitioning analysis (RPA), with progression-free survival (PFS) and overall survival (OS) as the primary end point [65]. An RPA classification was carried out to test how histone modification might influence prognosis (Fig. 9). Patients with astrocytoma were classified into two separate groups based on acetylation of H3K9. Patients whose tumors expressed H3K9Ac in <88% of tumor cells (group 3) had a reduced survival rate compared with patients whose tumors had at least 88% of cells expressing H3K9Ac (group 2). In WHO grade 3 tumors, patients whose tumors expressed H3K4diMe in <64% of tumor cells (group 6) had a reduced survival rate compared with patients whose tumors had at least 64%

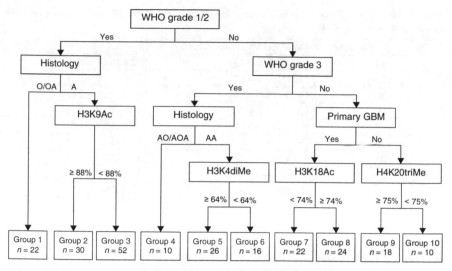

Fig. 9 RPA results individualizing 10 different prognostic groups among the 230 samples from glioma patients who underwent resection included. Each node, where the branches of the RPA tree bifurcate, divides patients according to whether the value of a specific feature (predictor) is above or below a selected cutoff value. The first node is represented by the tumor grade. In low-grade glioma patients, histologic subtype provides the second node, and histone modifications (e.g., the percentage of cells stained positively for H3K9Ac) provide the third node. High-grade glioma patients were further divided into WHO grade 3 and 4 ones. Histologic subtype and pathogenesis provide the third node, respectively, and histone modifications of H3K4me2, H3K18Ac, or H4K20me3 provide the fourth node (Adapted by Liu et al. [39])

of cells expressing H3K4me2 (group 5). Acetylation of H3K18 also significantly influenced the survival of primary glioblastoma patients. Patients whose tumor expressed lower levels (<74% of tumor cells) of H3K18Ac (group 7 *vs.* group 8) experienced a greater survival rate. Meanwhile, trimethylation of H4K20 significantly influenced the survival of secondary glioblastoma patients; with a greater survival for patients whose tumor expressed higher levels (≥75% of tumor cells) of H4K20me3 (group 9 *vs.* group 10). Conclusively, these data suggest that the 10 groups defined the terminal classification of the 230 patients and were associated with significantly different PFS ($p < 0.0001$) and OS ($p < 0.0001$; Table 7) [65].

4.4 Potential Epigenetic-Based Therapies for GBM

Epigenetic-based therapies, such as the DNMT inhibitor Decitabine (5-aza-2′-deoxycytidine) and the HDACi suberoylanilide hydroxamic acid (SAHA; Vorinostat), are currently being tested in multiple cancers, although only HDACi is

Table 7 Median progression-free survival and overall survival of the different groups of glioma patients established by RPA

Group	# of patients	Median PFS month (95% CI)	Median OS month (95% CI)
1	22	51.8 (46.1–57.5)	52.4 (48.4–56.4)
2	30	36.0 (27.2–44.8)	57.6 (49.9–65.3)
3	52	31.9 (29.4–34.4)	32.0 (21.5–42.5)
4	10	35.9 (29.7–42.1)	28.5 (22.2–34.8)
5	26	14.0 (10.8–17.2)	18.6 (15.9–21.3)
6	16	9.2 (8.3–10.0)	11.3 (10.0–12.6)
7	22	11.6 (7.8–15.4)	14.0 (10.9–17.1)
8	24	7.9 (4.9–10.9)	10.1 (9.0–11.2)
9	18	7.9 (5.1–10.7)	9.7 (6.2–13.2)
10	10	6.2 (4.4–8.0)	6.5 (4.6–8.4)

$p < 0.0001$

in trials for GBM [22]. In contrast to genetic mutations, which are "hard-wired" once mutated, epigenetic mutations, such as promoter hypermethylation and histone acetylation status, are theoretically reversible through drug treatment or changes in the diet.

A major unresolved issue with epigenetic therapy for cancer is target specificity. First, some genes that require DNA methylation or histone deacetylation for silencing in normal cells could be unintentionally activated by agents that inhibit DNMTs or HDACs. Second, cancer genomes are characterized by both DNA hyper- and hypomethylation. Therefore, using drugs that reactivate silenced tumor suppressors may have the undesired effect of further activating oncogenes through hypomethylation. These problems should be addressed to gain a more complete understanding of the molecular events that may result from epigenetic-based therapy.

5 Future Directions for Histone Modifications in GBM

Epigenetic studies of GBM are poised to (i) make substantial contributions to the understanding of GBM biology, (ii) identify new predictive biomarkers and (iii) discover novel targets for therapy. New models, such as GBM patient-derived tumor stem cells grown in neurosphere culture, may be a valuable addition to epigenetic research into GBM, particularly if the epigenetic profiles of the corresponding primary tumors are retained, as has been shown in gene expression patterns and invasive growth patterns of these cells [38]. Epigenomic profiling of DNA methylation, histone modifications and non-coding RNAs (such as microRNAs) in primary tumors, orthotopic xenografts, and tumor neurospheres are strategies that will likely uncover many additional epigenetic alterations in GBMs, and potential targets for therapy.

There are still many questions remaining about the role of epigenetics in GBM. The causes and consequences of epigenetic alterations are still mostly unknown, and the relative contributions of genetic and environmental factors to epigenetic alterations have not been quantified. It is still unclear as to why some genes or pathways are more affected by epigenetic alterations than they are by genetic alterations (or vice versa). It is clear, however, that simultaneously examining both genetic and epigenetic defects, complemented with functional studies, will be essential in answering these questions. It will also be important to understand the effects of HDACi on the entire cancer acetylome to elucidate the molecular consequences of this treatment strategy.

Therapies that combine both DNMT and HDAC inhibitors may be an effective strategy against GBM. A dual treatment approach may have a synergistic effect on gene activation, and could allow lower doses of each drug to be used. Such a strategy is being tested in a clinical trial for myelodysplastic syndrome (MDS) and acute myelogenous leukemia (AML) using the DNMT inhibitor Decitabine with or without valproic acid (clinicaltrials.gov ID NCT00414310).

An area that is mostly unexplored in GBM is the development and testing of drugs directed against histone modifications other than acetylation. H3K27 methylation at promoter regions of silenced tumor suppressors could be targeted to reactivate these genes by, for example, using the S-adenosylhomocysteine hydrolase inhibitor 3-Deazaneplanocin A (DZNep) [38]. However, it should be noted that the degree of specificity of DZNep for inhibiting H3K27me3 has not yet been fully determined because of its strong toxicity. As epigenetic modifications are better understood and more types are discovered, additional epigenetic drug targets can be tested in GBMs and other cancers.

Acknowledgements I would like to thank Min Gyu Lee, Ph.D. (mglee@mdanderson.org) whose recent affiliation is the Department of Molecular and Cellular Oncology, The University of Texas MD Anderson Cancer Center for reviewing this manuscript sincerely. Recently, Sung-Hun Lee moved to Plumbline Life Science Inc., whose affiliation is Department of Research and Development, Plumbline Life Science Inc., Ansan, Gyeonggi-do, South Korea.

Declarations The author has no conflicts of interests.

References

1. Anand R, Marmorstein R (2007) Structure and mechanism of lysine-specific demethylase enzymes. J Biol Chem 282:35425–35429
2. Ancelin K, Lange UC, Hajkova P, Schneider R, Bannister AJ, Kouzarides T, Surani MA (2006) Blimp1 associates with Prmt5 and directs histone arginine methylation in mouse germ cells. Nat Cell Biol 8:623–630
3. Benetatos L, Vartholomatos G, Hatzimichael E (2011) MEG3 imprinted gene contribution in tumorigenesis. Int J Cancer 129(4):773–779
4. Bernstein BE, Mikkelsen TS, Xie X, Kamal M, Huebert DJ, Cuff J, Fry B, Meissner A, Wernig M, Plath K, Jaenisch R, Wagschal A, Feil R, Schreiber SL, Lander ES (2006) A bivalent chromatin structure marks key developmental genes in embryonic stem cells. Cell 125:315–326

5. Botuyan MV, Lee J, Ward IM, Kim JE, Thompson JR, Chen J, Mer G (2006) Structural basis for the methylation state-specific recognition of histone H4-K20 by 53BP1 and Crb2 in DNA repair. Cell 127:1361–1373

6. Burke TW, Cook JG, Asano M, Nevins JR (2001) Replication factors MCM2 and ORC1 interact with the histone acetyltransferase HBO1. J Biol Chem 276:15397–15408

7. Campos B, Bermejo JL, Han L, Felsberg J, Ahmadi R, Grabe N, Reifenberger G, Unterberg A, Herold-Mende C (2011) Expression of nuclear receptor corepressors and class I histone deacetylases in astrocytic gliomas. Cancer Sci 102:387–392

8. Cao R, Wang L, Wang H, Xia L, Erdjument-Bromage H, Tempst P, Jones RS, Zhang Y (2002) Role of histone H3 lysine 27 methylation in Polycomb-group silencing. Science 298:1039–1043

9. Cimbora DM, Schubeler D, Reik A, Hamilton J, Francastel C, Epner EM, Groudine M (2000) Long-distance control of origin choice and replication timing in the human beta-globin locus are independent of the locus control region. Mol Cell Biol 20:5581–5591

10. Clark SJ, Harrison J, Frommer M (1995) CpNpG methylation in mammalian cells. Nat Genet 10:20–27

11. Clarke S (1993) Protein methylation. Curr Opin Cell Biol 5:977–983

12. Dacwag CS, Ohkawa Y, Pal S, Sif S, Imbalzano AN (2007) The protein arginine methyltransferase Prmt5 is required for myogenesis because it facilitates ATP-dependent chromatin remodeling. Mol Cell Biol 27:384–394

13. Di Croce L (2005) Chromatin modifying activity of leukaemia associated fusion proteins. Hum Mol Genet 14:R77–R84

14. Downs JA, Cote J (2005) Dynamics of chromatin during the repair of DNA double-strand breaks. Cell Cycle 4:1373–1376

15. Downs JA, Allard S, Jobin-Robitaille O, Javaheri A, Auger A, Bouchard N, Kron SJ, Jackson SP, Côté J (2004) Binding of chromatin-modifying activities to phosphorylated histone H2A at DNA damage sites. Mol Cell 16:979–990

16. Doyon Y, Cayrou C, Ullah M, Landry AJ, Côté V, Selleck W, Lane WS, Tan S, Yang XJ, Côté J (2006) ING tumor suppressor proteins are critical regulators of chromatin acetylation required for genome expression and perpetuation. Mol Cell 21:51–64

17. Eden A, Gaudet F, Waghmare A, Jaenisch R (2003) Chromosomal instability and tumors promoted by DNA hypomethylation. Science 300:455

18. Esteller M (2007) Cancer epigenomics: DNA methylomes and histone-modification maps. Nat Rev Genet 8:286–298

19. Feng Q, Wang H, Ng HH, Erdjument-Bromage H, Tempst P, Struhl K, Zhang Y (2002) Methylation of H3-lysine 79 is mediated by a new family of HMTases without a SET domain. Curr Biol 12:1052–1058

20. Fouse SD, Shen Y, Pellegrini M, Cole S, Meissner A, Van Neste L, Jaenisch R, Fan G (2008) Promoter CpG methylation contributes to ES cell gene regulation in parallel with Oct4/Nanog, PcG complex, and histone H3 K4/K27 trimethylation. Cell Stem Cell 2:160–169

21. Gary JD, Clarke S (1998) RNA and protein interactions modulated by protein arginine methylation. Prog Nucleic Acid Res Mol Biol 61:65–131

22. Gimsing P, Hansen M, Knudsen LM, Knoblauch P, Christensen IJ, Ooi CE, Buhl-Jensen P (2008) A phase I clinical trial of the histone deacetylase inhibitor belinostat in patients with advanced hematological neoplasia. Eur J Haematol 81:170–176

23. Guccione E, Bassi C, Casadio F, Martinato F, Cesaroni M, Schuchlautz H, Luscher B, Amati B (2007) Methylation of histone H3R2 by PRMT6 and H3K4 by an MLL complex are mutually exclusive. Nature 449:933–937

24. Hakimi MA, Dong Y, Lane WS, Speicher DW, Shiekhattar R (2003) A candidate X-linked mental retardation gene is a component of a new family of histone deacetylase-containing complexes. J Biol Chem 278:7234–7239

25. Hamada S, Kim TD, Suzuki T, Itoh Y, Tsumoto H, Nakagawa H, Janknecht R, Miyata N (2009) Synthesis and activity of Noxalylglycine and its derivatives as Jumonji C-domain containing histone lysine demethylase inhibitors. Bioorg Med Chem Lett 19:2852–2855

26. Hansen RS, Gartler SM (1990) 5-Azacytidine-induced reactivation of the human X chromosome-linked PGK1 gene is associated with a large region of cytosine demethylation in the 5′ CpG island. Proc Natl Acad Sci U S A 87:4174–4178

27. Hayry V, Tanner M, Blom T, Tynninen O, Roselli A, Ollikainen M, Sariola H, Wartiovaara K, Nupponen NN (2008) Copy number alterations of the polycomb gene BMI1 in gliomas. Acta Neuropathol 116:97–102

28. Henikoff S, Ahmad K (2005) Assembly of variant histones into chromatin. Annu Rev Cell Dev Biol 21:133–153

29. Hirota T, Lipp JJ, Toh BH, Peters JM (2005) Histone H3 serine 10 phosphorylation by Aurora B causes HP1 dissociation from heterochromatin. Nature 438:1176–1180

30. Huang J, Berger SL (2008) The emerging field of dynamic lysine methylation of non-histone proteins. Curr Opin Genet Dev 18:152–158

31. Jenuwein T, Allis CD (2001) Translating the histone code. Science 293:1074–1080

32. Jung KW, Ha JH, Lee SH, Won YJ, Yoo H (2013) An updated nationwide epidemiology of primary brain tumors in republic of Korea. Brain Tumor Res Treat 1:16–23

33. Kampranis SC, Tsichlis PN (2009) Histone demethylases and cancer. Adv Cancer Res 102:103–169

34. Kornberg RD, Lorch Y (1999) Twenty-five years of the nucleosome, fundamental particle of the eukaryote chromosome. Cell 98:285–294

35. Kouzarides T (2002) Histone methylation in transcriptional control. Curr Opin Genet Dev 12(2):198–209

36. Kouzarides T (2007) Chromatin modifications and their function. Cell 128:693–705

37. Li E, Beard C, Jaenisch R (1993) Role for DNA methylation in genomic imprinting. Nature 366:362–365

38. Li A, Walling J, Kotliarov Y, Center A, Steed ME, Ahn SJ, Rosenblum M, Mikkelsen T, Zenklusen JC, Fine HA (2008) Genomic changes and gene expression profiles reveal that established glioma cell lines are poorly representative of primary human gliomas. Mol Cancer Res 6:21–30

39. Liu BL, Cheng JX, Zhang X, Wang R, Zhang W, Lin H, Xiao X, Cai S, Chen XY, Cheng H (2010) Global histone modification patterns as prognostic markers to classify glioma patients. Cancer Epidemiol Biomark Prev 19(11):2888–2896

40. Lucio-Eterovic AK, Cortez MA, Valera ET, Motta FJ, Queiroz RG, Machado HR, Carlotti CG Jr, Neder L, Scrideli CA, Tone LG (2008) Differential expression of 12 histone deacetylase (HDAC) genes in astrocytomas and normal brain tissue: class II and IV are hypoexpressed in glioblastomas. BMC Cancer 8:243

41. Masumoto H, Hawke D, Kobayashi R, Verreault A (2005) A role for cell-cycle-regulated histone H3 lysine 56 acetylation in the DNA damage response. Nature 436:294–298

42. McBride AE, Silver PA (2001) State of the Arg: protein methylation at arginine comes of age. Cell 106:5–8

43. Mercurio C, Plyte S, Minucci S (2012) Alterations of histone modifications in cancer. Epigenet Hum Dis 4:53–87

44. Metzger E, Wissmann M, Yin N, Müller JM, Schneider R, Peters AH, Günther T, Buettner R, Schüle R (2005) LSD1 demethylates repressive histone marks to promote androgen-receptor-dependent transcription. Nature 437:436–439

45. Metzger E, Imhof A, Patel D, Kahl P, Hoffmeyer K, Friedrichs N, Müller JM, Greschik H, Kirfel J, Ji S, Kunowska N, Beisenherz-Huss C, Günther T, Buettner R, Schüle R (2010) Phosphorylation of histone H3T6 by PKC-beta(I) controls demethylation at histone H3K4. Nature 464:792–796

46. Mills KD, Ferguson DO, Alt FW (2003) The role of DNA breaks in genomic instability and tumorigenesis. Immunol Rev 194:77–95

47. Milne TA, Briggs SD, Brock HW, Martin ME, Gibbs D, Allis CD, Hess JL (2002) MLL targets SET domain methyltransferase activity to Hox gene promoters. Mol Cell 10:1107–1117

48. Murr R, Vaissiere T, Sawan C, Shukla V, Herceg Z (2007) Orchestration of chromatin-based processes: mind the TRRAP. Oncogene 26:5358–5372

49. Murray K (1964) The occurrence of Epsilon-N-methyl lysine in histones. Biochemistry 3:10–15
50. Nishioka K, Rice JC, Sarma K, Erdjument-Bromage H, Werner J, Wang Y, Chuikov S, Valenzuela P, Tempst P, Steward R, Lis JT, Allis CD, Reinberg D (2002) PR-Set7 is a nucleo-some-specific methyltransferase that modifies lysine 20 of histone H4 and is associated with silent chromatin. Mol Cell 9:1201–1213
51. Norton VG, Imai BS, Yau P, Bradbury EM (1989) Histone acetylation reduces nucleosome core particle linking number change. Cell 57:449–457
52. Ohm JE, McGarvey KM, Yu X, Cheng L, Schuebel KE, Cope L, Mohammad HP, Chen W, Daniel VC, Yu W, Berman DM, Jenuwein T, Pruitt K, Sharkis SJ, Watkins DN, Herman JG, Baylin SB (2007) A stem cell-like chromatin pattern may predispose tumor suppressor genes to DNA hypermethylation and heritable silencing. Nat Genet 39:237–242
53. Okano M, Xie S, Li E (1998) Cloning and characterization of a family of novel mammalian DNA (cytosine-5) methyltransferases. Nat Genet 19:219–220
54. Pal S, Vishwanath SN, Erdjument-Bromage H, Tempst P, Sif S (2004) Human SWI/SNF-associated PRMT5 methylates histone H3 arginine 8 and negatively regulates expression of ST7 and NM23 tumor suppressor genes. Mol Cell Biol 24:9630–9645
55. Parsons DW, Jones S, Zhang X, Lin JC, Leary RJ, Angenendt P, Mankoo P, Carter H, Siu IM, Gallia GL, Olivi A, McLendon R, Rasheed BA, Keir S, Nikolskaya T, Nikolsky Y, Busam DA, Tekleab H, Diaz LA Jr, Hartigan J, Smith DR, Strausberg RL, Marie SK, Shinjo SM, Yan H, Riggins GJ, Bigner DD, Karchin R, Papadopoulos N, Parmigiani G, Vogelstein B, Velculescu VE, Kinzler KW (2008) An integrated genomic analysis of human glioblastoma multiforme. Science 321(5897):1807–1812
56. Peterson CL, Laniel MA (2004) Histones and histone modifications. Curr Biol 14:R546–R551
57. Petrij F, Giles RH, Dauwerse HG, Saris JJ, Hennekam RC, Masuno M, Tommerup N, van Ommen GJ, Goodman RH, Peters DJ (1995) Rubinstein-Taybi syndrome caused by mutations in the transcriptional coactivator CBP. Nature 376(6538):348–351
58. Rea S, Eisenhaber F, O'Carroll D, Strahl BD, Sun ZW, Schmid M, Opravil S, Mechtler K, Ponting CP, Allis CD, Jenuwein T (2000) Regulation of chromatin structure by site-specific histone H3 methyltransferases. Nature 406:593–599
59. Sanders SL, Portoso M, Mata J, Bahler J, Allshire RC, Kouzarides T (2004) Methylation of histone H4 lysine 20 controls recruitment of Crb2 to sites of DNA damage. Cell 119:603–614
60. Santos-Rosa H, Kirmizis A, Nelson C, Bartke T, Saksouk N, Cote J, Kouzarides T (2009) Histone H3 tail clipping regulates gene expression. Nat Struct Mol Biol 16:17–22
61. Sawan C, Herceg Z (2010) Histone modifications and cancer. Adv Genet 70:57–85
62. Schmidt N, Windmann S, Reifenberger G, Riemenschneider MJ (2012) DNA hypermethyl-ation and histone modifications down-regulate the candidate tumor suppressor gene RRP22 on 22q12 in human gliomas. Brain Pathol 22:17–25
63. Schulte JH, Lim S, Schramm A, Friedrichs N, Koster J, Versteeg R, Ora I, Pajtler K, Klein-Hitpass L, Kuhfittig-Kulle S, Metzger E, Schüle R, Eggert A, Buettner R, Kirfel J (2009) Lysine-specific demethylase 1 is strongly expressed in poorly differentiated neuroblastoma: implications for therapy. Cancer Res 69:2065–2071
64. Schurter BT, Koh SS, Chen D, Bunick GJ, Harp JM, Hanson BL, Henschen-Edman A, Mackay DR, Stallcup MR, Aswad DW (2001) Methylation of histone H3 by coactivator-associated arginine methyltransferase 1. Biochemistry 40:5747–5756
65. Schwartzentruber J, Korshunov A, Liu XY, Jones DT, Pfaff E, Jacob K, Sturm D, Fontebasso AM, Quang DA, Tönjes M, Hovestadt V, Albrecht S, Kool M, Nantel A, Konermann C, Lindroth A, Jäger N, Rausch T, Ryzhova M, Korbel JO, Hielscher T, Hauser P, Garami M, Klekner A, Bognar L, Ebinger M, Schuhmann MU, Scheurlen W, Pekrun A, Frühwald MC, Roggendorf W, Kramm C, Dürken M, Atkinson J, Lepage P, Montpetit A, Zakrzewska M, Zakrzewski K, Liberski PP, Dong Z, Siegel P, Kulozik AE, Zapatka M, Guha A, Malkin D, Felsberg J, Reifenberger G, von Deimling A, Ichimura K, Collins VP, Witt H, Milde T, Witt O, Zhang C, Castelo-Branco P, Lichter P, Faury D, Tabori U, Plass C, Majewski J, Pfister SM,

Jabado N (2012) Driver mutations in histone H3.3 and chromatin remodelling genes in paediatric glioblastoma. Nature 482:226–231

66. Shahbazian MD, Grunstein M (2007) Functions of site-specific histone acetylation and deacetylation. Annu Rev Biochem 76:75–100

67. Shi Y (2007) Histone lysine demethylases: emerging roles in development, physiology and disease. Nat Rev Genet 8:829–833

68. Shi Y, Lan F, Matson C, Mulligan P, Whetstine JR, Cole PA, Casero RA, Shi Y (2004) Histone demethylation mediated by the nuclear amine oxidase homolog LSD1. Cell 119:941–953

69. Shilatifard A (2006) Chromatin modifications by methylation and ubiquitination: implications in the regulation of gene expression. Annu Rev Biochem 75:243–269

70. Shroff R, Arbel-Eden A, Pilch D, Ira G, Bonner WM, Petrini JH, Haber JE, Lichten M (2004) Distribution and dynamics of chromatin modification induced by a defined DNA double-strand break. Curr Biol 14:1703–1711

71. Sims RJ 3rd, Reinberg D (2006) Histone H3 Lys 4 methylation: caught in a bind? Genes Dev 20:2779–2786

72. Sims RJ 3rd, Nishioka K, Reinberg D (2003) Histone lysine methylation: a signature for chromatin function. Trends Genet 19:629–639

73. Strahl BD, Grant PA, Briggs SD, Sun ZW, Bone JR, Caldwell JA, Mollah S, Cook RG, Shabanowitz J, Hunt DF, Allis CD (2002) Set2 is a nucleosomal histone H3-selective methyltransferase that mediates transcriptional repression. Mol Cell Biol 22:1298–1306

74. Sun ZW, Allis CD (2002) Ubiquitination of histone H2B regulates H3 methylation and gene silencing in yeast. Nature 418:104–108

75. Sun Y, Jiang X, Xu Y, Ayrapetov MK, Moreau LA, Whetstine JR, Price BD (2009) Histone H3 methylation links DNA damage detection to activation of the tumour suppressor Tip60. Nat Cell Biol 11:1376–1382

76. Tachibana M, Sugimoto K, Nozaki M, Ueda J, Ohta T, Ohki M, Fukuda M, Fukuda M, Takeda N, Niida H, Kato H, Shinkai Y (2002) G9a histone methyltransferase plays a dominant role in euchromatic histone H3 lysine 9 methylation and is essential for early embryogenesis. Genes Dev 16:1779–1791

77. Tachibana M, Ueda J, Fukuda M, Takeda N, Ohta T, Iwanari H, Sakihama T, Kodama T, Hamakubo T, Shinkai Y (2005) Histone methyltransferases G9a and GLP form heteromeric complexes and are both crucial for methylation of euchromatin at H3-K9. Genes Dev 19:815–826

78. Torres-Padilla ME, Parfitt DE, Kouzarides T, Zernicka-Goetz M (2007) Histone arginine methylation regulates pluripotency in the early mouse embryo. Nature 445:214–218

79. Tsukada Y, Fang J, Erdjument-Bromage H, Warren ME, Borchers CH, Tempst P, Zhang Y (2006) Histone demethylation by a family of JmjC domain-containing proteins. Nature 439:811–816

80. Turner BM (2005) Reading signals on the nucleosome with a new nomenclature for modified histones. Nat Struct Mol Biol 12:110–112

81. Ueda R, Suzuki T, Mino K, Tsumoto H, Nakagawa H, Hasegawa M, Sasaki R, Mizukami T, Miyata N (2009) Identification of cell-active lysine specific demethylase 1-selective inhibitors. J Am Chem Soc 131:17536–17537

82. Unnikrishnan A, Gafken PR, Tsukiyama T (2010) Dynamic changes in histone acetylation regulate origins of DNA replication. Nat Struct Mol Biol 17:430–437

83. van Attikum H, Gasser SM (2005) The histone code at DNA breaks: a guide to repair? Nat Rev 6:757–765

84. van Leeuwen F, Gafken PR, Gottschling DE (2002) Dot1p modulates silencing in yeast by methylation of the nucleosome core. Cell 109:745–756

85. Vermeulen M, Mulder KW, Denissov S, Pijnappel WW, van Schaik FM, Varier RA, Baltissen MP, Stunnenberg HG, Mann M, Timmers HT (2007) Selective anchoring of TFIID to nucleosomes by trimethylation of histone H3 lysine 4. Cell 131:58–69

86. Vissers JH, Nicassio F, van Lohuizen M, Di Fiore PP, Citterio E (2008) The many faces of ubiquitinated histone H2A: insights from the DUBs. Cell Div 3:8
87. Wang H, Cao R, Xia L, Erdjument-Bromage H, Borchers C, Tempst P, Zhang Y (2001) Purification and functional characterization of a histone H3-lysine 4-specific methyltransferase. Mol Cell 8:1207–1217
88. Weiss VH, McBride AE, Soriano MA, Filman DJ, Silver PA, Hogle JM (2000) The structure and oligomerization of the yeast arginine methyltransferase, Hmt1. Nat Struct Biol 7:1165–1171
89. Wen PY, Kesari S (2008) Malignant gliomas in adults. N Engl J Med 359:492–507
90. Whetstine JR, Nottke A, Lan F, Huarte M, Smolikov S, Chen Z, Spooner E, Li F, Zhang G, Colaiacovo M, Shi Y (2006) Reversal of histone lysine trimethylation by the JMJD2 family of histone demethylases. Cell 125:467–481
91. Yang M, Culhane JC, Szewczuk LM, Jalili P, Ball HL, Machius M, Cole PA, Yu H (2007) Structural basis for the inhibition of the LSD1 histone demethylase by the antidepressant trans-2-phenylcyclopropylamine. Biochemistry 46:8058–8065
92. Zaidi SK, Young DW, Montecino M, Lian JB, Stein JL, van Wijnen AJ, Stein GS (2010) Architectural epigenetics: mitotic retention of mammalian transcriptional regulatory information. Mol Cell Biol 30(20):4758–4766
93. Zhang J, Xu F, Hashimshony T, Keshet I, Cedar H (2002) Establishment of transcriptional competence in early and late S phase. Nature 420:198–202

DNA and Histone Methylation in Gastric Cancer

Keisuke Matsusaka and Atsushi Kaneda

Abstract Two unique pathogens play crucial roles in gastric carcinogenesis, namely *Helicobacter pylori* (*H. pylori*) and Epstein-Barr virus (EBV). Gastric cancer is frequently associated with aberrant DNA hypermethylation as well as genetic alterations, and the both these infectious agents are involved in various molecular events. This chapter focuses on epigenetic aberrations in gastric cancer, including hypermethylation and its correlations with the two infectious agents as well as the recently reported histone modifications.

Keywords Gastric cancer • DNA methylation • Epstein-Barr virus • *Helicobacter pylori* • Histone modification

1 Introduction

Gastric cancer is one of the most common and lethal malignant tumors worldwide. Two unique pathogens play crucial roles in the etiology of gastric cancer, namely *Helicobacter pylori* (*H. pylori*) and Epstein-Barr virus (EBV). From the molecular viewpoint, gastric cancer is frequently associated with aberrant DNA hypermethylation as well as genetic alterations, and the both these infectious agents are involved in these and other molecular events. This chapter focuses on epigenetic aberrations in gastric cancer, including hypermethylation and its correlations with the two infectious agents as well as the recently reported histone modifications.

K. Matsusaka (✉)
Department of Molecular Oncology, Graduate School of Medicine, Chiba University, Chiba, Japan
e-mail: ksk.matsusaka@chiba-u.jp

A. Kaneda
Graduate School of Medicine, Chiba University, Chiba, Japan

© Springer International Publishing AG 2017
A. Kaneda, Y.-i. Tsukada (eds.), *DNA and Histone Methylation as Cancer Targets*, Cancer Drug Discovery and Development, DOI 10.1007/978-3-319-59786-7_13

2 Gastric Cancer and Two Unique Pathogens that Induce DNA Hypermethylation

Gastric cancer is one of the major causes of cancer-related death worldwide [65]. Two unique pathogens, *H. pylori* and EBV, are known to participate in gastric carcinogenesis. In this section, we review these two infectious agents.

H. pylori is a helix-shaped Gram-negative bacterium that infects the surface of gastric mucosa. It was first reported by Marshall BJ and Warren JR in 1983 [39]. About half the world's population is infected with *H. pylori* [53, 57]. *H. pylori* infection triggers chronic active gastritis and is characterized by persistent infiltration of plasma cells and neutrophils into the gastric mucosa, accompanied by sustained injury to epithelial cells [39]. If the infection persists for decades, the proper gastric glands, i.e. fundic and pyloric glands, become atrophied, causing a decrease in the gland volume and a replacement of the intestinal metaplasia; this condition is called chronic atrophic gastritis [11, 12, 58]. Before the discovery of *H. pylori*, the gastric lumen was assumed to be sterile because of its highly acidic nature, and the atrophic changes were explained as age-related phenomena. The unexpected discovery of *H. pylori* was a revolutionary event in the field of gastroenterology and caused a drastic paradigm shift in the attitude towards gastric disorders. Many subsequent exploratory studies demonstrated that *H. pylori* was associated with chronic atrophic gastritis and played a crucial role in gastric carcinogenesis [55, 71]. After consistent accumulation of such epidemiological proof, the World Health Organization finally concluded that, "*H. pylori* is a definite carcinogen" [53, 57].

EBV is another infectious agent associated with gastric cancer. EBV belongs to the subfamily *Gammaherpesvirinae* and has a double-stranded DNA genome. EBV was the first virus to be isolated from a human malignant tumor, Burkitt lymphoma, in 1964 by Epstein MA and Barr Y [15]. It was later found to be the cause of infectious mononucleosis, which causes severe symptoms such as fatigue, fever, pharyngitis, and lymphadenopathy in post-pubertal patients [50]. EBV is usually retained inside inactivated memory B-lymphocytes in a latent form. However, it occasionally switches into a lytic form and produces infectious viral particles in pharyngeal tonsils, which are transmitted via saliva. Eventually, more than 90% of adults become EBV carriers and do not exhibit any symptoms. Thus, EBV is one of the most successful infectious agents to survive in humans. EBV has also been reported to be associated with several kinds of malignant cancers including gastric cancer [6], Hodgkin's lymphoma [81], opportunistic lymphoma in immunocompromised hosts [13, 48], and nasopharyngeal carcinoma [84].

Generally, gastric cancer is characterized by complicated clinicopathological features; based on the histopathology, gastric cancers were even classified into several types [30]. Furthermore, intratumoral heterogeneity is frequently observed [59]. This clinicopathological diversity may be responsible for the long-term chronic gastritis induced by *H. pylori* infection, causing large-scale molecular damage. While gastric cancer is generally characterized by a variety of properties, EBV+ gastric cancer has been shown to be a distinguished subgroup from a clinicopathological as well as a molecular viewpoint. The following sections illustrate the correlations between molecular aberration and *H. pylori* or EBV.

3   *H. pylori* Infection and Gastric Cancer

H. pylori exerts its pathogenic effects via two pathways. One is direct interaction with gastric epithelial cells, and the other is indirect interference mediated by non-specific chronic inflammation. These pathways are not always independent and facilitate each other, resulting in gastric carcinogenesis.

3.1   Direct Interaction of **H. pylori** for DNA Hypermethylation

Most Gram-negative bacteria have an innate capacity to acquire exogenous gene clusters, called pathogenicity islands (PAI), and this often accounts for their pathogenicity. *H. pylori* can also acquire PAI and it was reported that it directly interacts with gastric epithelial cells through a PAI encoding about 30 genes, including a type IV secretion system [5]. The pathogenicity of *H. pylori* depends on its ability to produce the cytotoxin-associated gene A (CagA) protein. Almost all strains in East Asia and about half the strains in the west can produce CagA protein; this biased distribution is reflected on the incidence of gastric cancer. *H. pylori* directly injects the CagA protein into gastric epithelial cells through the type IV secretion system. This protein invasion affects the host cells in different ways by causing enhancement of cell motility (so-called hummingbird) [62], disruption of the epithelial apical-junctional complex [3], and epithelial proliferation [66]. CagA was proven to possess oncogenic properties when a transgenic mouse model expressing CagA developed gastric adenocarcinoma [55]. However, its direct contribution to the induction of aberrant DNA hypermethylation remains unknown.

3.2   Indirect Effect of **H. pylori** Through Chronic Inflammation

The indirect interference of *H. pylori* mediated by chronic inflammation plays a more crucial role in the induction of aberrant DNA hypermethylation [35, 51]. Chronic persisting injuries that cause inflammation can stimulate cell-cycle progression and induce molecular damage by producing free radicals [68] or causing aberrant expression of activation-induced cytidine deaminases [40]. In a Mongolian gerbil model, aberrant DNA hypermethylation was suppressed by a demethylating agent 5-aza-2-deoxycytidine, and this resulted in a decrease in incidence of *H. pylori*-induced gastric cancer although it was not completely prevented [52]. While this result indicates that aberrant DNA hypermethylation promotes the risk of *H. pylori*-related gastric cancer, it is possible that *H. pylori* itself plays an important role in the carcinogenesis.

Long-term persistent gastritis caused by *H. pylori* causes aberrant hypermethylation in promoters of many genes including tumor-suppressor genes ($p16^{INK4A}$ and *LOX*) [32, 73]. Thus, chronic damage to the gastric mucosa leads to field cancerization, in which vast areas of the gastric mucosa is at risk of tumorigenesis because of accumulation of genetic or epigenetic alterations. Therefore, the incidence of gastric cancer could be reduced by eradication of *H. pylori*. At present, *H. pylori* can be eradicated through standard protocols of polypharmacy, with the use of antibiotics and proton pump inhibitors. However, once a promoter gets aberrantly hypermethylated, eradication of *H. pylori* will not help, as a certain amount of methylation is retained [47, 51]. This suggests that aberrant hypermethylation might occur at the stem cell or progenitor cell level. Upregulation of inflammatory genes like *IL-1β*, *IL-8*, *NOS2*, and *TNF* was assumed to induce aberrant hypermethylation during chronic inflammation in inflammatory disorders like human ulcerative colitis or hepatitis [8, 37, 43, 44]. *IL-1β* was reported to be a significant factor for the induction of aberrant hypermethylation in the promoter regions during gastric carcinogenesis [9, 14]. The role of *IL-1β* in *H. pylori*-induced gastritis was demonstrated using mice in which the IL-1 receptor type 1 was knocked out [24].

4   EBV⁺ Gastric Cancer and Epigenetic Alterations

In 1990, the EBV genome was detected by PCR in a gastric cancer tissue showing lymphoepithelial features [6]. Advances in *in situ* hybridization methods for detecting EBV-encoded small RNAs (EBERs) have enabled the high-throughput detection of EBV-infected cells in tissue specimens. Subsequently, intensive surveys were carried out and the results have revealed that EBV-positive (EBV⁺) gastric cancer (or EBV-associated gastric cancer) is distributed worldwide with very low endemic deviation rates of 7–15% [17, 63, 64, 67], unlike other cancers like Burkitt lymphoma in equatorial Africa or nasopharyngeal carcinoma in southern China. Other meta-analyses report an overall frequency of 8.2–8.7% [7, 46]. EBV⁺ gastric cancer is characterized by unique histopathological features such as poorly differentiated adenocarcinoma and marked lymphocyte infiltration in the cancer stromas; it has therefore been called "gastric cancer with lymphoid stroma" [76]. Moreover, EBV⁺ gastric cancer shows distinct clinicopathological features such as predominance in males, proximal location, post-operative recurrent gastric cancer, synchronous or metachronous multiple occurrences, and relatively favorable prognoses with reduced frequency of lymph node metastases [7, 17]. These features serve to distinguish EBV⁺ gastric cancers from other gastric cancers. This was validated through molecular approaches, as discussed below.

4.1   Characteristics of EBV⁺ Gastric Cancer

Evidence from a number of studies suggests that EBV is associated with gastric carcinogenesis for three reasons. Firstly, the EBV genome isolated from many cases demonstrated mono- or oligoclonality, regardless of the tumor stage [18, 25, 72]. Secondly, all the cells in each EBV⁺ gastric cancer tissue tested positive for the presence of EBER-ISH [17, 64]. Finally, the incidence of EBV⁺ gastric cancer does not show any significant difference between early and advanced stages [17, 64]. EBV has a double-strand DNA genome with about 170,000 bp. In the infectious viral particles, the DNA takes a linear form. After it enters the host cells, it takes a circular form by the fusion of its two ends with terminal repeats. The length of the terminal repeats in the circular EBV genome is maintained inside the nuclei of the host cells because integration into the host genome does not occur [36]. The clonality of the EBV genome inside the host cells could be evaluated by a Southern blot analysis, which can estimate the lengths of terminal repeats showing single or oligo bands. The investigation of clonality of the EBV genome in EBV$^+$ gastric cancer revealed that the infection was established at an initial or very early stage before clonal expansion of tumor cells.

The in vivo mechanism by which EBV establishes its infection in the gastric epithelial cells is still unknown. The innate receptor for EBV infection is CR2 (CD21), which is expressed on the cell membrane of B lymphocytes. However, gastric epithelial cells do not express this receptor [80], and EBV by itself cannot infect unintended host cells. This issue could be explained by a cell-to-cell contact model for in vitro infection called the Akata system. The Akata cell line is a floating cell line derived from EBV-infected Burkitt lymphoma tissues and usually exists in the latent infection form without virus production. Akata cells express the IgG receptor on the cell surface and so, stimulation of this receptor using anti-IgG antibodies could induce the switch to lytic form and the production of infectious viral particles. Co-culturing of these lytic Akata cells with adhesive epithelial cells can facilitate EBV infection of the epithelial cell through cell-to-cell contact [26]. The mucosa surrounding EBV$^+$ gastric cancer tissues often shows chronic gastritis with atrophic changes caused by *H. pylori* infection [31]. This non-physiological inflammatory condition caused by *H. pylori* might provide the opportunity for EBV to infect the epithelial cells, which are usually not present in the EBV lifecycle. Recently, interaction between *H. pylori* and EBV in gastric carcinogenesis was reported at the molecular level [60]. The CagA protein undergoes tyrosine phosphorylation, and the tyrosine-phosphorylated CagA then binds to the pro-oncogenic protein tyrosine phosphatase SHP2, which is considered to play significant roles in gastric carcinogenesis. SHP1, an SHP2 homologue, is involved in tumor-suppression and specifically interacts with CagA to dephosphorylate it. EBV infection, however, induces aberrant hypermethylation of the SHP1 promoter, thereby silencing its expression. EBV thus strengthens the phosphorylation-dependent CagA action.

4.2 DNA Hypermethylation in EBV$^+$ Gastric Cancer

EBV$^+$ gastric cancer was reported to be associated with a high frequency of promoter hypermethylation [10, 34, 74]; however, previous analyses were limited to known cancer-related genes. A genome-wide DNA methylation analysis in clinical gastric cancers was performed to reveal the methylation epigenotype (ME) of gastric cancer. Gastric cancers were classified into three distinct groups based on MEs: low-ME, high-ME, and extremely high-ME [42]. The EBV$^+$ gastric cancer was classified as having an extremely high-ME. The methylation pattern in EBV$^+$ gastric cancer is characterized by two features. Firstly, non-specific genes, which are methylated in EBV-negative cases as well, are also methylated. Secondly, excess hypermethylation is observed specifically in EBV⁺ gastric cancer; this characterizes the EBV⁺ ME. Generally, aberrant promoter hypermethylation in cancer is significantly higher in the target genes of the Polycomb repressive complex (PRC) in embryonic stem cells [54, 61, 77]. Commonly methylated genes in gastric cancer showed a significantly higher level of methylation in PRC-target genes, similar to other kinds of tumors. However, genes specifically methylated in EBV⁺ gastric cancers extended to non PRC-target genes, which are rarely methylated in other cells [42]. This implies the presence of some unique mechanism to induce excessive DNA hypermethylation in EBV⁺ gastric cancer cells. The high-ME group contained some cases in which the mismatch repair gene *MLH1* was methylated, while EBV⁺ gastric cancer was free from *MLH1*-methylation, implying the presence of a different mechanism.

In vitro EBV infection experiments were performed using the Akata system to clarify the causal relationship between EBV infection and extremely high-ME. Surprisingly, EBV infection in low-methylation gastric cancer cells, MKN7, induced genome-wide de novo DNA methylation in the host cellular genome. De novo methylation extended into the specifically methylated genes as well as the commonly methylated genes in EBV⁺ gastric cancer tissues, which suggested that EBV infection itself could be the definite cause of extremely high-ME. The methylated genes actually caused the downregulation of various genes including tumor-suppressor genes, which suggests that EBV plays a key role in gastric carcinogenesis [42].

The mechanism of induction of de novo DNA methylation has not been fully elucidated. The unmethylated genes in the EBV-uninfected state can be subdivided into three categories according to behavior during de novo DNA methylation [41]. The first category includes methylation-resistant genes, which show partial methylation but are resistant to methylation around the transcription start site (TSS). The second category includes methylation-sensitive genes, which show complete methylation in promoter regions. The last category includes the non-methylated genes, which show no de novo methylation. The identification of methylation-resistant genes helps us perceive the EBV-induced de novo methylation as a competition between methylation-induction and -suppression. Recently, the TET (ten-eleven-translocation)-family gene *TET2* was identified as a resistance factor against DNA methylation during EBV infection [49]. The TET family genes encode DNA demethylases that oxidize 5-methylcytosine to 5-hydroxymethylcytosine, 5-formyl-cytosine, and 5-carboxylcytosine [20, 27]. The TET family genes, especially *TET2*, are downregulated during EBV infection. This could be reproduced by a few EBV transcripts and human miRNAs against *TET2*, which were upregulated by EBV infection. EBV infection induced de novo methylation in a greater number of genes *TET2* was knocked out by shRNA.

The candidate factors of methylation-induction should be separately studied in EBV and host cells. EBV shows three types of latent forms, based on the expression pattern of latent genes. The lymphoblastoid cell line (LCL), which is transformed by EBV infection into primary B lymphocytes, expresses all types of latent genes, and is called type III latency. Other examples include latent membrane proteins

(LMPs) (-1, -2A, and -2B), EBV nuclear antigens (EBNAs) (-1, -2, -3A, -3B, -3C, and -LP), EBV-encoded small RNAs (EBERs) (-1 and -2), and BARTs. Whereas, Burkitt lymphoma shows type I latency, with only EBNA-1, EBERs, and BARTs expressed during latent infection. Type II latency is intermediate to Type I and III and is exhibited by EBV-associated Hodgkin lymphoma, peripheral natural killer/T-cell lymphoma, and nasopharyngeal carcinoma. In this pattern, LMP-1 and LMP-2 are expressed in addition to the Type I latency genes. The EBV+ gastric cancer shows either latency I or II and expresses EBNA-1, EBERs, BARTs, and/or LMP2A [18, 19, 81]. From the viewpoint of the epigenome, a well-ordered mechanism for the interaction between host cell and EBV could be highlighted. In latent infection, the EBV genome is modified by dense DNA methylation and histone modification to suppress most of viral genes unnecessary maintenance of the latent form. Thus, EBV takes advantage of the host cellular mechanism to control its gene expression. During DNA methylation in the most restricted type I latency, the host genome itself is synchronously extensively hypermethylated [16, 33]. In the least restricted type III latency, the host genome also shows methylation levels as low as those seen in peripheral blood cells [33]. This parallel behavior of the methylome of host cell and EBV implies that the host-driven mechanism to induce DNA methylation in viral genome may extensively affect even host genome.

Many studies have been performed to investigate the methylation-inducer among EBV factors. LMP-1 was found to be expressed in nasopharyngeal carcinomas. It was reported that *CDH1* was downregulated *via* aberrant promoter hypermethylation and that this downregulation induced cell migration activity [69, 70]. LMP-2A expressed in gastric cancer induced promoter hypermethylation for *PTEN* [22]. EBER1 and EBER2 are small non-coding RNAs of about 170 bp length and are expressed abundantly in the nuclei of infected cells (up to 10^7 copies per cell). Their role in the induction of epigenetic modification has remained unclear; however, some oncogenic features of EBERs were reported, such as the ability to increase the transformation efficiency of B-lymphocytes [78, 79] or the induction of insulin-like growth factor 1, which functioned as an autocrine growth factor in gastric cancers and nasopharyngeal carcinoma cells [28, 29]. While these viral factors may affect the local epigenetic modifications, the alteration of genome-wide DNA methylome observed in EBV infection could not be reproduced by forced expression of these viral factors [42].

Recent comprehensive analyses have revealed various genetic alterations, and EBV+ gastric cancer showed particular genetic mutations, notably in chromatin remodeling factors like *ARID1A* [1, 75, 82]. *ARID1A* consists of SWI/SNF complex as the chromatin-remodeling factor; however, it remains unclear whether impairment of these genes causally affects epigenetic alteration in EBV+ gastric cancers. Further investigation is necessary to clarify the roles of host cellular factors in the induction of methylation.

5 Histone Modification

Along with DNA methylation, histone modification is one of the major events associated with epigenetic regulation. However, because DNA methylation is easier to study with high reliability and reproducibility, studies concerning histone modification have been lagging. Mainstream research on epigenetic alterations in gastric cancer has focused only on hypermethylation in promoters of tumor-suppressor genes so far. However, comprehensive analyses of histone modifications are rapidly gaining popularity because of the advances in the chromatin immunoprecipitation with high-throughput sequencer (ChIP-seq) methods. These analyses have highlighted the significance of histone modification in tumorigenicity and cellular development [2, 21, 45]. Analyzing histone modifications is a better way to measure transcriptional status than RNA sequencing because histone modifications are more stable than RNA transcripts [83].

Epigenetic profiling of primary gastric cancers as well as cell lines has been performed, with the focus on histone modifications in enhancer regions [56]. Enhancers are distal regulatory elements. They can be modified by histone H3 lysine 4 monomethylation (H3K4me1) as a location marker, actively regulated by H3 lysine 27 acetylation (H3K27ac), or repressed by H3K27me3 [4, 21]. Super-enhancers are larger than typical enhancers, and are often associated with multiple factors that decide cellular identity or disease properties [23, 38]. It has been reported that a genome-wide reprogramming of enhancers and super-enhancers occur during gastric carcinogenesis, and that it contributes to the dysregulation of local and regional gene expression in a heterogeneous manner [56]. Today, molecular analysis techniques are sufficiently developed to enable genome-wide studies of histone modification even in primary samples; therefore, further studies can be expected.

6 Summary

In this chapter, the correlations between gastric cancer and two unique infectious agents, *H. pylori* and EBV, were discussed, with a focus on epigenetic alterations. Inadequate downregulation of tumor-suppressor genes because of aberrant epigenetic modifications can be used as a target for therapy. The primary DNA sequence remains intact and physiological gene expression could be recovered with adequate control. Furthermore, as the EBV genome is also regulated by epigenetic modifications, it might present an attractive target for antitumor activity. A better understanding of the molecular events in the development of various tumors is required to develop improved treatment strategies.

References

1. Abe H, Maeda D, Hino R, Otake Y, Isogai M, Ushiku AS, Matsusaka K, Kunita A, Ushiku T, Uozaki H, Tateishi Y, Hishima T, Iwasaki Y, Ishikawa S, Fukayama M (2012) ARID1A expression loss in gastric cancer: pathway-dependent roles with and without Epstein-Barr virus infection and microsatellite instability. Virchows Archiv 461(4):367–377. doi:10.1007/s00428-012-1303-2

2. Akhtar-Zaidi B, Cowper-Sal-lari R, Corradin O, Saiakhova A, Bartels CF, Balasubramanian D, Myeroff L, Lutterbaugh J, Jarrar A, Kalady MF, Willis J, Moore JH, Tesar PJ, Laframboise T, Markowitz S, Lupien M, Scacheri PC (2012) Epigenomic enhancer profiling defines a signature of colon cancer. Science 336(6082):736–739. doi:10.1126/science.1217277

3. Amieva MR, Vogelmann R, Covacci A, Tompkins LS, Nelson WJ, Falkow S (2003) Disruption of the epithelial apical-junctional complex by Helicobacter pylori CagA. Science 300(5624):1430–1434. doi:10.1126/science.1081919

4. Bernstein BE, Kamal M, Lindblad-Toh K, Bekiranov S, Bailey DK, Huebert DJ, McMahon S, Karlsson EK, Kulbokas EJ 3rd, Gingeras TR, Schreiber SL, Lander ES (2005) Genomic maps and comparative analysis of histone modifications in human and mouse. Cell 120(2):169–181. doi:10.1016/j.cell.2005.01.001

5. Bourzac KM, Guillemin K (2005) Helicobacter pylori-host cell interactions mediated by type IV secretion. Cell Microbiol 7(7):911–919. doi:10.1111/j.1462-5822.2005.00541.x

6. Burke AP, Yen TS, Shekitka KM, Sobin LH (1990) Lymphoepithelial carcinoma of the stomach with Epstein-Barr virus demonstrated by polymerase chain reaction. Mod Pathol 3(3):377–380

7. Camargo MC, Kim WH, Chiaravalli AM, Kim KM, Corvalan AH, Matsuo K, Yu J, Sung JJ, Herrera-Goepfert R, Meneses-Gonzalez F, Kijima Y, Natsugoe S, Liao LM, Lissowska J, Kim S, Hu N, Gonzalez CA, Yatabe Y, Koriyama C, Hewitt SM, Akiba S, Gulley ML, Taylor PR, Rabkin CS (2014) Improved survival of gastric cancer with tumour Epstein-Barr virus positivity: an international pooled analysis. Gut 63(2):236–243. doi:10.1136/gutjnl-2013-304531

8. Cappello M, Keshav S, Prince C, Jewell DP, Gordon S (1992) Detection of mRNAs for macrophage products in inflammatory bowel disease by in situ hybridisation. Gut 33(9):1214–1219

9. Chan AO, Chu KM, Huang C, Lam KF, Leung SY, Sun YW, Ko S, Xia HH, Cho CH, Hui WM, Lam SK, Rashid A (2007) Association between Helicobacter pylori infection and interleukin 1beta polymorphism predispose to CpG island methylation in gastric cancer. Gut 56(4):595–597. doi:10.1136/gut.2006.113258

10. Chang MS, Uozaki H, Chong JM, Ushiku T, Sakuma K, Ishikawa S, Hino R, Barua RR, Iwasaki Y, Arai K, Fujii H, Nagai H, Fukayama M (2006) CpG island methylation status in gastric carcinoma with and without infection of Epstein-Barr virus. Clin Cancer Res 12(10):2995–3002. doi:10.1158/1078-0432.CCR-05-1601

11. Craanen ME, Dekker W, Blok P, Ferwerda J, Tytgat GN (1992) Intestinal metaplasia and Helicobacter pylori: an endoscopic bioptic study of the gastric antrum. Gut 33(1):16–20

12. Dixon MF, Genta RM, Yardley JH, Correa P (1996) Classification and grading of gastritis. The updated Sydney System. International Workshop on the Histopathology of Gastritis, Houston 1994. Am J Surg Pathol 20(10):1161–1181

13. Duval A, Raphael M, Brennetot C, Poirel H, Buhard O, Aubry A, Martin A, Krimi A, Leblond V, Gabarre J, Davi F, Charlotte F, Berger F, Gaidano G, Capello D, Canioni D, Bordessoule D, Feuillard J, Gaulard P, Delfau MH, Ferlicot S, Eclache V, Prevot S, Guettier C, Lefevre PC, Adotti F, Hamelin R (2004) The mutator pathway is a feature of immunodeficiency-related lymphomas. Proc Natl Acad Sci U S A 101(14):5002–5007. doi:10.1073/pnas.0400945101

14. El-Omar EM, Carrington M, Chow WH, McColl KE, Bream JH, Young HA, Herrera J, Lissowska J, Yuan CC, Rothman N, Lanyon G, Martin M, Fraumeni JF Jr, Rabkin CS (2000) Interleukin-1 polymorphisms associated with increased risk of gastric cancer. Nature 404(6776):398–402. doi:10.1038/35006081

15. Epstein MA, Barr YM (1964) Cultivation in vitro of human lymphoblasts from Burkitt's malignant lymphoma. Lancet 1(7327):252–253

16. Fernandez AF, Rosales C, Lopez-Nieva P, Grana O, Ballestar E, Ropero S, Espada J, Melo SA, Lujambio A, Fraga MF, Pino I, Javierre B, Carmona FJ, Acquadro F, Steenbergen RD, Snijders PJ, Meijer CJ, Pineau P, Dejean A, Lloveras B, Capella G, Quer J, Buti M, Esteban JI, Allende H, Rodriguez-Frias F, Castellsague X, Minarovits J, Ponce J, Capello D, Gaidano G, Cigudosa JC, Gomez-Lopez G, Pisano DG, Valencia A, Piris MA, Bosch FX, Cahir-McFarland E, Kieff E, Esteller M (2009) The dynamic DNA methylomes of double-stranded DNA viruses associated with human cancer. Genome Res 19(3):438–451

17. Fukayama M, Ushiku T (2011) Epstein-Barr virus-associated gastric carcinoma. Pathol Res Pract 207(9):529–537. doi:10.1016/j.prp.2011.07.004

18. Fukayama M, Hayashi Y, Iwasaki Y, Chong J, Ooba T, Takizawa T, Koike M, Mizutani S, Miyaki M, Hirai K (1994) Epstein-Barr virus-associated gastric carcinoma and Epstein-Barr virus infection of the stomach. Lab Invest 71(1):73–81

19. Fukayama M, Hino R, Uozaki H (2008) Epstein-Barr virus and gastric carcinoma: virus-host interactions leading to carcinoma. Cancer Sci 99(9):1726–1733. doi:10.1111/j.1349-7006.2008.00888.x

20. He YF, Li BZ, Li Z, Liu P, Wang Y, Tang Q, Ding J, Jia Y, Chen Z, Li L, Sun Y, Li X, Dai Q, Song CX, Zhang K, He C, Xu GL (2011) Tet-mediated formation of 5-carboxylcytosine and its excision by TDG in mammalian DNA. Science 333(6047):1303–1307. doi:10.1126/science.1210944

21. Heintzman ND, Stuart RK, Hon G, Fu Y, Ching CW, Hawkins RD, Barrera LO, Van Calcar S, Qu C, Ching KA, Wang W, Weng Z, Green RD, Crawford GE, Ren B (2007) Distinct and predictive chromatin signatures of transcriptional promoters and enhancers in the human genome. Nat Genet 39(3):311–318. doi:10.1038/ng1966

22. Hino R, Uozaki H, Murakami N, Ushiku T, Shinozaki A, Ishikawa S, Morikawa T, Nakaya T, Sakatani T, Takada K, Fukayama M (2009) Activation of DNA methyltransferase 1 by EBV latent membrane protein 2A leads to promoter hypermethylation of PTEN gene in gastric carcinoma. Cancer Res 69(7):2766–2774

23. Hnisz D, Abraham BJ, Lee TI, Lau A, Saint-Andre V, Sigova AA, Hoke HA, Young RA (2013) Super-enhancers in the control of cell identity and disease. Cell 155(4):934–947. doi:10.1016/j.cell.2013.09.053

24. Huang FY, Chan AO, Lo RC, Rashid A, Wong DK, Cho CH, Lai CL, Yuen MF (2013) Characterization of interleukin-1beta in Helicobacter pylori-induced gastric inflammation and DNA methylation in interleukin-1 receptor type 1 knockout (IL-1R1(−/−)) mice. Eur J Cancer 49(12):2760–2770. doi:10.1016/j.ejca.2013.03.031

25. Imai S, Koizumi S, Sugiura M, Tokunaga M, Uemura Y, Yamamoto N, Tanaka S, Sato E, Osato T (1994) Gastric carcinoma: monoclonal epithelial malignant cells expressing Epstein-Barr virus latent infection protein. Proc Natl Acad Sci U S A 91(19):9131–9135

26. Imai S, Nishikawa J, Takada K (1998) Cell-to-cell contact as an efficient mode of Epstein-Barr virus infection of diverse human epithelial cells. J Virol 72(5):4371–4378

27. Ito S, Shen L, Dai Q, Wu SC, Collins LB, Swenberg JA, He C, Zhang Y (2011) Tet proteins can convert 5-methylcytosine to 5-formylcytosine and 5-carboxylcytosine. Science 333(6047):1300–1303. doi:10.1126/science.1210597

28. Iwakiri D, Eizuru Y, Tokunaga M, Takada K (2003) Autocrine growth of Epstein-Barr virus-positive gastric carcinoma cells mediated by an Epstein-Barr virus-encoded small RNA. Cancer Res 63(21):7062–7067

29. Iwakiri D, Sheen TS, Chen JY, Huang DP, Takada K (2005) Epstein-Barr virus-encoded small RNA induces insulin-like growth factor 1 and supports growth of nasopharyngeal carcinoma-derived cell lines. Oncogene 24(10):1767–1773. doi:10.1038/sj.onc.1208357

30. Japanese Gastric Cancer A (2011) Japanese classification of gastric carcinoma: 3rd English edition. Gastric Cancer 14(2):101–112. doi:10.1007/s10120-011-0041-5

31. Kaizaki Y, Sakurai S, Chong JM, Fukayama M (1999) Atrophic gastritis, Epstein-Barr virus infection, and Epstein-Barr virus-associated gastric carcinoma. Gastric Cancer 2(2):101–108. doi:10.1007/s101209900003

32. Kaneda A, Wakazono K, Tsukamoto T, Watanabe N, Yagi Y, Tatematsu M, Kaminishi M, Sugimura T, Ushijima T (2004) Lysyl oxidase is a tumor suppressor gene inactivated by methylation and loss of heterozygosity in human gastric cancers. Cancer Res 64(18):6410–6415. doi:10.1158/0008-5472.CAN-04-1543

33. Kaneda A, Matsusaka K, Aburatani H, Fukayama M (2012) Epstein-barr virus infection as an epigenetic driver of tumorigenesis. Cancer Res 72(14):3445–3450. doi:10.1158/0008-5472. CAN-11-3919

34. Kang GH, Lee S, Kim WH, Lee HW, Kim JC, Rhyu MG, Ro JY (2002) Epstein-Barr virus-positive gastric carcinoma demonstrates frequent aberrant methylation of multiple genes and constitutes CpG island methylator phenotype-positive gastric carcinoma. Am J Pathol 160(3):787–794. doi:10.1016/S0002-9440(10)64901-2

35. Kondo Y, Kanai Y, Sakamoto M, Mizokami M, Ueda R, Hirohashi S (2000) Genetic instability and aberrant DNA methylation in chronic hepatitis and cirrhosis--a comprehensive study of loss of heterozygosity and microsatellite instability at 39 loci and DNA hypermethylation on 8 CpG islands in microdissected specimens from patients with hepatocellular carcinoma. Hepatology 32(5):970–979. doi:10.1053/jhep.2000.19797

36. Kutok JL, Wang F (2006) Spectrum of Epstein-Barr virus-associated diseases. Annu Rev Pathol 1:375–404. doi:10.1146/annurev.pathol.1.110304.100209

37. Llorent L, Richaud-Patin Y, Alcocer-Castillejos N, Ruiz-Soto R, Mercado MA, Orozco H, Gamboa-Dominguez A, Alcocer-Varela J (1996) Cytokine gene expression in cirrhotic and non-cirrhotic human liver. J Hepatol 24(5):555–563

38. Loven J, Hoke HA, Lin CY, Lau A, Orlando DA, Vakoc CR, Bradner JE, Lee TI, Young RA (2013) Selective inhibition of tumor oncogenes by disruption of super-enhancers. Cell 153(2):320–334. doi:10.1016/j.cell.2013.03.036

39. Marshall BJ, Warren JR (1984) Unidentified curved bacilli in the stomach of patients with gastritis and peptic ulceration. Lancet 1(8390):1311–1315

40. Matsumoto Y, Marusawa H, Kinoshita K, Endo Y, Kou T, Morisawa T, Azuma T, Okazaki IM, Honjo T, Chiba T (2007) Helicobacter pylori infection triggers aberrant expression of activation-induced cytidine deaminase in gastric epithelium. Nat Med 13(4):470–476. doi:10.1038/nm1566

41. Matsusaka K, Funata S, Fukuyo M, Seto Y, Aburatani H, Fukayama M, Kaneda A (2017) Epstein-Barr virus infection induces genome-wide de novo DNA methylation in non-neoplastic gastric epithelial cells. J Pathol. doi:10.1002/path.4909

42. Matsusaka K, Kaneda A, Nagae G, Ushiku T, Kikuchi Y, Hino R, Uozaki H, Seto Y, Takada K, Aburatani H, Fukayama M (2011) Classification of Epstein-Barr virus-positive gastric cancers by definition of DNA methylation epigenotypes. Cancer Res 71(23):7187–7197. doi:10.1158/0008-5472.CAN-11-1349

43. McLaughlan JM, Seth R, Vautier G, Robins RA, Scott BB, Hawkey CJ, Jenkins D (1997) Interleukin-8 and inducible nitric oxide synthase mRNA levels in inflammatory bowel disease at first presentation. J Pathol 181(1):87–92. doi:10.1002/ (SICI)1096-9896(199701)181:1<87::AID-PATH736>3.0.CO;2-J

44. Mihm S, Fayyazi A, Ramadori G (1997) Hepatic expression of inducible nitric oxide synthase transcripts in chronic hepatitis C virus infection: relation to hepatic viral load and liver injury. Hepatology 26(2):451–458. doi:10.1002/hep.510260228

45. Muratani M, Deng N, Ooi WF, Lin SJ, Xing M, Xu C, Qamra A, Tay ST, Malik S, Wu J, Lee MH, Zhang S, Tan LL, Chua H, Wong WK, Ong HS, Ooi LL, Chow PK, Chan WH, Soo KC, Goh LK, Rozen S, Teh BT, Yu Q, Ng HH, Tan P (2014) Nanoscale chromatin profiling of gastric adenocarcinoma reveals cancer-associated cryptic promoters and somatically acquired regulatory elements. Nat Commun 5:4361. doi:10.1038/ncomms5361

46. Murphy G, Pfeiffer R, Camargo MC, Rabkin CS (2009) Meta-analysis shows that prevalence of Epstein-Barr virus-positive gastric cancer differs based on sex and anatomic location. Gastroenterology 137(3):824–833. doi:10.1053/j.gastro.2009.05.001

47. Nakajima T, Enomoto S, Yamashita S, Ando T, Nakanishi Y, Nakazawa K, Oda I, Gotoda T, Ushijima T (2010) Persistence of a component of DNA methylation in gastric mucosae after Helicobacter pylori eradication. J Gastroenterol 45(1):37–44. doi:10.1007/s00535-009-0142-7

48. Nalesnik MA, Jaffe R, Starzl TE, Demetris AJ, Porter K, Burnham JA, Makowka L, Ho M, Locker J (1988) The pathology of posttransplant lymphoproliferative disorders occurring in the setting of cyclosporine A-prednisone immunosuppression. Am J Pathol 133(1):173–192

49. Namba-Fukuyo H, Funata S, Matsusaka K, Fukuyo M, Rahmutulla B, Mano Y, Fukayama M, Aburatani H, Kaneda A (2016) TET2 functions as a resistance factor against DNA methylation acquisition during Epstein-Barr virus infection. Oncotarget. doi:10.18632/oncotarget.13130

50. Niedobitek G, Agathanggelou A, Steven N, Young LS (2000) Epstein-Barr virus (EBV) in infectious mononucleosis: detection of the virus in tonsillar B lymphocytes but not in desquamated oropharyngeal epithelial cells. Mol Pathol 53(1):37–42

51. Niwa T, Tsukamoto T, Toyoda T, Mori A, Tanaka H, Maekita T, Ichinose M, Tatematsu M, Ushijima T (2010) Inflammatory processes triggered by Helicobacter pylori infection cause aberrant DNA methylation in gastric epithelial cells. Cancer Res 70(4):1430–1440. doi:10.1158/0008-5472.CAN-09-2755

52. Niwa T, Toyoda T, Tsukamoto T, Mori A, Tatematsu M, Ushijima T (2013) Prevention of Helicobacter pylori-induced gastric cancers in gerbils by a DNA demethylating agent. Cancer Prev Res (Phila) 6(4):263–270. doi:10.1158/1940-6207.CAPR-12-0369

53. Nomura A, Stemmermann GN, Chyou PH, Kato I, Perez-Perez GI, Blaser MJ (1991) Helicobacter pylori infection and gastric carcinoma among Japanese Americans in Hawaii. N Engl J Med 325(16):1132–1136. doi:10.1056/NEJM199110173251604

54. Ohm JE, McGarvey KM, Yu X, Cheng L, Schuebel KE, Cope L, Mohammad HP, Chen W, Daniel VC, Yu W, Berman DM, Jenuwein T, Pruitt K, Sharkis SJ, Watkins DN, Herman JG, Baylin SB (2007) A stem cell-like chromatin pattern may predispose tumor suppressor genes to DNA hypermethylation and heritable silencing. Nat Genet 39(2):237–242. doi:10.1038/ng1972

55. Ohnishi N, Yuasa H, Tanaka S, Sawa H, Miura M, Matsui A, Higashi H, Musashi M, Iwabuchi K, Suzuki M, Yamada G, Azuma T, Hatakeyama M (2008) Transgenic expression of Helicobacter pylori CagA induces gastrointestinal and hematopoietic neoplasms in mouse. Proc Natl Acad Sci U S A 105(3):1003–1008

56. Ooi WF, Xing M, Xu C, Yao X, Ramlee MK, Lim MC, Cao F, Lim K, Babu D, Poon LF, Lin Suling J, Qamra A, Irwanto A, Qu Zhengzhong J, Nandi T, Lee-Lim AP, Chan YS, Tay ST, Lee MH, Davies JO, Wong WK, Soo KC, Chan WH, Ong HS, Chow P, Wong CY, Rha SY, Liu J, Hillmer AM, Hughes JR, Rozen S, Teh BT, Fullwood MJ, Li S, Tan P (2016) Epigenomic profiling of primary gastric adenocarcinoma reveals super-enhancer heterogeneity. Nat Commun 7:12983. doi:10.1038/ncomms12983

57. Parsonnet J, Friedman GD, Vandersteen DP, Chang Y, Vogelman JH, Orentreich N, Sibley RK (1991) Helicobacter pylori infection and the risk of gastric carcinoma. N Engl J Med 325(16):1127–1131. doi:10.1056/NEJM199110173251603

58. Rugge M, Cassaro M, Leandro G, Baffa R, Avellini C, Bufo P, Stracca V, Battaglia G, Fabiano A, Guerini A, Di Mario F (1996) Helicobacter pylori in promotion of gastric carcinogenesis. Dig Dis Sci 41(5):950–955

59. Saito A, Shimoda T, Nakanishi Y, Ochiai A, Toda G (2001) Histologic heterogeneity and mucin phenotypic expression in early gastric cancer. Pathol Int 51(3):165–171

60. Saju P, Murata-Kamiya N, Hayashi T, Senda Y, Nagase L, Noda S, Matsusaka K, Funata S, Kunita A, Urabe M, Seto Y, Fukayama M, Kaneda A, Hatakeyama M (2016) Host SHP1 phosphatase antagonizes Helicobacter pylori CagA and can be downregulated by Epstein-Barr virus. Nat Microbiol 1:16026. doi:10.1038/nmicrobiol.2016.26

61. Schlesinger Y, Straussman R, Keshet I, Farkash S, Hecht M, Zimmerman J, Eden E, Yakhini Z, Ben-Shushan E, Reubinoff BE, Bergman Y, Simon I, Cedar H (2007) Polycomb-mediated methylation on Lys27 of histone H3 pre-marks genes for de novo methylation in cancer. Nat Genet 39(2):232–236. doi:10.1038/ng1950

62. Segal ED, Cha J, Lo J, Falkow S, Tompkins LS (1999) Altered states: involvement of phosphorylated CagA in the induction of host cellular growth changes by Helicobacter pylori. Proc Natl Acad Sci U S A 96(25):14559–14564
63. Shibata D, Weiss LM, Hernandez AM, Nathwani BN, Bernstein L, Levine AM (1993) Epstein-Barr virus-associated non-Hodgkin's lymphoma in patients infected with the human immuno-deficiency virus. Blood 81(8):2102–2109
64. Shinozaki-Ushiku A, Kunita A, Fukayama M (2015) Update on Epstein-Barr virus and gastric cancer (review). Int J Oncol 46(4):1421–1434. doi:10.3892/ijo.2015.2856
65. Siegel RL, Miller KD, Jemal A (2016) Cancer statistics, 2016. CA Cancer J Clin 66(1):7–30. doi:10.3322/caac.21332
66. Suzuki M, Mimuro H, Kiga K, Fukumatsu M, Ishijima N, Morikawa H, Nagai S, Koyasu S, Gilman RH, Kersulyte D, Berg DE, Sasakawa C (2009) Helicobacter pylori CagA phosphorylation-independent function in epithelial proliferation and inflammation. Cell Host Microbe 5(1):23–34. doi:10.1016/j.chom.2008.11.010
67. Tokunaga M, Land CE, Uemura Y, Tokudome T, Tanaka S, Sato E (1993) Epstein-Barr virus in gastric carcinoma. Am J Pathol 143(5):1250–1254
68. Tretyakova NY, Burney S, Pamir B, Wishnok JS, Dedon PC, Wogan GN, Tannenbaum SR (2000) Peroxynitrite-induced DNA damage in the supF gene: correlation with the mutational spectrum. Mutat Res 447(2):287–303
69. Tsai CN, Tsai CL, Tse KP, Chang HY, Chang YS (2002) The Epstein-Barr virus oncogene product, latent membrane protein 1, induces the downregulation of E-cadherin gene expression via activation of DNA methyltransferases. Proc Natl Acad Sci U S A 99(15):10084–10089
70. Tsai CL, Li HP, Lu YJ, Hsueh C, Liang Y, Chen CL, Tsao SW, Tse KP, Yu JS, Chang YS (2006) Activation of DNA methyltransferase 1 by EBV LMP1 Involves c-Jun NH(2)-terminal kinase signaling. Cancer Res 66(24):11668–11676
71. Uemura N, Okamoto S, Yamamoto S, Matsumura N, Yamaguchi S, Yamakido M, Taniyama K, Sasaki N, Schlemper RJ (2001) Helicobacter pylori infection and the development of gastric cancer. N Engl J Med 345(11):784–789. doi:10.1056/NEJMoa001999
72. Uozaki H, Fukayama M (2008) Epstein-Barr virus and gastric carcinoma--viral carcinogenesis through epigenetic mechanisms. Int J Clin Exp Pathol 1(3):198–216
73. Ushijima T, Nakajima T, Maekita T (2006) DNA methylation as a marker for the past and future. J Gastroenterol 41(5):401–407. doi:10.1007/s00535-006-1846-6
74. Ushiku T, Chong JM, Uozaki H, Hino R, Chang MS, Sudo M, Rani BR, Sakuma K, Nagai H, Fukayama M (2007) p73 gene promoter methylation in Epstein-Barr virus-associated gastric carcinoma. Int J Cancer 120(1):60–66
75. Wang K, Kan J, Yuen ST, Shi ST, Chu KM, Law S, Chan TL, Kan Z, Chan AS, Tsui WY, Lee SP, Ho SL, Chan AK, Cheng GH, Roberts PC, Rejto PA, Gibson NW, Pocalyko DJ, Mao M, Xu J, Leung SY (2011) Exome sequencing identifies frequent mutation of ARID1A in molecular subtypes of gastric cancer. Nat Genet 43(12):1219–1223. doi:10.1038/ng.982
76. Watanabe H, Enjoji M, Imai T (1976) Gastric carcinoma with lymphoid stroma. Its morphologic characteristics and prognostic correlations. Cancer 38(1):232–243
77. Widschwendter M, Fiegl H, Egle D, Mueller-Holzner E, Spizzo G, Marth C, Weisenberger DJ, Campan M, Young J, Jacobs I, Laird PW (2007) Epigenetic stem cell signature in cancer. Nat Genet 39(2):157–158. doi:10.1038/ng1941
78. Wu Y, Maruo S, Yajima M, Kanda T, Takada K (2007) Epstein-Barr virus (EBV)-encoded RNA 2 (EBER2) but not EBER1 plays a critical role in EBV-induced B-cell growth transformation. J Virol 81(20):11236–11245. doi:10.1128/JVI.00579-07
79. Yajima M, Kanda T, Takada K (2005) Critical role of Epstein-Barr Virus (EBV)-encoded RNA in efficient EBV-induced B-lymphocyte growth transformation. J Virol 79(7):4298–4307. doi:10.1128/JVI.79.7.4298-4307.2005
80. Yoshiyama H, Imai S, Shimizu N, Takada K (1997) Epstein-Barr virus infection of human gastric carcinoma cells: implication of the existence of a new virus receptor different from CD21. J Virol 71(7):5688–5691

81. Young LS, Rickinson AB (2004) Epstein-Barr virus: 40 years on. Nat Rev Cancer 4(10):757–768. doi:10.1038/nrc1452
82. Zang ZJ, Cutcutache I, Poon SL, Zhang SL, McPherson JR, Tao J, Rajasegaran V, Heng HL, Deng N, Gan A, Lim KH, Ong CK, Huang D, Chin SY, Tan IB, Ng CC, Yu W, Wu Y, Lee M, Wu J, Poh D, Wan WK, Rha SY, So J, Salto-Tellez M, Yeoh KG, Wong WK, Zhu YJ, Futreal PA, Pang B, Ruan Y, Hillmer AM, Bertrand D, Nagarajan N, Rozen S, Teh BT, Tan P (2012) Exome sequencing of gastric adenocarcinoma identifies recurrent somatic mutations in cell adhesion and chromatin remodeling genes. Nat Genet 44(5):570–574. doi:10.1038/ng.2246
83. Zhang JA, Mortazavi A, Williams BA, Wold BJ, Rothenberg EV (2012) Dynamic transformations of genome-wide epigenetic marking and transcriptional control establish T cell identity. Cell 149(2):467–482. doi:10.1016/j.cell.2012.01.056
84. zur Hausen H, Schulte-Holthausen H, Klein G, Henle W, Henle G, Clifford P, Santesson L (1970) EBV DNA in biopsies of Burkitt tumours and anaplastic carcinomas of the nasopharynx. Nature 228(5276):1056–1058

DNA and Histone Methylation in Hematopoietic Malignancy

Biology of Epigenetic Regulators in Hematological Malignancies as Basis of Therapeutic Targets

Kimihito Cojin Kawabata and Toshio Kitamura

Abstract Recent advances in next-generation sequencing technologies have revealed frequent somatic mutations in hematological malignancies. As the epigenetic landscapes of hematological malignancies are unveiled, epigenetic regulatory processes have become therapeutic targets. After the success of hypomethylating agents, azacitidine and decitabine for myelodysplastic syndrome (both FDA-approved), inhibitors of other epigenetic regulators have become candidate agents for next-generation therapy against refractory hematological malignancies. In addition to tyrosine kinase inhibitors and immunotherapeutic agents, inhibitors of epigenetic regulators have been used either in a salvage monotherapy regimen or in combination therapy with conventional chemotherapy. In this chapter, alterations in DNA cytosine methylation and histone methylation as targets of therapeutics for hematological malignancies are discussed with outlines of clinical trials.

Keywords DNA cytosine methylation • Post-translational histone modifications • Epigenetic writers/erasers/readers

K.C. Kawabata (✉)
Division of Hematology-Medical Oncology, Department of Medicine, Weill-Cornell Medicine, Cornell University, 413E 69th Street, New York, NY 10065, USA

Division of Cellular Therapy, Institute of Medical Science, The University of Tokyo, 4-6-1, Shirokanedai, Minato-city, Tokyo 1088639, Japan
e-mail: kkawabata-tky@umin.net

T. Kitamura
Division of Cellular Therapy, Institute of Medical Science, The University of Tokyo, 4-6-1, Shirokanedai, Minato-city, Tokyo 1088639, Japan

© Springer International Publishing AG 2017
A. Kaneda, Y.-i. Tsukada (eds.), *DNA and Histone Methylation as Cancer Targets*, Cancer Drug Discovery and Development, DOI 10.1007/978-3-319-59786-7_14

1 Epigenetic Regulators in Hematopoietic Malignancies

While the word epigenetics generally represents all the mechanisms that regulate the expression of genes without changes in DNA sequences or the inheritable phenotypes as a result of those mechanisms [1], the epigenetic biological processes include non-coding RNA, RNA splicing, as well as chemical modifications of DNA or histone. Among those epigenetic processes, DNA methylation and histone methylation are the most profoundly investigated in detail. In hematological malignancy, epigenetic regulators have been identified as novel classes of somatic mutations in myeloid malignancies [2]. Studies on epigenetics in hematological malignancies began with the next-generation whole exome and whole genome sequencing of large acute myeloid leukemia (AML) cohorts [3–5]. These findings were followed by sequencing of other myeloid tumors, including myeloproliferative neoplasm (NPM), MDS, and myelofibrosis (MF) [6–8]. Moreover, T-cell acute lymphoblastic leukemia (T-ALL) was found to be associated with somatic mutations in genes encoding epigenetic regulators [9, 10]. As shown in Tables 1 and 2, both myeloid malignancies and T-ALL harbor mutations in

Table 1 Somatic mutations in genes encoding epigenetic molecules observed in myeloid malignancies

Genes	Frequency in diseases
DNMT3A	AML; 26%
	MDS; 5–10%
ASXL1	AML; 17–19%
TET2	AML; 8–27%
IDH1	AML; 8–9%
	MDS; 6%
IDH2	AML; 8–9%
	MDS; 9%
MLL-PTD	AML; 5%
MLL-fusion	AML; 5%
EZII2	AML; 2%
	EZH2; 5%
PHF6	AML; 3%
SF3B1	MDS; 20%, MDS-RS; 65%
U2AF1	MDS; 7%
SRSF2	MDS; 12%
ZRSR2	MDS; 3%

Based on the data introduced in Refs. [2, 4, 6, 8], frequently observed somatic mutations are listed with their frequency in myeloid malignancies. Abbreviations of genes or mutational status not mentioned in the paragraphs are as follows; MLL-PTD MLL-partial tandem duplication, PHF6 plant homeodomain finger 6, SF3B1, U2AF1 U2-associated factor 1, SRSF2 serine and arginine rich splicing factor 2, ZRSR2 zinc finger CCCH-type, RNA binding motif and serine/arginine rich 2

Table 2 Somatic mutations in genes encoding epigenetic molecules observed in T-ALL

Genes	Frequency in diseases
PHF6	16–38%
DNMT3A	4–18%
TET1	6–14%
IDH1	2–6%
IDH2	5–9%
EZH2	11–18%
SUZ12	6–11%
EED	10%
UTX	5%
JMJD3	NA
MLL1	5%
MLL2	ETP-all; 10%
DOT1L	10%
SETD2	ETP-all; 8%
EP300	2%
NCOA2	NA
HDAC5	1%
HDAC7	4%
USP7	8%

Based on the data introduced in Refs. [9, 10], frequently observed somatic mutations are listed with their frequency in T-ALL. EED Embryonic Ectoderm Development, UTX Ubiquitously transcribed tetratricopeptide repeat, X chromosome, SETD2 SET Domain Containing 2, EP300 E1A Binding Protein P300, NCOA2 Nuclear Receptor Coactivator 2, USP7 Ubiquitin Specific Peptidase 7

various epigenetic factors. In this chapter, epigenetic regulators as targets of novel therapies for hematological malignancies are reviewed together with considerations of their functions (Table 3).

2 DNA Methylation as a Therapeutic Target

In myeloid malignancies, DNA-methyltransferase 3A (DNMT3A) is mutated in 26% of AML cases and 5–10% of MDS [3, 8, 11, 12]. Its major role is cytosine methylation of DNA (5-methyl-cytosine (5mC)), and it is required for the self-renewal of normal hematopoietic stem cells [3, 13]. In malignancy, the loss of DNMTs is associated with global loss of 5mC and epigenetic instability [14, 15]. In general, attenuation of the functions of DNMT3A is thought to be caused by truncation or missense point mutation occurring at R882. In T-ALL, DNMT3A mutations

Table 3 Inhibitors for epigenetic regulators in clinical use

Molecules	Inhibitors (clinical studies for hematological malignancies)
DNMT3A	Azacitidine (approved), Decitabine (approved), SGI-110 (NCT02935361)
IDH1/2	AG-221 (NCT01915498, NCT02632708, NCT02677922, NCT02577406), IDH305 (NCT02826642, NCT02381886), AG120 (NCT02632708, NCT02677922), AG881 (NCT02492737, NCT02481154)
EZH2	EPZ-6438 (NCT01897571), CPI-1205 (NCT02395601), GSK2816126 (NCT02082977), MAK683 (NCT02900651)
JMJD3	GSKJ4
MLL-fusion (DOT1L)	EPZ004777, EPZ-5676 (NCT02141828)
HDAC	Vorinostat (FDA approved), Romidepsin (FDA approved), Panobinostat (NCT00967044)
BET	FT-1101 (NCT02543879), CPI-0610 (NCT01949883), MK-8628 (NCT02698189)

Inhibitors of epigenetic regulators either in regular clinical use or in clinical trial are listed. ClinicalTrials.gov numbers are added in parentheses

are present in up to 18% of patients. In these T-ALL patients, R882 is also mutated and inactivation of DNMT3A has been predicted [9, 14–17]. Overexpression or truncated form mutant proteins of DNMT3B are detected in adult T-ALL cases [18]. While DNMT3A and DNMT3B, which are 'writers' of cytosine DNA methylation, are mutated in hematological malignancies, 'erasers' are also mutated. The erasers include tet methylcytosine dioxygenase 1 and 2 (TET1 and TET2) or isocitrate dehydrogenase 1 and 2 (IDH1 and IDH2). TET2 mutations are observed in approximately 20% of AML and MDS patients, respectively. IDH1 mutations are observed in 6% of MDS patients and 8–9% of AML patients, whereas IDH2 mutations affect 9% of MDS patients and 8–9% of AML patients [3, 8, 19–25]. In T-ALL patients, TET1 mutations are present in 6–14% of the patients, and IDH1 and IDH2 are observed in 2–6%, and 5–9 of patients, respectively [17, 19, 20, 26, 27]. The gene products of both groups function to decrease 5mC DNA. The initiation of 5mC reduction begins with the oxidation of 5mC, yielding 5-hydroxymethyl-cytosine (5hmC). TET1 and TET2 are enzymes with hydroxylmethyltransferase activity. 5hmC is an intermediate product that is converted into unmethylated cytosine. The initial processes mediated by TET1/2 depend on the existence of oxygen, iron, and α-ketoglutarate (α-KG) [3, 5, 8, 28–31]. For the production of α-KG, isocitrate is subjected to oxidative decarboxylation. Homodimeric enzymes encoded by *IDH1* or *IDH2* normally catalyze this reaction. Mutations found in AML occur in gain-of-function manners. IDH1 mutations occur at arginine R132 (predominantly R132H), whereas IDH2 mutations occur at homologous arginine R172 (predominantly R172K) and arginine R140 (R140Q). These mutations are mutually exclusive in AML clinical samples [2, 4, 32]. Mutant IDH1/2 lead to a neomorphic enzymatic reaction to produce 2-hydroxyglutarate (2-HG) from isocitrate. Consequently, IDH1/2 mutations inhibit TET1/2-mediated oxidation of 5mC. Mutations in genes encoding writers of DNA cytosine methylation are associated with genome-wide alterations in cytosine methylation status [32–34]. The epigenetic landscapes cluster AML into 16 distinct subgroups based on methylome analysis [32, 35]. Epigenetic landscapes may function as clinical biomarkers to predict the prognosis or drug sensitivity of novel AML cases [32].

In T-ALL, inactivating mutations of TET1, IDH1, and IDH2 have been documented [17, 26, 27, 36, 37]. Their prognostic significance requires further investigation. IDH1/2 mutations are observed exclusively in adult T-ALL cases, as well as DNMT3A [9].

In the age of molecular targeting therapy and ongoing studies to determine the significance of epigenetic alterations in various types of cancer, epigenetic molecules have been targeted for AML treatment [2, 3, 28]. Among them, DNA-hypomethylating agents (HMA) were one of the earliest agents employed for clinical use [30]. Based on studies of decitabine and azacitidine *in vitro* and *in vivo* [38–42], clinical trials targeting MDS or MDS/AML cases that are not indicated for hematopoietic stem cell transplantations were conducted to compare their benefits to those of conventional chemotherapy (CCR). Several multicenter randomized studies were conducted, including trials of D-007, AZA-001, CALGB-9221, and EORTC-06011. Data from these trials revealed improvement in progression-free-survival ranging from 3 to 8 months. Currently, decitabine, azacitidine and lenalidmide are FDA-approved drugs for MDS [43]. Until late 2016, there were more than 20 clinical studies using HMAs (NCT01595295, NCT02863458, NCT02721875). In a meta-analysis including five randomized clinical trials using HMA for myeloid malignancies, significant benefits in overall survival were observed only in the azacitidine, but not decitabine group [30]. Further studies are needed to evaluate the use of HMAs depending on clinical profiles, timings, and doses. Additionally, guadecitabine (SGI-110), a second-generation HMA, is in a phase I/II clinical trial (NCT02935361) [44–51].

Mutant IDH1/2 inhibitors are also in phase I/II clinical trials. AG-221 is an inhibitor of IDH2 and the first IDH inhibitor to be evaluated in clinical trials (NCT01915498, NCT02632708, NCT02677922, NCT02577406). In late 2016, interim reports of phase I/II trials became available. The interim report revealed striking effects, including a 45% overall response rate (OR rate) for refractory/relapsed AML [52, 53]. For mutant IDH1, AG120 and IDH305 are specific inhibitors used in clinical trials (NCT02632708, NCT02826642, NCT02381886). The results of these interim reports are comparable to those of IDH2 inhibitors [53]. An IDH1/2 dual inhibitor currently being examined in clinical trials is AG881 (NCT02492737, NCT02481154).

3   Histone Methylation as a Therapeutic Target

Octamers of histone proteins (two copies of H2A, H2B, H3, and H4) are subjected to post-translational modifications (PTMs). The PTMs of histone proteins include acetylation, methylation, phosphorylation, and ubiquitination [29, 31, 54]. The chromatin codes composed of those PTMs appear to contribute to the accessibility of the transcriptional machinery to chromatin, resulting in the regulation of gene expression. Enzymes catalyzing this process mediate each of the modifications. These enzymes are known as epigenetic writers, whereas those that eliminate the modifications are known as epigenetic erasers. Proteins to recognize PTMs and contribute to the regulation of transcription, DNA replication, DNA repair are referred to as epigenetic readers. [31, 54].

Histone H3 lysin 27 (H3K27) methylation is catalyzed by Polycomb repressive comprex 2 (PRC2). EZH2 is a catalytic subunit of the PRC2 complex. Trimethylation of H3K27 is referred to as a suppressive histone mark, as it is associated with decreased expression of genes [3, 4, 55]. Mutations in EZH2 are rare in AML (1–2%), but occur in 5% of MDS or MPN cases [8]. While EZH2 mutations occur mostly as loss-of-function mutations in myeloid malignancies, activation of EZH2 has been observed in B cell non-Hodgkin lymphoma (B-NHL) [7, 56, 57]. Therefore, inhibitors of EZH2 began to be used clinically for B-NHL in advance. In late 2016, various selective EZH2-inhibitors, including EPZ-6438 (NCT01897571) and GSK126 (NCT02082977), were evaluated in clinical trials [58]. However, in myeloid malignancies, some experimental data has shown that inhibition of EZH2 can antagonize tumor progression [4]. Although mutations in EZH2 and other PRC2 components (EED, SUZ12, RBAP48) occur less frequently in myeloid malignancies, mutations in ASXL1, occurring in 15–20% of myeloid malignancies, result in inactivation or truncation of ASXL protein and suppress the function of PRC2 [59, 60]. Therefore, to use EZH1/2 inhibitors against AML, careful selection of indicated cases based on biological markers is required. To date, it was reported that in germinal center (GC) B cells, EZH2 and BCL6, a transcriptional repressor cooperate to stabilize non-canonical polycomb repressor complex (PRC)1 including CBX8-BOCR. Those mechanisms are also associated with tumorigenesis of B-NHL [61]. Moreover, inhibitions of BCL6 in B-NHL have been reported in many articles [62–65].

While methylation of H3K27 catalyzed by EZH2 is a suppressive histone mark, methylation of H3K4 is an active histone mark. Mixed-lineage leukemia 1 (MLL1) is a histone methylansferase that catalyzes H3K4 methylation. In AML, translocations involving MLL or partial tandem duplication are observed in 5% of patients [3, 28, 31]. In T-ALL, MLL1 alterations are observed in 5% of patients, while mutations in MLL2 are observed in 10% of early T-cell precursor (ETP) ALL [9, 66–68]. In AML, MLL1 is involved in translocation with multiple fusion partners, including AF4, AF9, AF10, and ENL. In MLL-fusion proteins, the H3K4 methyltransferase domain is absent. However, a complex including DOT1L, an H3K79 methyltransferase, binds to MLL-fusion proteins. In MLL-induced leukemia, DOT1L is required for leukemogenesis [69–71]. Inhibitors of DOT1L showed anti-leukemic effects in mouse xenograft models using MLL-fusion AML cells [70, 72, 73]. In a clinical study of EPZ-5676, high OR rate and acceptable safety were reported (NCT02141828).

Histone demethylase, erasers of epigenetic processes, are also targets of leukemia treatments. Jumonji C (JmjC) domain-containing proteins, JMJD3 and UTX, are demethylases for H3K27 methylation [74, 75]. The use of inhibitors for these demethylases is justified by mutations in the PRC2 complex or ASXL1 in hematological malignancies. Lysine-specific demethylase (LSD1) was found to be overexpressed in multiple types of tumors, including hematological malignancies. LSD1 promotes demethylation of H3K4 and H3K9 [76–80]. The roles of LSD1 in leukemogenesis have been determined in various contexts, including MLL-fusion leukemia. Additionally, pro-differentiational effects of LSD1 inhibition were suggested in experiments using all-trans retinoic acid(ATRA) [76]. Currently, phase I clinical studies of LSD1 inhibitors are ongoing. Tranylcypromine (NCT02261779) and GSK2879552 (NCT02177812) are used against AML.

4 Future Perspectives

Novel therapeutic strategies for targeting epigenetic regulators will expand as further additional knowledge on epigenetics of hematological malignancy is accumulated [33, 35, 81, 82]. Not only for DNA cytosine or histone methylation, but inhibitors of histone deacetylase (HDAC), bromodomain, and extraterminal-family (BET) proteins recognizing acetyl-lysine have also been proposed as novel therapeutic agents for hematological malignancies [3, 31]. While HDAC is an eraser of the acetylated histone, BET proteins are epigenetic reader, as they recognize acetylated histone. Histone acetylation is associated with chromatin structure and determines accessibility of DNA, regulating transcriptions. As shown in Table 3, inhibitors for these targets are in clinical trials. JQ-1 and I-BET762 (GSK525762) are the earliest BET inhibitors that went on the clinical trials [83]. Thus using the integrated information for the inhibitors reviewed in this chapter, either from research or clinical fields, combination therapy using conventional chemotherapy and inhibitors for epigenetic regulators have been considered. Next-generation therapeutics against hematological malignancies will be developed.

References

1. Feinberg AP, Tycko B (2004) The history of cancer epigenetics. Nat Rev Cancer 4(2):143–153
2. Shih AH, Abdel-Wahab O, Patel JP, Levine RL (2012) The role of mutations in epigenetic regulators in myeloid malignancies. Nat Rev Cancer 12(9):599–612
3. Coombs CC, Tallman MS, Levine RL (2016) Molecular therapy for acute myeloid leukaemia. Nat Rev Clin Oncol 13(5):305–318
4. Pastore F, Levine RL (2016) Epigenetic regulators and their impact on therapy in acute myeloid leukemia. Haematologica 101(3):269–278
5. Kitamura T, Inoue D, Okochi-Watanabe N, Kato N, Komeno Y, Lu Y et al (2014) The molecular basis of myeloid malignancies. Proc Jpn Acad Ser B Phys Biol Sci 90(10):389–404
6. Bejar R, Stevenson K, Abdel-Wahab O, Galili N, Nilsson B, Garcia-Manero G et al (2011) Clinical effect of point mutations in myelodysplastic syndromes. N Engl J Med 364(26):2496–2506

7. Nikoloski G, Langemeijer SM, Kuiper RP, Knops R, Massop M, Tonnissen ER et al (2010) Somatic mutations of the histone methyltransferase gene EZH2 in myelodysplastic syndromes. Nat Genet 42(8):665–667

8. Raza A, Galili N (2012) The genetic basis of phenotypic heterogeneity in myelodysplastic syndromes. Nat Rev Cancer 12(12):849–859

9. Peirs S, Van der Meulen J, Van de Walle I, Taghon T, Speleman F, Poppe B et al (2015) Epigenetics in T-cell acute lymphoblastic leukemia. Immunol Rev 263(1):50–67

10. You MJ, Medeiros LJ, Hsi ED (2015) T-lymphoblastic leukemia/lymphoma. Am J Clin Pathol 144(3):411–422

11. Walter MJ, Ding L, Shen D, Shao J, Grillot M, McLellan M et al (2011) Recurrent DNMT3A mutations in patients with myelodysplastic syndromes. Leukemia 25(7):1153–1158

12. Ewalt M, Galili NG, Mumtaz M, Churchill M, Rivera S, Borot F et al (2011) DNMT3a mutations in high-risk myelodysplastic syndrome parallel those found in acute myeloid leukemia. Blood Cancer J 1(3):e9

13. Tadokoro Y, Ema H, Okano M, Li E, Nakauchi H (2007) De novo DNA methyltransferase is essential for self-renewal, but not for differentiation, in hematopoietic stem cells. J Exp Med 204(4):715–722

14. Illingworth RS, Bird AP (2009) CpG islands—'a rough guide'. FEBS Lett 583(11):1713–1720

15. Bird AP (1986) CpG-rich islands and the function of DNA methylation. Nature 321(6067):209–213

16. Grossmann V, Haferlach C, Weissmann S, Roller A, Schindela S, Poetzinger F et al (2013) The molecular profile of adult T-cell acute lymphoblastic leukemia: mutations in RUNX1 and DNMT3A are associated with poor prognosis in T-ALL. Genes Chromosomes Cancer 52(4):410–422

17. Van Vlierberghe P, Ambesi-Impiombato A, Perez-Garcia A, Haydu JE, Rigo I, Hadler M et al (2011) ETV6 mutations in early immature human T cell leukemias. J Exp Med 208(13):2571–2579

18. Ostler KR, Davis EM, Payne SL, Gosalia BB, Exposito-Cespedes J, Le Beau MM et al (2007) Cancer cells express aberrant DNMT3B transcripts encoding truncated proteins. Oncogene 26(38):5553–5563

19. Rhyasen GW, Starczynowski DT (2012) Deregulation of microRNAs in myelodysplastic syndrome. Leukemia 26(1):13–22

20. Raaijmakers MH, Mukherjee S, Guo S, Zhang S, Kobayashi T, Schoonmaker JA et al (2010) Bone progenitor dysfunction induces myelodysplasia and secondary leukaemia. Nature 464(7290):852–857

21. Cancer Genome Atlas Research Network, Ley TJ, Miller C, Ding L, Raphael BJ et al (2013) Genomic and epigenomic landscapes of adult de novo acute myeloid leukemia. N Engl J Med 368(22):2059–2074

22. Mardis ER, Ding L, Dooling DJ, Larson DE, McLellan MD, Chen K et al (2009) Recurring mutations found by sequencing an acute myeloid leukemia genome. N Engl J Med 361(11):1058–1066

23. Yamaguchi S, Iwanaga E, Tokunaga K, Nanri T, Shimomura T, Suzushima H et al (2014) IDH1 and IDH2 mutations confer an adverse effect in patients with acute myeloid leukemia lacking the NPM1 mutation. Eur J Haematol 92(6):471–477

24. Weissmann S, Alpermann T, Grossmann V, Kowarsch A, Nadarajah N, Eder C et al (2012) Landscape of TET2 mutations in acute myeloid leukemia. Leukemia 26(5):934–942

25. Ganguly BB, Kadam NN (2016) Mutations of myelodysplastic syndromes (MDS): an update. Mutat Res Rev Mutat Res 769:47–62

26. Sasaki M, Knobbe CB, Munger JC, Lind EF, Brenner D, Brustle A et al (2012) IDH1(R132H) mutation increases murine haematopoietic progenitors and alters epigenetics. Nature 488(7413):656–659

27. Simon C, Chagraoui J, Krosl J, Gendron P, Wilhelm B, Lemieux S et al (2012) A key role for EZH2 and associated genes in mouse and human adult T-cell acute leukemia. Genes Dev 26(7):651–656

28. Abdel-Wahab O, Patel J, Levine RL (2011) Clinical implications of novel mutations in epigenetic modifiers in AML. Hematol Oncol Clin North Am 25(6):1119–1133
29. Fong CY, Morison J, Dawson MA (2014) Epigenetics in the hematologic malignancies. Haematologica 99(12):1772–1783
30. Yun S, Vincelette ND, Abraham I, Robertson KD, Fernandez-Zapico ME, Patnaik MM (2016) Targeting epigenetic pathways in acute myeloid leukemia and myelodysplastic syndrome: a systematic review of hypomethylating agents trials. Clin Epigenetics 8:68
31. Gallipoli P, Giotopoulos G, Huntly BJ (2015) Epigenetic regulators as promising therapeutic targets in acute myeloid leukemia. Ther Adv Hematol 6(3):103–119
32. Li S, Mason CE, Melnick A (2016) Genetic and epigenetic heterogeneity in acute myeloid leukemia. Curr Opin Genet Dev 36:100–106
33. Figueroa ME, Abdel-Wahab O, Lu C, Ward PS, Patel J, Shih A et al (2010) Leukemic IDH1 and IDH2 mutations result in a hypermethylation phenotype, disrupt TET2 function, and impair hematopoietic differentiation. Cancer Cell 18(6):553–567
34. Rampal R, Alkalin A, Madzo J, Vasanthakumar A, Pronier E, Patel J et al (2014) DNA hydroxymethylation profiling reveals that WT1 mutations result in loss of TET2 function in acute myeloid leukemia. Cell Rep 9(5):1841–1855
35. Figueroa ME, Lugthart S, Li Y, Erpolinok Verschueren C, Deng X, Christos PJ et al (2010) DNA methylation signatures identify biologically distinct subtypes in acute myeloid leukemia. Cancer Cell 17(1):13–27
36. De Keersmaecker K, Atak ZK, Li N, Vicente C, Patchett S, Girardi T et al (2013) Exome sequencing identifies mutation in CNOT3 and ribosomal genes RPL5 and RPL10 in T-cell acute lymphoblastic leukemia. Nat Genet 45(2):186–190
37. Van Vlierberghe P, Ambesi-Impiombato A, De Keersmaecker K, Hadler M, Paietta E, Tallman MS et al (2013) Prognostic relevance of integrated genetic profiling in adult T-cell acute lymphoblastic leukemia. Blood 122(1):74–82
38. Lyko F, Brown R (2005) DNA methyltransferase inhibitors and the development of epigenetic cancer therapies. J Natl Cancer Inst 97(20):1498–1506
39. Jones PA, Taylor SM, Mohandas T, Shapiro LJ (1982) Cell cycle-specific reactivation of an inactive X-chromosome locus by 5-azadeoxycytidine. Proc Natl Acad Sci U S A 79(4):1215–1219
40. Nieto M, Samper E, Fraga MF, Gonzalez de Buitrago G, Esteller M, Serrano M (2004) The absence of p53 is critical for the induction of apoptosis by 5-aza-2′-deoxycytidine. Oncogene 23(3):735–743
41. Juttermann R, Li E, Jaenisch R (1994) Toxicity of 5-aza-2′-deoxycytidine to mammalian cells is mediated primarily by covalent trapping of DNA methyltransferase rather than DNA demethylation. Proc Natl Acad Sci U S A 91(25):11797–11801
42. Di Croce L, Raker VA, Corsaro M, Fazi F, Fanelli M, Faretta M et al (2002) Methyltransferase recruitment and DNA hypermethylation of target promoters by an oncogenic transcription factor. Science 295(5557):1079–1082
43. DeZern AE (2015) Nine years without a new FDA-approved therapy for MDS: how can we break through the impasse? Hematology Am Soc Hematol Educ Program 2015:308–316
44. Tellez CS, Grimes MJ, Picchi MA, Liu Y, March TH, Reed MD et al (2014) SGI-110 and entinostat therapy reduces lung tumor burden and reprograms the epigenome. Int J Cancer 135(9):2223–2231
45. Srivastava P, Paluch BE, Matsuzaki J, James SR, Collamat-Lai G, Karbach J et al (2014) Immunomodulatory action of SGI-110, a hypomethylating agent, in acute myeloid leukemia cells and xenografts. Leuk Res 38(11):1332–1341
46. Kuang Y, El-Khoueiry A, Taverna P, Ljungman M, Neamati N (2015) Guadecitabine (SGI-110) priming sensitizes hepatocellular carcinoma cells to oxaliplatin. Mol Oncol 9(9):1799–1814
47. Kharfan-Dabaja MA (2015) Guadecitabine for AML and MDS: hype or hope? Lancet Oncol 16(9):1009–1011
48. Jueliger S, Lyons J, Cannito S, Pata I, Pata P, Shkolnaya M et al (2016) Efficacy and epigenetic interactions of novel DNA hypomethylating agent guadecitabine (SGI-110) in preclinical models of hepatocellular carcinoma. Epigenetics 11:1–12

49. Issa JP, Roboz G, Rizzieri D, Jabbour E, Stock W, O'Connell C et al (2015) Safety and tolerability of guadecitabine (SGI-110) in patients with myelodysplastic syndrome and acute myeloid leukaemia: a multicentre, randomised, dose-escalation phase 1 study. Lancet Oncol 16(9):1099–1110

50. Griffiths EA, Choy G, Redkar S, Taverna P, Azab M, Karpf AR (2013) SGI-110: DNA methyltransferase inhibitor oncolytic. Drugs Future 38(8):535–543

51. Fang F, Munck J, Tang J, Taverna P, Wang Y, Miller DF et al (2014) The novel, small-molecule DNA methylation inhibitor SGI-110 as an ovarian cancer chemosensitizer. Clin Cancer Res 20(24):6504–6516

52. Stein EM, Altman JK, Collins R, DeAngelo DJ, Fathi AT, Flinn I et al (2014) AG 221, an oral, selective, first-in-class, potent inhibitor of the IDH2 mutant metabolic enzyme, induces durable remissions in a phase I study in patients with IDH2 mutation positive advanced hematologic malignancies. Blood 124(21):115

53. Stein EM, Tallman MS (2015) Emerging therapeutic drugs for AML. Blood 125:2923–2932

54. Dawson MA, Kouzarides T (2012) Cancer epigenetics: from mechanism to therapy. Cell 150(1):12–27

55. Takamatsu-Ichihara E, Kitabayashi I (2016) The roles of Polycomb group proteins in hematopoietic stem cells and hematological malignancies. Int J Hematol 103(6):634–642

56. Morin RD, Johnson NA, Severson TM, Mungall AJ, An J, Goya R et al (2010) Somatic mutations altering EZH2 (Tyr641) in follicular and diffuse large B-cell lymphomas of germinal-center origin. Nat Genet 42(2):181–185

57. Ernst T, Chase AJ, Score J, Hidalgo-Curtis CE, Bryant C, Jones AV et al (2010) Inactivating mutations of the histone methyltransferase gene EZH2 in myeloid disorders. Nat Genet 42(8):722–726

58. Kim KH, Roberts CW (2016) Targeting EZH2 in cancer. Nat Med 22(2):128–134

59. Abdel-Wahab O, Adli M, LaFave LM, Gao J, Hricik T, Shih AH et al (2012) ASXL1 mutations promote myeloid transformation through loss of PRC2-mediated gene repression. Cancer Cell 22(2):180–193

60. Inoue D, Kitaura J, Togami K, Nishimura K, Enomoto Y, Uchida T et al (2013) Myelodysplastic syndromes are induced by histone methylation-altering ASXL1 mutations. J Clin Invest 123(11):4627–4640

61. Beguelin W, Teater M, Gearhart MD, Calvo Fernandez MT, Goldstein RL, Cardenas MG et al (2016) EZH2 and BCL6 cooperate to assemble CBX8-BCOR complex to repress bivalent promoters, mediate germinal center formation and lymphomagenesis. Cancer Cell 30(2):197–213

62. Cerchietti LC, Ghetu AF, Zhu X, Da Silva GF, Zhong S, Matthews M et al (2010) A small-molecule inhibitor of BCL6 kills DLBCL cells in vitro and in vivo. Cancer Cell 17(4):400–411

63. Cerchietti LC, Hatzi K, Caldas-Lopes E, Yang SN, Figueroa ME, Morin RD et al (2010) BCL6 repression of EP300 in human diffuse large B cell lymphoma cells provides a basis for rational combinatorial therapy. J Clin Invest 120(12):4569–4582

64. Cardenas MG, Yu W, Beguelin W, Teater MR, Geng H, Goldstein RL et al (2016) Rationally designed BCL6 inhibitors target activated B cell diffuse large B cell lymphoma. J Clin Invest 126(9):3351–3362

65. Dupont T, Yang SN, Patel J, Hatzi K, Malik A, Tam W et al (2016) Selective targeting of BCL6 induces oncogene addiction switching to BCL2 in B-cell lymphoma. Oncotarget 7(3):3520–3532

66. Moorman AV, Richards S, Harrison CJ (2002) Involvement of the MLL gene in T-lineage acute lymphoblastic leukemia. Blood 100(6):2273–2274

67. Neumann M, Heesch S, Schlee C, Schwartz S, Gokbuget N, Hoelzer D et al (2013) Whole-exome sequencing in adult ETP-ALL reveals a high rate of DNMT3A mutations. Blood 121(23):4749–4752

68. Yang W, Ernst P (2016) SET/MLL family proteins in hematopoiesis and leukemia. Int J Hematol 105:7–16

69. Nguyen AT, Taranova O, He J, Zhang Y (2011) DOT1L, the H3K79 methyltransferase, is required for MLL-AF9-mediated leukemogenesis. Blood 117(25):6912–6922

70. Jo SY, Granowicz EM, Maillard I, Thomas D, Hess JL (2011) Requirement for Dot1l in murine postnatal hematopoiesis and leukemogenesis by MLL translocation. Blood 117(18):4759–4768
71. Bernt KM, Zhu N, Sinha AU, Vempati S, Faber J, Krivtsov AV et al (2011) MLL-rearranged leukemia is dependent on aberrant H3K79 methylation by DOT1L. Cancer Cell 20(1):66–78
72. Daigle SR, Olhava EJ, Therkelsen CA, Majer CR, Sneeringer CJ, Song J et al (2011) Selective killing of mixed lineage leukemia cells by a potent small-molecule DOT1L inhibitor. Cancer Cell 20(1):53–65
73. Yu W, Chory EJ, Wernimont AK, Tempel W, Scopton A, Federation A et al (2012) Catalytic site remodelling of the DOT1L methyltransferase by selective inhibitors. Nat Commun 3:1288
74. Hong S, Cho YW, Yu LR, Yu H, Veenstra TD, Ge K (2007) Identification of JmjC domain-containing UTX and JMJD3 as histone H3 lysine 27 demethylases. Proc Natl Acad Sci U S A 104(47):18439–18444
75. Accari SL, Fisher PR (2015) Emerging roles of JmjC domain-containing proteins. Int Rev Cell Mol Biol 319:165–220
76. Schenk T, Chen WC, Gollner S, Howell L, Jin L, Hebestreit K et al (2012) Inhibition of the LSD1 (KDM1A) demethylase reactivates the all-trans-retinoic acid differentiation pathway in acute myeloid leukemia. Nat Med 18(4):605–611
77. Lokken AA, Zeleznik-Le NJ (2012) Breaking the LSD1/KDM1A addiction: therapeutic targeting of the epigenetic modifier in AML. Cancer Cell 21(4):451–453
78. Hayami S, Kelly JD, Cho HS, Yoshimatsu M, Unoki M, Tsunoda T et al (2011) Overexpression of LSD1 contributes to human carcinogenesis through chromatin regulation in various cancers. Int J Cancer 128(3):574–586
79. Berglund L, Bjorling E, Oksvold P, Fagerberg L, Asplund A, Szigyarto CA et al (2008) A gene-centric Human Protein Atlas for expression profiles based on antibodies. Mol Cell Proteomics 7(10):2019–2027
80. Niebel D, Kirfel J, Janzen V, Holler T, Majores M, Gutgemann I (2014) Lysine-specific demethylase 1 (LSD1) in hematopoietic and lymphoid neoplasms. Blood 124(1):151–152
81. Melnick AM (2010) Epigenetics in AML. Best Pract Res Clin Haematol 23(4):463–468
82. Pan H, Jiang Y, Boi M, Tabbo F, Redmond D, Nie K et al (2015) Epigenomic evolution in diffuse large B-cell lymphomas. Nat Commun 6:6921
83. Ferri E, Petosa C, McKenna CE (2016) Bromodomains: structure, function and pharmacology of inhibition. Biochem Pharmacol 106:1–18

DNA and Histone Methylation in Lung Cancer

Sophia Mastoraki and Evi Lianidou

Abstract Oncogenesis is driven by the accumulation of genetic and epigenetic alterations that result in dysregulation of key oncogenes, tumor suppressor genes, and DNA repair/housekeeping genes. One of the major clinical needs is the discovery and clinical validation of new molecular biomarkers using non-or minimally invasive procedures to assist early diagnosis, prognosis and prediction of response to treatment. Histone methylation has profound effects on nuclear functions such as transcriptional regulation, maintenance of genome integrity and epigenetic inheritance. On the other hand, aberrant DNA methylation can be detected in several biological fluids of patients and could be served as a potential tumor biomarker. In the present chapter we describe latest developments on histone and DNA methylation based biomarkers in Lung cancer.

Keywords DNA methylation • Epigenetic silencing • Lung cancer • miRNAs methylation • DNA methylation biomarkers • Liquid biopsy • ctDNA

1 Introduction

Lung cancer remains the second leading cause of death worldwide, after heart disease with more than 200,000 new cases and 160,000 deaths each year. The high incidence of lung cancer in combination with the very low 5-year survival rate of 17% is the main cause of high mortality rate in this type of cancer [188]. The main subtypes of lung cancer are small cell lung cancer carcinoma (SCLC) and non-small cell lung carcinoma (NSCLC), which includes squamous cell carcinoma, adenocarcinoma, and large cell carcinoma subtypes [38]. NSCLC is the most common type, accounting for approximately 85% of all lung cancer cases. Although smoking remains the major risk factor for all histologies (especially small cell and squamous cell carcinoma), it is important to note that only around 10% of smokers will

S. Mastoraki • E. Lianidou (✉)
Analysis of Circulating Tumor Cells, Lab of Analytical Chemistry, Department of Chemistry, University Campus, University of Athens, 15771 Athens, Greece
e-mail: lianidou@chem.uoa.gr

© Springer International Publishing AG 2017
A. Kaneda, Y.-i. Tsukada (eds.), *DNA and Histone Methylation as Cancer Targets*, Cancer Drug Discovery and Development, DOI 10.1007/978-3-319-59786-7_15

ultimately develop lung cancer [134]. Globally, an estimated 15% of men and 53% of women with lung cancer are never-smokers. This fact indicates additional risk factors for the disease. Adenocarcinoma, for example, is the most common form among nonsmokers. Other risk factors include exposure to radon, asbestos, and environmental/occupational exposure to polycyclic aromatic hydrocarbons and other pollutants [177]. However, as with smoking, not all exposed to these environmental factors develop lung cancer.

The carcinogenic process is driven by the accumulation of genetic and epigenetic alterations that result in dysregulation of key oncogenes, tumor suppressor genes, and DNA repair/housekeeping genes. The probability that these pathologically important events will occur is not only dependent on the individual's exposure but also on interpersonal phenotypic variability. Although genetic heterogeneity accounts for some of the variable risk, it does not totally explain this phenomenon [107]. Epigenetic variability, including DNA methylation, histone modifications, and noncoding RNA expression, also contribute to the phenotype of an individual and, accordingly, to the risk of malignancy [108].

Early detection of lung carcinoma could change the disease outcome; in fact, the survival rate can increase dramatically. In the effort to improve early detection, many imaging and cytology-based strategies have been employed; however, none has yet been highly effective, mainly because of limited sensitivity and the huge cost they bear to public health systems [7]. It is now widely accepted that epidemiological risk modeling is required for stratification of individuals for CT screening for early detection of lung cancer [161]. In addition to CT, one of the major clinical needs is now the inclusion of new molecular biomarkers detected in clinical samples using non-or minimally invasive procedures to assist early diagnosis, prognosis and prediction of response to treatment. Understanding the molecular pathways within lung cancer, and focusing on their molecular heterogeneity, is the most effective way towards the development of novel diagnostic and therapeutic tools. In the last decade, a plethora of molecular factors all involved in lung carcinogenesis have been evaluated as prognostic biomarkers [8].

2   Histone Methylation

Histone post-translational modifications include methylation, acetylation, phosphorylation and ubiquitination; through the modulation of chromatin structure, histones play a significant role in creating gene transcriptional activation or repression [224]. Their role is crucial for precise coordination and organization of the open and closed chromatin structure during many dynamic processes such as DNA replication, repair, recombination, and transcription. Changes in local or global chromatin structure have been found to be the key features of many if not all tumors, indicating that such epigenetic changes may make a potential contribution to carcinogenesis [184, 207].

Histone methylation has profound effects on nuclear functions such as transcriptional regulation, maintenance of genome integrity and epigenetic inheritance [132]. For example, histone methylation on arginine or lysine residues can either activate or repress gene transcription, depending on which particular arginine or lysine residue become modified [103]. Methylation and demethylation on arginine or lysine residues in histone tails are reversible modifications that are tightly controlled by histone methyltransferases and histone demethylases. Such dynamic balance of methylation and demethylation is frequently altered in tumorigenesis and pathogenesis of other disorders as well [31, 45, 87, 220].

There are three histone methylation states: monomethyl (me1), dimethyl (me2) or trimethyl (me3) [162]. In general, methylation of H3K4, H3K36 and H3K79 is generally considered to activate genes while methylation of H3K9, H3K27, H3K56, H4K20 and H1.4K26 causes transcriptional repression [105]. H3K4me1 is related with enhancer functions and participates in gene repression in metazoans [30, 66], nucleosome dynamics and chromatin regulation of yeast stress-responsive genes [141]. H3K4me2 is connected to gene repression and transcription in yeast [130, 151], whereas H3K4me3 is linked to active transcription and is present around transcriptional start sites [14, 219].

Lysine-specific demethylation is facilitated by two families of enzymes, of which the JmjC (JumonjiC) domain-containing family of histone demethylases (JHDMs) is the major one. KDM proteins are divided in two subgroups; KDM1 and KDM 2-7 [201]. Unfortunately, there are few studies on KDM demethylases in lung tumors. KDM5B (lysine-specific demethylase 5B), also known as JARID1B (jumonji AT-rich interactive domain 1B) or PLU-1, is one member of the JHDMs subfamily which has recently attracted much attention [64]. Famous oncogenes such as E2F1 and E2F2 are downstream genes in the KDM5B pathway [65, 114]. Recently, KDM5B was found to stimulate NSCLC cell proliferation and invasion by affecting p53 expression [183]. KDM4A and KDM4B remove the tri- and dimethylated marks from H3K9 and H3K36 thus leading to gene repression while KDM4D can only move a methyl group from a trimethylated mark of H3K36. In non-neoplastic tissues, expression of KDM- 4C is especially high in the testes and expression in the lung is very low. KDM4A and KDM4B have a generally higher expression in non-neoplastic tissues the highest levels being found in ovary and spleen, but they are moderately expressed also in the lung [105]. Another recent study was undertaken to investigate the immunohistochemical expression of KDM4A, KDM4B and KDM4D in a set of 188 lung carcinomas. The results were associated with tumor histology, parameters describing the spread of the tumors, and survival of the patients. As an additional marker, the antibody to H3 trimethylated state was used. KDM4A and KDM4D play a role in spread of the lung carcinomas. Further, cytoplasmic KDM4A positivity associates with patient survival. These results are in line with the supposed role of KDMs in epigenetic regulation of cancer cells, affecting proliferation, apoptosis and DNA repair mechanisms [192].

In lung cancer, several global histone modifications have been associated with survival; in particular, decreased levels of H3K4diMe have been associated with poor outcome [178]. Furthermore, the combination of several histone modifications have been reported to predict survival (H3K4me2, H3K9ac, and H2AK5ac) [13], and H4K20me3 downregulation has been associated with poor prognosis in patients with stage I lung adenocarcinoma [210].

Over the last decade, many studies have revealed epigenetic aberrations involving histone modifications in lung cancer. Miyanaga et al. [139] treated 16 NSCLC cell lines with HDAC inhibitors and both displayed antitumor activities in 50% of the cell lines tested. They also conducted gene expression profiling and created a nine-gene classifier which predicts HDAC inhibitor drug sensitivities. Another group compared lung cancer cells with normal lung cells, and they found that lung cancer cells displayed aberrant histone H4 modification patterns with hyperacetylation of H4K5/H4K8, hypoacetylation of H4K12/H4K16, and loss of H4K20 trimethylation [210]. These findings indicate an important role for histone H4 modifications and highlight H4K20me3 as a potential diagnostic biomarker and therapeutic target for lung cancer. Another study has shown that lower global levels of histone modifications are predictive of a more aggressive cancer phenotype in lung adenocarcinoma [178].

Additionally, the differential expression pattern of HATs and HDACs in the tumor samples, as compared to normals, may have important implications for the management of the patients [147]. HDAC1 gene expression appears to correlate with lung cancer progression; overexpression of HDAC1 and HDAC3 correlates with poor prognosis in pulmonary adebocarcinoma patients [137, 138, 171]. HDAC3 was also found in elevated levels in 92% cases of SCC tumors using antibody microarrays for detection of target proteins [15].

Histone deacetylase inhibitors (HDIs) might beneficially contribute to tumor treatment, by reducing the responsiveness of tumor cells to the TNF mediated activation of the NF-B pathway. This is shown in NSCLC cells treated with HDIs which down-regulated TNF-receptor-1 mRNA, protein levels, and surface protein expression, and consequently responded to TNF-treatment with attenuated NF-B nuclear translocation and DNA binding [78]. Treatment with trichostatin A (TSA) resulted in a dose dependent reduction of H157 lung cancer cells by apoptosis with nuclear fragmentation and an increase in the sub-G0/ G1 fraction. TSA initiated apoptosis by activation of the intrinsic mitochondrial and extrinsic/Fas/FasL system death pathways [93–95]. TSA is also a powerful NSCLC cell radiosensitizer, enhancing G2/M cell cycle arrest, promoting apoptosis, interfering with DNA damage repair and synergistically causing cell death when combined with other HDAC inhibitors, such as vorinostat [180, 231]. It has been shown that vorinostat inhibits telomerase activity by reducing hTERT expression [113] and decreases bcl-2 expression [100].

The first compound clinically used as an LSD1 inhibitor is tranylcypromine, a monoamine oxidase inhibitor approved more than 50 years ago for treatment-refractory depression. More potent and specific LSD1 inhibitors are presently under preclinical and early clinical development. The methylation of lysine 27 of histone

H3, H3K27, is regulated by the enhancer of zeste homolog 2 (EZH2), the catalytic domain of the polycomb repressive complex 2 (PRC2). Trimethylation of H3K27 by EZH2 leads to silencing of PRC2 target genes that are involved in stem cell differentiation and embryonic development. EZH2 is overexpressed in a variety of cancers, including NSCLC. 3-Deazaneplanocin A (DZNep) is an EZH2 inhibitor that leads to reduced trimethylated H3K27 levels in breast cancer cells and the derepression of aberrantly silenced genes [172].

Aberrant histone methylation is a relatively recently discovered feature in NSCLC, which is reflected in the scarceness of studies using agents affecting histone methylation. It was recently shown that EZH2 knockdown as well as indirect EZH2 inhibition using 3-deazaneplanocin A (DZNep) could prime NSCLC cell lines to the effect of the topoisomerase inhibitor etoposide [53]. Aberrant histone demethylation in NSCLC however is not extensively studied so far in NSCLC. LSD1 knockdown as well as LSD1 inhibition using pargyline suppressed invasion, migration, and proliferation in lung cancer specimens [211]. To our knowledge, there are as yet no studies investigating combination therapies for lung cancer using LSD1 inhibitors [172].

Changes in the number of methyl residues in lysine residues of H3K9, H3K27 and H3K36 through lysine methylation/demethylation is very important since it affects the expression of genes by loosening or tightening the attachment of DNA to the nucleosome [98].

3   DNA Methylation in Lung Cancer

DNA methylation is the most studied epigenetic regulatory mechanism. CpG island methylation is mediated by different DNA methyltransferases (DNMTs) that can lead to gene silencing. Three active DNMTs (DNMT1, DNMT3a, and DNMT3b) are in charge to transfer a methyl group from S-adenosyl-L-methionine to the CpG islands 5′-cytosine carbon [32, 55, 150] DNMT1 is primarily involved in the maintenance methylation after DNA replication, while DNMT3a and b are responsible of de novo DNA methylation [47, 118, 119, 235]. During the last years DNA methylation is gaining ground as a potential biomarker for diagnosis, staging, prognosis, and monitoring of response to therapy. The field of DNA methylation based markers for prognosis and diagnosis is still emerging and its widespread use in clinical practice needs to be implemented [83]. As DNA methylation is often considered an early event in carcinogenesis, tumor-specific methylation has a great potential to be used as a screening and/or diagnostic tool in a non-invasive and cost-effective way.

Hypermethylation includes tumor suppressor gene inactivation through promoter methylation, is a hallmark of lung cancer and tends to occur as an early event in carcinogenesis [21, 236]. Tumor suppressor genes can be inactivated through a combined ation of promoter methylation in one allele and the presence of mutation or deletion in the other; in dominantly acting suppressor gene loci inactivation of one allele is generally insufficient to lead to clonal selection, since the protein can still be produced from the other normal allele. However, there is also evidence that in some cases partial inactivation of one allele by promoter methylation can contribute to carcinogenesis and be sufficient for clonal selection [24].

Lung cancer involves an accumulation of genetic and epigenetic events in the respiratory epithelium. Mutations and copy number alterations play a well-known role in oncogenesis, though epigenetic alterations are, in fact, more frequent than somatic aberrations in lung cancer [28]. During the neoplastic progression from hyperplasia to adenocarcinoma, promoter methylation of specific tumor suppressor genes, along with the overall number of hypermethylated genes seems to be increased [115].

3.1 Tumor Suppressor Gene Inactivation Through Gene Promoter Methylation

Many of the tumor suppressor genes that are hypermethylated in lung cancer are found to be hypermethylated in other types of solid tumors as well. Moreover, some are specific, although many are not. In premalignant and malignant states, promoter methylation is commonly observed in genes involved with crucial functions, including cell cycle control, proliferation, apoptosis, cellular adhesion, motility, and DNA repair [108]. Up to now, there is some evidence for a CpG island methylator phenotype (CIMP), a tumor phenotype characterized by widespread hypermethylation of a panel of genes, in lung cancer [124–126, 131, 186]. This is not wholly surprising, since the group of enzymes that catalyze the covalent attachment of the methyl group to the cytosine base (DNMTs), are upregulated in NSCLC [93–95, 116].

3.2 lncRNAs and miRNAs Methylation in Lung Cancer

It has been recently shown that abnormal promoter methylation does not affect only protein coding genes but can also affect various noncoding RNAs that may play a role in malignant growth [128]. To identify which long non-coding RNAs (lncRNAs) are involved in non-small cell lung cancer (NSCLC), *Feng et al.* analyzed microarray data on gene expression and methylation and identified 8500 lncRNAs that are expressed differentially between tumor and non-malignant tissues; 1504 of these were correlated with mRNA expression. Two of the lncRNAs, LOC146880 and ENST00000439577, were positively correlated with expression of two cancer-related genes, KPNA2 and RCC2, respectively. High expression of these two lncRNAs was also associated with poor survival. Analysis of lncRNA expression in relation to DNA methylation has shown that LOC146880 expression was down-regulated by DNA methylation in its promoter [51].

MicroRNAs (miRNAs) also play an important role in cancer development and progression, altering several biological functions by affecting targets through either their degradation or suppression of protein encoded. It has been recently shown that miR-1247, is downregulated in various cancers, but its biological role in non-small-cell lung cancer (NSCLC) is unknown. Furthermore, Stathmin 1 (STMN1) was found to be an immediate and functional target of miR-1247. The expression of *STMN1* was significantly increased in NSCLC cell lines but was decreased by 5-Aza treatment. In addition, miR-1247 upregulation partially inhibited STMN1-induced promotion of migration and invasion of A549 and H1299 cells. These results indicate that miR-1247 was silenced by DNA methylation. Therefore, miR-1247 and its downstream target gene *STMN1* may be a future target for the treatment of NSCLC [234].

3.3   Genomic Hypomethylation

DNA hypomethylation at CpG dinucleotides was the first epigenetic abnormality to be identified in cancer cells, over three decades ago. The degree of hypomethylation of genomic DNA was shown to correlate with the severity of the cancer; genome-wide DNA methylation decreased as the tumor progressed from a benign proliferating mass to metastatic invasive cancer [217].

A possible explanation for the mechanism of reduced DNA methylation contribution to carcinogenesis is that hypomethylation of genomic DNA favors mitotic recombination between repetitive sequences resulting in chromosomal instability. Mitotic recombination normally occurs at a high frequency in human cells [60, 69]. Since recombination depends on the homology between nucleotide sequences, repetitive sequences are especially permissive to recombination events, resulting in gross chromosomal anomalies, including chromosomal rearrangements, deletions, and/or translocations [217].

Another mechanism through which DNA hypomethylation contributes to carcinogenesis is reactivation of transposable elements. It was shown already many years ago that SINEs and LINEs together make up approximately 45% of the human genome [106] and are usually methylated in normal tissues. LINEs belong to the class of transposable elements that lack LTRs at their ends. LINEs, which are part of the LINE-1 (or L1) family, constitute approximately 17% of the human genome and are the only transposable elements capable of autonomous transposition [17].

In lung cancer, genomic hypomethylation may be a late event in tumorigenesis in contrast to gene-specific hypermethylation, which can occur early during cancer development. However, currently there is not a clear consensus on the timing, as Anisowicz et al. [4] found that hypomethylation was associated with NSCLC progression from normal to lung cancer. DNA hypomethylation in lung cancers, as this was shown by high-resolution CpG methylation mapping, occur specifically at repetitive sequences [166], including heterochromatin repeats (e.g., satellite DNA), SINEs (short interspersed nuclear elements), LINEs (long interspersed nuclear elements), LTR (long terminal repeat) elements, and segmental duplications in subtelomeric regions. However cancer-specific hypomethylation at repeat regions was not conserved between the individual tumors indicating randomness for targeting repeat sequences for demethylation in cancer [57]. In NSCLC widespread hypomethylation has been associated with genomic instability [35] that could result in oncogene activation [49] and loss of imprinting [101]. In lung cancer, hypomethylation tends to occur at nuclear elements, long terminal repeat (LTR) elements, segmental duplicates, and subtelomeric regions. On the contrary, loss of methylation is much less common at non-repetitive sequences [166].

In addition to the genomic loss of methyl content, gene-specific hypomethylation has been reported for several loci, including MAGEA [58, 97], TKTL1 [86], BORIS [70, 167], DDR131 14-3-3s [160, 185], and TMSB10 [60]. MAGE overexpression with an associated loss of methylation is a common event in lung cancer, as it has been observed in 75–80% of NSCLC [81].

3.4   EMT and DNA Methylation

EMT is a fundamental and conserved process characterized by loss of cell adhesion and increased cell motility. EMT is essential for numerous developmental processes including mesoderm formation and neural tube formation and wound healing. However, initiation of metastasis involves invasion, which has many phenotypic similarities to EMT, including a loss of cell-cell adhesion and an increase in cell mobility [200].

EMT is regulated by a variety of growth factors including epidermal growth factor (EGF), platelet derived growth factors (PDGFs), fibroblast growth factor-2 (FGF-2), and transforming growth factor-beta (TGF-β) [85] and is characterized by the loss of CDH1 (E-cadherin), a trans-membrane protein that is required for adherent junctions [109]. Following the loss of epithelial markers, there is a corresponding increase in mesenchymal markers, for example VIM (vimentin), CDH12 (N-cadherin) FN1 (fibronectin), ACTA2 (alpha-smooth muscle actin), and increased activity of MMP (matrix metalloproteinases) [168, 221]. Recent studies have shown that a multilayer regulatory network of transcription factors controls EMT. The most studied network is the regulation through SNAIL (SNAI1 and SNAI2), ZEB (ZEB1 and ZEB2), and TWIST (TWIST1) family members, which are referred as EMT transcription factors (EMT-TF) [190].

In NSCLC, DNA methylation of a subset of genes related to EMT leads to their transcriptional inactivation [120]. One of the master regulators of EMT, TWIST, binds to the CDH1 promoter and recruits the CHD4/nucleosome remodeling and deacetylase complex (CHD4/NuRD complex, also known as Mi2/NuRD complex) by direct interaction to several of its components as MTA2, CHD4, and RBBP7 [56]. In addition, MTA2 directly recruits the histone deacetylase HDAC2. The TWIST/CHD4/NuRD complex represses CHD1 expression by nucleosome remodeling as well as deacetylation of histones. The biological relevance of this mechanism of transcription regulation was demonstrated within the context of metastasis of two types of cancers, lung and breast cancer, since depletion of the components of the TWIST/CHD4/ NuRD complex suppressed cell migration and invasion in cell culture and murine models of cancer metastasis. This work [56] shows that not only DNA methylation but also other chromatin modifications, as nucleosome remodeling and histone modifications, play a role during cancer metastasis.

4 Smoking and DNA Methylation

Some epigenetic alterations reported for lung cancer may be smoking-specific, since they occur at greater frequency in smokers and increase with increasing smoking duration and intensity [90, 123, 202]. Genes reported to undergo smoking specific promoter hypermethylation include APC, FHIT, RASSF1A, and CCND2 [50, 203]. Also, the frequency of promoter hypermethylation of p16INK4a, MGMT, RASSF1A, MTHFR, and FHIT is greater in the NSCLC tumors of smokers relative to nonsmokers [91, 123, 209]. Moreover, RARb, p16INK4a, FHIT, and RASSF1A promoter hypermethylation increases with increasing smoking intensity [3, 71, 228].

DNMT1 expression is elevated in smokers with lung cancer, likely due to tobacco-specific nitrosamines that reduce DNMT1 ubiquitination and degradation [118, 119]. Additionally, it is widely accepted tha smoking-induced chronic inflammation and increased reactive oxygen species generation lead to increased DNA methylation [144].

Damiani et al. [34] developed an in vitro model that mimics the field cancerization observed in chronic smokers and identified several epigenetic changes and their kinetics. More specifically, immortalized normal human bronchial epithelial cells (HBECs) were exposed for 12 weeks to two cigarette carcinogens; methylnitrosurea (MNU) and benzo(a)pyrenediolepoxide 1 (BPDE). Stable knockdown of DNMT1, but not DNMT3 prevented cell transformation after exposure to these carcinogens. HBECs transform to a fibroblast like mesenchymal form after 4 weeks of carcinogen exposure. Significant reductions in miR-200b and miR-200c, were observed at 4 weeks exposure and was sustained upon cell transformation at 12 weeks. Interestingly, these two microRNAs are involved in regulating and inhibiting the EMT. Further studies revealed that expression of these EMT-regulating microRNAs are initially reduced by transcriptionally inactive chromatin at 4 weeks, followed by cytosine methylation-mediated repression at their promoters [19].

Interestingly long-term exposure to carcinogenic stimuli would imply a later selection of existing clones, thus genes that are silenced due to the duration or amount of tobacco smoking, are likely later stage contributors to this disease. Experimentally, wide genomic hypomethylation and promoter hypermethylation of RASSF1A and RARb were observed when normal small-airway epithelial cells and immortalized bronchial epithelial cells were exposed to cigarette smoke condensate [125, 126]. There is also experimental evidence indicating that cigarette condensate decreases nuclear levels of H4K16ac and H4K2me3 in respiratory epithelial cells [133].

Conversely, RASSF2, TNFRSF10, BHLHB5, and BOLL have been reported to be hypermethylated more frequently in NSCLC of patients who never smoked [108]. Moreover, chronic inflammation, which occurs in response to cigarette smoking, also plays an important role in lung cancer development, stimulating cellular turnover and proliferation. Inflammation has long been associated with DNA methylation in lung cancer [11, 136]. There is evidence that reactive oxygen species, generated during chronic inflammation, target transcriptional repressors and lead to increased levels of DNA methylation [144].

Cigarette smoke also inhibits the metabolism and storage of folate [143]. It has been shown on studies based in experimental models, that nitrates, nitrous oxide, cyanates, and isocyanates found in tobacco smoke transform folate, a major source of methyl groups for 1-carbon metabolism, into a biologically inactive compound [1, 89]. In additional support of this, reduced serum folate levels have been observed in smokers relative to nonsmokers [145, 152]. One-carbon metabolism is a critical pathway in the DNA methylation process, and depletion of folate can impact negatively the availability of s-adenosylmethionine, the primary methyl donor in the cytosine methylation reaction. Consequently, folate deficiency can result in chromosomal damage through impaired nucleotide synthesis and aberrant DNA methylation [25, 48].

5   Hypermethylated Genes in Lung Cancer

DNA 5'-cytosine hypermethylation is an early event in lung carcinogenesis [28, 83]. Many genes are hypermethylated in lung cancer including p16, PAK3, NISCH, KIF1A, OGDHL, BRMS1, FHIT, CTSZ, CCNA1, NRCAM, LOX, MGMT, DOK1, SOX15, TCF21, DAPK, RAR, RASSF1, CYGB, MSX1, BNC1, CTSZ, and CDKN2A [6, 44, 46, 72, 80, 82, 140, 149, 176, 182, 191, 205, 215].

The percent of hypermethylation for each gene varies, for example p16 and MGMT are hypermethylated in 100% of patients with pulmonary SqCC up the 3 years before cancer diagnosis. p16 inhibits cyclin-dependent kinases 4 and 6, which after binding cyclin D1, phosphorylate and inactivate the retinoblastoma (Rb) tumor suppressor gene, blocking cell cycle progression [218]. p16 is lost in ~70% of lung cancer cases, often by promoter methylation, promoting the G1 to S phase transition [181]. Interestingly, p16 methylation occurs in normal-appearing epithelium from smokers and precursors lesions, and increases as the disease progresses [20]. The specific mechanisms by which each gene hypermethylation event promotes cancer vary, but most of them include repression of tumor suppressor genes with subsequent activation of genes promoting cell growth and cell cycle progression [6, 44, 46, 72, 80, 82, 140, 149, 176, 191, 205, 215].

Some of the most often studied hypermethylated genes in lung cancer include p16INK4a, RASSF1A, APC, RARb, CDH1, CDH13, DAPK, FHIT, and MGMT. Although p16INK4a is hypermethylated, mutated, or deleted frequently in NSCLC, with estimates for the prevalence of alteration of this gene around 60%, p14arf, which is also encoded on the CDKN2A gene, is inactivated much less commonly (8–30% of NSCLC) [54, 204]. On the other hand, p16INK4a is disrupted in less than 10% of SCLC patients. In addition, RASSF1A is deleted or hypermethylated in 30–40% of NSCLC and 70–100% of SCLC, FHIT is deleted or hypermethylated in 40–70% of NSCLC and 50–80% of SCLC and finally TSLC1 is hypermethylated in an estimated 85% of NSCLC [204].

Hypermethylation of CDKN2A has been identified in premalignant lesions, thus may occur early in the tumorigenesis of some lung cancers types [18]. Promoter methylation of RASSF1A, APC, ESR1, ABCB1, MT1G, and HOXC9 have been associated with stage I NSCLC [117] suggesting they also are an early event in lung cancer. CpG island methylation of homeobox-associated genes is also common in stage I lung cancer, appearing in nearly all early-stage tumors [165]. Conversely, other commonly hypermethylated genes, such as hDAB2IP, H-Cadherin, DAL-1, and FBN2, have been associated with advanced stage NSCLC [29, 229], suggesting these changes may occur at a later point during cancer progression. However, it is important to note that later involvement does not preclude the importance of the modification in the development of the disease, as these modifications may play key roles in the ability of the cancer to continue to develop in its advanced state, to slide over host immunity or exogenous cancer treatments, or to metastasize locally. Furthermore, due to the heterogeneity and the unique molecular signature of lung cancer, it is critical that these generalized "temporal" observations are kept in perspective; an early event in 1 tumor may not occur until later on in another [108].

Promoter methylation of CDKN2A and PTPRN2 has been shown to be one of the earliest events in cellular hyperplasia. Subsequently, studies have shown aberrant promoter hypermethylation of RASSF1A, CDH13, MGMT, and APC in lung cancer [92, 117, 158, 226]. Methylation of SHOX2, in bronchial aspirates as a biomarker, was identified in a 250-patient case-control study with 78% sensitivity and 96% specificity [99]. Hypermethylation of each CDKN2A, CDX2, HOXA1, and OPCML individually distinguished lung adenocarcinoma from healthy donors with a sensitivity of 67–86% and a specificity of 74–82% and showed significant DNA methylation even in stage I tumor samples [206]. Moreover, hypermethylation of the DAPK promoter was found in 34% of lung cancer samples. Taking into consideration the different histological subtypes of NSCLC, DAPK promoter methylation was more frequently observed in squamous cell carcinoma than in adenocarcinoma and large cell carcinoma; however, these differences were not statistically significant [142].

In sputum, tumor cells can be identified by atypical cell morphology. Sputum collection is a procedure that can be done easily and non-invasively by the patient. However, sampling may be inadequate because of the presence of epithelial cells resulting in underestimation of the methylation level in cancer cells. Sputum cytology is still implemented as standard diagnostic tool for lung cancer diagnosis, although in developed countries, it was replaced by tumor biopsies/ tumor cytology. Over the last decade, research on sputum cytology for risk assessment and recurrence of early lung cancer brought new insights and advanced highly sensitive molecular techniques [135].

Analysis of the RASSF1A and 3OST2 promoters methylation in sputum specimen demonstrated a combined sensitivity of 85% with a specificity of 74% [77].
Promoter methylation of 31 genes was also analyzed in sputum of lung cancer
patients in two independent cohorts to define a gene unique methylation signature
for lung cancer risk assessment [111]. Accurate diagnosis was made for 71–77% of
the patients using the promoter methylation signature of seven of these genes
(PAX5β, PAX5α, Dal-1, GATA5, SULF2, and CXCL14). *Whang et al.* observed
55% MLH1 promoter hypermethylation of the tumor samples obtained from stage
I and II patients. Further evaluation demonstrated a similar promoter
hypermethylation in 38% of the sputum samples. Finally, they reported a 72%
concordance of sputum samples matched to tissue biopsies [213]. A different study
found that CDKN2A was methylated in 80.2% of tumor tissues and showed a frequency of 74.7% in sputum specimens. Several studies have evaluated the correlation between tissue and sputum samples. Hypermethylation of the best studied
gene, CDKN2A, seems to be higher in tumor samples than in sputum with an
interquartile range of 84–37% to 74–32%, respectively [33, 40, 122].

In serum and plasma of cancer patients cell free DNA from necrotic and apoptotic cancer cells have been detected [12]. A lot of genes have been evaluated in lung
cancer patients to identify specific and sensitive targets for early lung cancer detection in clinical trials. In NSCLC, 75–87% of serum samples corresponding to their
matched tissue samples for promoter hypermethylation of RASSF1A, CDKN2A,
RARb, CDH13, FHIT, and BLU. In a study evaluating lung cancer risk using this
panel of six genes, a sensitivity of 73% and a specificity of 82% were reported, with
a concordance between tumor tissues and corresponding matched plasma samples,
of 75% [74]. Promoter methylation of CDKN2A, DAPK, PAX5b, and GATA5 was
analyzed in blood but it was 0.2–0.6-fold lower than in tissue biopsy samples [23].
Subsequent studies have shown CDKN2A methylation in blood, but the results
given are very different in different studies, varying from 22.2% to 75.7% [16, 195].
Hypermethylation for DAPK was found in 35% of the bronchial epithelium and in
41% of blood samples from smokers whereas the remaining samples from nonsmokers were unaffected, showing smoking–/lung cancer-associated methylation
changes [169].

In a very recent study, Daugaard I et al. compared the genome-wide methylation
pattern in tumor and tumor adjacent normal lung tissues from four lung adenocarcinoma patients using DNA methylation microarrays and identified 74 differentially
methylated regions (DMRs), 15 of which were validated and can be targeted as
biomarkers in LAC [36]. Another study demonstrated that SPAG6 and L1TD1 are
tumor-specifically methylated in NSCLC DNA methylation is involved in the transcriptional regulation of these genes and tumor-cell growth suppressing properties
of L1TD1 in NSCLC cells [2].

In the past, abberant estrogen receptor (ER) regulation has been associated with
various lung pathologies, but so far its involvement in lung cancer initiation and/or
progression has remained unclear. *Tekpli et al.*, aimed to assess in vivo and in vitro
ER expression and its possible epigenetic regulation in non-small cell lung cancer
(NSCLC) samples and their corresponding normal tissues and cells, and they reported

significantly lower ERα and ERβ expression levels in the NSCLC tissue samples compared to their normal adjacent tissue samples. They also found that in tumor and normal lung tissues, smoking was associated with decreased ER expression and that normal lung tissues with a low ERβ expression level exhibited increased smoking-related DNA adducts. Taken together, these results indicate that decreased ER expression mediated by DNA methylation may play a role in NSCLC development [199].

6 DNA Methylation Based Biomarkers

The virtually universal presence of DNA hypermethylation in all types of cancer makes it an ideal candidate tumor biomarker. Compared with other molecular marker classes such as mRNA and proteins, DNA methylation has many advantages. First, DNA methylation is a covalent modification of DNA, so it is chemically stable and can survive harsh conditions for long periods of time. Second, through simple procedures it can be readily amplifiable and easily detectable. In addition, contrary to cancer-specific mutations, which are relatively rare and present in different gene positions, the incidence of aberrant methylation of specific CGIs is much higher, and moreover such methylation can be discovered by genome-wide screening procedures. Finally, DNA methylation has been detected in a number of body fluids of patients with cancer. In lung cancer, aberrant DNA methylation can be detected in the ctDNA, in sputum, in bronchoalveolar lavage and saliva of patients [8].

DNA hypermethylation in lung cancer patients can be detected in a plethora of biological samples, including bronchoscopic washings/brushings, sputum samples, and blood (plasma and serum), all of which are less invasive and easier on the patient than a tumor biopsy [5]. The clinical significance of detecting methylation biomarkers in blood could facilitate the evaluation of tumor progression next to routine screening. Nevertheless, it could be an indication of invasiveness, reflecting an advanced tumor stage [135].

6.1 Early Detection

Lung cancer mortality could be reduced significantly with the early detection of the disease. However, only about 15% of lung tumors are localized in the time of diagnosis, with the majority presenting at an advanced stage [38]. Five-year survival for lung cancer is markedly better for early-stage patients, with a less than 10% 5-year survival for advanced-stage patients vs greater than 70% for early-stage patients [68]. Cytology is by far the gold standard method for lung cancer diagnosis in minimally-invasive respiratory samples, despite its low sensitivity. Spiral computed tomography has shown promise for the early detection of lung cancer, but it has a high false positive rate [52], with as many as 30% of indeterminate nodules identified by computed tomography found ultimately to be benign [79], indicating that there is a need for development of additional markers to increase specificity. As discussed previously, promoter hypermethylation can be an early event in lung carcinogenesis and, as such, may have utility in early detection of the disease.

Promoter hypermethylation of p16INK4a has been observed in NSCLC precursor lesions [115], and PTPRN2 promoter methylation is reported to be an early event in pulmonary adenocarcinoma, with detectable changes in the premalignant atypical adenomatous hyperplasia [177].

More important, some of these early epigenetic events can be detected by non- or minimally invasive sample collection techniques, the most important characteristic for cancer-screening applications. For example, aberrant DNA methylation can be detected in sputum [109, 127], bronchoalveolar aspirate/lavage [37, 43, 175] and saliva [75, 189] in patients with lung cancer. For example, CDKN2A and MGMT promoter methylation was detected in sputum as long as 3-years before lung cancer diagnosis [148] and promoter methylation of p16INK4a, MGMT, PAX5b, DAPK, GATA5, and in another study RASSF1A was detected in sputum 18 months before lung cancer diagnosis [22].

Diaz et al. aimed to identify epigenetic biomarkers with clinical utility for cancer diagnosis in minimally or non-invasive specimens to improve the accuracy of current technologies. They identified nine cancer-specific hypermethylated genes in early-stage lung primary tumors, four of which (*BCAT1, CDO1, TRIM58* and *ZNF177*) presented consistent CpG island-hypermethylation compared to nonmalignant tissue and were associated with transcriptional silencing. It was shown that this epigenetic signature achieved higher diagnostic efficacy in bronchial fluids as compared with conventional cytology for lung cancer diagnosis, indicating that minimally-invasive epigenetic biomarkers have emerged as promising tools for cancer diagnosis [41].

However, specificity can be an issue for some of these early markers; they can also be detected in individuals who never developed the disease, something that underscores the importance of multimarker panels. Interestingly, promoter methylation of p16INK4a has been detected in sputum from former and current smokers [21]. However, not all single markers are nonspecific, as exemplified by SHOX2 promoter methylation, which has demonstrated good sensitivity (68–78%) and specificity (95–96%) for NSCLC in bronchial aspirates (AUC, 86–94%) samples [43].

Breath capture methods are also evaluated for early detection of lung cancer. Breath capture methods can be based on direct breathing into an analysis platform or on the collection of exhaled breath through cooling devices (exhaled breath condensates, EBCs) [164]. EBC-based lung cancer diagnosis has recently become more relevant, especially since studies have reported that EBCs can also be used to detect DNA mutations and DNA methylation patterns in lung cancer patients [39]. A recent study demonstrated promoter hypermethylation of CDKN2A in EBC of 40% of the NSCLC patients that were analyzed using fluorescent quantitative methylation-specific PCR (F-MSP) [222]. However, DNA methylation of DAPK, PAX5beta, and RASSF1A has been also assayed in EBCs of lung cancer patients showing high variability between each individual [62]. The discrepancies between different reports might be explained through the fact that EBC is a highly diluted mixtures of compounds. Thus, EBC-based diagnosis of lung cancer requires appropriate stringent standardization protocols in order to reduce variability and increase sensitivity of the technique. Nevertheless, collecting EBCs is a promising new strategy of diagnosis of lung diseases, including lung cancer [135].

Three studies reported methylation of p16 and RARbata; two studies showed methylation of APC, RASSF1A, DAPK, SHP1P2, DLEC1, KLK10, and SFRP1. The other genes were reported to be methylated only once. The genes found to be hypermethylated in over 30% of NSCLC (based on at least two independent studies) were APC and RASSF1A. The methylation frequency of DAPK between different studies varied from 26.1% to 68.4%. Except for DAPK, the methylation frequencies of other genes had little differences across studies. Most of the studies involved controls; therefore, comparison of the data across cases and controls was possible. Methylation-specific PCR techniques have been employed by most of the studies to quantify the methylation statues of genes [104].

Many studies have demonstrated that hypermethylation in promoter region of RARb gene could be found with high prevalence in tumor tissue and autologous controls such as corresponding non-tumor lung tissue, sputum and plasma of the NSCLC patients, but due to the small number of subjects included in the individual study, the statistical power is limited. *Hua et al.* performed a meta-analysis using a systematic search strategy in PubMed, EMBASE and CNKI databases and calculated the pooled odds ratio (OR) of RARb promoter methylation in lung cancer tissue versus autologous controls. The results show a strong and significant correlation between tumor tissue and autologous controls of RARb gene promoter hypermethylation prevalence across studies, indicating that RARb promoter methylation may play an important role in carcinogenesis of the NSCLC [76].

Another team performed a meta-analysis to review the diagnostic ability of *CDH13* methylation in NSCLC as well as in its subsets. Thirteen studies, including 1850 samples were included in this meta-analysis. In a validation stage, 126 paired samples from TCGA were analyzed and 5 out of the 6 CpG sites in the CpG island of *CDH13* were significantly hypermethylated in lung adenocarcinoma tissues but none of the 6 CpG sites was hypermethylated in squamous cell carcinoma tissues. These pooled data showed that the methylation status of the *CDH13* promoter is strongly associated with lung adenocarcinoma. The *CDH13* methylation status could be a promising diagnostic biomarker for diagnosis of lung adenocarcinoma [157].

Han et al. investigated the correlation of hMLH1 promoter hypermethylation and NSCLC using 13 studies by comprising 1056 lung cancer patients via a meta-analysis. Initially, they observed that loss of hMLH1 protein expression was significantly associated with its promoter hypermethylation, hMLH1 gene inactivation through hypermethylation contributed to the tumorigenesis of NSCLC, and that there is a correlation between histologic subtypes/disease stages (TNM I + II vs III + IV) and hypermethylation status of hMLH1 gene.Finally, they found that NSCLC patients with hMLH1 hypermethylation and subsequent low expression levels of hMLH1 have a short overall survival period than those patients with normal expression of hMLH1 gene. Thus, they concluded that hMLH1 hypermethylation should be an early diagnostic marker for NSCLC and also a prognostic index for NSCLC. hMLH1 is an interesting therapeutic target in human lung cancers [63].

Abnormal miRNA expression and promoter methylation of genes detected in sputum may provide biomarkers for non-small lung cancer (NSCLC). In a recent study, they evaluated the individual and combined analysis of the two classes of sputum molecular biomarkers for NSCLC detection and they found that integrated analysis of 2 miRNAs (miR-31 and miR-210) and 2 genes (RASSF1A and 3OST2) yields higher sensitivity (87.3%) and specificity (90.3%) compared with the individual panels of the biomarkers ($P < 0.05$) [194].

6.2 Prognostic Biomarkers

Promoter methylation of RASSF1A [214, 227], PTEN, DAPK[198], p16INK4a [59, 93–95, 146], Wif-1, CXCL12 [197], DLEC1, MLH1 [179], CDH1, CDH [96], APC [26, 208], RUNX3 [227], SPARC and DAL1 have all been associated with NSCLC outcome [27, 196, 230]. In addition, DNMT1 overexpression in NSCLC is associated with decreased survival [93–95, 116] and DNMT3b, only in patients younger than 65 years [223]. Along similar lines, the CpG island methylator phenotype has also been correlated with prognosis in NSCLC. Relative to advanced-stage lung cancers, chemotherapeutic recommendations are not as clear for earlystage disease, with no true consensus regarding the optimal approach [193]. Early-stage lung cancer can be controlled locally, but exhibits a high recurrence rate. Completely resected stage IB and II tumors have a near-50% recurrence rate, with a median time to recurrence of 1 year [88]. Patients with stage IA tumors are less likely to experience a recurrence, although certain IA subsets have high recurrence rates [187]. Methylation of p16INK4a, RASSF1A, CDH13, and APC has been associated with early recurrence in surgically treated stage I NSCLCs [27]. The combination of FHIT and p16INK4a promoter methylation has also been associated with recurrence in stage I NSCLC [93–95].

The results of a metaanalysis suggest that *FHIT* hypermethylation is associated with an increased risk and worse survival in NSCLC patients. *FHIT* hypermethylation, which induces the inactivation of *FHIT* gene, plays an important role in the carcinogenesis and clinical outcome and may serve as a potential drug target of NSCLC [225]. Another recent study was the first to investigate SFRP3 expression and its potential clinical impact on non-small cell lung carcinoma (NSCLC). WNT signaling components present on NSCLC subtypes were preliminary elucidated by expression data of The Cancer Genome Atlas (TCGA). They identified a distinct expression signature of relevant WNT signaling components that differ between adenocarcinoma (LUAD) and squamous cell carcinoma (LUSC). Of interest, canonical WNT signaling is predominant in LUAD samples and non-canonical WNT signaling is predominant in LUSC. In line, high SFRP3 expression resulted in beneficial clinical outcome for LUAD but not for LUSC patients. Moreover, DNA hypermethylation of SFRP3 was evaluated in the TCGA methylation dataset resulting in epigenetic inactivation of SFRP3 expression in LUAD, but not in LUSC, and was validated by pyrosequencing of our NSCLC tissue cohort and in vitro demethylation experiments. Immunohistochemistry confirmed SFRP3 protein downregulation in primary NSCLC and indicated abundant expression in normal lung tissue. Thus, the above results indicate that SFRP3 acts as a novel putative tumor suppressor gene in adenocarcinoma of the lung possibly regulating canonical WNT signaling [173]. Functional analysis revealed that overexpressed *STXBP6* in A549 and H1299 cells significantly decreased cell proliferation, colony formation, and migration, and increased apoptosis. Finally, significantly lower survival rates ($P < 0.05$) were observed when expression levels of *STXBP6* were low, providing a basis for the genetic etiology of lung adenocarcinoma [112]. Moreover, recently *Zhang et al.* found that PAX6 gene was specifically methylated in NSCLC, and demonstrated the effect of promoter methylation of PAX6 gene on clinical outcome in NSCLC, indicating the methylated PAX6 may be useful biomarkers for prognostic evaluation in NSCLC [233]. Interestingly, it is found for the first time that *TMEM196* acts as a novel functional tumour suppressor inactivated by DNA methylation and is an independent prognostic factor of lung cancer. Multivariate analysis showed that patients with *TMEM196* expression had a better overall survival [127].

Targeted therapies can be successfully used in a subset of patients with lung adenocarcinomas (ADC), but they are not appropriate for patients with squamous cell carcinomas (SCC). In addition, there is a need for the identification of prognostic biomarkers that can select patients at risk of relapse in early stages. It has been shown that a high prometastatic serine protease TMPRSS4 expression is an independent prognostic factor in SCC. Similarly, aberrant hypomethylation in tumors correlates with high TMPRSS4 expression and could be used as an independent prognostic predictor in SCC. The inverse correlation between expression and methylation status was also observed in cell lines. *In vitro* studies showed that treatment of cells lacking TMPRSS4 expression with a demethylating agent significantly increased TMPRSS4 levels. In conclusion, TMPRSS4 is a novel independent prognostic biomarker regulated by epigenetic changes in SCC and a potential therapeutic target in this tumor type, where targeted therapy is still underdeveloped [212].

6.3 Methylated ctDNA as a Biomarker in Liquid Biopsy

Several studies have reported the potential of investigating tumor-specific methylation in blood for the screening and diagnosis of lung cancer. Determination of the methylation patterns of multiple genes to obtain complex ctDNA methylation signatures can contribute importantly to cancer development and/or progression. In recent years, methylation specific PCR has been successfully applied in the area of evaluating gene hypermethylation in the ctDNA, leading to highly sensitive and specific methodologies for NSCLC diagnosis.

6.3.1 Methylated ctDNA as a Marker for Early Diagnosis

Various gene promoters were found to be differentially methylated in ctDNA of lung cancer patients and healthy controls. These differences have been evaluated towards early detection of lung cancer and are summarized in Table 1. Epigenetically regulated genes have been evaluated for this purpose, such as Short stature homebox 2 (*SHOX2*) [100, 103], doublecortin like kinase 1 (*DCLK1*) [156], septin9 (*SEPT9*) [155], ras association domain family 1 isoform A (*RASSF1A*) and retinoic acid receptor B2 (*RARB2*) [154]. It is important to note that a large proportion of cases in these studies are late-stage cancers. Therefore, it has to be an inclusion of patients amenable to therapy in order to validate a biomarker useful for the screening and diagnosis of lung cancer [121].

Zhang Y et al. evaluated the methylation status of 20 tumor-suppressor genes in serum of NSCLC patients using methylation-specific PCR [232]. They report that nine genes (APC, CDH13, KLK10, DLEC1, RASSF1A, EFEMP1, SFRP1, RARbeta, and p16 (INK4A) were hypermethylated in NSCLC patients. The methylation frequencies in the plasma were consistent with those in the paired tumor tissues. The above results indicated that methylated alteration of multiple genes played important roles in NSCLC pathogenesis and the methylated genes in ctDNA might be potential candidate epigenetic biomarkers for NSCLC detection [54]. As the human 8-oxoguanine DNA glycosylase (hOGG1) gene promoter is frequently methylated in NSCLC, *Qin et al.* evaluated whether genetic or epigenetic alterations of hOGG1 are associated with increased risk of non-small cell lung cancer. The methylation profiles of peripheral blood mononuclear cell specimens from 121 NSCLC patients and 121 controls were determined through methylation-specific PCR of hOGG1. hOGG1 methylation-positive carriers had a 2.25-fold greater risk of developing NSCLC than methylation-free subjects. Furthermore, the demethylating agent 5 aza-2′-deoxycytidine restored hOGG1 expression in NSCLC cell lines. These data provide strong evidence of an association between peripheral blood mononuclear cell hOGG1 methylation and the risk of NSCLC in a Chinese population [159].

6.3.2 Methylated ctDNA as a Prognostic Marker

DNA methylation can be indicative of tumor aggressiveness and risk of cancer recurrence due to residual disease after surgical resection and/or chemotherapy. ctDNA has a short half-life (~2 h), and its persistence in the blood following surgery has been linked to poor prognosis [42]. In the context of early stage malignancies, prognostic biomarkers are urgently needed to distinguish patients who are cured with surgery alone, from those at high risk of disease recurrence who may benefit from adjuvant chemotherapy. The prognostic significance of gene promoter ctDNA methylation has been described in several studies, although most of them evaluate late-stage cancers, as summarized in Table 2.

Table 1 DNA methylation as a diagnostic biomarker in lung cancer

Study, year/ref	Gene	Sample	Patients	Controls	Biomarker classification
Palmisano et al. [148]	P16 and MGMT	Sputum	21 sputum samples and matched SCC tissues	123 cancer-free sputum samples	Diagnostic
Belinsky et al. [21]	*p16*	Sputum, plasma	56 plasma samples 56 sputum samples	195 normal plasma samples 121 sputum samples	Diagnostic
Belinsky et al. [22]	p16INK4a, MGMT, PAX5b, DAPK, GATA5, and RASSF1A	Sputum	98	92	Diagnostic
Licchesi et al. [115]	p16INK4a *TIMP3, DAPK, MGMT, RARβ, RASSF1A,* and *hTERT*	FFPEs	19 primary lung carcinomas	56 AAHs 46 histologically normal lung samples	Diagnostic
Selamat et al. [177]	PTPRN2	FFPEs	50 adenocarcinomas, 16 AIS	41 AAHs, 63 adjacent normal tissue	Diagnostic
Zhang et al. [232]	*APC, CDH13, KLK10, DLEC1, RASSF1A, EFEMP1, SFRP1, RARbeta,* and *p16 (INK4A)*	FFPEs, plasma	78 NSCLC FFPEs 110 NSCLC plasma samples	78 adjacent normal tissue 50 cancer-free plasma samples	Diagnostic
Dietrich et al. [43]	*SHOX2*	BAS	125	125	Diagnostic
Lee et al. [110]	*TMEFF2*	Serum	316	50	Diagnostic
Ponomaryova et al. [154]	*RASSF1A* and *RARB2*	Plasma	60	32	Diagnostic
Powrózek et al. [155]	*SEPT9*	Plasma	70	100	Diagnostic

(continued)

Table 1 (continued)

Study, year/ref	Gene	Sample	Patients	Controls	Biomarker classification
Diaz-Lagares et al. [41]	BCAT1, CDO1, TRIM58 and ZNF177	FFPEs, BAS, BAL, sputum	122 FFPEs, 51 BAS, 82 BAL, 72 sputum samples Discovery cohort: 237 FFPEs (181 lung adenocarcinomas and 56 SCCs)	79 FFPEs, 29 BAS, 29 BAL, 26 sputum samples Discovery cohort: 25 FFPEs	Diagnostic
Pu et al. [157]	CDH13 (meta-analysis)	Tissue/ serum	1206 in total; 1113 NSCLC tissue samples 93 serum samples	644 in total; 589 normal tissue samples 55 normal serum samples	Diagnostic
Han et al. [63]	hMLH1 (meta-analysis)	Tissue	912 lung cancer tissues	666 non-malignant lung tissues	Diagnostic
Konecny et al. [102]	SHOX2	Plasma	38	31	Diagnostic
Powrózek et al. [156]	DCLK1	Plasma	65	95	Diagnostic
Qin et al. [159]	hOGG1	Peripheral blood (PBMCs)	121	121	Diagnostic

AAH atypical adenomatous hyperplasia, *AIS* adenocarcinoma in situ, *FFPEs* formalin-fixed paraffin-embedded tissues, *SCC* squamous cell carcinoma, *NSCLC* non-small cell lung cancer, *BAS* bronchial aspirates, *BAL* bronchioalveoar lavages, *NM* not mentioned

Detection of methylated breast cancer metastasis suppressor-1 (*BRMS1*) and (sex determining region Y)-box 17 (*SOX17*) in operable and advanced NSCLC, was shown to have a negative impact on survival [9, 10]. In contrast, *SFN* (14–3-3 Sigma) promoter methylation was correlated with a reduced risk of death [163].

In SCLC evaluation of doublecortin-like kinase 1 (DCLK1) promoter region methylation may be useful in both early diagnosis and prediction of the course of lung cancer [156].

6.3.3 Methylated ctDNA in the Prediction and Monitoring of Response to Therapy

Several studies have reported the detection of tumor-specific methylation in plasma for tracking a patient's response to therapy as summarized in Table 3. The value of methylated ctDNA in plasma to predict response to therapy has also been investigated, although it is important to distinguish cfDNA from leukocytic DNA, because

Table 2 DNA methylation as a prognostic biomarker in lung cancer

Study, year/ref	Gene	Sample	Patients	Controls	Biomarker classification
Yanagawa et al. [227]	RASSF1A, RUNX3	Tissue	101	101 non-neoplastic lung tissues	Prognostic
Kim et al. [96]	CDH1, CDH	Tissue	88	88 adjacent normal tissues	Prognostic
Suzuki et al. [197]	CXCL12	Tissue	236	163 tissues adjacent to resected tumors	Prognostic
Seng et al. [179]	DLEC1, MLH1	FFPEs	239	200	Prognostic
Brock et al. [27]	p16INK4a, RASSF1A, CDH13, and APC, SPARC, and DAL1	FFPEs	71	116	Prognostic
Balgkouranidou et al. [9]	BRMS1	Plasma	122	24	Prognostic
Zhang et al. [233]	PAX6	Tissue	143	143 adjacent normal tissues	Prognostic
Liu et al. [127]	TMEM196	Tissue	85	20	Prognostic
Yan et al. [225]	FHIT (meta-analysis)	Tissue	735	708	Prognostic
Schlensog et al. [173]	SFRP3	Tissue	15	12	Prognostic
Villalba et al. [212]	TMPRSS4	Tissue	88	66	Prognostic
Balgkouranidou et al. [10]	SOX17	Plasma	122	49	Prognostic
Powrozek et al. [156]	DCLK1	Plasma	32	8	Prognostic

DNA methylation marks are coupled tightly to cellular differentiation and vary by cell type [73].

Wang and colleagues observed that there is an elevated level of adenomatous polyposis coli (APC) and RASSF1A promoter methylation in ctDNA within 24 h after cisplatin-based therapy, consistent with chemotherapy-induced cell death [216]. Moreover, methylation status of SHOX2, RASSF1A and RARB2 has shown potential to monitor disease recurrence after surgery and chemotherapy [174]. A recent manuscript addresses the role of O6-methylguanine-DNA methyltransferase (MGMT) as a biomarker in the oncogenesis of cancer and the opportunity of turning this gene into a drugable target in neuroendocrine tumours of the lung. Studies in brain tumours conclude that MGMT promoter methylation is considered

Table 3 DNA methylation as a predictive biomarker in lung cancer

Study, year/ref	Gene	Sample	Patients	Biomarker classification	Treatment
Ramirez et al. [163]	*14-3-3 sigma*	Serum	99 NSCLC	Predictive	Cisplatin plus gemcitabine
Salazar et al. [170]	*CHFR*	Serum	179	Predictive	EGFR tyrosine kinase inhibitors as second-line treatment
Wang et al. [216]	*APC* and *RASSF1A*	Plasma	216	Predictive	24 h after cisplatin-based therapy, consistent with chemotherapy-induced cell death
Schmidt et al. [174]	*SHOX2*, *RASSF1A* and *RARB2*	Plasma	31	Predictive	Clinical course of late stage lung cancer patients receiving a systemic treatment
Poirier et al. [153]	*EZH2*	Tissue	SCLC PDX	Predictive	EPZ-6438 inhibits tumor growth *in vivo* in SCLC PDX
Hiddinga et al. [67]	*MGMT*	Plasma	89 SCLC	Predictive	Temozolomide

SCLC PDX small cell lung cancer patient derived xenograft

a strong predictive factor for a favourable outcome for treatment with temozolomide, e.g. alkylating agent. In NSCLC MGMT promoter methylation is not a prognostic and predictive factor, hence temozolomide has no place. Temozolomide can be considered a 'personalized' treatment if the predictive role of the gene is further confirmed [67]. Another example of the use of DNA methylation as a predictive biomarker, are patients with unmethylated checkpoint with forkhead and ring finger domains (*CHFR*) promoter who survived longer when receiving EGFR tyrosine kinase inhibitors as second-line treatment, compared to conventional chemotherapy [170]. Furthermore, *Ramirez et al.* found that 14-3-3 sigma methylation in pretreatment serum may be an important predictor of NSCLC outcome in patients treated with platinum based chemotherapy [163]. Another study profiled DNA methylation in SCLC, patient-derived xenografts (PDX) and cell lines at single-nucleotide resolution. DNA methylation patterns of primary samples are distinct from those of cell lines, whereas PDX maintain a pattern closely consistent with primary samples. Clustering of DNA methylation and gene expression of primary SCLC revealed distinct disease subtypes among primary patient samples with similar genetic alterations which were histologically indistinguishable. SCLC is notable for dense clustering of high-level methylation in discrete promoter CpG islands, in a pattern clearly distinct from other lung cancers and strongly correlated with high expression of the E2F target and histone methyltransferase gene EZH2. Pharmacologic inhibition of EZH2 in a SCLC PDX markedly inhibited tumor growth [153]. Finally, with the demonstration that combined epigenetic therapy has efficacy in lung cancer patients [84], future applications of methylated ctDNA for monitoring the activity of demethylating agents will soon come to the forefront [121]. Thus, without careful study design, blood-based methylation profiles can be confounded by variation in relative circulating proportions of leukocyte types associated with outcome, such as immune response [107].

7 Conclusions

DNA methylation is a very early step in tumorigenesis and analysis of DNA methylation in clinical samples is very informative. DNA methylation markers have potential as prognostic markers and, accordingly, have been studied and reported widely in the literature. It is now known that a variety of hypermethylated tumor suppressor genes is implicated in lung cancer oncogenesis and have been associated with prognosis. Moreover, detection of DNA methylated sequences in plasma samples is a very important liquid biopsy approach that allows continuous monitoring of tumor evolution in real ime, in a non-invasive way.

Acknowledgements This manuscript was supported by the IMI contract no. 115749 CANCER-ID (E.L, S.M).

References

1. Abu Khaled M, Watkins CL, Krumdieck CL (1986) Inactivation of B12 and folate coenzymes by butyl nitrite as observed by NMR: implications on one-carbon transfer mechanism. Biochem Biophys Res Commun 135:201–207
2. Altenberger C, Heller C, Ziegler B, Tomasich E, Marhold M, Topakian T et al (2017) SPAG6 and L1TD1 are transcriptionally regulated by DNA methylation in non-small cell lung cancers. Mol Cancer 16:1
3. Andujar P, Wang J, Descatha A, Galateau-Sallé F, Abd-Alsamad I, Billon-Galland MA et al (2010) p16INK4A inactivation mechanisms in non-small-cell patients with lung cancer occupationally exposed to asbestos. Lung Cancer 67:23–30
4. Anisowicz A, Huang H, Braunschweiger KI, Liu Z, Giese H, Wang H et al (2008) A highthroughput and sensitive method to measure global DNA methylation: application in lung cancer. BMC Cancer 8:222
5. Ansari J, Shackelford RE, El-Osta H (2016) Epigenetics in non-small cell lung cancer: from basics to therapeutics. Transl Lung Cancer Res 5(2):155–171
6. Bailey-Wilson JE, Amos CI, Pinney SM, Petersen GM, de Andrade M, Wiest JS et al (2004) A major lung cancer susceptibility locus maps to chromosome 6q23-25. Am J Hum Genet 75:460–474
7. Baldwin DR, Duffy SW, Wald NJ, Page R, Hansell DM, Field JK (2011) UK lung screen (UKLS) nodule management protocol: modelling of a single screen randomised controlled trial of low-dose CT screening for lung cancer. Thorax 66(4):308–313
8. Balgkouranidou I, Liloglou T, Lianidou ES (2013) Lung cancer epigenetics: emerging biomarkers. Biomark Med 7(1):49–58
9. Balgkouranidou I, Chimonidou M, Milaki G, Tsarouxa EG, Kakolyris S, Welch DR et al (2014) Breast cancer metastasis suppressor-1 promoter methylation in cell-free DNA provides prognostic information in non-small cell lung cancer. Br J Cancer 110:2054–2062

10. Balgkouranidou I, Chimonidou M, Milaki G, Tsaroucha E, Kakolyris S, Georgoulias V et al (2016) SOX17 promoter methylation in plasma circulating tumor DNA of patients with non-small cell lung cancer. Clin Chem Lab Med 54:1385–1393
11. Balkwill F, Coussens LM (2004) Cancer: an inflammatory link. Nature 431:405–406
12. Bardelli A, Pantel K (2017) Liquid biopsies, what we do not know (yet). Cancer Cell 31(2):172–179
13. Barlesi F, Giaccone G, Gallegos-Ruiz MI, Loundou A, Span SW, Lefesvre P et al (2007) Global histone modifications predict prognosis of resected non small-cell lung cancer. J Clin Oncol 25(28):4358–4364
14. Barski A, Cuddapah S, Cui K, Roh TY, Schones DE, Wang Z et al (2007) High-resolution profiling of histone methylations in the human genome. Cell 129:823–837
15. Bartling B, Hofmann HS, Boettger T, Hansen G, Burdach S, Silber RE et al (2005) Comparative application of antibody and gene array for expression profiling in human squamous cell lung carcinoma. Lung Cancer 49:145–154
16. Bearzatto A, Conte D, Frattini M, Zaffaroni N, Andriani F, Balestra D et al (2002) p16(INK4A) Hypermethylation detected by fluorescent methylation-specific PCR in plasmas from non-small cell lung cancer. Clin Cancer Res 8(12):3782–3787
17. Beck CR, Garcia-Perez JL, Badge RM, Moran JV (2011) LINE-1 elements in structural variation and disease. Annu Rev Genomics Hum Genet 12:187–215
18. Belinsky SA (2005) Silencing of genes by promoter hypermethylation: key event in rodent and human lung cancer. Carcinogenesis 26:1481–1487
19. Belinsky SA (2015) Unmasking the lung cancer epigenome. Annu Rev Physiol 77:453–474
20. Belinsky SA, Nikula KJ, Palmisano WA, Michels R, Saccomanno G, Gabrielson E et al (1998) Aberrant methylation of p16(INK4a) is an early event in lung cancer and a potential biomarker for early diagnosis. Proc Natl Acad Sci U S A 95:11891–11896
21. Belinsky SA, Klinge DM, Dekker JD, Smith MW, Bocklage TJ, Gilliland FD et al (2005) Gene promoter methylation in plasma and sputum increases with lung cancer risk. Clin Cancer Res 11:6505–6511
22. Belinsky SA, Liechty KC, Gentry FD, Wolf HJ, Rogers J, Vu K et al (2006) Promoter hypermethylation of multiple genes in sputum precedes lung cancer incidence in a high-risk cohort. Cancer Res 66:3338–3344
23. Belinsky SA, Grimes MJ, Casas E, Stidley CA, Franklin WA, Bocklage TJ et al (2007) Predicting gene promoter methylation in non-small-cell lung cancer by evaluating sputum and serum. Br J Cancer 96(8):1278–1283
24. Berger AH, Knudson AG, Pandolfi PP (2011) A continuum model for tumour suppression. Nature 476:163–169
25. Blount BC, Mack MM, Wehr CM, MacGregor JT, Hiatt RA, Wang G et al (1997) Folate deficiency causes uracil misincorporation into human DNA and chromosome breakage: implications for cancer and neuronal damage. Proc Natl Acad Sci U S A 94:3290–3295
26. Brabender J, Usadel H, Danenberg KD, Metzger R, Schneider PM, Lord RV et al (2001) Adenomatous polyposis coli gene promoter hypermethylation in non-small cell lung cancer is associated with survival. Oncogene 20:3528–3532
27. Brock MV, Hooker CM, Ota-Machida E, Han Y, Guo M, Ames S et al (2008) DNA methylation markers and early recurrence in stage I lung cancer. N Engl J Med 358:1118–1128
28. Brzezianska E, Dutkowska A, Antczak A (2013) The significance of epigenetic alterations in lung carcinogenesis. Mol Biol Rep 40:309–325
29. Chen H, Suzuki M, Nakamura Y, Ohira M, Ando S, Iida T et al (2005) Aberrant methylation of FBN2 in human non-small cell lung cancer. Lung Cancer 50:43–49
30. Cheng J, Blum R, Bowman C, Hu D, Shilatifard A, Shen S et al (2014) A role for H3K4 mono-methylation in gene repression and partitioning of chromatin readers. Mol Cell 53:979–992
31. Chi P, Allis CD, Wang GG (2010) Covalent histone modifications – miswritten, misinterpreted and mis-erased in human cancers. Nat Rev Cancer 10:457–469
32. Christman JK (2002) 5-Azacytidine and 5-aza-2'-deoxycytidine as inhibitors of DNA methylation: mechanistic studies and their implications for cancer therapy. Oncogene 21:5483–5495

33. Cirincione R, Lintas C, Conte D, Mariani L, Roz L, Vignola AM et al (2006) Methylation profile in tumor and sputum samples of lung cancer patients detected by spiral computed tomography: a nested case–control study. Int J Cancer 118(5):1248–1253

34. Damiani LA, Yingling CM, Leng S, Romo PE, Nakamura J, Belinsky SA (2008) Carcinogeninduced gene promoter hypermethylation is mediated by DNMT1 and causal for transformation of immortalized bronchial epithelial cells. Cancer Res 68:9005–9014

35. Daskalos A, Logotheti S, Markopoulou S, Xinarianos G, Gosney JR, Kastania AN et al (2011) Global DNA hypomethylation-induced deltaNp73 transcriptional activation in non-small cell lung cancer. Cancer Lett 300:79–86

36. Daugaard I, Dominguez D, Kjeldsen TE, Kristensen LS, Hager H, Wojdacz TK et al (2016) Identification and validation of candidate epigenetic biomarkers in lung adenocarcinoma. Sci Rep 6:35807

37. de Fraipont F, Moro-Sibilot D, Michelland S, Brambilla E, Brambilla C, Favrot MC (2005) Promoter methylation of genes in bronchial lavages: a marker for early diagnosis of primary and relapsing non-small cell lung cancer? Lung Cancer 50:199–209

38. Dela Cruz CS, Tanoue LT, Matthay RA (2011) Lung cancer: epidemiology, etiology, and prevention. Clin Chest Med 32:605–644

39. Dent AG, Sutedja TG, Zimmerman PV (2013) Exhaled breath analysis for lung cancer. J Thorac Dis 5(Suppl 5):S540–S550

40. Destro A, Bianchi P, Alloisio M, Laghi L, Di Gioia S, Malesci A et al (2004) K-ras and p16(INK4A)alterations in sputum of NSCLC patients and in heavy asymptomatic chronic smokers. Lung Cancer 44(1):23–32

41. Diaz-Lagares J, Mendez-Gonzalez D, Hervas M, Saigi MJ, Pajares D, Garcia AB et al (2016) A novel epigenetic signature for early diagnosis in lung cancer. Clin Cancer Res 22(13):3361–3371

42. Diehl F, Schmidt K, Choti MA, Romans K, Goodman S, Li M et al (2008) Circulating mutant DNA to assess tumor dynamics. Nat Med 14:985–990

43. Dietrich D, Kneip C, Raji O, Liloglou T, Seegebarth A, Schlegel T et al (2012) Performance evaluation of the DNA methylation biomarker SHOX2 for the aid in diagnosis of lung cancer based on the analysis of bronchial aspirates. Int J Oncol 40:825–832

44. Eckhardt F, Lewin J, Cortese R, Rakyan VK, Attwood J, Burger M et al (2006) DNA methylation profiling of human chromosomes 6, 20 and 22. Nat Genet 38:1378–1385

45. Ellinger J, Kahl P, von der Gathen J, Rogenhofer S, Heukamp LC, Gutgemann I et al (2010) Global levels of histone modifications predict prostate cancer recurrence. Prostate 70:61–69

46. Estécio MR, Yan PS, Ibrahim AE, Tellez CS, Shen L, Huang TH et al (2007) High-throughput methylation profiling by MCA coupled to CpG island microarray. Genome Res 17:1529–1536

47. Fabbri M, Garzon R, Cimmino A, Liu Z, Zanesi N, Callegari E et al (2007) MicroRNA-29 family reverts aberrant methylation in lung cancer by targeting DNA methyltransferases 3A and 3B. Proc Natl Acad Sci U S A 104:15805–15810

48. Fang JY, Xiao SD (2003) Folic acid, polymorphism of methyl-group metabolism genes, and DNA methylation in relation to GI carcinogenesis. J Gastroenterol 38:821–829

49. Feinberg AP, Vogelstein B (1983) Hypomethylation distinguishes genes of some human cancers from their normal counterparts. Nature 301:89–92

50. Feng Q, Hawes SE, Stern JE, Wiens L, Lu H, Dong ZM et al (2008) DNA methylation in tumor and matched normal tissues from non-small cell patients with lung cancer. Cancer Epidemiol Biomarkers Prev 17:645–654

51. Feng N, Ching T, Wang Y, Liu B, Lin H, Shi O et al (2016) Analysis of microarray data on gene expression and methylation to identify long non-coding RNAs in non-small cell lung cancer. Sci Rep 6:37233

52. Field JK, Baldwin D, Brain K, Devaraj A, Eisen T, Duffy SW et al (2011) CT screening for lung cancer in the UK: position statement by UKLS investigators following the NLST report. Thorax 66:736–737

53. Fillmore CM, Xu C, Desai PT, Berry JM, Rowbotham SP, Lin Y-J et al (2015) EZH2 inhibition sensitizes BRG1 and EGFR mutant lung tumours to TopoII inhibitors. Nature 520:239–242

54. Fischer JR, Ohnmacht U, Rieger N, Zemaitis M, Stoffregen C, Manegold C et al (2007) Prognostic significance of RASSF1A promoter methylation on survival of non-small cell patients with lung cancer treated with gemcitabine. Lung Cancer 56:115–123
55. Forde PM, Brahmer JR, Kelly RJ (2014) New strategies in lung cancer: epigenetic therapy for non-small cell lung cancer. Clin Cancer Res 20:2244–2248
56. Fu J, Qin L, He T, Qin J, Hong J, Wong J et al (2011) The TWIST/Mi2/NuRD protein complex and its essential role in cancer metastasis. Cell Res 21(2):275–289
57. Gaudet F, Hodgson JG, Eden A, Jackson-Grusby L, Dausman J, Gray JW et al (2003) Induction of tumors in mice by genomic hypomethylation. Science 300(5618):489–492
58. Glazer CA, Smith IM, Ochs MF, Begum S, Westra W, Chang SS et al (2009) Integrative discovery of epigenetically derepressed cancer testis antigens in NSCLC. PLoS One 4:e8189
59. Gu J, Berman D, Lu C, Wistuba II, Roth JA, Frazier M et al (2006) Aberrant promoter methylation profile and association with survival in patients with non-small cell lung cancer. Clin Cancer Res 12:7329–7338
60. Gu Y, Wang C, Wang Y, Qiu X, Wang E (2009) Expression of thymosin beta10 and its role in non-small cell lung cancer. Hum Pathol 40:117–124
61. Gupta PK, Sahota A, Boyadjiev SA, Bye S, Shao C, O'Neill JP et al (1997) High frequency in vivo loss of heterozygosity is primarily a consequence of mitotic recombination. Cancer Res 57(6):1188–1193
62. Han W, Wang T, Reilly AA, Keller SM, Spivack SD (2009) Gene promoter methylation assayed in exhaled breath, with differences in smokers and lung cancer patients. Respir Res 10:86
63. Han Y, Shi K, Zhou SJ, Yu DP, Liu ZD (2016) The clinicopathological significance of *hMLH1* hypermethylation in non-small-cell lung cancer: a meta-analysis and literature review. Onco Targets Ther 9:5081–5090
64. Han M, Xu W, Cheng P, Jin H, Wang X (2017) Histone demethylase lysine demethylase 5B in development and cancer. Oncotarget 8(5):8980–8991
65. Hayami S, Yoshimatsu M, Veerakumarasivam A, Unoki M, Iwai Y, Tsunoda T et al (2010) Overexpression of the JmjC histone demethylase KDM5B in human carcinogenesis: involvement in the proliferation of cancer cells through the E2F/RB pathway. Mol Cancer 9:59
66. Heintzman ND, Stuart RK, Hon G, Fu Y, Ching CW, Hawkins RD et al (2007) Distinct and predictive chromatin signatures of transcriptional promoters and enhancers in the human genome. Nat Genet 39:311–318
67. Hiddinga BI, Pauwels P, Janssens A, van Meerbeeck JP (2016) O6-Methylguanine-DNA methyltransferase (MGMT): a drugable target in lung cancer? Lung Cancer. pii:S0169-5002(16)30412-3
68. Hoffman PC, Mauer AM, Vokes EE (2000) Lung cancer. Lancet 355:479–485
69. Holt D, Dreimanis M, Pfeiffer M, Firgaira F, Morley A, Turner D (1999) Interindividual variation in mitotic recombination. Am J Hum Genet 65(5):1423–1427
70. Hong JA, Kang Y, Abdullaev Z et al (2005) Reciprocal binding of CTCF and BORIS to the NY-ESO-1 promoter coincides with derepression of this cancer-testis gene in lung cancer cells. Cancer Res 65:7763–7774
71. Hong YS, Roh MS, Kim NY et al (2007) Hypermethylation of p16INK4a in Korean non-small cell patients with lung cancer. J Korean Med Sci 22:S32–S37
72. Hoque MO, Kim MS, Ostrow KL et al (2008) Genomewide promoter analysis uncovers portions of the cancer methylome. Cancer Res 68:2661–2670
73. Houseman EA, Accomando WP, Koestler DC et al (2012) DNA methylation arrays as surrogate measures of cell mixture distribution. BMC Bioinformatics 13:86
74. Hsu HS, Chen TP, Hung CH, Wen CK, Lin RK, Lee HC et al (2007) Characterization of a multiple epigenetic marker panel for lung cancer detection and risk assessment in plasma. Cancer 110(9):2019–2026
75. Hu YC, Sidransky D, Ahrendt SA (2002) Molecular detection approaches ⱴfor smoking associated tumors. Oncogene 21:ⱴ7289–ⱴ7297

76. Hua F, Fang N, Li X, Zhu S, Zhang W, Gu J (2014) A meta analysis of the relationship between RARb Gene promoter methylation and non-small cell lung cancer. PLoS One 9(5):e96163

77. Hubers AJ, Brinkman P, Boksem RJ, Rhodius RJ, Witte BI, Zwinderman AH et al (2014) Combined sputum hypermethylation and eNose analysis for lung cancer diagnosis. J Clin Pathol 67(8):707–711

78. Imre G, Gekeler V, Leja A et al (2006) Histone deacetylase inhibitors suppress the inducibility of nuclear factor kappaB by tumor necrosis factor-alpha receptor-1 downregulation. Cancer Res 66:5409–5418

79. Isbell JM, Deppen S, Putnam JB Jr et al (2011) Existing general population models inaccurately predict lung cancer risk in patients referred for surgical evaluation. Ann Thorac Surg 91:227–233

80. Ito M, Ito G, Kondo M et al (2005) Frequent inactivation of RASSF1A, BLU, and SEMA3B on 3p21.3 by promoter hypermethylation and allele loss in non-small cell lung cancer. Cancer Lett 225:131–139

81. Jang SJ, Soria JC, Wang L et al (2001) Activation of melanoma antigen tumor antigens occurs early in lung carcinogenesis. Cancer Res 61:7959–7963

82. Johnstone RW (2002) Histone-deacetylase inhibitors: novel drugs for the treatment of cancer. Nat Rev Drug Discov 1:287–299

83. Jones PA, Baylin SB (2002) The fundamental role of epigenetic events in cancer. Nat Rev Genet 3:415–428

84. Juergens RA, Wrangle J, Vendetti FP et al (2011) Combination epigenetic therapy has efficacy in patients with refractory advanced non-small cell lung cancer. Cancer Discov 1:598–607

85. Kalluri R, Weinberg RA (2009) The basics of epithelialmesenchymal transition. J Clin Invest 119(6):1420–1428

86. Kayser G, Sienel W, Kubitz B et al (2011) Poor outcome in primary non-small cell lung cancers is predicted by transketolase TKTL1 expression. Pathology 43:719–724

87. Ke XS, Qu Y, Rostad K, Li WC, Lin B, Halvorsen OJ et al (2009) Genome-wide profiling of histone h3 lysine 4 and lysine 27 trimethylation reveals an epigenetic signature in prostate carcinogenesis. PLoS One 4:e4687

88. Kelsey CR, Marks LB, Hollis D et al (2009) Local recurrence after surgery for early stage lung cancer: an 11-year experience with 975 patients. Cancer 115:5218–5227

89. Khaled MA, Krumdieck CL (1985) Association of folate molecules as determined by proton NMR: implications on enzyme binding. Biochem Biophys Res Commun 130:1273–1280

90. Kim DH, Nelson HH, Wiencke JK et al (2001) p16(INK4a) and histology-specific methylation of CpG islands by exposure to tobacco smoke in non-small cell lung cancer. Cancer Res 61:3419–3424

91. Kim H, Kwon YM, Kim JS et al (2004) Tumor-specific methylation in bronchial lavage for the early detection of non-small-cell lung cancer. J Clin Oncol 22:2363–2370

92. Kim JS, Han J, Shim YM, Park J, Kim DH (2005) Aberrant methylation of H-cadherin (CDH13) promoter is associated with tumor progression in primary nonsmall cell lung carcinoma. Cancer 104(9):1825–1833

93. Kim H, Kwon YM, Kim JS et al (2006a) Elevated mRNA levels of DNA methyltransferase-1 as an independent prognostic factor in primary nonsmall cell lung cancer. Cancer 107:1042–1049

94. Kim HR, Kim EJ, Yang SH et al (2006b) Trichostatin A induces apoptosis in lung cancer cells via simultaneous activation of the death receptor-mediated and mitochondrial pathway? Exp Mol Med 38:616–624

95. Kim JS, Kim JW, Han J, Shim YM, Park J, Kim DH (2006c) Cohypermethylation of p16 and FHIT promoters as a prognostic factor of recurrence in surgically resected stage I non-small cell lung cancer. Cancer Res 66:4049–4054

96. Kim DS, Kim MJ, Lee JY, Kim YZ, Kim EJ, Park JY (2007) Aberrant methylation of E-cadherin and H-cadherin genes in nonsmall cell lung cancer and its relation to clinicopathologic features. Cancer 110:2785–2792

97. Kim SH, Lee S, Lee CH et al (2009) Expression of cancer-testis antigens MAGE-A3/6 and NY-ESO-1 in non-small-cell lung carcinomas and their relationship with immune cell infiltration. Lung 187:401–411

98. Kimura H (2013) Histone modifications for human epigenome analysis. J Hum Genet 58:439–445

99. Kneip C, Schmidt B, Seegebarth A et al (2011) SHOX2 DNA methylation is a biomarker for the diagnosis of lung cancer in plasma. J Thorac Oncol 6:1632–1638

100. Komatsu N, Kawamata N, Takeuchi S et al (2006) SAHA, a HDAC inhibitor, has profound anti-growth activity against non-small cell lung cancer cells. Oncol Rep 15:187–191

101. Kondo M, Suzuki H, Ueda R et al (1995) Frequent loss of imprinting of the H19 gene is often associated with its overexpression in human lung cancers. Oncogene 10:1193–1198

102. Konecny M, Markus J, Waczulikova I et al (2016) The value of SHOX2 methylation test in peripheral blood samples used for the differential diagnosis of lung cancer and other lung disorders. Neoplasma 63:246–253

103. Kristensen LH, Nielsen AL, Helgstrand C, Lees M, Cloos P, Kastrup JS et al (2012) Studies of H3K4me3 demethylation by KDM5B/Jarid1B/PLU1 reveals strong substrate recognition *in vitro* and identifies 2,4-pyridine-dicarboxylic acid as an *in vitro* and in cell inhibitor. FEBS J 279:1905–1914

104. Kun N, Yujie J, Xuezhu Z (2015) Cell-free circulating tumor DNA in plasma/serum of non-small cell lung cancer. Tumour Biol 36(1):7–19

105. Labbé RM, Holowatyj A, Yang ZQ (2013) Histone lysine demethylase (KDM) subfamily 4: structures, functions and therapeutic potential. Am J Transl Res 6:1–15

106. Lander ES, Linton LM, Birren B et al (2009) Initial sequencing and analysis of the human genome. Nature 409(6822):860–921

107. Langevin SM, Kelsey KT (2013) The fate is not always written in the genes: epigenomics in epidemiologic studies. Environ Mol Mutagen 54:533–541

108. Langevin SM, Kratzke RA, Kelsey KT (2015) Epigenetics of lung cancer. Transl Res 165(1):74–90

109. Le Bras GF, Taubenslag KJ, Andl CD (2012) The regulation of cell-cell adhesion during epithelial-mesenchymal transition, motility and tumor progression. Cell Adh Migr 6(4):365–373

110. Lee SM, Park JY, Kim DS (2012 Aug) Methylation of TMEFF2 gene in tissue and serum DNA from patients with non-small cell lung cancer. Mol Cells 34(2):171–176

111. Leng S, Do K, Yingling CM et al (2012) Defining a gene promoter methylation signature in sputum for lung cancer risk assessment. Clin Cancer Res 18:3387–3395

112. Lenka G, Tsai MH, Lin HC, Hsiao JH, Lee YC, Lu TP et al (2017) Identification of methylation- driven, differentially expressed STXBP6 as a novel biomarker in lung adenocarcinoma. Sci Rep 7:42573

113. Li CT, Hsiao YM, Wu TC et al (2011) Vorinostat, SAHA, represses telomerase activity via epigenetic regulation of telomerase reverse transcriptase in non-small cell lung cancer cells. J Cell Biochem 112:3044–3053

114. Li X, Su Y, Pan J, Zhou Z, Song B, Xiong E et al (2013) Connexin 26 is down-regulated by KDM5B in the progression of bladder cancer. Int J Mol Sci 14:7866–7879

115. Licchesi JD, Westra WH, Hooker CM, Herman JG (2008) Promoter hypermethylation of hallmark cancer genes in atypical adenomatous hyperplasia of the lung. Clin Cancer Res 14:2570–2578

116. Lin RK, Hsu HS, Chang JW, Chen CY, Chen JT, Wang YC (2007) Alteration of DNA methyltransferases contributes to 5'CpG methylation and poor prognosis in lung cancer. Lung Cancer 55:205–213

117. Lin Q, Geng J, Ma K, Yu J, Sun J, Shen Z et al (2009) RASSF1A, APC, ESR1, ABCB1 and HOXC9, but not p16INK4A, DAPK1, PTEN and MT1G genes were frequently methylated in the stage I non-small cell lung cancer in China. J Cancer Res Clin Oncol 135(12):1675–1684

118. Lin RK, Hsieh YS, Lin P et al (2010a) The tobacco-specific carcinogen NNK induces DNA methyltransferase 1 accumulation and tumor suppressor gene hypermethylation in mice and lung cancer patients. J Clin Invest 120:521–532

119. Lin RK, Wu CY, Chang JW et al (2010b) Dysregulation of p53/Sp1 control leads to DNA methyltransferase-1 overexpression in lung cancer. Cancer Res 70:5807–5817
120. Lin SH, Wang J, Saintigny P, Wu CC, Giri U, Zhang J et al (2014) Genes suppressed by DNA methylation in non-small cell lung cancer reveal the epigenetics of epithelialmesenchymal transition. BMC Genomics 15:1079
121. Lissa D, Robles AI (2016) Methylation analyses in liquid biopsy. Transl Lung Cancer Res 5(5):492–504
122. Liu Y, An Q, Li L, Zhang D, Huang J, Feng X et al (2003) Hypermethylation of p16INK4a in Chinese lung cancer patients: biological and clinical implications. Carcinogenesis 24(12):1897–1901
123. Liu Y, Lan Q, Siegfried JM, Luketich JD, Keohavong P (2006) Aberrant promoter methylation of p16 and MGMT genes in lung tumors from smoking and never-smoking patients with lung cancer. Neoplasia 8:46–51
124. Liu Z, Zhao J, Chen XF et al (2008) CpG island methylator phenotype involving tumor suppressor genes located on chromosome 3p in non-small cell lung cancer. Lung Cancer 62:15–22
125. Liu F, Killian JK, Yang M et al (2010a) Epigenomic alterations and gene expression profiles in respiratory epithelia exposed to cigarette smoke condensate. Oncogene 29:3650–3664
126. Liu Z, Li W, Lei Z et al (2010b) CpG island methylator phenotype involving chromosome 3p confers an increased risk of nonsmall cell lung cancer. J Thorac Oncol 5:790–797
127. Liu WB, Han F, Jiang X, Chen HQ, Zhao H, Liu Y et al (2015) *TMEM196* acts as a novel functional tumour suppressor inactivated by DNA methylation and is a potential prognostic biomarker in lung cancer. Oncotarget 6(25):21225–21239
128. Lujambio A, Portela A, Liz J, Melo SA, Rossi S, Spizzo R et al (2010) CpG island hypermethylation-associated silencing of non-coding RNAs transcribed from ultraconserved regions in human cancer. Oncogene 29(48):6390–6401
129. Machida EO, Brock MV, Hooker CM et al (2006) Hypermethylation of ASC/TMS1 is a sputum marker for late-stage lung cancer. Cancer Res 66:6210–6218
130. Margaritis T, Oreal V, Brabers N, Maestroni L, Vitaliano-Prunier A, Benschop JJ et al (2012) Two distinct repressive mechanisms for histone 3 lysine 4 methylation through promoting 3'-end antisense transcription. PLoS Genet 8:e1002952
131. Marsit CJ, Houseman EA, Christensen BC et al (2006) Examination of a CpG island methylator phenotype and implications of methylation profiles in solid tumors. Cancer Res 66:10621–10629
132. Martin C, Zhang Y (2005) The diverse functions of histone lysine methylation. Nat Rev Mol Cell Biol 6:838–849
133. Marwick JA, Kirkham PA, Stevenson CS et al (2004) Cigarette smoke alters chromatin remodeling and induces proinflammatory genes in rat lungs. Am J Respir Cell Mol Biol 31:633–642
134. Massion PP, Carbone DP (2003) The molecular basis of lung cancer: molecular abnormalities and therapeutic implications. Respir Res 4:12
135. Mehta A, Dobersch S, Romero-Olmedo AJ, Barreto G (2015) Epigenetics in lung cancer diagnosis and therapy. Cancer Metastasis Rev 34:229–241
136. Meng X, Riordan NH (2006) Cancer is a functional repair tissue. Med Hypotheses 66:486–490
137. Minamiya Y, Ono T, Saito H et al (2010) Strong expression of HDAC3 correlates with a poor prognosis in patients with adenocarcinoma of the lung. Tumour Biol 31:533–539
138. Minamiya Y, Ono T, Saito H et al (2011) Expression of histone deacetylase 1 correlates with a poor prognosis in patients with adenocarcinoma of the lung. Lung Cancer 74:300–304
139. Miyanaga A, Gemma A, Noro R et al (2008) Antitumor activity of histone deacetylase inhibitors in non-small cell lung cancer cells: development of a molecular predictive model. Mol Cancer Ther 7:1923–1930
140. Mungall AJ, Palmer SA, Sims SK et al (2003) The DNA sequence and analysis of human chromosome 6. Nature 425:805–811

141. Nadal-Ribelles M, Mas G, Millan-Zambrano G, Sole C, Ammerer G, Chavez S et al (2015) H3K4 monomethylation dictates nucleosome dynamics and chromatin remodeling at stress-responsive genes. Nucleic Acids Res 43:4937–4949

142. Niklinska W, Naumnik W, Sulewska A, Kozłowski M, Pankiewicz W, Milewski R (2009) Prognostic significance of DAPK and RASSF1A promoter hypermethylation in non-small cell lung cancer (NSCLC). Folia Histochem Cytobiol 47(2):275–280

143. Northrop-Clewes CA, Thurnham DI (2007) Monitoring micronutrients in cigarette smokers. Clin Chim Acta 377:14–38

144. O'Hagan HM, Wang W, Sen S et al (2011) Oxidative damage targets complexes containing DNA methyltransferases, SIRT1, and polycomb members to promoter CpG Islands. Cancer Cell 20:606–619

145. Ortega RM, Lopez-Sobaler AM, Gonzalez-Gross MM et al (1994) Influence of smoking on folate intake and blood folate concentrations in a group of elderly Spanish men. J Am Coll Nutr 13:68–72

146. Ota N, Kawakami K, Okuda T et al (2006) Prognostic significance of p16(INK4a) hypermethylation in non-small cell lung cancer is evident by quantitative DNA methylation analysis. Anticancer Res 26:3729–3732

147. Ozdağ H, Teschendorff AE, Ahmed AA et al (2006) Differential expression of selected histone modifier genes in human solid cancers. BMC Genomics 7:90

148. Palmisano WA, Divine KK, Saccomanno G et al (2000) Predicting lung cancer by detecting aberrant promoter methylation in sputum. Cancer Res 60:5954–5958

149. Palmisano WA, Crume KP, Grimes MJ et al (2003) Aberrant promoter methylation of the transcription factor genes PAX5 alpha and beta in human cancers. Cancer Res 63:4620–4625

150. Patel K, Dickson J, Din S et al (2010) Targeting of 5-aza-2'- deoxycytidine residues by chromatin-associated DNMT1 induces proteasomal degradation of the free enzyme. Nucleic Acids Res 38:4313–4324

151. Pinskaya M, Morillon A (2009) Histone H3 lysine 4 di-methylation: a novel mark for transcriptional fidelity? Epigenetics 4:302–306

152. Piyathilake CJ, Macaluso M, Hine RJ, Richards EW, Krumdieck CL (1994) Local and systemic effects of cigarette smoking on folate and vitamin B-12. Am J Clin Nutr 60:559–566

153. Poirier JT, Gardner EE, Connis N, Moreira AL, de Stanchina E, Hann CL et al (2015) DNA methylation in small cell lung cancer defines distinct disease subtypes and correlates with high expression of EZH2. Oncogene 34(48):5869–5878

154. Ponomaryova AA, Rykova EY, Cherdyntseva NV et al (2013) Potentialities of aberrantly methylated circulating DNA for diagnostics and post-treatment follow-up of lung cancer patients. Lung Cancer 81:397–403

155. Powrózek T, Krawczyk P, Kucharczyk T et al (2014) Septin 9 promoter region methylation in free circulating DNA-potential role in noninvasive diagnosis of lung cancer: preliminary report. Med Oncol 31:917

156. Powrozek T, Krawczyk P, Nicos M, Kuznar-Kaminska B, Batura-Gabryel H, Milanowski J (2016) Methylation of the DCLK1 promoter region in circulating free DNA and its prognostic value in lung cancer patients. Clin Transl Oncol 18:398–404

157. Pu W, Geng X, Chen S, Tan L, Tan Y, Wang A et al (2016) Aberrant methylation of CDH13 can be a diagnostic biomarker for lung adenocarcinoma. J Cancer 7(15):2280–2289

158. Pulling LC, Divine KK, Klinge DM, Gilliland FD, Kang T, Schwartz AG et al (2003) Promoter hypermethylation of the O6- methylguanine-DNA methyltransferase gene: more common in lung adenocarcinomas from never-smokers than smokers and associated with tumor progression. Cancer Res 63(16):4842–4848

159. Qin H, Zhu J, Zeng Y et al (2017) Aberrant promoter methylation of hOGG1 may be associated with increased risk of non-small cell lung cancer. Oncotarget 8(5):8330–8341

160. Radhakrishnan VM, Jensen TJ, Cui H, Futscher BW, Martinez JD (2011) Hypomethylation of the 14-3-3sigma promoter leads to increased expression in non-small cell lung cancer. Genes Chromosom Cancer 50:830–836

161. Raji OY, Duffy SW, Agbaje OF et al (2012) Predictive accuracy of the Liverpool lung project risk model for stratifying patients for computed tomography screening for lung cancer: a case–control and cohort validation study. Ann Intern Med 157(4):242–250
162. Ramakrishnan S, Pokhrel S, Palani S, Pflueger C, Parnell TJ, Cairns BR et al (2016) Counteracting H3K4 methylation modulators Set1 and Jhd2 co-regulate chromatin dynamics and gene transcription. Nat Commun 7:11949
163. Ramirez JL, Rosell R, Taron M et al (2005) 14-3-3sigma methylation in pretreatment serum circulating DNA of cisplatin-plus-gemcitabine-treated advanced non-small-cell lung cancer patients predicts survival: the Spanish Lung Cancer Group. J Clin Oncol 23:9105–9112
164. Rattray NJ, Hamrang Z, Trivedi DK, Goodacre R, Fowler SJ (2014) Taking your breath away: metabolomics breathes life in to personalized medicine. Trends Biotechnol 32(10):538–548
165. Rauch T, Wang Z, Zhang X et al (2007) Homeobox gene methylation in lung cancer studied by genome-wide analysis with a microarray-based methylated CpG island recovery assay. Proc Natl Acad Sci U S A 104:5527–5532
166. Rauch TA, Zhong X, Wu X et al (2008) High-resolution mapping of DNA hypermethylation and hypomethylation in lung cancer. Proc Natl Acad Sci U S A 105:252–257
167. Renaud S, Pugacheva EM, Delgado MD et al (2007) Expression of the CTCF-paralogous cancer-testis gene, brother of the regulator of imprinted sites (BORIS), is regulated by three alternative promoters modulated by CpG methylation and by CTCF and p53 transcription factors. Nucl Acids Res 35:7372–7388
168. Richardson F, Young GD, Sennello R, Wolf J, Argast GM, Mercado P et al (2012) The evaluation of E-Cadherin and vimentin as biomarkers of clinical outcomes among patients with non-small cell lung cancer treated with erlotinib as second- or third-line therapy. Anticancer Res 32(2):537–552
169. Russo AL, Thiagalingam A, Pan H, Califano J, Cheng KH, Ponte JF et al (2005) Differential DNA hypermethylation of critical genes mediates the stage-specific tobacco smoke-induced neoplastic progression of lung cancer. Clin Cancer Res 11(7):2466–2470
170. Salazar F, Molina MA, Sanchez-Ronco M et al (2011) First-line therapy and methylation status of CHFR in serum influence outcome to chemotherapy versus EGFR tyrosine kinase inhibitors as second-line therapy in stage IV non-small-cell lung cancer patients. Lung Cancer 72:84–91
171. Sasaki H, Moriyama S, Nakashima Y et al (2004) Histone deacetylase 1 mRNA expression in lung cancer. Lung Cancer 46:171–178
172. Schiffmann I, Greve G, Jung M, Lübbert M (2016) Epigenetic therapy approaches in non-small cell lung cancer: update and perspectives. Epigenetics 11(12):858–870
173. Schlensog M, Magnus L, Heide T, Eschenbruch J, Steib F, Tator M et al (2016) Epigenetic loss of putative tumor suppressor SFRP3 correlates with poor prognosis of lung adenocarcinoma patients. Epigenetics
174. Schmidt B, Beyer J, Dietrich D et al (2015) Quantification of cell-free mSHOX2 plasma DNA for therapy monitoring in advanced stage non-small cell (NSCLC) and small-cell lung cancer (SCLC) patients. PLoS One 10:e0118195
175. Schmiemann V, Bocking A, Kazimirek M et al (2005) Methylation assay for the diagnosis of lung cancer on bronchial aspirates: a cohort study. Clin Cancer Res 11:7728–7734
176. Schuebel KE, Chen W, Cope L et al (2007) Comparing the DNA hypermethylome with gene mutations in human colorectal cancer. PLoS Genet 3:1709–1723
177. Selamat SA, Galler JS, Joshi AD et al (2011) DNA methylation changes in atypical adenomatous hyperplasia, adenocarcinoma in situ, and lung adenocarcinoma. PLoS One 6:e21443
178. Seligson DB, Horvath S, McBrian MA et al (2009) Global levels of histone modifications predict prognosis in different cancers. Am J Pathol 174:1619–1628
179. Seng TJ, Currey N, Cooper WA et al (2008) DLEC1 and MLH1 promoter methylation are associated with poor prognosis in non-small cell lung carcinoma. Br J Cancer 99:375–382
180. Seo SK, Jin HO, Woo SH et al (2011) Histone deacetylase inhibitors sensitize human non-small cell lung cancer cells to ionizing radiation through acetyl p53-mediated c-myc down-regulation. J Thorac Oncol 6:1313–1319

181. Shackelford RE, Kaufmann WK, Paules RS (1999) Cell cycle control, checkpoint mechanisms, and genotoxic stress. Environ Health Perspect 107(Suppl 1):5–24
182. Shames DS, Girard L, Gao B et al (2006) A genome-wide screen for promoter methylation in lung cancer identifies novel methylation markers for multiple malignancies. PLoS Med 3:e486
183. Shen X, Zhuang Z, Zhang Y, Chen Z, Shen L, Pu W et al (2015) JARID1B modulates lung cancer cell proliferation and invasion by regulating p53 expression. Tumour Biol 36:7133–7142
184. Shi Y, Lan F, Matson C, Mulligan P, Whetstine JR, Cole PA et al (2004) Histone demethylation mediated by the nuclear amine oxidase homolog LSD1. Cell 119.941–953
185. Shiba-Ishii A, Noguchi M (2012) Aberrant stratifin overexpression is regulated by tumor-associated CpG demethylation in lung adenocarcinoma. Am J Pathol 180:1653–1662
186. Shinjo K, Okamoto Y, An B et al (2012) Integrated analysis of genetic and epigenetic alterations reveals CpG island methylator phenotype associated with distinct clinical characters of lung adenocarcinoma. Carcinogenesis 33:1277–1285
187. Shoji F, Haro A, Yoshida T et al (2010) Prognostic significance of intratumoral blood vessel invasion in pathologic stage IA non-small cell lung cancer. Ann Thorac Surg 89:864–869
188. Siegel R, Naishadham D, Jemal A (2013) Cancer statistics, 2013. CA Cancer J Clin 63:11–30
189. Simkin M, Abdalla M, El-Mogy M, Haj-Ahmad Y (2012) Differences in the quantity of DNA found in the urine and saliva of smokers versus nonsmokers: implications for the timing of epigenetic events. Epigenomics 4:343–352
190. Singh A, Settleman J (2010) EMT, cancer stem cells and drug resistance: an emerging axis of evil in the war on cancer. Oncogene 29(34):4741–4751
191. Smith LT, Lin M, Brena RM et al (2006) Epigenetic regulation of the tumor suppressor gene TCF21 on 6q23-q24 in lung and head and neck cancer. Proc Natl Acad Sci U S A 103:982–987
192. Soini Y, Kosma VM, Pirinen R (2015) KDM4A, KDM4B and KDM4C in non-small cell lung cancer. Int J Clin Exp Pathol 8(10):12922–12928
193. Strauss GM, Herndon JE 2nd, Maddaus MA et al (2008) Adjuvant paclitaxel plus carboplatin compared with observation in stage IB non-small-cell lung cancer: CALGB 9633 with the Cancer and Leukemia Group B, Radiation Therapy Oncology Group, and North Central Cancer Treatment Group Study Groups. J Clin Oncol 26:5043–5051
194. Su Y, Fang HB, Jiang F (2016) Integrating DNA methylation and microRNA biomarkers in sputum for lung cancer detection. Clin Epigenetics 8:109
195. Suga Y, Miyajima K, Oikawa T, Maeda J, Usuda J, Kajiwara N et al (2008) Quantitative p16 and ESR1 methylation in the peripheral blood of patients with non-small cell lung cancer. Oncol Rep 20(5):1137–1142
196. Suzuki M, Hao C, Takahashi T et al (2005) Aberrant methylation of SPARC in human lung cancers. Br J Cancer 92:942–948
197. Suzuki M, Mohamed S, Nakajima T et al (2008) Aberrant methylation of CXCL12 in non-small cell lung cancer is associated with an unfavorable prognosis. Int J Oncol 33:113–119
198. Tang X, Khuri FR, Lee JJ et al (2000) Hypermethylation of the deathassociated protein (DAP) kinase promoter and aggressiveness in stage I non-small-cell lung cancer. J Natl Cancer Inst 92:1511–1516
199. Tekpli X, Skaug V, Bæra R, Phillips DH, Haugen A, Mollerup S (2016) Estrogen receptor expression and gene promoter methylation in non-small cell lung cancer – a short report. Cell Oncol (Dordr) 39(6):583–589
200. Thiery JP, Acloque H, Huang RY et al (2009) Epithelial-mesenchymal transitions in development and disease. Cell 139(5):871–890
201. Thinnes CC, England KS, Kawamura A, Chowdhury R, Schofield CJ, Hopkinson RJ (2014) Targeting histone lysine demethylases-progress, challenges, and the future. Biochim Biophys Acta 1839:1416–1432
202. Toyooka S, Maruyama R, Toyooka KO et al (2003) Smoke exposure, histologic type and geography-related differences in the methylation profiles of non-small cell lung cancer. Int J Cancer 103:153–160

203. Toyooka S, Suzuki M, Tsuda T et al (2004) Dose effect of smoking on aberrant methylation in non-small cell lung cancers. Int J Cancer 110:462–464
204. Toyooka S, Mitsudomi T, Soh J et al (2011) Molecular oncology of lung cancer. Gen Thorac Cardiovasc Surg 59:527–537
205. Toyota M, Ahuja N, Ohe-Toyota M et al (1999) CpG island methylator phenotype in colorectal cancer. Proc Natl Acad Sci U S A 96:8681–8686
206. Tsou JA, Galler JS, Siegmund KD, Laird PW, Turla S, Cozen W et al (2007) Identification of a panel of sensitive and specific DNA methylation markers for lung adenocarcinoma. Mol Cancer 6:70
207. Tsukada Y, Fang J, Erdjument-Bromage H, Warren ME, Borchers CH, Tempst P et al (2006) Histone demethylation by a family of JmjC domain-containing proteins. Nature 439:811–816
208. Usadel H, Brabender J, Danenberg KD et al (2002) Quantitative adenomatous polyposis coli promoter methylation analysis in tumor tissue, serum, and plasma DNA of patients with lung cancer. Cancer Res 62:371–375
209. Vaissiere T, Hung RJ, Zaridze D et al (2009) Quantitative analysis of DNA methylation profiles in lung cancer identifies aberrant DNA methylation of specific genes and its association with gender and cancer risk factors. Cancer Res 69:243–252
210. Van Den Broeck A, Brambilla E, Moro-Sibilot D et al (2008) Loss of histone H4K20 trimethylation occurs in preneoplasia and influences prognosis of non-small cell lung cancer. Clin Cancer Res 14:7237–7245
211. Vasilatos SN, Katz T, Oesterreich S, Wan Y, Davidson NE, Huang Y (2013) Crosstalk between lysine-specific demethylase 1 (LSD1) and histone deacetylases mediates antineoplastic efficacy of HDAC inhibitors in human breast cancer cells. Carcinogenesis 34:1196–1207
212. Villalba M, Diaz-Lagares A, Redrado M, de Aberasturi AL, Segura V, Bodegas ME et al (2016) Epigenetic alterations leading to TMPRSS4 promoter hypomethylation and protein overexpression predict poor prognosis in squamous lung cancer patients. Oncotarget 7(16):22752–22769
213. Wang YC, Lu YP, Tseng RC, Lin RK, Chang JW, Chen JT et al (2003) Inactivation of hMLH1 and hMSH2 by promoter methylation in primary non-small cell lung tumors and matched sputum samples. J Clin Invest 111(6):887–895
214. Wang J, Lee JJ, Wang L et al (2004) Value of p16INK4a and RASSF1A promoter hypermethylation in prognosis of patients with resectable non-small cell lung cancer. Clin Cancer Res 10:6119–6125
215. Wang M, Vikis HG, Wang Y et al (2007) Identification of a novel tumor suppressor gene p34 on human chromosome 6q25.1. Cancer Res 67:93–99
216. Wang H, Zhang B, Chen D et al (2015) Real-time monitoring efficiency and toxicity of chemotherapy in patients with advanced lung cancer. Clin Epigenetics 7:119
217. Weber M, Davies JJ, Wittig D, Oakeley EJ, Haase M, Lam WL et al (2005) Chromosome-wide and promoter-specific analyses identify sites of differential DNA methylation in normal and transformed human cells. Nat Genet 37(8):853–862
218. Weinberg RA (1995) The retinoblastoma protein and cell cycle control. Cell 81:323–330
219. Weiner A, Hsieh TH, Appleboim A, Chen HV, Rahat A, Amit I et al (2015) High-resolution chromatin dynamics during a yeast stress response. Mol Cell 58:371–386
220. Xiang Y, Zhu Z, Han G, Ye X, Xu B, Peng Z et al (2007) JARID1B is a histone H3 lysine 4 demethylase up-regulated in prostate cancer. Proc Natl Acad Sci U S A 104:19226–19231
221. Xiao D, He J (2010) Epithelial mesenchymal transition and lung cancer. J Thorac Dis 2(3):154–159
222. Xiao P, Chen JR, Zhou F, Lu CX, Yang Q, Tao GH et al (2014) Methylation of P16 in exhaled breath condensate for diagnosis of non-small cell lung cancer. Lung Cancer 83(1):56–60
223. Xing J, Stewart DJ, Gu J, Lu C, Spitz MR, Wu X (2008) Expression of methylation-related genes is associated with overall survival in patients with non-small cell lung cancer. Br J Cancer 98:1716–1722
224. Yamane K, Tateishi K, Klose RJ, Fang J, Fabrizio LA, Erdjument-Bromage H et al (2007) PLU-1 is an H3K4 demethylase involved in transcriptional repression and breast cancer cell proliferation. Mol Cell 25:801–812

225. Yan W, Xu N, Han X, Zhou XM, He B (2016) The clinicopathological significance of FHIT hypermethylation in non-small cell lung cancer, a meta-analysis and literature review. Sci Rep 6:19303
226. Yanagawa N, Tamura G, Oizumi H et al (2003) Promoter hypermethylation of tumor suppressor and tumor-related genes in non-small cell lung cancers. Cancer Sci 94(7):589–592
227. Yanagawa N, Tamura G, Oizumi H et al (2007) Promoter hypermethylation of RASSF1A and RUNX3 genes as an independent prognostic prediction marker in surgically resected non-small cell lung cancers. Lung Cancer 58:131–138
228. Yanagawa N, Tamura G, Oizumi H, Endoh M, Sadahiro M, Motoyama T (2011) Inverse correlation between EGFR mutation and FHIT, RASSF1A and RUNX3 methylation in lung adenocarcinoma: relation with smoking status. Anticancer Res 31:1211–1214
229. Yano M, Toyooka S, Tsukuda K et al (2005) Aberrant promoter methylation of human DAB2 interactive protein (hDAB2IP) gene in lung cancers. Int J Cancer 113:59–66
230. Yoshino M, Suzuki M, Tian L et al (2009) Promoter hypermethylation of the p16 andWif-1 genes as an independent prognostic marker in stage IA non-small cell lung cancers. Int J Oncol 35:1201–1209
231. Zhang F, Zhang T, Teng ZH et al (2009) Sensitization to gamma-irradiation-induced cell cycle arrest and apoptosis by the histone deacetylase inhibitor trichostatin A in nonsmall cell lung cancer (NSCLC) cells. Cancer Biol Ther 8:823–831
232. Zhang Y, Wang R, Song H, Huang G, Yi J, Zheng Y et al (2011) Methylation of multiple genes as a candidate biomarker in non-small cell lung cancer. Cancer Lett 303(1):21–28
233. Zhang X, Yang X, Wang J, Liang T, Gu Y, Yang D (2015) Down-regulation of *PAX6* by promoter methylation is associated with poor prognosis in non small cell lung cancer. Int J Clin Exp Pathol 8(9):11452–11457
234. Zhang J, Fu J, Pan Y, Zhang X, Shen L (2016) Silencing of miR-1247 by DNA methylation promoted non-small-cell lung cancer cell invasion and migration by effects of STMN1. Onco Targets Ther 9:7297–7307
235. Zhou Q, Agoston AT, Atadja P et al (2008) Inhibition of histone deacetylases promotes ubiquitin-dependent proteasomal degradation of DNA methyltransferase 1 in human breast cancer cells. Mol Cancer Res 6:873–883
236. Zochbauer-Muller S, Minna JD, Gazdar AF (2002) Aberrant DNA methylation in lung cancer: biological and clinical implications. Oncologist 7:451–457

DNA and Histone Methylation in Liver Cancer

Eri Arai, Takuya Yotani, and Yae Kanai

Abstract Epigenetic alterations, such as alterations of histone modification and DNA methylation, occur in a genome-wide manner under precancerous conditions resulting from hepatitis B virus (HBV) or hepatitis C virus (HCV) infection followed by chronic hepatitis and cirrhosis, or aberrant lipogenesis and abnormal metabolism of reactive oxygen species that characterize the pathophysiology of non-alcoholic steatohepatitis (NASH). Once DNA methylation alterations occur at the precancerous stage, they are stably preserved on DNA double strands through methylation maintenance by DNA methyltransferase 1 (*DNMT1*). DNA methylation alterations associated with abnormalities of DNA methyltransferase, such as overexpression of DNMT1 and splicing alterations of DNMT3B, participate in multistage hepatocarcinogenesis from the precancerous stage to the malignant progression stage and are correlated with aggressiveness of hepatocellular carcinomas (HCCs) and poorer outcome of affected patients. A number of tumor-related genes, such as *ATK3, APC, BMP4, CCL20, CDH1, CDKN2A, CDKN2B, CSPG2, DAB2IP, DCC, DLC1, DPT, DPYSL3, EMILIN2, FZD7, GRASP, GSTP1, HIST1H4F, IGFALS, MGMT, MZB1, NAT2, NEFH, NFATC1, PAX4, PDSS2, PER3, PROZ, PYCARD, RASSF1A, SPDY1, RUNX3, SCGB1D1, SFN, SMPD3, SOCS1, TIMP3, TLX3, TM6SF1, TRIM33, TRIM58, WFDC6, WNK2* and *ZFP41*, are known to be silenced by DNA hypermethylation in human HCCs. It is believed that DNA methylation alterations could be excellent biomarkers for carcinogenetic risk estimation and prognostication. To facilitate clinical application of DNA methylation diagnosis, a scaled-down device that allows quick and accurate analysis, even in small hospitals and clinics, is now being developed. One therapeutic strategy against HCC

E. Arai • Y. Kanai (✉)
Department of Pathology, Keio University School of Medicine,
35 Shinanomachi, Shinjuku-ku, Tokyo 160-8582, Japan
e-mail: ykanai@keio.jp

T. Yotani
Department of Pathology, Keio University School of Medicine,
35 Shinanomachi, Shinjuku-ku, Tokyo 160-8582, Japan

Tsukuba Research Institute, Research and Development Division, Sekisui Medical Co., Ltd,
Ibaraki 301-0852, Japan

© Springer International Publishing AG 2017
A. Kaneda, Y.-i. Tsukada (eds.), *DNA and Histone Methylation as Cancer Targets*,
Cancer Drug Discovery and Development, DOI 10.1007/978-3-319-59786-7_16

proliferation could involve a combination of epigenetic modifiers, such as a DNA methylation inhibitor, a histone deacetylase inhibitor and an S-adenosylhomocysteine hydrolase inhibitor, to sensitize cancer cells to conventional chemotherapies, in addition to eradication of hepatitis viruses for personalized and/or pre-emptive medical care.

Keywords DNA methylation • DNMT1 • DNMT3B • Hepatitis virus infection • Histone modification • Non-alcoholic steatohepatitis • Precancerous condition • Prognostication • Risk estimation

1 Introduction: Epigenomic Mechanism of Multistage Carcinogenesis

Epigenetic processes are defined as heritable alterations to biological information without changes in the DNA sequence. Such processes go beyond DNA-stored information and are essential for interpretation of the genome [32]. The modulation of epigenetic profiles contributes to embryonic development and differentiation, and underlies responses to environmental signals such as nutrients and inflammation [13]. Histone modification and DNA methylation are both key elements of epigenetic mechanisms and cooperatively determine chromatin configuration and regulate the levels of gene expression [32].

In vitro analysis using cultured cells or in vivo analysis using animal models is very important for clarifying the impact of epigenetic abnormalities on human carcinogenesis, but these alone are insufficient, and detailed analysis of human tissue specimens from large cohorts of clinical cases is essential. In addition, there has been insufficient accumulation of data from histone modification analyses (chromatin-immunoprecipitation [ChIP]) of human tissue specimens, probably due to the difficulty involved in achieving stable and reproducible fixation and fragmentation of large numbers of surgical specimens. On the other hand, DNA methylation analyses have been conducted using both the candidate-gene and genome-wide approaches, using techniques such as methylation-specific PCR [25], combined-bisulfite and restriction enzyme analysis [96], pyrosequencing [14], MassARAAY [34] and various methylation array systems, for large series of tissue specimens, including microdissected materials. Moreover, whole-genome bisulfite sequencing (WGBS) has been applied even for analysis of clinical tissue specimens. Therefore, the significance of DNA methylation alterations during human carcinogenesis is becoming better understood [33].

The most striking feature of DNA methylation alterations during human carcinogenesis is that they frequently occur even in precancerous conditions and early-stage cancers, suggesting that epigenetic alterations may precede mutations of tumor-suppressor genes, amplification of oncogenes and chromosomal instability.

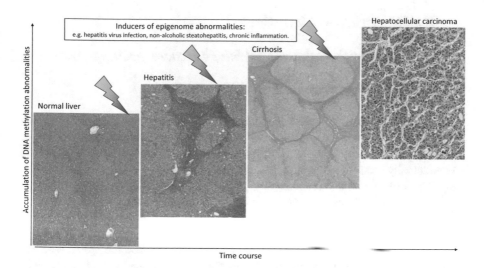

Fig. 1 DNA methylation alterations during multistage hepatocarcinogenesis. DNA methylation alterations occur in precancerous conditions due to hepatitis virus infection followed by chronic hepatitis and cirrhosis, or due to aberrant lipogenesis and aberrant metabolism of reactive oxygen species, which are the pathophysiologic hallmark of non-alcoholic steatohepatitis. Once DNA methylation alterations occur at the precancerous stage, they are inherited by or strengthened in hepatocellular carcinomas (HCCs) and determine tumor aggressiveness and patient outcome

Environmental factors including exposure to carcinogens influence epigenetic profiles. Thus, aberrant DNA methylation may be especially associated with precancerous conditions such as chronic inflammation and persistent viral infection [35]. In addition, DNA methylation alterations are frequently and significantly correlated with tumor aggressiveness and poorer outcome of patients with cancers. Therefore, on the basis of DNA methylation analysis, various biomarkers and therapeutic targets are now being explored [1].

In the case of hepatocarcinogenesis, the majority of hepatocellular carcinomas (HCCs) are known to be associated with hepatitis B virus (HBV) or hepatitis C virus (HCV) infection. Clonal expansion of hepatocytes is initiated during chronic hepatitis and liver cirrhosis, which are widely considered to be precancerous conditions. Small nodular lesions of early-stage HCC may develop in liver affected by chronic hepatitis and cirrhosis [86], and after further progression HCCs often emerge as nodule-in-nodule-type lesions in which the progressed HCC component is surrounded by the early HCC component [58]. Ordinary HCCs showing increased cell proliferation and neovascularization are then formed. Therefore, HCC can be considered a typical model of multistage carcinogenesis [28]. The significance of DNA methylation alterations during multistage carcinogenesis has been well studied using human liver tissue specimens at various steps of multistage hepatocarcinogenesis (Fig. 1).

2   DNA Methylation Alterations

2.1   *Viral Hepatitis-Related Multistage Hepatocarcinogenesis*

2.1.1   Early Findings at the Dawn of Epigenetics Research

In the early 1990s, various genetic alterations were revealed using classical techniques such as Southern blotting, especially in HCCs that were poorly differentiated, large in size, and associated with metastasis [28, 86]. However, only a few of the genetic events actually occurring in the earlier stage of hepatocarcinogenesis were detectable. Since DNA methylation alterations may be correlated with chromosomal instability, in 1996 we used Southern blotting with DNA methylation-sensitive restriction enzymes to examine DNA methylation status on chromosome 16, which is known to be a hot spot for loss of heterozygosity (LOH) in HCCs. In comparison with normal liver tissue samples obtained from patients without HCCs, DNA methylation alterations at multiple loci on chromosome 16 were frequently revealed, even in samples of non-cancerous liver tissue showing chronic hepatitis or cirrhosis with HBV or HCV infection. This was one of the earliest reports of DNA methylation alterations in liver at the precancerous stage [37]. In addition, the incidence of DNA methylation alterations on chromosome 16 was significantly correlated with higher histological grade, portal vein involvement and intrahepatic metastasis of HCCs. Since DNA methylation alterations were observed in both precancerous conditions and advanced HCCs, we speculated that such alterations at the precancerous stage might rapidly generate more malignant cancers [37].

The *CDH1* tumor suppressor gene is located on 16q22.1 near the hot spots for both DNA hypermethylation and LOH in HCC and encodes the E-cadherin Ca^{2+}-dependent cell-cell adhesion molecule that functions in the adherens junctions of epithelial cells. When *RB* and *VHL* were the only two genes known to be tumor suppressor genes silenced by DNA methylation, we demonstrated a significant correlation between DNA hypermethylation around the promoter region of the *CDH-1* gene and reduced expression of E-cadherin [99]. Reduction of E-cadherin expression may result in loss of intercellular adhesiveness and destruction of tissue morphology, which are the histological hallmarks of HCCs [38]. On the basis of our data, the E-cadherin gene was confirmed to be the third chronological example of a tumor suppressor gene silenced by DNA methylation, suggesting that LOH and DNA hypermethylation constitute another example of "two hits" that are capable of initiating cancers, in addition to the classical two-hit mechanism involving LOH and mutation.

In the late 1990s, microdissection techniques and PCR using microsatellite markers were developed for detecting LOH in small numbers of cells from paraffin-embedded tissue samples. This allowed us to examine microdissected specimens obtained from lobules, pseudo-lobules and regenerative nodules in non-cancerous liver tissue from patients with HCCs, and also the HCCs themselves. The incidence of DNA hypermethylation on CpG islands overwhelmed that of LOH at all stages of chronic hepatitis, liver cirrhosis and HCC, indicating that aberrant DNA methylation is an earlier event preceding chromosomal instability during hepatocarcinogenesis [45].

2.1.2 Abnormalities of DNA Methyltransferases (DNMTs) and Ten-Eleven Translocation Family Enzymes (TETs)

Abnormalities of DNMTs during hepatocarcinogenesis are considered likely to explain the molecular backgrounds of DNA methylation alterations. The major DNMT, DNMT1, shows a preference for hemimethylated over unmethylated substrates in vitro, and targets replication foci by binding to proliferating cell nuclear antigen (PCNA) [26]. Thus, DNMT1 has been recognized as a "maintenance" DNMT that allows copying of the DNA methylation pattern on the parental strand to the newly synthesized daughter DNA strand. Mutational inactivation of the *DNMT1* gene is not a major event in HCCs [39]. On the other hand, levels of *DNMT1* mRNA and protein are significantly higher in samples of non-cancerous liver tissue showing chronic hepatitis or cirrhosis than in normal liver tissue, and are even higher in HCCs [71, 80]. The incidence of *DNMT1* overexpression in HCCs is significantly correlated with histological features reflecting tumor aggressiveness, such as poorer tumor differentiation and portal vein involvement [73]. Moreover, the recurrence-free and overall survival rates of patients with HCCs showing *DNMT1* overexpression are significantly lower than those of patients with HCCs that do not [73].

The expression levels of *miR-200b* are significantly reduced in HCC tissue samples relative to normal liver tissue. Levels of *DNMT3A* expression are significantly higher in samples of HCC tissue, and *DNMT3A* is proposed to be a possible target gene for *miR-200b* [49]. In addition, a connection between HBV x protein (HBx) and DNMTs has been reported [69]. HBx upregulates the expression of *DNMT1* and *DNMT3A*, and selectively facilitates regional DNA hypermethylation around the promoter region of tumor suppressor genes [87]. Direct interaction between HBx and DNMT3A reportedly promotes recruitment of DNMT3A to the promoters of specific target genes, such as *MT1F* and *IL4*, or prevents DNMT3A recruitment to specific genomic loci, such as *CDH6* and *IGFBP3* [102].

On the other hand, germline mutations of the *DNMT3B* gene have been reported in patients with immunodeficiency, centromeric instability, and facial anomalies (ICF) syndrome, a rare recessive autosomal disorder characterized by DNA hypomethylation of pericentromeric satellite regions [24]. In HCCs, DNA hypomethylation of these regions is correlated with copy number alterations on chromosome 1, where satellite regions are rich [92]. Moreover, the major splice variant of *DNMT3B* in normal liver tissue is *DNMT3B3*, which possesses the conserved catalytic domains, whereas *DNMT3B4* lacks them while retaining the N-terminal domain required for targeting to heterochromatin sites. The level of *DNMT3B4* mRNA expression and the ratio of *DNMT3B4* mRNA to *DNMT3B3* mRNA in samples of non-cancerous liver tissue obtained from patients with HCCs, and in the HCCs themselves, were significantly correlated with the degree of DNA hypomethylation in pericentromeric satellite regions [72]. DNA demethylation on satellite 2 was observed in DNMT3B4-transfected human epithelial cells [72]. Since *DNMT3B4* lacking DNMT activity competes with *DNMT3B3* for targeting to pericentromeric satellite regions, *DNMT3B4* overexpression may lead to chromosomal instability through induction of DNA hypomethylation in such regions.

Furthermore, the growth rate of *DNMT3B4* transfectants was increased to a greater degree than in mock-transfectants at an early stage, when chromosomal instability may not yet have accumulated. Furthermore, an effector of interferon signaling, *STAT1*, was upregulated in *DNMT3B4* transfectants relative to mock-transfectants [72]. Later, it was reported that inhibition of DNA methylation in cultured human cancer cells by 5-aza-2′-deoxycytidine induced a set of genes implicated in interferon signaling, primarily via overexpression of *STAT1, 2* and *3* [40]. Thus, overexpression of *DNMT3B4* plays a role in multistage carcinogenesis not only by inducing chromosomal instability but also by affecting the expression of specific genes.

Recently, conversion of 5-methylcytosine to 5-hydroxymethylcytosine by TET family enzymes has attracted a great deal of attention as a mechanism of DNA demethylation. The level of 5-hydroxymethylcytosine was reportedly decreased in HCC tissues relative to non-tumorous tissues, and this decrease was associated with a larger tumor size, a higher alpha fetoprotein level and poorer patient outcome [53]. Moreover, a decreased level of 5-hydroxymethylcytosine in non-tumorous tissue was associated with tumor recurrence in the first year after surgical resection. Even in a diethylnitrosamine-induced animal model of HCC, the level of 5-hydroxymethylcytosine in the liver gradually fell during the period of induction [53]. A further reduction in tumorous tissues associated with an increase in the level of 5-methylcytosine was associated with capsular invasion, vascular thrombosis, tumor recurrence and overall survival. Expression of *TET1*, but not *TET2* and *TET3*, was downregulated in the HCCs, indicating that decreased expression of *TET1* is probably one of the mechanisms underlying the reduction of 5-hydroxymethylcytosine during hepatocarcinogenesis [53].

2.1.3   Genome-Wide DNA Methylation Analysis

For genome-wide profiling and stratification of patients with HCCs, we first employed bacterial artificial chromosome (BAC) array-based methylated CpG island amplification (BAMCA) [30]. Unlike promoter arrays, which can only examine regions directly participating in the regulation of expression, BAC array makes it possible to examine genomic regions in which DNA hypomethylation affects chromosomal instability and which are regulated in a coordinated manner in human cancers through a process of long-range epigenetic silencing [19]. In fact, using BAMCA, we have successfully identified many BAC clones showing DNA hypo- or hypermethylation in non-cancerous liver tissue from patients with HCCs in comparison with normal liver tissue from patients without HCCs. Patients showing

DNA hypo- or hypermethylation on more BAC clones in their non-cancerous liver tissue samples frequently developed metachronous or recurrent HCCs after hepatectomy, suggesting that DNA methylation alterations at the precancerous stage may render the liver prone to potential development of more malignant HCCs through induction of chromosomal instability and silencing of tumor-suppressor genes [2]. In HCCs themselves, more BAC clones showed DNA hypo- or hypermethylation, the degree of which was further increased in comparison with noncancerous liver tissue obtained from the same patients.

Recently, the Infinium Methylation Assay (Illumina) has facilitated quantitative measurement of methylation at the single-CpG-site level [8]. The Infinium assay employs a variety of probes, the most recently released being the MethylationEPIC BeadChip, covering a unique combination of over 850,000 methylation sites, including 99% of RefSeq genes, 95% of CpG islands, and the Encyclopedia of DNA Elements (ENCODE) enhancer regions. We have confirmed the reproducibility of the results of independently performed Infinium assays using the same human genomic DNA samples, and observed a good correlation between the results of WGBS and the Infinium assay. We have also verified the quantitative accuracy of the Infinium assay using pyrosequencing and the MassARRAY system [75]. Therefore, the Infinium assay is currently one of the most ideal techniques for analysis of many human tissue specimens from large cohorts [3]. Using the Infinium array, we have shown that DNA methylation levels on numerous probes are already altered in non-cancerous liver tissues with chronic hepatitis or cirrhosis, which are considered to be HBV or HCV viral hepatitis-related precancerous stages, and the HCCs themselves, relative to specimens of normal liver from patients without hepatitis virus infection, chronic hepatitis, liver cirrhosis or HCCs (unpublished data). Moreover, the Jonckheere-Terpstra trend test revealed that ordered differences in the levels of DNA methylation from normal liver tissue to liver tissues at the viral hepatitis-related precancerous stages, and then to HCCs themselves, occurred on about 21,000 probes, indicating that DNA methylation alterations were present even at these precancerous stages and were inherited by, or strengthened in HCCs. The DNA methylation alterations on these probes may continuously participate in multistage hepatocarcinogenesis from the precancerous to established cancer stage. Unsupervised hierarchical clustering using 21,000 such probes accurately classified all of the examined tissue samples into a cluster consisting mainly of normal liver tissue, a cluster consisting mainly of liver tissue at the precancerous stage, and a cluster consisting mainly of HCC, indicating that stepwise alterations of DNA methylation actually underlie multistage hepatocarcinogenesis (unpublished data).

When Infinium probes on which DNA methylation alterations were revealed even at precancerous stages and inherited by HCCs were separately identified in HBV-positive patients and HCV-positive patients, such alterations frequently occurred in gene bodies and non-coding regions in both HBV- and HCV-positive patients. The incidence of significant DNA methylation alterations was higher in HCV-positive than in HBV-positive patients. DNA hypermethylation appeared to be predominant in HCV-positive patients, whereas DNA hypomethylation was predominant in HBV-positive patients (unpublished data).

2.1.4   Epigenetically Regulated Tumor-Related Genes Participating in Hepatocarcinogenesis

Genome-wide procedures for analysis of DNA methylation status, such as array-based technologies and WGBS, have revealed many tumor-related genes whose expression levels are altered due to DNA hyper- or hypomethylation. For example, in HCCs, DNA hypermethylation-mediated silencing has been reported for cell cycle regulators such as *CDKN2A* [54] and *CDKN2B* [91], proapoptotic proteins such as *PYCARD* [46], matrix metalloproteinase inhibitor *TIMP3* [100] and DNA repair protein *MGMT* [56], and multifunctional tumor suppressor proteins such as *RASSF1A* [76], *SFN* [31] and *RUNX3* [60, 61]. DNA hypermethylation of *DLC1* (deleted in human liver cancer), located at chromosome 8p21.3–22 (a region frequently lost in various cancers including HCCs; [101]), significantly contributes to its silencing in primary HCCs [44, 52, 93]. DNA methylation of the cytokine mediator gene *SOCS1* [66] has attracted attention because it may activate the JAK/STAT signaling pathway and mediate the molecular link between inflammation and hepatocarcinogenesis. Recently, DNA hypermethylation of CpG islands in the *TRIM33* gene (transcriptional intermediary factor 1 gamma) has been reported to be responsible for its downregulation [15]. The expression level of *TRIM33* is decreased in HCC and this is associated with tumor stage and patient outcome. *TRIM33* reportedly inhibits the invasion and metastasis of HCC cells through suppression of TGF-β/Smad signaling. *DPYSL3* (dihydropyrimidinase-like 3), a cell adhesion molecule, is downregulated in HCC cell lines due to DNA hypermethylation. Knockdown of *DPYSL3* has been shown to enhance the migration and invasion of HCC cells. Moreover, patients with recurrence exhibited a significantly lower expression level of *DPYSL3* mRNA in their HCCs relative to those without recurrence [68]. *DPT* (dermatopontin), an acidic extracellular matrix protein that binds to α3β1 integrin, has also been shown to be silenced due to DNA hypermethylation. Downregulation of *DPT* was frequently observed in HCC tissues and was significantly associated with metastasis and poorer patient outcome [20]. Moreover, it was shown that inhibition of *DPT* resulted in dysregulation of focal adhesion assembly and a decrease of FAK phosphorylation via integrin signaling [20]. *PDSS2* (prenyl diphosphate synthase subunit 2), an essential enzyme involved in the biosynthesis of coenzyme Q10, may be possibly silenced by DNA hypermethylation in human HCCs. Aberrant expression of *PDSS2* in the liver may cause DNA damage and disrupt the cell cycle through inhibition of CoQ10 synthesis, resulting in poorer patient outcome [41]. In HBV-related HCC cells, silencing of *WNK2, EMILIN2, TRIM58, GRASP, TM6SF1, HIST1H4F,* and *TLX3* due to DNA hypermethylation has been reported [84].

In a study involving array-based analysis, Hernandez-Vargas et al. [27] demonstrated that a panel of hypermethylated gene promoters (*APC, RASSFIA, CDKN2A* and *FZD7*) were able to discriminate HCC tumors from paired surrounding nontumor liver tissues. Another set of hypermethylated genes (*e.g., NAT2, CSPG2* and *DCC*) were associated with HBV-related HCC [27]. Song et al. [79] found that *BMP4, CDKN2A, GSTP1,* and *NFATC1* were among a variety of genes with significant enrichment of promoter CpG island DNA methylation. In a genome-wide methylation study using plasma DNA from a cohort consisting predominantly of

HBV-positive HCC patients, Shen et al. [77] found that the top five hypermethylated genes were *DAB2IP, BMP4, ZFP41, SPDY1* and *CDKN2A*, whereas the top five hypomethylated genes were *CCL20, ATK3, SCGB1D1, WFDC6* and *PAX4*. Neumann et al. [64] reported that three candidate tumor-suppressor genes, *PER3, PROZ*, and *IGFALS*, showed abnormal methylation in HCCs, loss of the corresponding chromosomal regions, and re-expression after treatment with a demethylating agent. Matsumura et al. [57] also performed CpG island microarray analysis accompanied by treatment with a demethylating agent and, on the basis of their results, proposed *MZB1* as a new tumor-suppressor gene of HCC: down-regulation of *MZB1* was significantly associated with patient survival. Revill et al. [70] showed that transfection of HCC cell lines with *SMPD3* and *NEFH*, which are possible tumor-related genes silenced by DNA hypermethylation, led to cell growth inhibition, and that knockdown of these genes by small interfering RNA induced tumor formation and invasiveness in nude mice, indicating that these were potential tumor-suppressor genes. It has also been reported that expression of *SMPD3* was associated with recurrence-free survival after curative resection of HCC [70].

The transcription of non-coding RNAs, such as microRNA (miRNA) and long non-coding RNA, is also known to be regulated by DNA methylation. The role of miRNA in carcinogenesis is particularly well recognized. Coding regions of miRNA are generally located within the introns of host genes, and abnormal methylation of host genes leads to transcriptional inactivation of miRNA. Recent comprehensive methylation analyses have indicated that DNA hypermethylation of the *HOXB4* gene (the host gene of *miR-10a* located 1.46 kb upstream) possibly induces activation of the NF-κB signaling pathway and participates in HCC development [78].

With regard to the diagnostic impact of DNA hypomethylation in patients with HCCs [103], it has been reported that long interspersed nuclear element-1 (LINE-1) is significantly hypomethylated in tumor tissues relative to non-tumor tissues. Patients with LINE-1 hypomethylation exhibited significantly poorer outcome, and multivariate analysis revealed that LINE-1 hypomethylation was an independent risk factor for poorer overall and disease-free survival. The expression level of the LINE-1-inserted c-MET (L1-MET) gene was inversely correlated with the level of LINE-1 methylation, and positively correlated with c-MET expression. LINE-1 hypomethylation has a prognostic impact in patients with HCC, possibly due to activation of c-MET expression.

2.1.5 Carcinogenetic Risk Estimation and Prognostication Based on DNA Methylation Profiles

The effectiveness of surgical resection for HCC is limited, unless the disease is diagnosed early. Therefore, it is anticipated that surveillance at the precancerous stage will become a priority. Carcinogenetic risk estimation using liver biopsy specimens for baseline microscopy examination prior to interferon therapy would be advantageous for close follow-up of patients who are at high risk of HCC development.

To estimate the degree of carcinogenetic risk based on DNA methylation profiles using BAMCA, we omitted potentially insignificant BAC clones associated only with inflammation and/or fibrosis and focused on BAC clones for which DNA methylation status was inherited by HCCs from the precancerous stage. The top 25 BAC clones for which DNA methylation status was able to discriminate non-cancerous liver tissue from patients with HCCs in the learning cohort from normal liver tissue with sufficient sensitivity and specificity were identified using a bioinformatics approach [2].

However, CpG sites that are of diagnostic importance are unclear on BAC clones with an average insert size of 170 kbp [67]. In order to identify precisely CpG sites having the largest diagnostic impact, we quantitatively evaluated the DNA methylation status of 203 CpG sites on the top 25 BAC clones using pyrosequencing in tissue specimens. This again confirmed the reliability of BAMCA, which was able to provide an overview of DNA methylation in large regions of chromosomes, especially alterations occurring in a coordinated manner in the entire BAC region. Pyrosequencing-based quantification revealed that combining 30 regions including 45 specific CpG sites had a large diagnostic impact: the sensitivity and specificity for discrimination between normal liver tissues and liver tissues that had already generated HCCs were both almost 100% in the learning and validation cohorts [63]. The majority of the 30 regions used for defining the carcinogenetic risk estimation criteria were located within the gene bodies, non-CpG islands, and non-coding regions [63]. Although gene bodies, non-CpG islands, and non-coding regions have tended to be overlooked as targets of DNA methylation alterations in human cancers, it is feasible that DNA methylation alterations do not expand immediately to the promoter regions of tumor-related genes at the risk stage, but not in established cancers. Our findings indicate that gene bodies, non-CpG islands, and non-coding regions are also important for establishment of optimal diagnostic indicators.

To establish criteria for prognostication of patients with HCCs, Arai [2] defined HCC samples from patients who had survived more than 4 years after hepatectomy as a favorable-outcome group and HCC samples from patients who had suffered recurrence within 6 months and died within a year after hepatectomy as a poor-outcome group. Using appropriate cut-off values for each of the 41 BAC clones, the prognostication criteria were set to discriminate between the two groups. Multivariate analysis revealed that satisfying the criteria for more BAC clones was a predictor of recurrence, and was independent of known clinicopathological parameters reflecting tumor aggressiveness, such as the degree of histological differentiation and the presence/absence of portal vein tumor thrombi, intrahepatic metastasis and multi-centricity [2]. Such prognostication using liver biopsy specimens obtained before transarterial embolization and radiofrequency ablation may be advantageous even for patients who undergo such therapies.

Alterations of DNA methylation profiles are stably preserved on DNA double strands by covalent bonds as a result of the substrate preferences of DNMT1. Therefore, such methylation can be detected using a sufficiently sensitive method, even from a small sample volume, and for this reason it is believed that DNA methylation would be a better biomarker for carcinogenetic risk estimation and

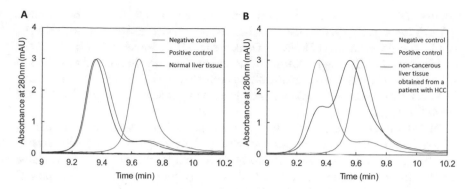

Fig. 2 Newly developed device for separating DNA fragments containing methylated-cytosine utilizing a high-performance liquid chromatography column. Representative chromatogram for normal liver tissue obtained from a patient without hepatocellular carcinoma (HCC) (**a**) and non cancerous liver tissue obtained from a patient with HCC (**b**). This newly developed technique is expected to facilitate quick and accurate analysis with a scaled-down model, even in small hospitals and clinics. Carcinogenetic risk estimation based on DNA methylation status in liver biopsy specimens may enable effective surveillance at the precancerous stage

prognostication than mRNA and protein expression profiles, which can be easily affected by the microenvironment of precursor cells [36]. Rapid and accurate quantification of methylated DNA is essential for application of DNA methylation diagnosis in hospitals and clinics. We are now developing a device based on polymer chemistry technology that can separate DNA fragments containing methylated cytosine: this optimizes the separation function of a high-performance liquid chromatography column for scaled-down implementation (unpublished data) (Fig. 2). This new approach is expected to facilitate quick and accurate analysis even in small hospitals and clinics, thus contributing to personalized and/or preemptive medical care.

2.2 Non-alcoholic Steatohepatitis (NASH)-Related Multistage Hepatocarcinogenesis

In addition to HBV or HCV infection followed by chronic hepatitis and liver cirrhosis, there has been an alarming increase in the incidence of NASH as a hepatic manifestation of metabolic syndrome, especially in developed countries [5]. NASH has become another precancerous condition for HCC via the development of liver cirrhosis. In addition, epigenomic alterations have recently attracted a great deal of attention as the molecular basis of not only cancer but also metabolic disorders [42]. In fact, studies using animal models of NASH have revealed a connection between the pathophysiological conditions for NASH and epigenome alterations [85]. For example, it has been shown that the ubiquitin-fold modifier 1 (Ufm1) conjugation pathway (Ufmylation), which is essential for protein degradation, protein quality control and signal transduction, was downregulated in 1,4-dihydro-2,4,6-trimethyl-3,5-pyridine-dicarboxylate (DDC)-fed NASH model mice and patients with NASH, resulting in the formation of Mallory-Denk bodies [10]. Moreover, levels of *DNMT1* and *DNMT3B* mRNA and DNA methylation levels in the promoter CpG region of *Ufm1*, *Ufc1* and *UfSP1* were markedly upregulated in NASH patients, suggesting that the maintenance of Ufmylation methylation might be mediated by *DNMT1* and *DNMT3B* together [10].

In order to clarify the significance of DNA methylation alterations, samples of normal liver tissue, non-cancerous liver tissue showing NASH, and NASH-related HCC were subjected to the Infinium assay. Even after Bonferroni correction, a large number of probes showed significant DNA methylation alterations in samples of non-cancerous liver tissue showing NASH relative to samples of normal liver tissue. The distinct DNA methylation profiles of NASH samples were clearly different from those of normal liver tissue samples and samples of non-cancerous liver tissue showing chronic hepatitis or cirrhosis associated with HBV or HCV infection (unpublished data). DNA methylation alterations in samples of non-cancerous liver tissue showing NASH were inherited by or strengthened in samples of NASH-related HCC (unpublished data). NASH- and NASH-related HCC-specific DNA methylation alterations, which were not evident in samples of non-cancerous liver tissue showing chronic hepatitis or cirrhosis, or in HCC associated with HBV or HCV infection, were observed in tumor-related genes and frequently associated with mRNA expression abnormalities, indicating that NASH-specific DNA methylation alterations may participate in NASH-related multistage hepatocarcinogenesis.

3   Histone Modification Alterations in HCCs

In addition to DNA methylation, histone modification is one of the key events of epigenetic alteration. Covalent histone modifications, especially histone methylation, mark active promoters (methylation of lysine 4 of histone H3 [H3K4]), active enhancers (H3K4 methylation), actively transcribed genes (H3K36 methylation), or heterochromatin regions (H3K9 methylation, H3K27 methylation) [23]. It has been reported that specific tumor-related genes are regulated by histone modification alterations. For example, generation of mouse HCC cells fused with mouse embryonic stem cells has revealed that enrichment of H3K27 trimethylation (me3), independent of H3K9 dimethylation (me2) and me3, associated with DNA methylation, is an early event in silencing of the *CDKN2A* gene during HCC development [97]. Another study has focused on suppression of the *CDKN2A* gene by HBx protein in hepatocarcinogenesis. Transfection of HCC cell lines with a HBx-expressing plasmid and immunohistochemistry of human HCCs with HBV infection have indicated that HBx can induce H3K9me3 in the promoter region of *CDKN2A* via a decrease in the expression of demethylase jumonji domain-containing protein 2B (JMJd2B) [89]. On the other hand, chromatin immunoprecipitation-sequencing (ChIP-seq) and gene expression profiling using microarray have identified *CLDN14* as a potential target for EZH2-mediated H3K27me3 in HCC [50]. Downregulation of *CLDN14* was significantly associated with advanced tumor stage and poorer outcome of HCC patients, probably due to enhancement of wnt/β-catenin signaling activity [50]. Epigenetic plasticity has an essential role in metabolic shift, i.e. from mitochondrial to glycolytic metabolism, in human HCC cells: during lysine-specific demethylase-1 (*LSD1*) inhibition in HCC cells, a set of mitochondrial metabolism genes was activated with concomitant increase of methylated histone H3K4 in the promoter regions [74].

Participation of histone methyltransferase in HCC development via a mechanism other than histone methylation has also been reported. *SETDB1* is a histone H3K9 methyltransferase located within a melanoma susceptibility locus. In HCCs, *SETDB1* is overexpressed with moderate copy number gain, together with mutation of the *TP53* gene, and the well-known hotspot gain-of-function mutation R249S associated with *SETDB1* overexpression [18]. Inactivation of *SETDB1* in HCC cell lines bearing the R249S mutation suppresses cell growth, and *TP53* mutation confers *SETDB1* dependence on cancer cells. Moreover, *SETDB1* forms a complex with *TP53* and catalyzes TP53K370me2, resulting in reduced recognition and degradation of TP53 by MDM2 [18].

In addition, a subset of histone deacetylases (HDACs) is increased in HCCs relative to normal liver tissues. It has been reported that *HDAC1* and *HDAC2* are upregulated from pre-neoplastic lesions to high-grade HCCs, whereas *HDAC6* is gradually downregulated [6]. Inactivation of *HDAC1* results in tumor cell regression and activation of caspase-independent autophagic cell death through activation of microtubule-associated protein 1 light chain 3 beta (MAP1LC3B) in HCCs cells [95]. On the other hand, depletion of *HDAC2* reportedly induces the expression of *CDKN1A* and *CDKN2A*, resulting in inhibition of G1/S cell cycle transition [65]. Thus, overexpression of *HDAC1* and *HDAC2*, which are class I HDACs, may play a pivotal role in the regulation of mitotic effectors during hepatocarcinogenesis. Treatment with the histone deacetylase inhibitor trichostatin A (TSA) and siRNA-knockdown of HDACs 1–3 in HCC cell lines followed by mRNA expression profiling have revealed that apoptotic protease-activating factor 1 (APAF1) is significantly upregulated after HDAC inhibition. The copy numbers of *HDAC3* and *HDAC5* DNA are altered, and their expression levels are significantly upregulated in HCC [9]. Moreover, the levels of *HDAC5* mRNA and protein are overexpressed in human HCC tissues, and inhibition of *HDAC5* represses the growth of HCC cell lines. Suppression of *HDAC5* induces apoptotic cell death and G1/S cell cycle arrest by regulating apoptosis-associated molecules and cell cycle regulators [16]. *HDAC8* is also overexpressed in HCCs and its knockdown represses tumor cell growth and induces apoptosis through p53 expression [94].

In NASH-related carcinogenesis, *HDAC8* is directly upregulated by the lipogenic transcription factor *SREBP-1* in dietary obesity models of NASH and HCC. Lentiviral-mediated *HDAC8* attenuation in vivo reverses insulin resistance and reduces tumorigenicity. *HDAC8* modulation has been shown to inhibit p53/p21-mediated apoptosis and G2-M phase cell-cycle arrest, and to stimulate β-catenin-dependent cell proliferation [85]. The molecular mechanism of this proliferation may involve physical interaction of *HDAC8* with the chromatin modifier EZH2, thus repressing Wnt antagonists via histone H4 deacetylation and H3K27me3 [85].

Components of chromatin-remodeling complexes are frequently mutated in HCC. *ARID1A*, a key component of the SWI/SNF chromatin-remodeling complex, is frequently mutated in HCC [104]. Huang et al. *[29]* have also shown that an aggressive cell line, HCC-LM6, contained *ARID1A* mutations that were absent from less metastatic cell lines. Knockdown of *ARID1A* promoted proliferation, migration and invasion. Mutations of genes such as *ARID2*, *MLL* and *MLL3*, encoding other epigenetic regulators, have also been reported. Fujimoto et al. [21] estimated that some form of chromatin regulator is mutated in about 50% of HCCs, indicating that aberrations in chromatin remodeling are a major hallmark of HCC.

4   Therapeutic Implications of Epigenetic Mechanisms in Patients with HCCs

DNA methylation has been shown to inactivate tumor-suppressor genes during hepatocarcinogenesis, suggesting a potential role of strong demethylating agents in the treatment of patients with HCCs. Combination of a DNA methylation inhibitor (5-aza-20- deoxycytidine [5-aza-dC]) with a histone deacetylase inhibitor (suberoylanilidehydroxamic acid [SAHA]) is considered to have potential clinical application [8]. On the other hand, increased expression of DNMTs in HBV-infected hepatocytes facilitates viral genome methylation and affects protein production and viral replication [87]. Therefore, potent demethylation treatment could lead to reactivation of HBV replication. In addition, dietary factors may also be potentially important for modulation of HBV replication, as deficiencies of folate, vitamin B12, choline and betaine can limit HBV methylation ability [90].

Histone deacetylase inhibitors (HDACs) such as TSA, panobinostat, valproic acid, belinostat and ITF2357 are known to have therapeutic activity against HCC cells [4, 22, 47, 55], and abexinostat, resminostat, givinostat, panobinostat, pracinostat, belinostat and CUDC-101 have yielded encouraging results as anti-cancer drugs in preclinical and clinical trials [62, 98].

3-Deazaneplanocin A (DZNep), an S-adenosylhomocysteine hydrolase inhibitor, has been shown to target polycomb proteins including EZH2 [82, 83]. Both loss of EZH2 and administration of DZNep have been shown to be effective in controlling the self-renewal and tumorigenic activity of tumor-initiating HCC [12]. EZH2 inhibitors, such as GSK126, EPZ005687, EI1, EPZ-6438 and EPZ011989, have been recently developed and may have the potential to target HCC tumorigenesis [43].

These epigenetic modifiers can act synergistically in combination with other traditional drugs. Inhibition of epigenetic regulators can sensitize cancer cells to conventional chemotherapies. Sorafenib, for example, has been shown to gain high effectiveness for control of HCC when used in combination with targeting *EZH2*, *ASH1L*, *C17ORF49* and *SETD4* [48, 88].

In addition, the limiting factor for elimination of HBV infection is clearance of the covalently closed circular DNA (cccDNA) pool from infected hepatocytes. Therefore, manipulation of the epigenetic regulation of the cccDNA minichromosome is a promising alternative therapeutic approach. Treatment with IFN-α has been shown to induce histone hypoacetylation of cccDNA and active recruitment of transcriptional co-repressors onto cccDNA in cultured cells [7]. IFN-α administration has also been shown to reduce binding of STAT1 and STAT2 transcription factors to active cccDNA [11]. Such cytokine treatment can activate the cellular response via epigenetic modification of cccDNA, which could mark the episome for selective eradication from infected cells or prevent cccDNA molecules from re-entering the nucleus after mitosis.

5 Analysis of the Hepatocyte Epigenome by the International Human Epigenome Consortium (IHEC)

On the basis of epigenome profiling of not only cancers but also neuronal, immune and metabolic disorders, attempts are now being made to elucidate the molecular pathogenesis of these diseases. In order to accurately identify disease-specific epigenome profiles, strict comparison with standard epigenome profiles of normal cells is indispensable. However, epigenome mechanisms show heterogeneity among various tissues and cell lineages. Therefore, it is not easy to obtain a comprehensive picture of the standard epigenome profiles of normal cells. Researchers and founding agencies from Canada, the EU, Germany, Hong Kong, Japan, Singapore, South Korea and the USA are now participating in the IHEC (http://ihec-epigenomes.org). At the establishment of the IHEC in 2010, an ambitious goal to decipher at least 1000 epigenomes within the next 7–10 years was declared. To achieve this goal, the consortium will use robust technologies to generate high-resolution maps of informative histone modifications, i.e. H3K4me3, H3K9me3, H3K27me3, H3K27ac, H3K4me1 and H3K36me3, high-resolution DNA methylation maps, and the entire catalogue of expression patterns including non-coding and small RNAs (Fig. 3). In Japan, three Japanese IHEC teams (http://crest-ihec.jp/) including our team are supported by the Core Research for Evolutional Science and Technology division of the Japan Agency for Medical Research and Development (AMED-CREST). To strengthen the research bases for HCCs, we have performed standard epigenome analyses of highly purified normal hepatocytes (Fig. 4). Samples of normal liver tissue were obtained distant from sites of liver metastases from primary colon cancers in partial hepatectomy specimens from patients without HBV or HCV infection, hepatitis or cirrhosis. To isolate hepatocytes, collagenase perfusion of cannulated branches of the hepatic vein was performed, followed by low-velocity centrifugation. Immunocytochemistry using Hep Par 1 antibody [17] has confirmed that the hepatocytes were more than 95% pure.

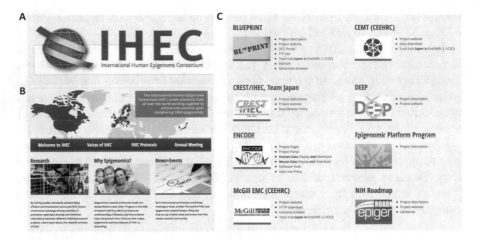

Fig. 3 International human epigenome consortium. (**a**) Logotype of the consortium. (**b**) Research outline of the IHEC from its webpage (http://ihec-epigenomes.org). (**c**) Individual research projects contributing to the IHEC appear on the website

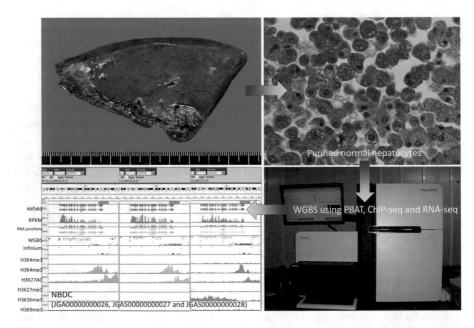

Fig. 4 Activities of our Japanese IHEC team (http://crest-ihec.jp/). To strengthen the research bases for HCCs, we have performed standard epigenome analyses of highly purified normal hepatocytes obtained from partial hepatectomy specimens of patients without hepatitis virus infection, chronic hepatitis or liver cirrhosis. The results of whole-genome bisulfite sequencing (WGBS) using post-bisulfite adaptor tagging (PBAT), chromatin immunoprecipitation-sequencing (ChIP-seq), and RNA-seq have been deposited in the National Bioscience Database Center (NBDC, http://humandbs.biosciencedbc.jp/en/, Accession number JGA00000000026, JGAS00000000027 and JGAS00000000028)

Hepatocytes of six Japanese patients were subjected to WGBS using post-bisulfite adaptor tagging (PBAT), CHIP-seq, RNA-seq and whole-genome sequencing. PBAT, an efficient library preparation method for WGBS, had been originally developed by members of our IHEC team [59]. The PBAT method minimally requires sub-microgram amounts of DNA for mammalian whole-genome bisulfite sequencing without global PCR amplification. A good correlation of the DNA methylation pattern was observed among PBAT, the standard Methyl C-seq methodology developed by Lister et al. [51], and the Infinium assay. Moreover, the PBAT method is advantageous in that it has good coverage of GC-rich regions, especially in CpG islands and gene-rich chromosomes.

Based on the epigenome landscape of human normal hepatocytes that we obtained, CpG methylation levels were low around the transcription start site and the first coding exon (unpublished data). Personal differentially methylated regions (pDMRs) were frequently observed in the vicinity of genetic variation loci, suggesting possible *cis*-acting genome-epigenome interaction (unpublished data). Genetic variations may induce epigenetic variations, generating individual differences in the phenotypes of normal hepatocytes through variations in expression.

6 Perspectives

Epigenome alterations, such as alterations of histone modification and DNA methylation, occur in precancerous conditions due to HBV or HCV infection followed by chronic hepatitis and cirrhosis, or due to aberrant lipogenesis and aberrant metabolism of reactive oxygen species, which are the pathophysiologic hallmark of NASH. DNA methylation alterations associated with DNA methyltransferase abnormalities participate in multistage hepatocarcinogenesis from the precancerous stage and may rapidly generate more malignant HCCs. Genome-wide DNA methylation profiling can provide optimal indicators for carcinogenetic risk estimation and prognostication. Comparison between IHEC reference epigenome profile data for normal hepatocytes and the epigenome profiles during viral hepatitis-related hepatocarcinogenesis and NASH-related hepatocarcinogenesis may facilitate accurate identification of disease-specific epigenome profiles, which would be indispensable to the development of more accurate disease biomarkers. Moreover, elucidation of the molecular backgrounds of DNA methylation alterations during hepatitis virus-related and NASH-related hepatocarcinogenesis may provide clues for epigenetic prevention and therapy of HCCs.

References

1. Arai E, Kanai Y (2010) DNA methylation profiles in precancerous tissue and cancers: carcinogenetic risk estimation and prognostication based on DNA methylation status. Epigenomics 2:467–481
2. Arai E, Ushijima S, Gotoh M, Ojima H, Kosuge T, Hosoda F, Shibata T, Kondo T, Yokoi S, Imoto I, Inazawa J, Hirohashi S, Kanai Y (2009) Genome-wide DNA methylation profiles in liver tissue at the precancerous stage and in hepatocellular carcinoma. Int J Cancer 125:2854–2862
3. Arai E, Chiku S, Mori T, Gotoh M, Nakagawa T, Fujimoto H, Kanai Y (2012) Single-CpG-resolution methylome analysis identifies clinicopathologically aggressive CpG island methylator phenotype clear cell renal cell carcinomas. Carcinogenesis 33:1487–1493
4. Armeanu S, Pathil A, Venturelli S, Mascagni P, Weiss TS, Göttlicher M, Gregor M, Lauer UM, Bitzer M (2005) Apoptosis on hepatoma cells but not on primary hepatocytes by histone deacetylase inhibitors valproate and ITF2357. J Hepatol 42:210–217
5. Asrih M, Jornayvaz FR (2015) Metabolic syndrome and nonalcoholic fatty liver disease: is insulin resistance the link? Mol Cell Endocrinol 418(Pt 1):55–65
6. Bae HJ, Jung KH, Eun JW, Shen Q, Kim HS, Park SJ, Shin WC, Yang HD, Park WS, Lee JY, Nam SW (2015) MicroRNA-221 governs tumor suppressor HDAC6 to potentiate malignant progression of liver cancer. J Hepatol 63:408–419
7. Belloni L, Allweiss L, Guerrieri F, Pediconi N, Volz T, Pollicino T, Petersen J, Raimondo G, Dandri M, Levrero M (2012) IFN-α inhibits HBV transcription and replication in cell culture and in humanized mice by targeting the epigenetic regulation of the nuclear cccDNA minichromosome. J Clin Invest 122:529–537
8. Bibikova M, Barnes B, Tsan C, Ho V, Klotzle B, Le JM, Delano D, Zhang L, Schroth GP, Gunderson KL, Fan JB, Shen R (2011) High density DNA methylation array with single CpG site resolution. Genomics 98:288–295
9. Buurman R, Sandbothe M, Schlegelberger B, Skawran B (2016) HDAC inhibition activates the apoptosome via Apaf1 upregulation in hepatocellular carcinoma. Eur J Med Res 21:26
10. Buzzanco A, Gomez A, Rodriguez E, French BA, Tillman BA, Chang S, Ganapathy E, Junrungsee S, Zarrinpar A, Agopian VG, Naini BV, French SW Jr, French SW Sr (2014) Digital quantitation of HCC-associated stem cell markers and protein quality control factors using tissue arrays of human liver sections. Exp Mol Pathol 97:399–410
11. Chen J, Wu M, Zhang X, Zhang W, Zhang Z, Chen L, He J, Zheng Y, Chen C, Wang F, Hu Y, Zhou X, Wang C, Xu Y, Lu M, Yuan Z (2013) Hepatitis B virus polymerase impairs interferon-α-induced STA T activation through inhibition of importin-α5 and protein kinase C-δ. Hepatology 57:470–482
12. Chiba T, Suzuki E, Negishi M, Saraya A, Miyagi S, Konuma T, Tanaka S, Tada M, Kanai F, Imazeki F, Iwama A, Yokosuka O (2012) 3-Deazaneplanocin A is a promising therapeutic agent for the eradication of tumor-initiating hepatocellular carcinoma cells. Int J Cancer 130:2557–2567
13. Claycombe KJ, Brissette CA, Ghribi O (2015) Epigenetics of inflammation, maternal infection, and nutrition. J Nutr 145:1109S–1115S
14. Colella S, Shen L, Baggerly KA, Issa JP, Krahe R (2003) Sensitive and quantitative universal pyrosequencing methylation analysis of CpG sites. BioTechniques 35:146–150
15. Ding ZY, Jin GN, Wang W, Chen WX, Wu YH, Ai X, Chen L, Zhang WG, Liang HF, Laurence A, Zhang MZ, Datta PK, Zhang B, Chen XP (2014) Reduced expression of transcriptional intermediary factor 1 gamma promotes metastasis and indicates poor prognosis of hepatocellular carcinoma. Hepatology 60:1620–1636
16. Fan J, Lou B, Chen W, Zhang J, Lin S, Lv FF, Chen Y (2014) Down-regulation of HDAC5 inhibits growth of human hepatocellular carcinoma by induction of apoptosis and cell cycle arrest. Tumour Biol 35:11523–11532
17. Fasano M, Theise ND, Nalesnik M, Goswami S (1998) Garcia de Davila MT, Finegold MJ, Greco MA. Immunohistochemical evaluation of hepatoblastomas with use of the

hepatocyte-specific marker, hepatocyte paraffin 1, and the polyclonal anti-carcinoembryonic antigen. Mod Pathol 11:934–938

18. Fei Q, Shang K, Zhang J, Chuai S, Kong D, Zhou T, Fu S, Liang Y, Li C, Chen Z, Zhao Y, Yu Z, Huang Z, Hu M, Ying H, Chen Z, Zhang Y, Xing F, Zhu J, Xu H, Zhao K, Lu C, Atadja P, Xiao ZX, Li E, Shou J (2015) Histone methyltransferase SETDB1 regulates liver cancer cell growth through methylation of p53. Nat Commun 6:8651

19. Frigola J, Song J, Stirzaker C, Hinshelwood RA, Peinado MA, Clark SJ (2006) Epigenetic remodeling in colorectal cancer results in coordinate gene suppression across an entire chromosome band. Nat Genet 38:540–549

20. Fu Y, Feng MX, Yu J, Ma MZ, Liu XJ, Li J, Yang XM, Wang YH, Zhang YL, Ao JP, Xue F, Qin W, Gu J, Xia Q, Zhang ZG (2014) DNA methylation-mediated silencing of matricellular protein dermatopontin promotes hepatocellular carcinoma metastasis by α3β1 integrin-Rho GTPase signaling. Oncotarget 5:6701–6715

21. Fujimoto A, Totoki Y, Abe T, Boroevich KA, Hosoda F, Nguyen HH, Aoki M, Hosono N, Kubo M, Miya F, Arai Y, Takahashi H, Shirakihara T, Nagasaki M, Shibuya T, Nakano K, Watanabe-Makino K, Tanaka H, Nakamura H, Kusuda J, Ojima H, Shimada K, Okusaka T, Ueno M, Shigekawa Y, Kawakami Y, Arihiro K, Ohdan H, Gotoh K, Ishikawa O, Ariizumi S, Yamamoto M, Yamada T, Chayama K, Kosuge T, Yamaue H, Kamatani N, Miyano S, Nakagama H, Nakamura Y, Tsunoda T, Shibata T, Nakagawa H (2012) Whole-genome sequencing of liver cancers identifies etiological influences on mutation patterns and recurrent mutations in chromatin regulators. Nat Genet 44:760–764

22. Gahr S, Mayr C, Kiesslich T, Illig R, Neureiter D, Alinger B, Ganslmayer M, Wissniowski T, Fazio PD, Montalbano R, Ficker JH, Ocker M, Quint K (2015) The pan–deacetylase inhibitor panobinostat affects angiogenesis in hepatocellular carcinoma models via modulation of CTGF expression. Int J Oncol 47:963–970

23. Gardner KE, Allis CD, Strahl BD (2011) Operating on chromatin, a colorful language where context matters. J Mol Biol 409:36–46

24. Hansen RS, Wijmenga C, Luo P, Stanek AM, Canfield TK, Weemaes CM, Gartler SM (1999) The DNMT3B DNA methyltransferase gene is mutated in the ICF immunodeficiency syndrome. Proc Natl Acad Sci U S A 96:14412–14417

25. Herman JG, Graff JR, Myöhänen S, Nelkin BD, Baylin SB (1996) Methylation-specific PCR: a novel PCR assay for methylation status of CpG islands. Proc Natl Acad Sci U S A 93:9821–9826

26. Hermann A, Gowher H, Jeltsch A (2004) Biochemistry and biology of mammalian DNA methyltransferases. Cell Mol Life Sci 61:2571–2587

27. Hernandez-Vargas H, Lambert MP, Le Calvez-Kelm F, Gouysse G, McKay-Chopin S, Tavtigian SV, Scoazec JY, Herceg Z (2010) Hepatocellular carcinoma displays distinct DNA methylation signatures with potential as clinical predictors. PLoS One 5:e9749

28. Hirohashi S (1991) Pathology and molecular mechanisms of multistage human hepatocarcinogenesis. Princess Takamatsu Symp 22:87–93

29. Huang J, Deng Q, Wang Q, Li KY, Dai JH, Li N, Zhu ZD, Zhou B, Liu XY, Liu RF, Fei QL, Chen H, Cai B, Zhou B, Xiao HS, Qin LX, Han ZG (2012) Exome sequencing of hepatitis B virus-associated hepatocellular carcinoma. Nat Genet 44:1117–1121

30. Inazawa J, Inoue J, Imoto I (2004) Comparative genomic hybridization (CGH)-arrays pave the way for identification of novel cancer-related genes. Cancer Sci 95:559–563

31. Iwata N, Yamamoto H, Sasaki S, Itoh F, Suzuki H, Kikuchi T, Kaneto H, Iku S, Ozeki I, Karino Y, Satoh T, Toyota J, Satoh M, Endo T, Imai K (2000) Frequent hypermethylation of CpG islands and loss of expression of the 14-3-3 sigma gene in human hepatocellular carcinoma. Oncogene 19:5298–5302

32. Jaenisch R, Bird A (2003) Epigenetic regulation of gene expression: how the genome integrates intrinsic and environmental signals. Nat Genet 33 Suppl:245–254

33. Jones PA, Issa J-P, Baylin S (2016) Targeting the cancer epigenome for therapy. Nat Rev Genet 17:630–641

34. Jurinke C, Denissenko MF, Oeth P, Ehrich M, van den Boom D, Cantor CR (2005) A single nucleotide polymorphism based approach for the identification and characterization of gene expression modulation using MassARRAY. Mutat Res 573:83–95
35. Kanai Y (2010) Genome-wide DNA methylation profiles in precancerous conditions and cancers. Cancer Sci 101:36–45
36. Kanai Y, Arai E (2014) Multilayer-omics analyses of human cancers: exploration of biomarkers and drug targets based on the activities of the International Human Epigenome Consortium. Front Genet 5:24
37. Kanai Y, Ushijima S, Tsuda H, Sakamoto M, Sugimura T, Hirohashi S (1996) Aberrant DNA methylation on chromosome 16 is an early event in hepatocarcinogenesis. Jpn J Cancer Res 87:1210–1217
38. Kanai Y, Ushijima S, Hui AM, Ochiai A, Tsuda H, Sakamoto M, Hirohashi S (1997) The E-cadherin gene is silenced by CpG methylation in human hepatocellular carcinomas. Int J Cancer 71:355–359
39. Kanai Y, Ushijima S, Nakanishi Y, Sakamoto M, Hirohashi S (2003) Mutation of the DNA methyltransferase (DNMT) 1 gene in human colorectal cancers. Cancer Lett 192:75–82
40. Kanai Y, Saito Y, Ushijima S, Hirohashi S (2004) Alterations in gene expression associated with the overexpression of a splice variant of DNA methyltransferase 3b, DNMT3b4, during human hepatocarcinogenesis. J Cancer Res Clin Oncol 130:636–644
41. Kanda M, Sugimoto H, Nomoto S, Oya H, Shimizu D, Takami H, Hashimoto R, Sonohara F, Okamura Y, Yamada S, Fujii T, Nakayama G, Koike M, Fujiwara M, Kodera Y (2014) Clinical utility of PDSS2 expression to stratify patients at risk for recurrence of hepatocellular carcinoma. Int J Oncol 45:2005–2012
42. Keating ST, El-Osta A (2015) Epigenetics and metabolism. Circ Res 116:715–736
43. Khan FS, Ali I, Afridi UK, Ishtiaq M, Mehmood R (2016) Epigenetic mechanisms regulating the developmentof hepatocellular carcinoma and their promise for therapeutics. Hepatol Int. doi:10.1007/s12072-016-9743-4
44. Kim TY, Jong HS, Song SH, Dimtchev A, Jeong SJ, Lee JW, Kim TY, Kim NK, Jung M, Bang YJ (2003) Transcriptional silencing of the DLC-1 tumor suppressor gene by epigenetic mechanism in gastric cancer cells. Oncogene 22:3943–3951
45. Kondo Y, Kanai Y, Sakamoto M, Mizokami M, Ueda R, Hirohashi S (2000) Genetic instability and aberrant DNA methylation in chronic hepatitis and cirrhosis – a comprehensive study of loss of heterozygosity and microsatellite instability at 39 loci and DNA hypermethylation on 8 CpG islands in microdissected specimens from patients with hepatocellular carcinoma. Hepatology 32:970–979
46. Kubo T, Yamamoto J, Shikauchi Y, Niwa Y, Matsubara K, Yoshikawa H (2004) Apoptotic speck protein-like, a highly homologous protein to apoptotic speck protein in the pyrin domain, is silenced by DNA methylation and induces apoptosis in human hepatocellular carcinoma. Cancer Res 64:5172–5177
47. Lachenmayer A, Toffanin S, Cabellos L, Alsinet C, Hoshida Y, Villanueva A, Minguez B, Tsai HW, Ward SC, Thung S, Friedman SL, Llovet JM (2012) Combination therapy for hepatocellular carcinoma: additive preclinical efficacy of the HDAC inhibitor panobinostat with sorafenib. J Hepatol 56:1343–1350
48. Li GM, Wang YG, Pan Q, Wang J, Fan JG, Sun C (2014) RNAi screening with shRNAs against histone methylation-related genes reveals determinants of sorafenib sensitivity in hepatocellular carcinoma cells. Int J Clin Exp Pathol 7:1085–1092
49. Li XY, Feng XZ, Tang JZ, Dong K, Wang JF, Meng CC, Wang J, Mo YW, Sun ZW (2016a) MicroRNA-200b inhibits the proliferation of hepatocellular carcinoma by targeting DNA methyltransferase 3a. Mol Med Rep 13:3929–3935
50. Li CP, Cai MY, Jiang LJ, Mai SJ, Chen JW, Wang FW, Liao YJ, Chen WH, Jin XH, Pei XQ, Guan XY, Zeng MS, Xie D (2016b) CLDN14 is epigenetically silenced by EZH2-mediated H3K27ME3 and is a novel prognostic biomarker in hepatocellular carcinoma. Carcinogenesis 37:557–566

51. Lister R, O'Malley RC, Tonti-Filippini J, Gregory BD, Berry CC, Millar AH, Ecker JR (2008) Highly integrated single-base resolution maps of the epigenome in Arabidopsis. Cell 133:523–536

52. Liu JB, Zhang YX, Zhou SH, Shi MX, Cai J, Liu Y, Chen KP, Qiang FL (2011) CpG island methylator phenotype in plasma is associated with hepatocellular carcinoma prognosis. World J Gastroenterol 17:4718–4724

53. Liu C, Liu L, Chen X, Shen J, Shan J, Xu Y, Yang Z, Wu L, Xia F, Bie P, Cui Y, Bian XW, Qian C (2013) Decrease of 5-hydroxymethylcytosine is associated with progression of hepatocellular carcinoma through downregulation of TET1. PLoS One 8:e62828

54. Matsuda Y, Ichida T, Matsuzawa J, Sugimura K, Asakura H (1999) p16(INK4) is inactivated by extensive CpG methylation in human hepatocellular carcinoma. Gastroenterology 116:394–400

55. Matsuda Y, Wakai T, Kubota M, Osawa M, Hirose Y, Sakata J, Kobayashi T, Fujimaki S, Takamura M, Yamagiwa S, Aoyagi Y (2014) Valproic acid overcomes transforming growth factor-β-mediated sorafenib resistance in hepatocellular carcinoma. Int J Clin Exp Pathol 7:1299–1313

56. Matsukura S, Soejima H, Nakagawachi T, Yakushiji H, Ogawa A, Fukuhara M, Miyazaki K, Nakabeppu Y, Sekiguchi M, Mukai T (2003) CpG methylation of MGMT and hMLH1 promoter in hepatocellular carcinoma associated with hepatitis viral infection. Br J Cancer 88:521–529

57. Matsumura S, Imoto I, Kozaki K, Matsui T, Muramatsu T, Furuta M, Tanaka S, Sakamoto M, Arii S, Inazawa J (2012) Integrative array-based approach identifies MZB1 as a frequently methylated putative tumor suppressor in hepatocellular carcinoma. Clin Cancer Res 18:3541–3551

58. Matsuno Y, Hirohashi S, Furuya S, Sakamoto M, Mukai K, Shimosato Y (1990) Heterogeneity of proliferative activity in nodule-in-nodule lesions of small hepatocellular carcinoma. Jpn J Cancer Res 81:1137–1140

59. Miura F, Enomoto Y, Dairiki R, Ito T (2012) Amplification-free whole-genome bisulfite sequencing by post-bisulfite adaptor tagging. Nucleic Acids Res 40:e136

60. Miyagawa K, Sakakura C, Nakashima S, Yoshikawa T, Kin S, Nakase Y, Ito K, Yamagishi H, Ida H, Yazumi S, Chiba T, Ito Y, Hagiwara A (2006) Down-regulation of RUNX1, RUNX3 and CBFbeta in hepatocellular carcinomas in an early stage of hepatocarcinogenesis. Anticancer Res 26:3633–3643

61. Mori T, Nomoto S, Koshikawa K, Fujii T, Sakai M, Nishikawa Y, Inoue S, Takeda S, Kaneko T, Nakao A (2005) Decreased expression and frequent allelic inactivation of the RUNX3 gene at 1p36 in human hepatocellular carcinoma. Liver Int 25:380–388

62. Mottamal M, Zheng S, Huang TL, Wang G (2015) Histone deacetylase inhibitors in clinical studies as templates for new anticancer agents. Molecules 20:3898–3941

63. Nagashio R, Arai E, Ojima H, Kosuge T, Kondo Y, Kanai Y (2011) Carcinogenetic risk estimation based on quantification of DNA methylation levels in liver tissue at the precancerous stage. Int J Cancer 129:1170–1179

64. Neumann O, Kesselmeier M, Geffers R, Pellegrino R, Radlwimmer B, Hoffmann K, Ehemann V, Schemmer P, Schirmacher P, Lorenzo Bermejo J, Longerich T (2012) Methylome analysis and integrative profiling of human HCCs identify novel protumorigenic factors. Hepatology 56:1817–1827

65. Noh JH, Jung KH, Kim JK, Eun JW, Bae HJ, Xie HJ, Chang YG, Kim MG, Park WS, Lee JY, Nam SW (2011) Aberrant regulation of HDAC2 mediates proliferation of hepatocellular carcinoma cells by deregulating expression of G1/S cell cycle proteins. PLoS One 6:e28103

66. Okochi O, Hibi K, Sakai M, Inoue S, Takeda S, Kaneko T, Nakao A (2003) Methylation-mediated silencing of SOCS-1 gene in hepatocellular carcinoma derived from cirrhosis. Clin Cancer Res 9:5295–5298

67. Osoegawa K, Mammoser AG, Wu C, Frengen E, Zeng C, Catanese JJ, de Jong PJ (2001) A bacterial artificial chromosome library for sequencing the complete human genome. Genome Res 11:483–496

68. Oya H, Kanda M, Sugimoto H, Shimizu D, Takami H, Hibino S, Hashimoto R, Okamura Y, Yamada S, Fujii T, Nakayama G, Koike M, Nomoto S, Fujiwara M, Kodera Y (2015) Dihydropyrimidinaselike 3 is a putative hepatocellular carcinoma tumor suppressor. J Gastroenterol 50:590–600

69. Park ES, Park YK, Shin CY, Park SH, Ahn SH, Kim DH, Lim KH, Kwon SY, Kim KP, Yang SI, Seong BL, Kim KH (2013) Hepatitis B virus inhibits liver regeneration via epigenetic regulation of urokinase-type plasminogen activator. Hepatology 58:762–776

70. Revill K, Wang T, Lachenmayer A, Kojima K, Harrington A, Li J, Hoshida Y, Llovet JM, Powers S (2013) Genome-wide methylation analysis and epigenetic unmasking identify tumor suppressor genes in hepatocellular carcinoma. Gastroenterology 145:1424–1435

71. Saito Y, Kanai Y, Sakamoto M, Saito H, Ishii H, Hirohashi S (2001) Expression of mRNA for DNA methyltransferases and methyl-CpG-binding proteins and DNA methylation status on CpG islands and pericentromeric satellite regions during human hepatocarcinogenesis. Hepatology 33:561–568

72. Saito Y, Kanai Y, Sakamoto M, Saito H, Ishii H, Hirohashi S (2002) Overexpression of a splice variant of DNA methyltransferase 3b, DNMT3b4, associated with DNA hypomethylation on pericentromeric satellite regions during human hepatocarcinogenesis. Proc Natl Acad Sci U S A 99:10060–10065

73. Saito Y, Kanai Y, Nakagawa T, Sakamoto M, Saito H, Ishii H, Hirohashi S (2003) Increased protein expression of DNA methyltransferase (DNMT) 1 is significantly correlated with the malignant potential and poor prognosis of human hepatocellular carcinomas. Int J Cancer 105:527–532

74. Sakamoto A, Hino S, Nagaoka K, Anan K, Takase R, Matsumori H, Ojima H, Kanai Y, Arita K, Nakao M (2015) Lysine Demethylase LSD1 coordinates glycolytic and mitochondrial metabolism in hepatocellular carcinoma cells. Cancer Res 75:1445–1456

75. Sato T, Arai E, Kohno T, Tsuta K, Watanabe S, Soejima K, Betsuyaku T, Kanai Y (2013) DNA methylation profiles at precancerous stages associated with recurrence of lung adenocarcinoma. PLoS One 8:e59444

76. Schagdarsurengin U, Wilkens L, Steinemann D, Flemming P, Kreipe HH, Pfeifer GP, Schlegelberger B, Dammann R (2003) Frequent epigenetic inactivation of the RASSF1A gene in hepatocellular carcinoma. Oncogene 22:1866–1871

77. Shen J, Wang S, Zhang YJ, Kappil M, Wu HC, Kibriya MG, Wang Q, Jasmine F, Ahsan H, Lee PH, Yu MW, Chen CJ, Santella RM (2012a) Genome-wide DNA methylation profiles in hepatocellular carcinoma. Hepatology 55:1799–1808

78. Shen J, Wang S, Zhang YJ, Kappil MA, Wu HC, Kibriya MG, Wang Q, Jasmine F, Ahsan H, Lee PH, Yu MW, Chen CJ, Santella RM (2012b) Genome-wide aberrant DNA methylation of microRNA host genes in hepatocellular carcinoma. Epigenetics 7:1230–1237

79. Song MA, Tiirikainen M, Kwee S, Okimoto G, Yu H, Wong LL (2013) Elucidating the landscape of aberrant DNA methylation in hepatocellular carcinoma. PLoS One 8:e55761

80. Sun L, Hui AM, Kanai Y, Sakamoto M, Hirohashi S (1997) Increased DNA methyltransferase expression is associated with an early stage of human hepatocarcinogenesis. Jpn J Cancer Res 88:1165–1170

81. Susanto JM, Colvin EK, Pinese M, Chang DK, Pajic M, Mawson A, Caldon CE, Musgrove EA, Henshall SM, Sutherland RL, Biankin AV, Scarlett CJ (2015) The epigenetic agents suberoylanilide hydroxamic acid and 5-AZA-2′ deoxycytidine decrease cell proliferation, induce cell death and delay the growth of MiaPaCa2 pancreatic cancer cells in vivo. Int J Oncol 46:2223–2230

82. Suva ML, Riggi N, Janiszewska M, Radovanovic I, Provero P et al (2009) EZH2 is essential for glioblastoma cancer stem cell maintenance. Cancer Res 69:9211–9218

83. Tan J, Yang X, Zhuang L, Jiang X, Chen W, Lee PL, Karuturi RK, Tan PB, Liu ET, Yu Q (2007) Pharmacologic disruption of Polycomb-repressive complex 2-mediated gene repression selectively induces apoptosis in cancer cells. Genes Dev 21:1050–1063

84. Tao R, Li J, Xin J, Wu J, Guo J, Zhang L, Jiang L, Zhang W, Yang Z, Li L (2011) Methylation profile of single hepatocytes derived from hepatitis B virus-related hepatocellular carcinoma. PLoS One 6:e19862

85. Tian Y, Wong VW, Wong GL, Yang W, Sun H, Shen J, Tong JH, Go MY, Cheung YS, Lai PB, Zhou M, Xu G, Huang TH, Yu J, To KF, Cheng AS, Chan HL (2015) Histone deacetylase HDAC8 promotes insulin resistance and β-catenin activation in NAFLD-associated hepatocellular carcinoma. Cancer Res 75:4803–4816

86. Tsuda H, Zhang WD, Shimosato Y, Yokota J, Terada M, Sugimura T, Miyamura T, Hirohashi S (1990) Allele loss on chromosome 16 associated with progression of human hepatocellular carcinoma. Proc Natl Acad Sci U S A 87:6791–6794

87. Vivekanandan P, Daniel HD, Kannangai R, Martinez-Murillo F, Torbenson M (2010) Hepatitis B virus vreplication induces methylation of both host and viral DNA. J Virol 84:4321–4329

88. Wang S, Zhu Y, He H, Liu J, Xu L, Zhang H, Liu H, Liu W, Liu Y, Pan D, Chen L, Wu Q, Xu J, Gu J (2013) Sorafenib suppresses growth and survival of hepatoma cells by accelerating degradation of enhancer of zeste homolog 2. Cancer Sci 104:750–759

89. Wang DY, Zou LP, Liu XJ, Zhu HG, Zhu R (2015) Hepatitis B virus X protein induces the histone H3 lysine 9 trimethylation on the promoter of p16 gene in hepatocarcinogenesis. Exp Mol Pathol 99:399–408

90. Waterland RA (2006) AssessingtheeffectsofhighmethionineintakeonDNA methylation. J Nutr 136:1706S–1710S

91. Wong IH, Lo YM, Yeo W, Lau WY, Johnson PJ (2000) Frequent p15 promoter methylation in tumor and peripheral blood from hepatocellular carcinoma patients. Clin Cancer Res 6:3516–3521

92. Wong N, Lam WC, Lai PB, Pang E, Lau WY, Johnson PJ (2001) Hypomethylation of chromosome 1 heterochromatin DNA correlates with q-arm copy gain in human hepatocellular carcinoma. Am J Pathol 159:465–471

93. Wong CM, Lee JM, Ching YP, Jin DY, Ng IO (2003) Genetic and epigenetic alterations of DLC-1 gene in hepatocellular carcinoma. Cancer Res 63:7646–7651

94. Wu J, Du C, Lv Z, Ding C, Cheng J, Xie H, Zhou L, Zheng S (2013) The up-regulation of histone deacetylase 8 promotes proliferation and inhibits apoptosis in hepatocellular carcinoma. Dig Dis Sci 58:3545–3553

95. Xie HJ, Noh JH, Kim JK, Jung KH, Eun JW, Bae HJ, Kim MG, Chang YG, Lee JY, Park H, Nam SW (2012) HDAC1 inactivation induces mitotic defect and caspase-independent autophagic cell death in liver cancer. PLoS One 7:e34265

96. Xiong Z, Laird PW (1997) COBRA: a sensitive and quantitative DNA methylation assay. Nucleic Acids Res 25:2532–2534

97. Yao JY, Zhang L, Zhang X, He ZY, Ma Y, Hui LJ, Wang X, Hu YP (2010) H3K27 trimethylation is an early epigenetic event of p16INK4a silencing for regaining tumorigenesis in fusion reprogrammed hepatoma cells. J Biol Chem 285:18828–18837

98. Yeo W, Chung HC, Chan SL, Wang LZ, Lim R, Picus J, Boyer M, Mo FK, Koh J, Rha SY, Hui EP, Jeung HC, Roh JK, Yu SC, To KF, Tao Q, Ma BB, Chan AW, Tong JH, Erlichman C, Chan AT, Goh BC (2012) Epigenetic therapy using belinostat for patients with unresectable hepatocellular carcinoma: a multicenter phase I/II study with biomarker and pharmacokinetic analysis of tumors from patients in the Mayo Phase II Consortium and the Cancer Therapeutics Research Group. J Clin Oncol 30:3361–3367

99. Yoshiura K, Kanai Y, Ochiai A, Shimoyama Y, Sugimura T, Hirohashi S (1995) Silencing of the E-cadherin invasion-suppressor gene by CpG methylation in human carcinomas. Proc Natl Acad Sci U S A 92:7416–7419

100. Yu J, Ni M, Xu J, Zhang H, Gao B, Gu J, Chen J, Zhang L, Wu M, Zhen S, Zhu J (2002) Methylation profiling of twenty promoter-CpG islands of genes which may contribute to hepatocellular carcinogenesis. BMC Cancer 2:29

101. Yuan BZ, Miller MJ, Keck CL, Zimonjic DB, Thorgeirsson SS, Popescu NC (1998) Cloning, characterization, and chromosomal localization of a gene frequently deleted in human liver cancer (DLC-1) homologous to rat RhoGAP. Cancer Res 58:2196–2199

102. Zheng DL, Zhang L, Cheng N, Xu X, Deng Q, Teng XM, Wang KS, Zhang X, Huang J, Han ZG (2009) Epigenetic modification induced by hepatitis B virus X protein via interaction with de novo DNA methyltransferase DNMT3A. J Hepatol 50:377–387

103. Zhu C, Utsunomiya T, Ikemoto T, Yamada S, Morine Y, Imura S, Arakawa Y, Takasu C, Ishikawa D, Imoto I, Shimada M (2014) Hypomethylation of long interspersed nuclear element-1 (LINE-1) is associated with poor prognosis via activation of c-MET in hepatocellular carcinoma. Ann Surg Oncol 21(Suppl 4):S729–S735

104. Zucman-Rossi J, Villanueva A, Nault JC, Llovet JM (2015) Genetic landscape and biomarkers of hepatocellular carcinoma. Gastroenterology 149:1226–1239

DNA and Histone Methylation in Colon Cancer

Its Biological Impact and Clinical Implications

Hiromu Suzuki, Eiichiro Yamamoto, Hiroshi Nakase, and Tamotsu Sugai

Abstract Colorectal cancers (CRCs) are thought to arise through accumulation of genetic and epigenetic alterations. CRC genomes exhibit dual-faceted DNA methylation abnormality, global hypomethylation with CpG island hypermethylation, and CRCs are classified into two groups based on whether their genomes exhibit microsatellite instability (MSI) or chromosomal instability (CIN). In addition, a subset of CRCs is characterized by concurrent hypermethylation of multiple CpG islands, known as the CpG island methylator phenotype (CIMP). Genomic instability and epigenetic alterations are tightly linked, and CRCs with MSI largely overlap CIMP-positive tumors, while CIN is associated with global DNA hypomethylation. Dysregulation of histone methylation and altered expression of histone modifying enzymes are also commonly observed in CRC, indicating their critical roles in CRC development. Evidence now suggests that DNA and histone methylation could potentially serve as biomarkers useful for CRC diagnosis, risk assessment and prediction of therapeutic effects and prognosis. Although many studies examining clinical applications are still at an early phase, it is anticipated that further investigation will lead to improved prevention and management of CRC.

H. Suzuki (✉)
Department of Molecular Biology, Sapporo Medical University School of Medicine, Sapporo, Japan
e-mail: hsuzuki@sapmed.ac.jp

E. Yamamoto
Department of Molecular Biology, Sapporo Medical University School of Medicine, Sapporo, Japan

Department of Gastroenterology and Hepatology, Sapporo Medical University School of Medicine, Sapporo, Japan

H. Nakase
Department of Gastroenterology and Hepatology, Sapporo Medical University School of Medicine, Sapporo, Japan

T. Sugai
Department of Molecular Diagnostic Pathology, Iwate Medical University, Morioka, Japan

© Springer International Publishing AG 2017
A. Kaneda, Y.-i. Tsukada (eds.), *DNA and Histone Methylation as Cancer Targets*, Cancer Drug Discovery and Development, DOI 10.1007/978-3-319-59786-7_17

Keywords Colorectal cancer • CpG island methylator phenotype • Microsatellite instability • Chromosomal instability • Biomarker

1 Introduction

Colorectal cancer (CRC) is the third most common cause of cancer and the fourth leading cause of cancer-related death in the world [1]. Much evidence suggests that CRCs develop through the accumulation of genetic and epigenetic alterations, which drives the progression from normal colorectal epithelium to adenoma, carcinoma and, eventually, metastatic disease. The sporadic form of CRC, which arises due to somatic mutations, accounts for approximately 70% of all CRCs, and up to one-third of CRCs show familial predisposition, although they do not present a Mendelian inheritance [2]. Only a small proportion of CRCs (2–5%) arise through well-defined inherited syndromes, including familial adenomatous polyposis (FAP), Lynch syndrome (hereditary nonpolyposis colorectal cancer, HNPCC) and MUTYH-associated polyposis [2]. Nonetheless, we have learned important lessons about the molecular abnormalities that lead to colorectal carcinogenesis from hereditary CRC syndromes [3]. For example, mutation of the *APC* gene, which is one of the most frequent genetic abnormalities in sporadic CRCs, was first discovered as the genetic cause of FAP [2]. Subsequent studies revealed that APC acts as a gatekeeper to CRC development by suppressing Wnt signaling [4]. Similarly, mutations in DNA mismatch repair (MMR) genes (*MLH1*, *MSH2*, *MSH6* and *PMS2*), which trigger microsatellite instability (MSI), were discovered as genetic causes of Lynch syndrome [5]. These findings later prompted the identification of promoter hypermethylation-associated silencing of *MLH1* in sporadic MSI-positive CRCs [6, 7]. The discovery of *MLH1* methylation in MSI tumors highlights the functional interaction between genomic and epigenomic abnormalities in CRC and facilitated the molecular subcategorization of CRC based on molecular characteristics. Thanks to remarkable advances in cancer genome analysis, we now understand that the CRC genome includes thousands of genetic and epigenetic abnormalities that affect the biological and clinical characteristics of this disease. In this review, we will focus on the contribution made by aberrant DNA and histone methylation events to CRC development and discuss their clinical application.

2 Aberrant DNA Methylation in CRC

CRC genomes generally show dual-faceted DNA methylation abnormality: global hypomethylation with regional hypermethylation [8–11]. Hypomethylation commonly occurs at repetitive genomic elements, including satellite DNA sequences and retrotransposons (LINEs, SINEs and Alu), and is thought to promote tumorigenesis though induction of chromosomal instability (CIN) and activation of proto-oncogenes [8, 10, 11]. Hypomethylation-induced loss of imprinting (LOI) is also frequently observed in CRC [11]. For instance, LOI of the insulin-like growth factor 2 gene (*IGF2*) results in abnormal expression of the maternal allele of the gene, which is normally epigenetically repressed. The upregulated *IGF2* expression leads to activation of IGF1 receptor and its downstream signaling pathways, which contributes to enhanced tumor growth [11–13].

By contrast, hypermethylation of CpG islands located at gene promoters is the major mechanism by which tumor suppressors and other tumor-related genes are silenced in cancer. The list of genes silenced by hypermethylation in CRC is rapidly growing and includes genes involved in virtually all key signaling pathways, including WNT, RAS and p53, as well as genes involved in regulating the cell cycle, apoptosis, DNA repair, immune system, angiogenesis, invasion and metastasis [9, 10, 14, 15] (Table 1). Recent studies also have shown that genes for noncoding RNA, including microRNAs (miRNAs) and long noncoding RNA, are also targets of methylation-associated silencing in CRC [15–17].

Recently, a new concept "CpG island shore" was proposed by Feinberg et al. [18]. CpG island shores refer to genomic areas within two kilobases of CpG islands, and methylation of this area is associated with gene transcriptional regulation. Patterns of CpG island shore methylation are tissue-specific and are altered in various malignancies, including CRC [9].

2.1 CpG Island Methylator Phenotype (CIMP) in CRC

Genomic instability is essential in the CRC development, and CRCs are thought to arise through two major forms of genomic instability: CIN and MSI [3] (Fig. 1). CIN is observed in the majority of CRCs (about 80–85%) and is associated with gains and losses of whole chromosomes or chromosomal regions [3, 15]. DNA methylation of LINE-1 is often used as a surrogate marker of global hypomethylation, and LINE-1 hypomethylation is frequently observed in CIN CRCs, whereas it is inversely associated with MSI [8, 19–21]. MSI, which is identified by the presence of frequent insertion and deletion mutations within repetitive DNA sequences, is found in approximately 15% of CRCs, among which about 3% are attributable to Lynch syndrome [3, 10]. The majority of sporadic CRCs with MSI exhibit biallelic hypermethylation of *MLH1* [10]. A recent comprehensive genomic analysis of CRC by The Cancer Genome Atlas project revealed that sporadic CRCs can be categorized as hypermutated (16%) or non-hypermutated (84%) tumors, which correspond to MSI and CIN, respectively [22].

In addition to those exhibiting genomic instabilities, a third subclass of CRCs characterized by concurrent hypermethylation of multiple CpG islands has been proposed. These tumors are defined as exhibiting a CpG island methylator phenotype (CIMP), the characteristic molecular and clinicopathological features of which suggest a distinct carcinogenic pathway [23] (Fig. 1). CIMP was initially identified

Table 1 Representative genes commonly hypermethylated in CRC

Categories	Genes
WNT signaling	*APC*
	SFRP1
	SFRP2
	SFRP5
	DKK1
	DKK2
	DKK3
	SOX17
	WIF1
RAS signaling	*RASSF1A*
	RASSF2
Growth factor signaling	*IGFBP3*
	IGFBP7
Cytokine signaling	*SOCS1*
Apoptosis	*BNIP3*
	DAPK1
	HRK
Cell cycle	*CHFR*
	CDKN2A/p16
	CDKN2A/p14
Chromatin remodeling	*HLTF*
DNA repair	*MLH1*
	MGMT
Calcium channel	*CACNA1G*
Inflammation	*COX2*
Invasion and metastasis	*CDH1*
	CDH13
	TIMP3
Transcription factor	*GATA4*
	GATA5
	HIC1
	ID4
	RUNX3
Putative tumor suppressor	*DCC*
	DFNA5
	NDRG4
	NEURL
	NEUROG1
	SLC5A8
	SYNE1
	TFPI2
miRNA	*miR-1-1*
	miR-9-1

Table 1 (continued)

Categories	Genes
	miR-9-2
	miR-9-3
	miR-34a
	miR-34b/c
	miR-124-1
	miR-124-2
	miR-124-3
	miR-127
	miR-129-2
	miR-137
	miR-148a
	miR-200c
	miR-345

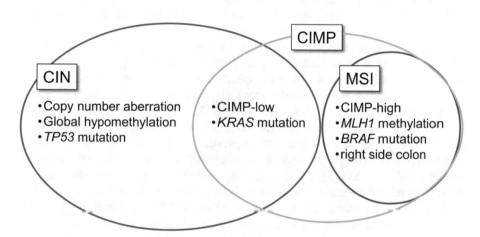

Fig. 1 Classification of CRCs based on genomic and epigenomic alterations

through a genome-wide DNA methylation analysis in CRC. By performing methyl-ated CpG amplification (MCA) coupled with representational difference analysis (RDA), Toyota and Issa compared the CpG island methylation statuses of CRC cells and normal colonic mucosa samples [24, 25]. This enabled them to isolate a series of CpG islands that were hypermethylated in CRC, which they termed MINT (methylated in tumor) sequences. They next analyzed the methylation status of 30 MINT clones from primary samples, and found that a majority (19/30) were meth-ylated in both tumoral and normal tissues in an age-related manner (type A methyla-tion), while a smaller number (7/30) were methylated in a cancer-specific pattern (type C methylation). By utilizing type C methylation markers (e.g. *MINT1*, *MINT2*, *MINT31*, *CDKN2A* (*p16*) and *MLH1*), they found that a subset of CRCs preferen-tially exhibited hypermethylation at multiple loci. Importantly, they also noted that CIMP-positive CRCs could be further subcategorized into two groups depending on the presence or absence of *MLH1* methylation and MSI. The CIMP phenotype was further confirmed in a number of subsequent studies, and CIMP CRCs were found to strongly associate with characteristic molecular and clinicopathological features, including a proximal colon location, older age, female sex, higher tumor grade, poor differentiation and mucinous histology, *KRAS/BRAF* mutations and wild-type *TP53* [26–29]. There is a strong overlap between CRCs with MSI and those with CIMP, whereas CIN is not often observed in CIMP tumors [30–32].

The CIMP hypothesis has been challenged by several groups who found that CRCs could not be clearly categorized as CIMP-positive or -negative [33, 34]. This ambiguity mainly reflects an absence of consistent criteria by which to define CIMP, and there is substantial inconsistency among studies with respect to the markers and techniques used to analyze DNA methylation [35]. For instance, Yamashita et al. reported that the numbers of methylated CpG islands vary gradually from a high methylation group to a low methylation group, which is in sharp contrast to the bimodal distribution of microsatellite mutations observed in MSI and microsatellite stable (MSS) tumors [33]. Importantly, they also showed that many of the hyper-methylation events are age-dependent, indicating that age-dependently methylated CpG islands are inappropriate as markers to define CIMP. In addition, many earlier studies used highly sensitive and qualitative methods to analyze DNA methylation of arbitrarily selected genes, which may lead to overestimation or incorrect catego-rization of CIMP tumors. By contrast, CIMP was originally defined through quan-titative DNA methylation analysis (COBRA assays), and subsequent studies confirmed that quantitative analysis is the key to accurate characterization of CIMP [25, 36, 37].

To address this controversy, substantial effort has been made to identify the best markers with which to define CIMP. Weisenberger et al. employed a quantitative MethyLight assay to analyze a series of 195 CpG islands in 295 primary CRC tumors [37]. They selected CpG islands that showed cancer-specific methylation, and carried out unsupervised clustering analysis, which confirmed the existence of CIMP-positive CRCs. As compared to the classic CIMP markers, CIMP tumors defined using the new markers identified in that study (*CACNA1G*, *IGF2*, *NEUROG1*, *RUNX3* and *SOCS1*) are more tightly associated with MSI and *BRAF* mutation.

2.2 Subclasses of CIMP in CRC

Since the first discovery of CIMP in CRC, a strong association between CIMP and MSI has been repeatedly documented, but results of many studies suggest that there are distinct subclasses of CIMP-positive CRCs (Fig. 1). For instance, Ogino et al. used a panel of 5 marker genes (*CACNA1G*, *CDKN2A*, *CRABP1*, *MLH1* and *NEUROG1*) to analyze 840 population-based CRC patients [38]. They found that CRCs with intermediate methylation, termed CIMP-low (defined by 1/5–3/5 methylated markers), are strongly associated with male sex and *KRAS* mutation, which are distinct from CIMP-high tumors (defined by 4/5 or 5/5 methylated markers). By performing unsupervised hierarchical clustering of 97 primary CRCs using 27 marker genes, Shen et al. showed that CRCs could be classified into 3 subclasses: CIMP1, which is tightly associated with MSI and *BRAF* mutation; CIMP2, which is characterized by frequent *KRAS* mutation; and CIMP-negative, which is associated with frequent *TP53* mutation [39]. Similarly, Yagi et al. used two marker panels to show that CRCs could be classified into high-, intermediate- and low-methylation epigenotypes [40]. Moreover, technical advances in recent years have enabled genome-wide DNA methylation analysis, and unsupervised clustering of the methylome data clearly delineated two subclasses of CIMP CRCs [22, 41].

CIMP-high (or CIMP1) CRCs show typical characteristics of the CIMP tumors: proximal colon location, older age, female sex, frequent *BRAF* mutation, *MLH1* methylation and MSI [39–41]. On the other hand, they rarely exhibit *KRAS* or *TP53* mutations. *IGFBP7* was recently found to be preferentially methylated in CIMP-high CRCs [42, 43]. Another study showed that *IGFBP7* is a downstream effector of oncogenic BRAF, which induces cellular senescence and apoptosis in melanocytes, and that inactivation of *IGFBP7* via CpG island methylation is a critical step in the development melanoma [44]. Thus, loss of *IGFBP7* may also be necessary to escape from oncogenic BRAF-induced senescence during the development of CIMP-high CRCs.

CIMP-low (or CIMP2) CRCs are strongly associated with *KRAS* mutation, while *BRAF* and *TP53* mutations and MSI are infrequently observed [38–41]. CIMP-low tumors are also preferentially located in the proximal colon, but they are slightly more common in males than females. Other biological and clinical characteristics of CIMP-low CRCs sometimes differ among studies, which may be due to an absence of commonly accepted criteria to define this subtype. Ogino et al. tested a set of 8 CIMP marker genes (Weisenberger's CIMP markers plus *CDKN2A*, *CRABP1* and *MLH1*), and again found that CIMP-low tumors (defined by 1/8–5/8 methylated markers) are associated *KRAS* mutation and male sex [45]. However, the differences between the CIMP-low and CIMP-negative groups are not large, indicating that these markers are more specific to CIMP-high. By contrast, Shen et al. reported that the single best marker for predicting CIMP2 (CIMP-low) is *KRAS* mutation [39]. To delineate CIMP subclasses more specifically, Hinoue et al. developed two panels of makers consisting of genes commonly methylated in CIMP-high and -low tumors and additional CIMP-high-specific genes [41]. Yagi et al. used a similar two-panel method to distinguish the three epigenotypes [40]. However, a recent study reported that intermediate- and low-methylation epigenotypes may not be equivalent to CIMP-low/−negative tumors, indicating that differences in marker genes can result in significant discrepancies among studies [46].

A recent large scale analysis using a series of gene expression datasets from primary CRCs concluded that CRCs can be classified into four consensus molecular subtypes (CMS): CMS1 (MSI immune, 14%), which exhibits MSI and strong immune activation; CMS2 (canonical, 37%), which is epithelial and exhibits marked WNT and MYC signal activation; CMS3 (metabolic, 13%), which is epithelial and exhibits metabolic dysregulation; and CMS4 (mesenchymal, 23%), which exhibits TGF-β activation, stromal invasion and angiogenesis [47]. CMS1 CRCs show frequent *BRAF* mutation and largely overlap CIMP-high tumors. CMS3 CRCs are characterized by *KRAS* mutation, which could induce prominent metabolic adaptation, and show fewer copy number alterations and a higher prevalence of CIMP-low. These results again indicate that DNA methylation is strongly associated with the molecular subtypes of CRC.

2.3   Serrated Lesions as Precursors of CIMP CRC

It is well known that aberrant DNA methylation, including both hypermethylation and hypomethylation, occurs early during colorectal tumorigenesis. Methylation of a number of cancer-related genes can be detected in premalignant lesions, including aberrant crypt foci and adenomas [9, 48–50]. It is noteworthy that the largest increase in the number of methylated genes occurs during the step from normal mucosa to adenoma [51, 52]. Multiple studies also have shown the presence of CIMP in adenomas and hyperplastic polyps (HPs) [25, 48, 53, 54]. For a long time, HPs were thought to be colorectal lesions with little neoplastic potential. However, a recently proposed "serrated pathway," via which lesions progress to CIMP-positive CRCs, challenges this view [55]. Serrated lesions include HPs, sessile serrated adenoma/polyps (SSA/Ps) and traditional serrated adenomas (TSAs) [56]. SSA/Ps preferentially occur in the proximal colon and frequently exhibit *BRAF* mutation and hypermethylation of multiple CpG islands, and they are considered to be precursor lesions of CIMP-high/MSI CRCs [55, 57] (Fig. 2).

When assessing the relationship between molecular features and locations of CRCs, most studies classify CRCs as proximal colonic, distal colonic and rectal. However, Yamauchi et al. showed that the incidence of CIMP-high, MSI-high and *BRAF* mutant tumors gradually increases along the bowel, from the rectum to the ascending colon, indicating that CRCs cannot be simply divided into proximal and distal colonic tumors [58]. Similarly, studies of colorectal serrated lesions revealed a gradual increase in the incidence of CIMP-high tumors from the rectum to the

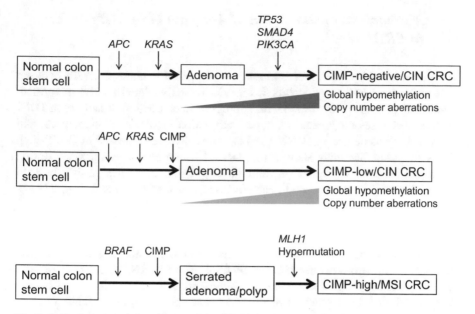

Fig. 2 Pathways of CRC development. Shown are the molecular carcinogenesis pathways of three representative CRC subclasses. CIMP-negative/CIN CRCs develop through the classical multistep carcinogenesis pathway, in which tumors develop through accumulation of multiple gene mutations. CIMP-low/CIN tumors are characterized by frequent *KRAS* mutation. CIN tumors are also associated with global hypomethylation and copy number aberrations. The CIMP-high/MSI tumor pathway is also known as the serrated pathway. These tumors are characterized by *BRAF* mutation, *MLH1* methylation and hypermutation

cecum, indicating a site-dependent difference in the susceptibility to CIMP and *BRAF* mutation in premalignant lesions [59, 60].

Detection and resection of SSA/Ps during colonoscopies would contribute to reducing CRC mortality, but it is often difficult to discriminate SSA/Ps from other HPs through colonoscopic observation, as neither exhibits the surface microstructures (pit patterns) specific to malignant lesions. A recent population-based study reported that use of colonoscopy could reduce both the incidence and mortality of CRC, but cancers diagnosed in patients within 5 years after colonoscopy are more likely to be CIMP and MSI tumors, which may reflect the difficulty of detecting SSA/Ps during colonoscopy [61]. Our group reported a SSA/P-specific pit pattern, Type II-O pits, which could improve colonoscopic detection of SSA/Ps [62]. We also performed genomic and epigenomic analysis of early colorectal lesions, and found that *BRAF* mutation and CIMP occur at the premalignant stage, while *MLH1* methylation and MSI are acquired during the progression from SSA/P to carcinoma [52]. We anticipate that further study of colorectal premalignant lesions will lead to better prevention and earlier detection of CRCs.

2.4 Mechanisms for Induction of Aberrant DNA Methylation in CRC

The mechanisms by which aberrant DNA methylation is induced in CRC are not fully understood, but several factors that may be causally related have been reported. It has been proposed, for example, that upregulated expression or activity of DNA methyltransferases are a cause of hypermethylation in various malignancies, and DNA methyltransferase 3B (DNMT3B) is reportedly overexpressed in CIMP-high CRCs [63]. Another study showed that DNMT3B expression is increased during colorectal neoplastic progression, and its expression correlates positively with methylation of CIMP-associated genes (NEUROG1, CACNA1G and CDKN2A) as well as SFRP2 [64].

Several lines of evidence indicate that dysregulation of miRNAs can lead to aberrant DNA methylation in cancer [16]. miRNAs are endogenous, small noncoding RNAs that function at the posttranscriptional level as negative regulators of gene expression. Numerous studies indicate that subsets of miRNAs act as tumor suppressor genes or oncogenes, and their dysregulation is a common feature of human cancers [65, 66]. Dysregulation of miRNAs that potentially target DNA methyltransferase genes is observed in various malignancies [67–70]. Among them, miR-342 is reportedly downregulated in CRC, and restoration of miR-342 in CRC cells leads to reactivation of the tumor suppressor genes ADAM23 and RASSF1A via promoter demethylation [71].

It has become evident in recent years that the ten-eleven translocation (TET) proteins are key mediators of active DNA demethylation. Members of the TET family (TET1–TET3) are oxoglutarate- and iron-dependent dioxygenases, which catalyze the oxidation of 5-mC to generate 5-hydroxymethylcytosine (5-hmC), which is in turn recognized by base excision repair proteins for removal and replacement with unmethylated cytosine [72]. Dysregulation of TET and thus 5-hmC levels can lead to carcinogenesis. Decreased TET expression and loss of 5-hmC are observed in various human malignancies including CRC [73]. Loss-of-function mutations in TET2 and the resultant reduction in 5-hmC are observed in myeloid malignancies [74, 75]. There is also an important relationship between TET dysfunction and mutations in isocitrate dehydrogenase (IDH) family genes in cancer. Somatic mutations in IDH1 or IDH2 result in the accumulation of an oncogenic metabolite, 2-hydroxyglutarate (2-HG), which can inhibit TET activity [76], and IDH1/2 mutations are strongly associated with the hypermethylator phenotype in glioma and AML [77–79]. There is at present no evidence of the association between aberrant DNA methylation and IDH or TET family genes mutation in CRC, but it was recently reported that TET1 is frequently silenced by CpG island methylation in CIMP-high CRCs [80]. Further study will be required to determine the biological significance of 5-hmC and TET proteins in the induction of aberrant DNA methylation in CRC.

The reason for frequent MLH1 methylation and BRAF mutation in CIMP-high CRCs is not fully understood, but several possible mechanisms have been proposed. For instance, a polymorphism in the promoter of MLH1 (c.-93G > A SNP) is reportedly associated with an increased risk of MSI-high CRC [81]. Later studies found a positive association between this polymorphism and *MLH1* methylation in CRC [82, 83], though conflicting results have also been reported [84]. Frequent *BRAF* mutation in SSA/P indicates that it may be causally related to the establishment of the CIMP phenotype, but an earlier study showed that ectopic expression of onco-genic BRAF (BRAF[V600E]) in CRC cells did not specifically induce CpG island methylation [42]. However, Fang et al. recently reported that activation of BRAF/MEK/ERK signaling by BRAF[V600E] leads to the activation of a transcriptional repressor, MAFG, in CRC cells [85]. MAFG recruits a corepressor complex that includes CHD8, BACH1 and DNMT3B to the promoters of *MLH1* and other CIMP-related genes and induces hypermethylation and transcriptional silencing. *CHD8* encodes a chromatin remodeling factor, and another recent study reported frequent mutation of *CHD7* and *CHD8* in CIMP1 (CIMP-high) CRCs, indicating a possible causal relationship between mutation of these genes and induction of CIMP [86].

The association of lifestyle and genetic factors with aberrant DNA methylation in CRC has also been investigated. Cigarette smoking is reportedly associated with CIMP-high and *BRAF* mutant CRCs [87, 88]. Dietary factors are believed to play important roles in CRC tumorigenesis, and a link between low folate status and increased risk of CRC has been shown in many studies [89]. Folate plays a crucial role in DNA metabolism and synthesis, and it is required to maintain an adequate cellular pool of the methyl donor S-adenosylmethionine (SAM). Folate deficiency leads to genomic DNA hypomethylation and defects in DNA synthesis, which increases the risk of colorectal tumorigenesis [90–92]. Possible association between low folate and high alcohol intake with the hypermethylation of tumor suppressor genes in CRC has been also reported [93]. Polymorphisms in genes encoding folate-metabolizing enzymes (e.g. *MTHFR*, *MTR* and *MTRR*) are also reportedly associated with CIMP status in CRC [94, 95]. Another study showed that a *MTHFR* polymorphism (*MTHFR* c.1298A > C) could be associated with the development of CIMP CRC in conjunction with a high-risk dietary pattern (low folate and methionine intake and high alcohol use) [96]. On the other hand, there is little evidence supporting an association between dietary folate, vitamin B6 and B12, methionine or alcohol intake with CIMP status in CRC [97, 98].

2.5 Epimutation of MMR Genes in Lynch Syndrome

As described above, *MLH1* methylation is a common feature of sporadic MSI-positive CRCs. However, germline mutations of MMR genes are undetectable in up to 30% of Lynch syndrome families, and some of the affected individuals exhibit "epimutation" of *MLH1*, which is characterized by monoallelic methylation throughout the normal somatic tissues [5, 99, 100]. Epimutations of *MLH1* are thought to account for 1–10% of MMR gene mutation-negative Lynch syndrome [101]. Hitchins et al. reported that the hypermethylated *MLH1* allele is maternally inherited, but the patient's mothers and siblings did not show the methylation, suggesting *MLH1* epimutation can arise as a *de novo* event [100]. They also showed that inheritance of *MLH1* epimutation occurs in a non-Mendelian pattern [102], and the epimutation was likened to polymorphisms in the 5′ untranslated region of the *MLH1* gene (*MLH1* c.−27C > A, *MLH1* c.85G > T) [103, 104].

In 2006, Chan et al. reported that heritable epimutation of *MSH2* could also cause Lynch syndrome [105]. A subsequent study demonstrated that germline deletion of the last exon of an adjacent gene, *TACSTD1* (also known as *EPCAM*), led to abnormal transcriptional elongation of *EPCAM* into *MSH2*, which could result in the methylation and silencing of *MSH2* [106]. Because *EPCAM* is expressed exclusively in epithelial tissues, *MSH2* methylation shows a mosaic pattern, in which the epimutation is observed only in epithelial tissues.

3   DNA Methylation Biomarkers

3.1   DNA Methylation as a Diagnostic Biomarker of CRC

Although treatment options for CRC have significantly improved in recent years, detection and removal of premalignant and early-stage lesions is essential for reducing CRC mortality. Large population-based studies have also shown that the fecal occult blood test (FOBT) and fecal immunological test (FIT) are highly cost-effective screening methods for CRC [107, 108]. However, there are limitations to the diagnostic accuracy of FOBT and FIT, especially for detection of early lesions. Fecal DNA tests are noninvasive and potentially effective methods for detecting CRCs, and because of its high frequency and early occurrence, aberrant DNA methylation could be a promising biomarker. Numerous studies have tested the usefulness of methylated genes as stool-based biomarkers. The genes tested include *APC* [109], *CDKN2A* [110], *GATA4* [111], *ITGA4* [112], *MGMT* [110], *miR-34b/c* [113], *NDRG4* [114], *RASSF2A* [115], *SFRP2* [116], *TFPI2* [117] and *VIM* [118]. For instance, an early study identified methylated *SFRP2* as a potential diagnostic biomarker with high sensitivity (77–90%) and specificity (77%) [116]. One of the most well studied marker genes is *VIM*, which encodes vimentin. *VIM* is frequently methylated in primary colonic neoplasms, and methylated *VIM* is detected in the fecal DNA of colon cancer patients with high sensitivity (46%) and specificity (90%) [118]. Subsequent studies confirmed the potential of *VIM* methylation as a diagnostic marker of CRC, and methylated *VIM* detection served as the basis for development of the first commercial fecal-DNA screening tests for CRC (ColoSure, Lab Corp) [8]. More recently, the effectiveness of multi-target stool DNA testing, which detects *BMP3* and *NDRG4* methylation and *KRAS* mutation, has been confirmed in a large study of nearly 10,000 participants [119]. This study demonstrated that the sensitivity for detecting CRC was 92.3% with DNA testing, while it was 73.8% with FIT. Moreover, the sensitivities for detecting precancerous lesions were 42.4% with DNA testing and 23.8% with FIT. These results led to the development of a FDA-approved stool-based CRC screening test, Cologuard (Exact Sciences Corporation) [8].

Blood is also an ideal material for detecting cancer biomarkers, and many groups have reported detecting aberrant DNA methylation in the serum or plasma of patients with CRC. The potential blood-based methylation marker genes identified to date include *ALX4* [120], *APC* [121], *FOXE1* [122], *MGMT* [121], *NEUROG1* [123], *RASSF2A* [121], *SEPT9* [124], *SYNE1* [122], *VIM* [125] and *WIF1* [121]. One of the most well studied marker genes is *SEPT9*, which encodes septin 9. Lofton-Day et al. first reported that detection of *SETP9* methylation in plasma samples achieved 69% sensitivity and 86% specificity for diagnosis of CRC [124]. Subsequent studies validated the clinical usefulness of *SEPT9* methylation as a biomarker for CRC screening, which led to the development of several commercially available blood-based screening tests, including Epi proColon (Epigenomics), ColoVantage (Quest Diagnostics) and RealTime mS9 (Abbott Laboratories) [8].

3.2 DNA Methylation as a Predictive Biomarker of Clinical Outcomes

DNA methylation may also be predictive of clinical outcome of CRC. The impact of CIMP on the outcome of CRC has been extensively analyzed in several studies. Although some conflicting results are seen among studies, much evidence suggests that CIMP is predictive of an unfavorable outcome in CRC. Ward et al. analyzed more than 600 CRC patients and found that no single marker is independently associated with prognosis [126]. However, when they divided the patients into MSI and MSS groups, methylation of multiple genes (>3/5) was significantly associated with a worse prognosis in the MSS group. A worse prognosis in patients with CIMP-positive and MSS CRCs was also shown in later studies [127, 128]. When CIMP tumors were divided into two subclasses, CIMP-high status in MSS tumors was again associated with shorter survival, whereas CIMP-low was a likely indicator of poor outcome, irrespective of MSI status [127, 129]. Similarly, the intermediate-methylation epigenotype with *KRAS* mutation was associated with poor outcome [40]. The association between CIMP and poor outcome in CRC patients was further validated in recent studies [130–133], though other lines of evidence suggest that the adverse effects may be attributable to *BRAF* mutation. Ogino et al. showed that CIMP-high is an independent predictor of low colon cancer-specific mortality, regardless of MSI or *BRAF* status, while *BRAF* mutation is strongly associated with high colon cancer-specific mortality [134]. Poor outcomes in patients with MSS and *BRAF* mutant CRCs were also reported in other independent studies [135, 136].

CIMP may also be a predictive biomarker for responses to treatment in CRC. An early report showed that CIMP is an independent predictor of survival benefit from 5-fluorouracil (5-FU) in stage III CRCs [137]. An association between CIMP status and survival benefit from 5-FU-based chemotherapy has been validated by multiple groups, but results are inconsistent among studies [138–140]. A more recent study reported that the addition of irinotecan to adjuvant 5-FU and leucovorin provides longer survival time to patients with stage III, CIMP-positive and MSS CRC [141]. Taken together, these results suggest that CIMP could be a useful biomarker for predicting outcome in CRC, and further studies testing its clinical application seem warranted.

Studies of pharmaco-epigenomics revealed that methylation of key regulator genes can be a predictive biomarker of chemoresistance or chemosensitivity in cancer cells [8]. An association between methylation of *MGMT*, which encodes O^6-methylguanine-DNA methyltransferase, and the therapeutic effects of alkylating agents (e.g. dacarbazine and temozolomide) in glioma is the most well known example [142]. A recent phase II study of dacarbazine in metastatic CRC found objective responses only in *MGMT* methylated tumors [143]. However, another phase II study of temozolomide in advanced CRCs showed only low response rates in *MGMT* methylated patients [144]. Recently, Ebert et al. recently reported that methylation of *TFAP2E*, which encodes transcription factor AP-2 epsilon, is associated with resistance to 5-FU based chemotherapy in CRC [145]. *DKK4* is a downstream target of *TFAP2E*, and *TFAP2E*-dependent chemoresistance is mediated through *DKK4* overexpression. Moreover, methylation of the BRCA1 interactor *SRBC* gene was discovered to be a predictive marker for oxaliplatin resistance in CRC [146].

Another form of aberrant DNA methylation that could potentially serve as a biomarker in CRC is global hypomethylation. Ogino et al. found that LINE-1 hypomethylation is independently associated with shorter survival among CRC patients in large prospective cohorts [147]. An association between poor clinical outcome and low levels of LINE-1 methylation was confirmed in subsequent studies [130, 148, 149]. It has been documented that aberrant DNA methylation is often observed in normal colonic mucosa adjacent to CRC, which is suggestive of an epigenetic field defect [50, 150]. Kamiyama et al. reported that levels of LINE-1 methylation are lower in noncancerous colonic mucosa from right-sided colon multiple cancer patients than colonic tissue from single cancer patients [151]. This suggests LINE-1 hypomethylation could be a predictive biomarker of the risk of multiple colon cancer.

4   Histone Methylation

4.1   Dysregulation of Histone Methylation in CRC

In addition to DNA methylation, an additional layer of epigenetic regulation of gene expression is mediated by covalent modification of histone tails. The most well characterized histone modifications in CRC are acetylation and methylation of lysine residues within histone tails; di- and trimethylation of histone H3 lysine 4 (H3K4me2/m3) and acetylation of histone H3 lysine 9 (H3K9ac) are associated with active transcription, while di- and trimethylation of histone H3 lysine 9 and lysine 27 (H3K9me2/me3 and H3K27me3) are marks of transcriptional silencing [152]. Histone modifications are tightly associated with DNA methylation-mediated gene silencing in cancer. For instance, CpG island hypermethylation of *MLH1* and *CDKN2A* is accompanied by low levels of histone H3K4 methylation and increased levels of H3K9 methylation in CRC cells [153, 154]. Pharmacological inhibition of DNMTs using 5-aza-2'-doxycytidine (5-aza-dC, decitabine) induces DNA demethylation as well as reversal of the histone code, which leads to reexpression of silenced genes [153, 154]. The concept that DNA methylation and histone modifications coordinately mediate gene silencing was further substantiated by a subsequent study. An earlier study showed that genetic disruption of *DNMT1* and *DNMT3B* in the HCT116 CRC cell line results in complete removal of DNA methylation and reexpression of the silenced genes [155]. Bachman et al. found that elimination of DNA methylation at the *CDKN2A* promoter was associated with loss of H3K9 methylation in the *DNMT1/DNMT3B* double knockout cells, while continued culture of the cells led to restoration of H3K9 methylation and re-silencing of the gene, and DNA demethylation subsequently occurred after a still longer time in culture [156]. A more recent study showed that DNA demethylation by 5-aza-dC is not sufficient to induce gene expression, and chromatin resetting to an active state, including nucleosome eviction is required for activation of protein expression in CRC cells [157].

The clinical application of histone methylation as a biomarker is hampered by the technical difficulty of analyzing histone modifications at specific gene loci in primary tumors [8]. Instead, global alterations in histone modification patterns in tumor tissues have been the focus for development of CRC biomarkers. Immunohistochemical analysis of H3K4me2, H3K9ac, H3K9me2 and H3K27me3 revealed higher levels of H3K9me2 in adenomas and CRCs than in normal colonic mucosa, suggesting that dysregulation of the global H3K9me2 level is an important epigenetic event during colorectal tumorigenesis [158]. Analyses using specimens of primary CRC and corresponding liver metastasis revealed that lower levels of H3K4me2 and H3K27me3 are potential prognostic factors of metachronous liver metastasis of CRC [159, 160]. Moreover, a recent study using a tissue microarray composed of 254 stage I–III CRC samples demonstrated that low levels of H3K4me3 and high levels of H3K9me3 and H4K20me3 are associated with a favorable prognosis in early-stage colon cancer [161]. These results suggest that global histone methylation status could be a potential biomarker for predicting outcomes in CRC.

4.2   Altered Expression of Histone Modifying Enzymes in CRC

Dysregulation of enzymes that catalyze histone modifications are also frequently observed in CRC. For instance, lysine-specific demethylase 1 (LSD1 also known as lysine-specific demethylase 1A, KDM1A) is a histone demethylase that specifically catalyzes demethylation of histone H3K4me1/me2. LSD1 is frequently upregulated in CRC, and expression of LSD1 is associated with low expression of CDH1 (E-cadherin), high TNM stage, distant metastasis and poor prognosis in CRC [162, 163]. LSD1 physically interacts with the *CDH1* promoter and decreases H3K4 methylation at that region, which suggests LSD1-mediated downregulation of *CDH1* contributes to CRC metastasis [162]. Expression of histone methyltransferase

(HMT) suppressor of variegation 3–9 homolog 1 (SUV39H1) is elevated in 25% of primary CRCs, and transcriptional activation of *SUV39H1* is positively associated with *DNMT1* mRNA levels [164]. This may indicate a functional interaction between SUV39H1 and DNMT1, though no association between SUV39H1 expression and hypermethylation of tumor-related genes was observed [164]. Overexpression of SUV39H1 induces high H3K9me3 levels and activates migration in CRC cells, and the presence of H3K9me3 in primary CRCs correlates positively with lymph node metastasis [165].

The histone H3K4-specific HMT SET domain-containing protein 1A (SETD1A) is also overexpressed in CRC cells, and its depletion suppresses CRC cell survival and xenograft formation in nude mice [166]. In addition, H3K4-specifc HMT SET and MYND domain-containing protein 3 (SMYD3) was originally identified as an oncogene overexpressed in CRC and hepatocellular carcinoma [167]. It was suggested that oncogenic RAS could alter global and gene-specific histone modification patterns in CRC cells [168]. Consistent with that idea, positive correlations between *KRAS* mutation and elevated *SMYD3* expression have been reported in primary CRCs [169, 170]. Multiple myeloma SET (MMSET also known as WHS candidate 1 gene, WHSC1), which is a H3K36-specific HMT, is highly expressed in colorectal premalignant lesions but its expression decreases with increased stage [171]. Interestingly, MMSET expression correlates with good prognostic factors at early stages of CRCs, whereas CRC patients exhibiting high MMSET expression showed poor 5-year survival [171]. Expression of H3K9-specific histone demethylase Jumonji domain containing 1A (JMJD1A, also known as lysine-specific demethylase 3A, KDM3A) is elevated in CRC cells under hypoxic conditions, and high JMJD1A expression is an independent prognostic factor for CRC [172]. Disruption of JMJD1A suppressed CRC cell proliferation in vitro and in vivo, suggesting it could be a potential therapeutic target [172].

Polycomb repressive complexes (PRCs), which consist of PRC1 and PRC2, mediate epigenetic gene silencing by modulating histone modification. The HMT enhancer of zeste homolog 2 (EZH2) is the central unit of PRC2, and it initiates methylation of H3K27. EZH2 is frequently overexpressed in CRC [173–175], and depletion of EZH2 blocks CRC cell proliferation [176]. PRC1 binds at H3K27me3 sites and catalyzes monoubiquitination of lysine 119 of histone H2A. Elevated expression of BMI1, which is a component of PRC1, is associated with a poor prognosis in CRC [177]. PRC-mediated epigenetic gene silencing is strongly implicated in various human malignancies. The polycomb group proteins, including EZH2 and CBX7, interact with DNA methyltransferases, and PRCs are thought to play key roles in DNA methylation-associated transcriptional silencing [178–180]. Moreover, many of the genes hypermethylated in cancer are pre-marked by H3K27me3 in embryonic stem cells, further substantiating the interaction between histone methylation and DNA methylation in cancer [181–183].

5 Concluding Remarks

We have presented an overview of the biological and clinical significance of aberrant DNA and histone methylation in CRC. Advances in the study of the CRC genome and epigenome have increased our understanding of the underlying molecular basis and subcategories of this disease. On the basis on that knowledge, substantial efforts have been made to develop new biomarkers for diagnosis, cancer risk assessment, prognosis and prediction of drug responses and patient outcome. Although the effects of current epigenetic drugs, including DNMT inhibitors, are limited in solid tumors such as CRC, epigenetic changes are promising therapeutic targets. That said, the majority of studies of the clinical application are at early phases, and we anticipate that further investigation will lead to greater prevention and better management of CRC.

Acknowledgements We thank Dr. William Goldman for editing the manuscript. This study was supported in part by Grants-in-Aid for Scientific Research (B) from the Japan Society for Promotion of Science (JSPS KAKENHI 15H04299, H. Suzuki).

References

1. Ferlay J, Soerjomataram I, Dikshit R, Eser S, Mathers C, Rebelo M et al (2015) Cancer incidence and mortality worldwide: sources, methods and major patterns in GLOBOCAN 2012. Int J Cancer 136:E359–E386
2. Jasperson KW, Tuohy TM, Neklason DW, Burt RW (2010) Hereditary and familial colon cancer. Gastroenterology 138:2044–2058
3. Carethers JM, Jung BH (2015) Genetics and genetic biomarkers in sporadic colorectal cancer. Gastroenterology 149:1177–1190. e3
4. Fodde R, Smits R, Clevers H (2001) APC, signal transduction and genetic instability in colorectal cancer. Nat Rev Cancer 1:55–67
5. Lynch HT, Snyder CL, Shaw TG, Heinen CD, Hitchins MP (2015) Milestones of Lynch syndrome: 1895–2015. Nat Rev Cancer 15:181–194
6. Kane MF, Loda M, Gaida GM, Lipman J, Mishra R, Goldman H et al (1997) Methylation of the hMLH1 promoter correlates with lack of expression of hMLH1 in sporadic colon tumors and mismatch repair-defective human tumor cell lines. Cancer Res 57:808–811
7. Herman JG, Umar A, Polyak K, Graff JR, Ahuja N, Issa JP et al (1998) Incidence and functional consequences of hMLH1 promoter hypermethylation in colorectal carcinoma. Proc Natl Acad Sci U S A 95:6870–6875
8. Okugawa Y, Grady WM, Goel A (2015) Epigenetic alterations in colorectal cancer: emerging biomarkers. Gastroenterology 149:1204–1225. e12
9. Lao VV, Grady WM (2011) Epigenetics and colorectal cancer. Nat Rev Gastroenterol Hepatol 8:686–700
10. Goel A, Boland CR (2012) Epigenetics of colorectal cancer. Gastroenterology 143:1442–1460. e1
11. Vaiopoulos AG, Athanasoula K, Papavassiliou AG (1842) Epigenetic modifications in colorectal cancer: molecular insights and therapeutic challenges. Biochim Biophys Acta 2014:971–980

12. Nakagawa H, Chadwick RB, Peltomaki P, Plass C, Nakamura Y, de La Chapelle A (2001) Loss of imprinting of the insulin-like growth factor II gene occurs by biallelic methylation in a core region of H19-associated CTCF-binding sites in colorectal cancer. Proc Natl Acad Sci U S A 98:591–596

13. Sakatani T, Kaneda A, Iacobuzio-Donahue CA, Carter MG, de Boom WS, Okano H et al (2005) Loss of imprinting of Igf2 alters intestinal maturation and tumorigenesis in mice. Science 307:1976–1978

14. Suzuki H, Tokino T, Shinomura Y, Imai K, Toyota M (2008) DNA methylation and cancer pathways in gastrointestinal tumors. Pharmacogenomics 9:1917–1928

15. Schnekenburger M, Diederich M (2012) Epigenetics offer new horizons for colorectal cancer prevention. Curr Colorectal Cancer Rep 8:66–81

16. Suzuki H, Maruyama R, Yamamoto E, Kai M (2012) DNA methylation and microRNA dysregulation in cancer. Mol Oncol 6:567–578

17. Kumegawa K, Maruyama R, Yamamoto E, Ashida M, Kitajima H, Tsuyada A et al (2016) A genomic screen for long noncoding RNA genes epigenetically silenced by aberrant DNA methylation in colorectal cancer. Sci Rep 6:26699

18. Irizarry RA, Ladd-Acosta C, Wen B, Wu Z, Montano C, Onyango P et al (2009) The human colon cancer methylome shows similar hypo- and hypermethylation at conserved tissue-specific CpG island shores. Nat Genet 41:178–186

19. Matsuzaki K, Deng G, Tanaka H, Kakar S, Miura S, Kim YS (2005) The relationship between global methylation level, loss of heterozygosity, and microsatellite instability in sporadic colorectal cancer. Clin Cancer Res 11:8564–8569

20. Estecio MR, Gharibyan V, Shen L, Ibrahim AE, Doshi K, He R et al (2007) LINE-1 hypomethylation in cancer is highly variable and inversely correlated with microsatellite instability. PLoS One 2:e399

21. Ogino S, Kawasaki T, Nosho K, Ohnishi M, Suemoto Y, Kirkner GJ et al (2008) LINE-1 hypomethylation is inversely associated with microsatellite instability and CpG island methylator phenotype in colorectal cancer. Int J Cancer 122:2767–2773

22. Cancer Genome Atlas Network (2012) Comprehensive molecular characterization of human colon and rectal cancer. Nature 487:330–337

23. Suzuki H, Yamamoto E, Maruyama R, Niinuma T, Kai M (2014) Biological significance of the CpG island methylator phenotype. Biochem Biophys Res Commun 455:35–42

24. Toyota M, Ho C, Ahuja N, Jair KW, Li Q, Ohe-Toyota M et al (1999) Identification of differentially methylated sequences in colorectal cancer by methylated CpG island amplification. Cancer Res 59:2307–2312

25. Toyota M, Ahuja N, Ohe-Toyota M, Herman JG, Baylin SB, Issa JP (1999) CpG island methylator phenotype in colorectal cancer. Proc Natl Acad Sci U S A 96:8681–8686

26. Toyota M, Ohe-Toyota M, Ahuja N, Issa JP (2000) Distinct genetic profiles in colorectal tumors with or without the CpG island methylator phenotype. Proc Natl Acad Sci U S A 97:710–715

27. van Rijnsoever M, Grieu F, Elsaleh H, Joseph D, Iacopetta B (2002) Characterisation of colorectal cancers showing hypermethylation at multiple CpG islands. Gut 51:797–802

28. Hawkins N, Norrie M, Cheong K, Mokany E, Ku SL, Meagher A et al (2002) CpG island methylation in sporadic colorectal cancers and its relationship to microsatellite instability. Gastroenterology 122:1376–1387

29. Samowitz WS, Albertsen H, Herrick J, Levin TR, Sweeney C, Murtaugh MA et al (2005) Evaluation of a large, population-based sample supports a CpG island methylator phenotype in colon cancer. Gastroenterology 129:837–845

30. Goel A, Nagasaka T, Arnold CN, Inoue T, Hamilton C, Niedzwiecki D et al (2007) The CpG island methylator phenotype and chromosomal instability are inversely correlated in sporadic colorectal cancer. Gastroenterology 132:127–138

31. Cheng YW, Pincas H, Bacolod MD, Schemmann G, Giardina SF, Huang J et al (2008) CpG island methylator phenotype associates with low-degree chromosomal abnormalities in colorectal cancer. Clin Cancer Res 14:6005–6013

32. Ogino S, Kawasaki T, Kirkner GJ, Ohnishi M, Fuchs CS (2007) 18q loss of heterozygosity in microsatellite stable colorectal cancer is correlated with CpG island methylator phenotype-negative (CIMP-0) and inversely with CIMP-low and CIMP-high. BMC Cancer 7:72

33. Yamashita K, Dai T, Dai Y, Yamamoto F, Perucho M (2003) Genetics supersedes epigenetics in colon cancer phenotype. Cancer Cell 4:121–131

34. Anacleto C, Leopoldino AM, Rossi B, Soares FA, Lopes A, Rocha JC et al (2005) Colorectal cancer "methylator phenotype": fact or artifact? Neoplasia 7:331–335

35. Issa JP (2004) CpG island methylator phenotype in cancer. Nat Rev Cancer 4:988–993

36. Ogino S, Cantor M, Kawasaki T, Brahmandam M, Kirkner GJ, Weisenberger DJ et al (2006) CpG island methylator phenotype (CIMP) of colorectal cancer is best characterised by quantitative DNA methylation analysis and prospective cohort studies. Gut 55:1000–1006

37. Weisenberger DJ, Siegmund KD, Campan M, Young J, Long TI, Faasse MA et al (2006) CpG island methylator phenotype underlies sporadic microsatellite instability and is tightly associated with BRAF mutation in colorectal cancer. Nat Genet 38:787–793

38. Ogino S, Kawasaki T, Kirkner GJ, Loda M, Fuchs CS (2006) CpG island methylator phenotype-low (CIMP-low) in colorectal cancer: possible associations with male sex and KRAS mutations. J Mol Diagn 8:582–588

39. Shen L, Toyota M, Kondo Y, Lin E, Zhang L, Guo Y et al (2007) Integrated genetic and epigenetic analysis identifies three different subclasses of colon cancer. Proc Natl Acad Sci U S A 104:18654–18659

40. Yagi K, Akagi K, Hayashi H, Nagae G, Tsuji S, Isagawa T et al (2010) Three DNA methylation epigenotypes in human colorectal cancer. Clin Cancer Res 16:21–33

41. Hinoue T, Weisenberger DJ, Lange CP, Shen H, Byun HM, Van Den Berg D et al (2012) Genome-scale analysis of aberrant DNA methylation in colorectal cancer. Genome Res 22:271–282

42. Hinoue T, Weisenberger DJ, Pan F, Campan M, Kim M, Young J et al (2009) Analysis of the association between CIMP and BRAF in colorectal cancer by DNA methylation profiling. PLoS One 4:e8357

43. Suzuki H, Igarashi S, Nojima M, Maruyama R, Yamamoto E, Kai M et al (2010) IGFBP7 is a p53-responsive gene specifically silenced in colorectal cancer with CpG island methylator phenotype. Carcinogenesis 31:342–349

44. Wajapeyee N, Serra RW, Zhu X, Mahalingam M, Green MR (2008) Oncogenic BRAF induces senescence and apoptosis through pathways mediated by the secreted protein IGFBP7. Cell 132:363–374

45. Ogino S, Kawasaki T, Kirkner GJ, Kraft P, Loda M, Fuchs CS (2007) Evaluation of markers for CpG island methylator phenotype (CIMP) in colorectal cancer by a large population-based sample. J Mol Diagn 9:305–314

46. Karpinski P, Walter M, Szmida E, Ramsey D, Misiak B, Kozlowska J et al (2013) Intermediate- and low-methylation epigenotypes do not correspond to CpG island methylator phenotype (low and -zero) in colorectal cancer. Cancer Epidemiol Biomark Prev 22:201–208

47. Guinney J, Dienstmann R, Wang X, de Reynies A, Schlicker A, Soneson C et al (2015) The consensus molecular subtypes of colorectal cancer. Nat Med 21:1350–1356

48. Rashid A, Shen L, Morris JS, Issa JP, Hamilton SR (2001) CpG island methylation in colorectal adenomas. Am J Pathol 159:1129–1135

49. Chan AO, Broaddus RR, Houlihan PS, Issa JP, Hamilton SR, Rashid A (2002) CpG island methylation in aberrant crypt foci of the colorectum. Am J Pathol 160:1823–1830

50. Suzuki H, Watkins DN, Jair KW, Schuebel KE, Markowitz SD, Chen WD et al (2004) Epigenetic inactivation of SFRP genes allows constitutive WNT signaling in colorectal cancer. Nat Genet 36:417–422

51. Kim YH, Petko Z, Dzieciatkowski S, Lin L, Ghiassi M, Stain S et al (2006) CpG island methylation of genes accumulates during the adenoma progression step of the multistep pathogenesis of colorectal cancer. Genes Chromosomes Cancer 45:781–789

52. Yamamoto E, Suzuki H, Yamano HO, Maruyama R, Nojima M, Kamimae S et al (2012) Molecular dissection of premalignant colorectal lesions reveals early onset of the CpG island methylator phenotype. Am J Pathol 181:1847–1861
53. Chan AO, Issa JP, Morris JS, Hamilton SR, Rashid A (2002) Concordant CpG island methylation in hyperplastic polyposis. Am J Pathol 160:529–536
54. Yagi K, Takahashi H, Akagi K, Matsusaka K, Seto Y, Aburatani H et al (2012) Intermediate methylation epigenotype and its correlation to KRAS mutation in conventional colorectal adenoma. Am J Pathol 180:616–625
55. Rex DK, Ahnen DJ, Baron JA, Batts KP, Burke CA, Burt RW et al (2012) Serrated lesions of the colorectum: review and recommendations from an expert panel. Am J Gastroenterol 107:1315–1329. quiz 4, 30
56. IJspeert JE, Vermeulen L, Meijer GA, Dekker E (2015) Serrated neoplasia-role in colorectal carcinogenesis and clinical implications. Nat Rev Gastroenterol Hepatol 12:401–409
57. Kambara T, Simms LA, Whitehall VL, Spring KJ, Wynter CV, Walsh MD et al (2004) BRAF mutation is associated with DNA methylation in serrated polyps and cancers of the colorectum. Gut 53:1137–1144
58. Yamauchi M, Morikawa T, Kuchiba A, Imamura Y, Qian ZR, Nishihara R et al (2012) Assessment of colorectal cancer molecular features along bowel subsites challenges the conception of distinct dichotomy of proximal versus distal colorectum. Gut 61:847–854
59. Burnett-Hartman AN, Newcomb PA, Potter JD, Passarelli MN, Phipps AI, Wurscher MA et al (2013) Genomic aberrations occurring in subsets of serrated colorectal lesions but not conventional adenomas. Cancer Res 73:2863–2872
60. Sawada T, Yamamoto E, Yamano HO, Nojima M, Harada T, Maruyama R et al (2016) Assessment of epigenetic alterations in early colorectal lesions containing BRAF mutations. Oncotarget 7:35106–35118
61. Nishihara R, Wu K, Lochhead P, Morikawa T, Liao X, Qian ZR et al (2013) Long-term colorectal-cancer incidence and mortality after lower endoscopy. N Engl J Med 369:1095–1105
62. Kimura T, Yamamoto E, Yamano HO, Suzuki H, Kamimae S, Nojima M et al (2012) A novel pit pattern identifies the precursor of colorectal cancer derived from sessile serrated adenoma. Am J Gastroenterol 107:460–469
63. Nosho K, Shima K, Irahara N, Kure S, Baba Y, Kirkner GJ et al (2009) DNMT3B expression might contribute to CpG island methylator phenotype in colorectal cancer. Clin Cancer Res 15:3663–3671
64. Ibrahim AE, Arends MJ, Silva AL, Wyllie AH, Greger L, Ito Y et al (2011) Sequential DNA methylation changes are associated with DNMT3B overexpression in colorectal neoplastic progression. Gut 60:499–508
65. Croce CM (2009) Causes and consequences of microRNA dysregulation in cancer. Nat Rev Genet 10:704–714
66. Esquela-Kerscher A, Slack FJ (2006) Oncomirs – microRNAs with a role in cancer. Nat Rev Cancer 6:259–269
67. Fabbri M, Garzon R, Cimmino A, Liu Z, Zanesi N, Callegari E et al (2007) MicroRNA-29 family reverts aberrant methylation in lung cancer by targeting DNA methyltransferases 3A and 3B. Proc Natl Acad Sci U S A 104:15805–15810
68. Huang J, Wang Y, Guo Y, Sun S (2010) Down-regulated microRNA-152 induces aberrant DNA methylation in hepatitis B virus-related hepatocellular carcinoma by targeting DNA methyltransferase 1. Hepatology 52:60–70
69. Zhang Z, Tang H, Wang Z, Zhang B, Liu W, Lu H et al (2011) MiR-185 targets the DNA methyltransferases 1 and regulates global DNA methylation in human glioma. Mol Cancer 10:124
70. Liu R, Gu J, Jiang P, Zheng Y, Liu X, Jiang X et al (2015) DNMT1-microRNA126 epigenetic circuit contributes to esophageal squamous cell carcinoma growth via ADAM9-EGFR-AKT signaling. Clin Cancer Res 21:854–863

71. Wang H, Wu J, Meng X, Ying X, Zuo Y, Liu R et al (2011) MicroRNA-342 inhibits colorectal cancer cell proliferation and invasion by directly targeting DNA methyltransferase 1. Carcinogenesis 32:1033–1042

72. Branco MR, Ficz G, Reik W (2012) Uncovering the role of 5-hydroxymethylcytosine in the epigenome. Nat Rev Genet 13:7–13

73. Kudo Y, Tateishi K, Yamamoto K, Yamamoto S, Asaoka Y, Ijichi H et al (2012) Loss of 5-hydroxymethylcytosine is accompanied with malignant cellular transformation. Cancer Sci 103:670–676

74. Delhommeau F, Dupont S, Della Valle V, James C, Trannoy S, Masse A et al (2009) Mutation in TET2 in myeloid cancers. N Engl J Med 360:2289–2301

75. Ko M, Huang Y, Jankowska AM, Pape UJ, Tahiliani M, Bandukwala HS et al (2010) Impaired hydroxylation of 5-methylcytosine in myeloid cancers with mutant TET2. Nature 468:839–843

76. Xu W, Yang H, Liu Y, Yang Y, Wang P, Kim SH et al (2011) Oncometabolite 2-hydroxyglutarate is a competitive inhibitor of alpha-ketoglutarate-dependent dioxygenases. Cancer Cell 19:17–30

77. Noushmehr H, Weisenberger DJ, Diefes K, Phillips HS, Pujara K, Berman BP et al (2010) Identification of a CpG island methylator phenotype that defines a distinct subgroup of glioma. Cancer Cell 17:510–522

78. Figueroa ME, Abdel-Wahab O, Lu C, Ward PS, Patel J, Shih A et al (2010) Leukemic IDH1 and IDH2 mutations result in a hypermethylation phenotype, disrupt TET2 function, and impair hematopoietic differentiation. Cancer Cell 18:553–567

79. Turcan S, Rohle D, Goenka A, Walsh LA, Fang F, Yilmaz E et al (2012) IDH1 mutation is sufficient to establish the glioma hypermethylator phenotype. Nature 483:479–483

80. Ichimura N, Shinjo K, An B, Shimizu Y, Yamao K, Ohka F et al (2015) Aberrant TET1 methylation closely associated with CpG island methylator phenotype in colorectal cancer. Cancer Prev Res (Phila) 8:702–711

81. Raptis S, Mrkonjic M, Green RC, Pethe VV, Monga N, Chan YM et al (2007) MLH1 -93G>A promoter polymorphism and the risk of microsatellite-unstable colorectal cancer. J Natl Cancer Inst 99:463–474

82. Samowitz WS, Curtin K, Wolff RK, Albertsen H, Sweeney C, Caan BJ et al (2008) The MLH1 -93 G>A promoter polymorphism and genetic and epigenetic alterations in colon cancer. Genes Chromosomes Cancer 47:835–844

83. Miyakura Y, Tahara M, Lefor AT, Yasuda Y, Sugano K (2014) Haplotype defined by the MLH1-93G/A polymorphism is associated with MLH1 promoter hypermethylation in sporadic colorectal cancers. BMC Res Notes 7:835

84. Wong JJ, Hawkins NJ, Ward RL, Hitchins MP (2011) Methylation of the 3p22 region encompassing MLH1 is representative of the CpG island methylator phenotype in colorectal cancer. Mod Pathol 24:396–411

85. Fang M, Ou J, Hutchinson L, Green MR (2014) The BRAF oncoprotein functions through the transcriptional repressor MAFG to mediate the CpG island methylator phenotype. Mol Cell 55:904–915

86. Tahara T, Yamamoto E, Madireddi P, Suzuki H, Maruyama R, Chung W et al (2014) Colorectal carcinomas with CpG island methylator phenotype 1 frequently contain mutations in chromatin regulators. Gastroenterology 146:530–538. e5

87. Samowitz WS, Albertsen H, Sweeney C, Herrick J, Caan BJ, Anderson KE et al (2006) Association of smoking, CpG island methylator phenotype, and V600E BRAF mutations in colon cancer. J Natl Cancer Inst 98:1731–1738

88. Limsui D, Vierkant RA, Tillmans LS, Wang AH, Weisenberger DJ, Laird PW et al (2010) Cigarette smoking and colorectal cancer risk by molecularly defined subtypes. J Natl Cancer Inst 102:1012–1022

89. Song M, Garrett WS, Chan AT (2015) Nutrients, foods, and colorectal cancer prevention. Gastroenterology 148:1244–1260. e16

90. Khosraviani K, Weir HP, Hamilton P, Moorehead J, Williamson K (2002) Effect of folate supplementation on mucosal cell proliferation in high risk patients for colon cancer. Gut 51:195–199

91. Pufulete M, Al-Ghnaniem R, Leather AJ, Appleby P, Gout S, Terry C et al (2003) Folate status, genomic DNA hypomethylation, and risk of colorectal adenoma and cancer: a case control study. Gastroenterology 124:1240–1248

92. Pufulete M, Al-Ghnaniem R, Khushal A, Appleby P, Harris N, Gout S et al (2005) Effect of folic acid supplementation on genomic DNA methylation in patients with colorectal adenoma. Gut 54:648–653

93. van Engeland M, Weijenberg MP, Roemen GM, Brink M, de Bruine AP, Goldbohm RA et al (2003) Effects of dietary folate and alcohol intake on promoter methylation in sporadic colorectal cancer: the Netherlands cohort study on diet and cancer. Cancer Res 63:3133–3137

94. de Vogel S, Wouters KA, Gottschalk RW, van Schooten FJ, de Goeij AF, de Bruine AP et al (2009) Genetic variants of methyl metabolizing enzymes and epigenetic regulators: associations with promoter CpG island hypermethylation in colorectal cancer. Cancer Epidemiol Biomark Prev 18:3086–3096

95. Hazra A, Fuchs CS, Kawasaki T, Kirkner GJ, Hunter DJ, Ogino S (2010) Germline polymorphisms in the one-carbon metabolism pathway and DNA methylation in colorectal cancer. Cancer Causes Control 21:331–345

96. Curtin K, Slattery ML, Ulrich CM, Bigler J, Levin TR, Wolff RK et al (2007) Genetic polymorphisms in one-carbon metabolism: associations with CpG island methylator phenotype (CIMP) in colon cancer and the modifying effects of diet. Carcinogenesis 28:1672–1679

97. Slattery ML, Curtin K, Sweeney C, Levin TR, Potter J, Wolff RK et al (2007) Diet and lifestyle factor associations with CpG island methylator phenotype and BRAF mutations in colon cancer. Int J Cancer 120:656–663

98. Schernhammer ES, Giovannucci E, Baba Y, Fuchs CS, Ogino S (2011) B vitamins, methionine and alcohol intake and risk of colon cancer in relation to BRAF mutation and CpG island methylator phenotype (CIMP). PLoS One 6:e21102

99. Gazzoli I, Loda M, Garber J, Syngal S, Kolodner RD (2002) A hereditary nonpolyposis colorectal carcinoma case associated with hypermethylation of the MLH1 gene in normal tissue and loss of heterozygosity of the unmethylated allele in the resulting microsatellite instability-high tumor. Cancer Res 62:3925–3928

100. Hitchins M, Williams R, Cheong K, Halani N, Lin VA, Packham D et al (2005) MLH1 germline epimutations as a factor in hereditary nonpolyposis colorectal cancer. Gastroenterology 129:1392–1399

101. Hitchins MP (2015) Constitutional epimutation as a mechanism for cancer causality and heritability? Nat Rev Cancer 15:625–634

102. Hitchins MP, Wong JJ, Suthers G, Suter CM, Martin DI, Hawkins NJ et al (2007) Inheritance of a cancer-associated MLH1 germ-line epimutation. N Engl J Med 356:697–705

103. Hitchins MP, Rapkins RW, Kwok CT, Srivastava S, Wong JJ, Khachigian LM et al (2011) Dominantly inherited constitutional epigenetic silencing of MLH1 in a cancer-affected family is linked to a single nucleotide variant within the 5'UTR. Cancer Cell 20:200–213

104. Kwok CT, Vogelaar IP, van Zelst-Stams WA, Mensenkamp AR, Ligtenberg MJ, Rapkins RW et al (2014) The MLH1 c.-27C>A and c.85G>T variants are linked to dominantly inherited MLH1 epimutation and are borne on a European ancestral haplotype. Eur J Hum Genet 22:617–624

105. Chan TL, Yuen ST, Kong CK, Chan YW, Chan AS, Ng WF et al (2006) Heritable germline epimutation of MSH2 in a family with hereditary nonpolyposis colorectal cancer. Nat Genet 38:1178–1183

106. Ligtenberg MJ, Kuiper RP, Chan TL, Goossens M, Hebeda KM, Voorendt M et al (2009) Heritable somatic methylation and inactivation of MSH2 in families with Lynch syndrome due to deletion of the 3' exons of TACSTD1. Nat Genet 41:112–117

107. Mandel JS, Church TR, Bond JH, Ederer F, Geisser MS, Mongin SJ et al (2000) The effect of fecal occult-blood screening on the incidence of colorectal cancer. N Engl J Med 343:1603–1607

108. van Rossum LG, van Rijn AF, Laheij RJ, van Oijen MG, Fockens P, van Krieken HH et al (2008) Random comparison of guaiac and immunochemical fecal occult blood tests for colorectal cancer in a screening population. Gastroenterology 135:82–90

109. Leung WK, To KF, Man EP, Chan MW, Hui AJ, Ng SS et al (2007) Detection of hypermethylated DNA or cyclooxygenase-2 messenger RNA in fecal samples of patients with colorectal cancer or polyps. Am J Gastroenterol 102:1070–1076

110. Petko Z, Ghiassi M, Shuber A, Gorham J, Smalley W, Washington MK et al (2005) Aberrantly methylated CDKN2A, MGMT, and MLH1 in colon polyps and in fecal DNA from patients with colorectal polyps. Clin Cancer Res 11:1203–1209

111. Hellebrekers DM, Lentjes MH, van den Bosch SM, Melotte V, Wouters KA, Daenen KL et al (2009) GATA4 and GATA5 are potential tumor suppressors and biomarkers in colorectal cancer. Clin Cancer Res 15:3990–3997

112. Ausch C, Kim YH, Tsuchiya KD, Dzieciatkowski S, Washington MK, Paraskeva C et al (2009) Comparative analysis of PCR-based biomarker assay methods for colorectal polyp detection from fecal DNA. Clin Chem 55:1559–1563

113. Kalimutho M, Di Cecilia S, Del Vecchio BG, Roviello F, Sileri P, Cretella M et al (2011) Epigenetically silenced miR-34b/c as a novel faecal-based screening marker for colorectal cancer. Br J Cancer 104:1770–1778

114. Melotte V, Lentjes MH, van den Bosch SM, Hellebrekers DM, de Hoon JP, Wouters KA et al (2009) N-Myc downstream-regulated gene 4 (NDRG4): a candidate tumor suppressor gene and potential biomarker for colorectal cancer. J Natl Cancer Inst 101:916–927

115. Nagasaka T, Tanaka N, Cullings HM, Sun DS, Sasamoto H, Uchida T et al (2009) Analysis of fecal DNA methylation to detect gastrointestinal neoplasia. J Natl Cancer Inst 101:1244–1258

116. Muller HM, Oberwalder M, Fiegl H, Morandell M, Goebel G, Zitt M et al (2004) Methylation changes in faecal DNA: a marker for colorectal cancer screening? Lancet 363:1283–1285

117. Glockner SC, Dhir M, Yi JM, McGarvey KE, Van Neste L, Louwagie J et al (2009) Methylation of TFPI2 in stool DNA: a potential novel biomarker for the detection of colorectal cancer. Cancer Res 69:4691–4699

118. Chen WD, Han ZJ, Skoletsky J, Olson J, Sah J, Myeroff L et al (2005) Detection in fecal DNA of colon cancer-specific methylation of the nonexpressed vimentin gene. J Natl Cancer Inst 97:1124–1132

119. Imperiale TF, Ransohoff DF, Itzkowitz SH, Levin TR, Lavin P, Lidgard GP et al (2014) Multitarget stool DNA testing for colorectal-cancer screening. N Engl J Med 370:1287–1297

120. Ebert MP, Model F, Mooney S, Hale K, Lograsso J, Tonnes-Priddy L et al (2006) Aristaless-like homeobox-4 gene methylation is a potential marker for colorectal adenocarcinomas. Gastroenterology 131:1418–1430

121. Lee BB, Lee EJ, Jung EH, Chun HK, Chang DK, Song SY et al (2009) Aberrant methylation of APC, MGMT, RASSF2A, and Wif-1 genes in plasma as a biomarker for early detection of colorectal cancer. Clin Cancer Res 15:6185–6191

122. Melotte V, Yi JM, Lentjes MH, Smits KM, Van Neste L, Niessen HE et al (2015) Spectrin repeat containing nuclear envelope 1 and forkhead box protein E1 are promising markers for the detection of colorectal cancer in blood. Cancer Prev Res (Phila) 8:157–164

123. Herbst A, Rahmig K, Stieber P, Philipp A, Jung A, Ofner A et al (2011) Methylation of NEUROG1 in serum is a sensitive marker for the detection of early colorectal cancer. Am J Gastroenterol 106:1110–1118

124. Lofton-Day C, Model F, Devos T, Tetzner R, Distler J, Schuster M et al (2008) DNA methylation biomarkers for blood-based colorectal cancer screening. Clin Chem 54:414–423

125. Li M, Chen WD, Papadopoulos N, Goodman SN, Bjerregaard NC, Laurberg S et al (2009) Sensitive digital quantification of DNA methylation in clinical samples. Nat Biotechnol 27:858–863

126. Ward RL, Cheong K, Ku SL, Meagher A, O'Connor T, Hawkins NJ (2003) Adverse prognostic effect of methylation in colorectal cancer is reversed by microsatellite instability. J Clin Oncol 21:3729–3736

127. Barault L, Charon-Barra C, Jooste V, de la Vega MF, Martin L, Roignot P et al (2008) Hypermethylator phenotype in sporadic colon cancer: study on a population-based series of 582 cases. Cancer Res 68:8541–8546

128. Kim JH, Shin SH, Kwon HJ, Cho NY, Kang GH (2009) Prognostic implications of CpG island hypermethylator phenotype in colorectal cancers. Virchows Arch 455:485–494

129. Dahlin AM, Palmqvist R, Henriksson ML, Jacobsson M, Eklof V, Rutegard J et al (2010) The role of the CpG island methylator phenotype in colorectal cancer prognosis depends on microsatellite instability screening status. Clin Cancer Res 16:1845–1855

130. Ahn JB, Chung WB, Maeda O, Shin SJ, Kim HS, Chung HC et al (2011) DNA methylation predicts recurrence from resected stage III proximal colon cancer. Cancer 117:1847–1854

131. Simons CC, Hughes LA, Smits KM, Khalid-de Bakker CA, de Bruine AP, Carvalho B et al (2013) A novel classification of colorectal tumors based on microsatellite instability, the CpG island methylator phenotype and chromosomal instability: implications for prognosis. Ann Oncol 24:2048–2056

132. Bae JM, Kim JH, Cho NY, Kim TY, Kang GH (2013) Prognostic implication of the CpG island methylator phenotype in colorectal cancers depends on tumour location. Br J Cancer 109:1004–1012

133. Juo YY, Johnston FM, Zhang DY, Juo HH, Wang H, Pappou EP et al (2014) Prognostic value of CpG island methylator phenotype among colorectal cancer patients: a systematic review and meta-analysis. Ann Oncol 25:2314–2327

134. Ogino S, Nosho K, Kirkner GJ, Kawasaki T, Meyerhardt JA, Loda M et al (2009) CpG island methylator phenotype, microsatellite instability, BRAF mutation and clinical outcome in colon cancer. Gut 58:90–96

135. Lee S, Cho NY, Choi M, Yoo EJ, Kim JH, Kang GH (2008) Clinicopathological features of CpG island methylator phenotype-positive colorectal cancer and its adverse prognosis in relation to KRAS/BRAF mutation. Pathol Int 58:104–113

136. Pai RK, Jayachandran P, Koong AC, Chang DT, Kwok S, Ma L et al (2012) BRAF-mutated, microsatellite-stable adenocarcinoma of the proximal colon: an aggressive adenocarcinoma with poor survival, mucinous differentiation, and adverse morphologic features. Am J Surg Pathol 36:744–752

137. Van Rijnsoever M, Elsaleh H, Joseph D, McCaul K, Iacopetta B (2003) CpG island methylator phenotype is an independent predictor of survival benefit from 5-fluorouracil in stage III colorectal cancer. Clin Cancer Res 9:2898–2903

138. Shen L, Catalano PJ, Benson AB 3rd, O'Dwyer P, Hamilton SR, Issa JP (2007) Association between DNA methylation and shortened survival in patients with advanced colorectal cancer treated with 5-fluorouracil based chemotherapy. Clin Cancer Res 13:6093–6098

139. Jover R, Nguyen TP, Perez-Carbonell L, Zapater P, Paya A, Alenda C et al (2011) 5-Fluorouracil adjuvant chemotherapy does not increase survival in patients with CpG island methylator phenotype colorectal cancer. Gastroenterology 140:1174–1181

140. Min BH, Bae JM, Lee EJ, Yu HS, Kim YH, Chang DK et al (2011) The CpG island methylator phenotype may confer a survival benefit in patients with stage II or III colorectal carcinomas receiving fluoropyrimidine-based adjuvant chemotherapy. BMC Cancer 11:344

141. Shiovitz S, Bertagnolli MM, Renfro LA, Nam E, Foster NR, Dzieciatkowski S et al (2014) CpG island methylator phenotype is associated with response to adjuvant irinotecan-based therapy for stage III colon cancer. Gastroenterology 147:637–645

142. Hegi ME, Diserens AC, Gorlia T, Hamou MF, de Tribolet N, Weller M et al (2005) MGMT gene silencing and benefit from temozolomide in glioblastoma. N Engl J Med 352:997–1003

143. Amatu A, Sartore-Bianchi A, Moutinho C, Belotti A, Bencardino K, Chirico G et al (2013) Promoter CpG island hypermethylation of the DNA repair enzyme MGMT predicts clinical response to dacarbazine in a phase II study for metastatic colorectal cancer. Clin Cancer Res 19:2265–2272

144. Hochhauser D, Glynne-Jones R, Potter V, Gravalos C, Doyle TJ, Pathiraja K et al (2013) A phase II study of temozolomide in patients with advanced aerodigestive tract and colorectal cancers and methylation of the O6-methylguanine-DNA methyltransferase promoter. Mol Cancer Ther 12:809–818

145. Ebert MP, Tanzer M, Balluff B, Burgermeister E, Kretzschmar AK, Hughes DJ et al (2012) TFAP2E-DKK4 and chemoresistance in colorectal cancer. N Engl J Med 366:44–53

146. Moutinho C, Martinez-Cardus A, Santos C, Navarro-Perez V, Martinez-Balibrea E, Musulen E et al (2014) Epigenetic inactivation of the BRCA1 interactor SRBC and resistance to oxaliplatin in colorectal cancer. J Natl Cancer Inst 106:djt322

147. Ogino S, Nosho K, Kirkner GJ, Kawasaki T, Chan AT, Schernhammer ES et al (2008) A cohort study of tumoral LINE-1 hypomethylation and prognosis in colon cancer. J Natl Cancer Inst 100:1734–1738

148. Antelo M, Balaguer F, Shia J, Shen Y, Hur K, Moreira L et al (2012) A high degree of LINE-1 hypomethylation is a unique feature of early-onset colorectal cancer. PLoS One 7:e45357

149. Rhee YY, Kim MJ, Bae JM, Koh JM, Cho NY, Juhnn YS et al (2012) Clinical outcomes of patients with microsatellite-unstable colorectal carcinomas depend on L1 methylation level. Ann Surg Oncol 19:3441–3448

150. Shen L, Kondo Y, Rosner GL, Xiao L, Hernandez NS, Vilaythong J et al (2005) MGMT promoter methylation and field defect in sporadic colorectal cancer. J Natl Cancer Inst 97:1330–1338

151. Kamiyama H, Suzuki K, Maeda T, Koizumi K, Miyaki Y, Okada S et al (2012) DNA demethylation in normal colon tissue predicts predisposition to multiple cancers. Oncogene 31:5029–5037

152. Baylin SB, Jones PA (2011) A decade of exploring the cancer epigenome – biological and translational implications. Nat Rev Cancer 11:726–734

153. Fahrner JA, Eguchi S, Herman JG, Baylin SB (2002) Dependence of histone modifications and gene expression on DNA hypermethylation in cancer. Cancer Res 62:7213–7218

154. Nguyen CT, Weisenberger DJ, Velicescu M, Gonzales FA, Lin JC, Liang G et al (2002) Histone H3-lysine 9 methylation is associated with aberrant gene silencing in cancer cells and is rapidly reversed by 5-aza-2'-deoxycytidine. Cancer Res 62:6456–6461

155. Rhee I, Jair KW, Yen RW, Lengauer C, Herman JG, Kinzler KW et al (2000) CpG methylation is maintained in human cancer cells lacking DNMT1. Nature 404:1003–1007

156. Bachman KE, Park BH, Rhee I, Rajagopalan H, Herman JG, Baylin SB et al (2003) Histone modifications and silencing prior to DNA methylation of a tumor suppressor gene. Cancer Cell 3:89–95

157. Si J, Boumber YA, Shu J, Qin T, Ahmed S, He R et al (2010) Chromatin remodeling is required for gene reactivation after decitabine-mediated DNA hypomethylation. Cancer Res 70:6968–6977

158. Nakazawa T, Kondo T, Ma D, Niu D, Mochizuki K, Kawasaki T et al (2012) Global histone modification of histone H3 in colorectal cancer and its precursor lesions. Hum Pathol 43:834–842

159. Tamagawa H, Oshima T, Shiozawa M, Morinaga S, Nakamura Y, Yoshihara M et al (2012) The global histone modification pattern correlates with overall survival in metachronous liver metastasis of colorectal cancer. Oncol Rep 27:637–642

160. Tamagawa H, Oshima T, Numata M, Yamamoto N, Shiozawa M, Morinaga S et al (2013) Global histone modification of H3K27 correlates with the outcomes in patients with metachronous liver metastasis of colorectal cancer. Eur J Surg Oncol 39:655–661

161. Benard A, Goossens-Beumer IJ, van Hoesel AQ, de Graaf W, Horati H, Putter H et al (2014) Histone trimethylation at H3K4, H3K9 and H4K20 correlates with patient survival and tumor recurrence in early-stage colon cancer. BMC Cancer 14:531

162. Ding J, Zhang ZM, Xia Y, Liao GQ, Pan Y, Liu S et al (2013) LSD1-mediated epigenetic modification contributes to proliferation and metastasis of colon cancer. Br J Cancer 109:994–1003

163. Jie D, Zhongmin Z, Guoqing L, Sheng L, Yi Z, Jing W et al (2013) Positive expression of LSD1 and negative expression of E-cadherin correlate with metastasis and poor prognosis of colon cancer. Dig Dis Sci 58:1581–1589

164. Kang MY, Lee BB, Kim YH, Chang DK, Kyu Park S, Chun HK et al (2007) Association of the SUV39H1 histone methyltransferase with the DNA methyltransferase 1 at mRNA expression level in primary colorectal cancer. Int J Cancer 121:2192–2197

165. Yokoyama Y, Hieda M, Nishioka Y, Matsumoto A, Higashi S, Kimura H et al (2013) Cancer-associated upregulation of histone H3 lysine 9 trimethylation promotes cell motility in vitro and drives tumor formation in vivo. Cancer Sci 104:889–895

166. Yadav S, Singhal J, Singhal SS, Awasthi S (2009) hSET1: a novel approach for colon cancer therapy. Biochem Pharmacol 77:1635–1641

167. Hamamoto R, Furukawa Y, Morita M, Iimura Y, Silva FP, Li M et al (2004) SMYD3 encodes a histone methyltransferase involved in the proliferation of cancer cells. Nat Cell Biol 6:731–740

168. Pelaez IM, Kalogeropoulou M, Ferraro A, Voulgari A, Pankotai T, Boros I et al (2010) Oncogenic RAS alters the global and gene-specific histone modification pattern during epithelial-mesenchymal transition in colorectal carcinoma cells. Int J Biochem Cell Biol 42:911–920

169. Gaedcke J, Grade M, Jung K, Camps J, Jo P, Emons G et al (2010) Mutated KRAS results in overexpression of DUSP4, a MAP-kinase phosphatase, and SMYD3, a histone methyltransferase, in rectal carcinomas. Genes Chromosomes Cancer 49:1024–1034

170. Watanabe T, Kobunai T, Yamamoto Y, Matsuda K, Ishihara S, Nozawa K et al (2011) Differential gene expression signatures between colorectal cancers with and without KRAS mutations: crosstalk between the KRAS pathway and other signalling pathways. Eur J Cancer 47:1946–1954

171. Hudlebusch HR, Santoni-Rugiu E, Simon R, Ralfkiaer E, Rossing HH, Johansen JV et al (2011) The histone methyltransferase and putative oncoprotein MMSET is overexpressed in a large variety of human tumors. Clin Cancer Res 17:2919–2933

172. Uemura M, Yamamoto H, Takemasa I, Mimori K, Hemmi H, Mizushima T et al (2010) Jumonji domain containing 1A is a novel prognostic marker for colorectal cancer: in vivo identification from hypoxic tumor cells. Clin Cancer Res 16:4636–4646

173. Fluge O, Gravdal K, Carlsen E, Vonen B, Kjellevold K, Refsum S et al (2009) Expression of EZH2 and Ki-67 in colorectal cancer and associations with treatment response and prognosis. Br J Cancer 101:1282–1289

174. Wang CG, Ye YJ, Yuan J, Liu FF, Zhang H, Wang S (2010) EZH2 and STAT6 expression profiles are correlated with colorectal cancer stage and prognosis. World J Gastroenterol 16:2421–2427

175. Takawa M, Masuda K, Kunizaki M, Daigo Y, Takagi K, Iwai Y et al (2011) Validation of the histone methyltransferase EZH2 as a therapeutic target for various types of human cancer and as a prognostic marker. Cancer Sci 102:1298–1305

176. Fussbroich B, Wagener N, Macher-Goeppinger S, Benner A, Falth M, Sultmann H et al (2011) EZH2 depletion blocks the proliferation of colon cancer cells. PLoS One 6:e21651

177. Du J, Li Y, Li J, Zheng J (2010) Polycomb group protein Bmi1 expression in colon cancers predicts the survival. Med Oncol 27:1273–1276

178. Vire E, Brenner C, Deplus R, Blanchon L, Fraga M, Didelot C et al (2006) The Polycomb group protein EZH2 directly controls DNA methylation. Nature 439:871–874

179. Mohammad HP, Cai Y, McGarvey KM, Easwaran H, Van Neste L, Ohm JE et al (2009) Polycomb CBX7 promotes initiation of heritable repression of genes frequently silenced with cancer-specific DNA hypermethylation. Cancer Res 69:6322–6330

180. Jin B, Yao B, Li JL, Fields CR, Delmas AL, Liu C et al (2009) DNMT1 and DNMT3B modulate distinct polycomb-mediated histone modifications in colon cancer. Cancer Res 69:7412–7421

181. Schlesinger Y, Straussman R, Keshet I, Farkash S, Hecht M, Zimmerman J et al (2007) Polycomb-mediated methylation on Lys27 of histone H3 pre-marks genes for de novo methylation in cancer. Nat Genet 39:232–236
182. Ohm JE, McGarvey KM, Yu X, Cheng L, Schuebel KE, Cope L et al (2007) A stem cell-like chromatin pattern may predispose tumor suppressor genes to DNA hypermethylation and heritable silencing. Nat Genet 39:237–242
183. Widschwendter M, Fiegl H, Egle D, Mueller-Holzner E, Spizzo G, Marth C et al (2007) Epigenetic stem cell signature in cancer. Nat Genet 39:157–158

DNA and Histone Methylation in Prostate Cancer

Kexin Xu

Abstract As a model of "epigenetic catastrophe", prostate cancer is driven by progressive epigenetic changes that arise early in carcinogenesis and persist throughout disease progression. In this chapter, two common epigenetic modifications, DNA methylation and histone methylation, are reviewed regarding their up-to-date roles in the disease. DNA hypermethylation at certain promoter regions is an early event during prostate tumorigenesis and epigenetically silences tumor suppressor genes. Genome-wide DNA hypomethylation is thought to activate oncogenes and becomes more extensive as the tumors become metastatic and aggressive. Dynamic regulation of histone methylation patterns leads to cancer-specific transcriptional profiles, and histone-modifying enzymes closely crosstalk with critical biological pathways such as the androgen receptor (AR) signaling. The functions and features of these two epigenetic programs make them highly promising as diagnostic and prognostic biomarkers or new therapeutic targets for prostate cancer. However, epigenetic therapy is still in its infancy and imposes a lot of challenging issues such as specificity, toxicity and potency. Therefore, we need to comprehensively understand the epigenetic regulatory mechanisms of prostate cancer development and progression, identify the pharmacodynamics and biomarkers of the epigenetic drugs targeting DNA methylation or histone methylation to better stratify patient populations who will likely benefit from the precision medicine.

Keywords Prostate cancer • Epigenetics • DNA methylation • Histone methylation • AR signaling • Gene expression regulation • Diagnostic/prognostic/predictive biomarkers • Epigenetic therapy

K. Xu (✉)
Department of Molecular Medicine/Institute of Biotechnology, University of Texas Health Science Center at San Antonio, 7703 Floyd Curl Drive, San Antonio 78229, TX, USA
e-mail: xuk3@uthscsa.edu

© Springer International Publishing AG 2017
A. Kaneda, Y.-i. Tsukada (eds.), *DNA and Histone Methylation as Cancer Targets*,
Cancer Drug Discovery and Development, DOI 10.1007/978-3-319-59786-7_18

1   The Prostate and Prostate Cancer

1.1   The Prostate and Prostate Epithelial Cells

The prostate is part of the mammalian reproductive system in males. It is a walnut-sized exocrine gland located in front of the rectum and just below the bladder. The main function of the organ is to discharge a clear, slightly alkaline solution that nourishes and protects sperm cells produced in the testicles [1]. During ejaculation, the muscles of the prostate help to squeeze this fluid into the urethra and expel it, together with sperms and fluids from other glands, as semen. Although the protein content of human prostatic secretions is less than 1%, it contains a very important clinical index for the pathological status of the organ, prostate-specific antigen (PSA). Male hormones, testosterone and predominantly its metabolite dihydrotestosterone (DHT), regulate the normal development, proper function as well as neoplastic transformation of the prostate cells through binding to and activating the nuclear receptor, the androgen receptor (AR).

There are two generic types of cells that form the prostate gland: epithelial and stromal [2]. The epithelial cells line the surfaces of the glandular ducts, and they are exclusively essential for the secretory activity and structural integrity of the gland. It goes without saying that the epithelium compartment is very important to the biology of prostate considering the fact that over 90% of the prostate tumors are adenocarcinomas [3]. Three prominent cell populations have been identified in prostate epithelium, which are the columnar luminal cells, the cuboidal basal cells, and the neuroendocrine (NE) cells [4]. These three cell types are quite distinguished in terms of their morphologies, molecular characteristics, functional significance, and relevance to carcinogenesis. The tall luminal cells are aligned along the inner layer of the prostate ducts and project inwards into the gland lumen. They express high levels of AR, so these cells require androgens for their survival and secret the AR-produced PSA into the fluid. The outer layer of the prostate ducts is lined up by the stretched basal cells that, together with an underlying basement membrane, divide the prostatic glands from the surrounding connective tissues. AR level in basal cells is low and even undetectable, so androgens are not essential for the growth of basal epithelial cells. It is generally believed that within the basal cell layer exist the prostate stem cells, which give rise to the terminally differentiated secretory cells [5]. Neuroendocrine (NE) cells constitute a small portion of cells within prostatic epithelium compartment. They are irregularly and sparsely scattered throughout the basal layer. Little is known about this type of cells, only that they are androgen-independent, non-proliferating and terminally differentiated. The exact origin and physiological function of the NE cells are not completely understood, but it is believed that they may play a role in the differentiation of growing prostate and have been implicated in the development of carcinogenesis. The stromal compartment is mainly composed of smooth muscle cells and also includes fibroblasts, nerves, blood vessels and various infiltrating immune and inflammatory cell types. Crosstalk between prostatic epithelium and the surrounding stroma has a profound effect on prostate organogenesis and development, maintenance of homeostasis of the organ, as well as the evolution of prostatic carcinogenesis and cancer progression [6].

1.2 Pathological Conditions of Prostate

As the largest accessory sex gland in men, the prostate, however, is not required for viability. Still, this organ has elicited great attention from biomedical researchers because of the high occurrence of prostate diseases. There are several common categories in prostate-related disorders: prostatitis, benign prostatic hyperplasia (BPH), prostate intraepithelial neoplasia (PIN), and cancer [7]. Prostatitis is actually inflammation and swelling of the gland, which can be caused by bacterial infection and therefore treated with antibiotics. Prostatitis can happen in men of all ages, and does not have a clear link with an increased risk of prostate malignancy. BPH is a specific term used to describe the condition of an enlarged prostate. It is the most common aging-related prostate problem, which occurs in up to 90% of men older than 80. The symptoms can be relieved by lifestyle management, medications, or surgery that removes part of the prostate. Again, having BPH does not necessarily lead to prostate cancer. PIN, however, is considered as a preliminary step in the development of prostate cancer. In this case, the epithelial cells lining the acini and ducts become abnormally shaped, their nuclei get enlarged and nucleoli darkened. PIN is recognized as a continuum between low-grade (LG) and high-grade (HG) forms according to increasing degrees of abnormality, with high-grade PIN considered as the immediate precursor of early invasive carcinoma. Currently, the only way to detect and diagnose PIN is to use the technique of transrectal ultrasonography-guided biopsy. When HGPIN is identified, follow-up care is necessary. If the lesions are present in multiple areas on the initial and subsequent biopsies, patients may be treated with inhibitors of the enzymes involved in androgen and estrogen metabolism, anti-androgens, or selective estrogen receptor modulators to eliminate HGPIN and to decrease the incidence of prostate cancer.

Carcinoma of prostate is for sure the most deleterious situation of the organ. For decades, prostate cancer has been the most prevalent non-dermatologic type of cancer in men in the Western countries, with death rates second only to lung cancer [8]. According to the American Cancer Society, about 1 man in 7 will be diagnosed with prostate cancer at some point during his lifetime, and this ratio is even higher in men aged 65 years or older, about 6 cases in 10. Every 20 min another American man dies from the disease. In the US, an estimated 180,890 men will be newly diagnosed with prostate cancer in 2016, and approximately 26,120 men will die from it [9]. The only established factors that may increase the risk of developing prostate cancer are age, race/ethnicity and family history. There are other factors that may also influence the risk, which include diet, exposures to endocrine disrupting chemicals, occupation, etc. [10]. Prostate cancer is intimately associated with aging. Statistic reports indicate that prostate cancer affects 1 in 44 males at the ages of 40–59, 1 in 7 males at 60–79 and over half of men over 80 years of age. These data clearly demonstrate that the risk of developing prostate cancer is significantly influenced by age. Racial disparity is another element critical for prostate cancer incidence and mortality. For example, the frequency of prostate carcinoma occurrence is the highest among African-American men and in Caribbean men of African ancestry, while

Asian men living in Asia have the lowest risk. The exact reasons for these ethnic differences are still not well understood, but may involve with the differences in genetic variations, lifestyles, and socioeconomic statuses, etc. About 20% of prostate cancer runs in a family, and a man having a first-degree relative (father or brother) who was diagnosed with the cancer is at least twice as likely to develop the disease other men in general. Studies have found some inherited gene changes, like mutations in the *BRCA1*, *BRCA2* and *HOXB13* genes, but they only account for about 5–10% of all prostate cancer cases [11]. Therefore, besides the shared genetic makeup, the familial prostate cancer may also be inherited due to similar living environment (e.g., diet, lifestyle, carcinogen exposures, etc.). There are still incomplete knowledge and several misconceptions regarding the risk factors for prostate cancer, therefore future work in prostate cancer etiology, especially understanding the gene-environment interaction, is necessary and will help to make more informed health care choices and personalized treatment of the disease.

1.3   Evolving Biology and Treatment of Prostate Cancer

High rates of incidence and mortality of prostate carcinoma lead to great interests and tremendous efforts in both basic research and clinical trials. Nearly every prostate cancer is adenocarcinoma, which starts in the glandular epithelial cells lining the prostate. The tumors display mainly a luminal phenotype as most prostate cancer cells express the steroid hormone receptor AR, which is only present in the luminal layer. It is now widely accepted that androgens-AR axis plays a pivotal role in almost every step of prostate cancer initiation and progression [12]. The male hormone binds to a specific protein module on AR, which is called ligand-binding domain (LBD), and activates the nuclear receptor by promoting its translocation from the cytosol into the nucleus. Once activated, AR binds to target DNA sequences, also known as androgen response elements (AREs), and results in up- or down-regulation of specific gene transcription, which will stimulate proliferation, inhibit apoptosis or maintain dedifferentiation status. Activation of AR signaling is a predominant driving force for the uncontrolled growth of cancerous prostate cells, thus AR-expressing luminal cells are targets of tumorigenic transformation. Prostate cancer is very multi-focal, and different foci of the carcinoma are anatomically distinct. Compared with other epithelial cancers, prostate carcinoma is unique in that it is a relatively slow growing malignancy and follows a multistage process. Finally, metastatic cascade of the tumors may precede clinical detection of indicative parameters and happen even without capsule perforation. All these factors make the behaviors of prostate cancer cells highly unpredictable. The disease is usually detected and monitored by measuring the amount and velocity of serum PSA, which is a secretory prostatic protein circulating in the blood. The quantity of PSA generally rises when prostate cancer occurs, and the upper limit of a normal situation is clinically set at 4.0 ng/ml. Any tumors with PSA levels between 4 and 10 ng/ml are usually considered at intermediate stage, and may or may not need a biopsy. Cases with PSA concentrations over 10 ng/ml in general indicate the presence of prostate cancer. The other diagnostic method to detect the tumor at its earliest stages is a digital rectal exam (DRE), which looks for any irregularities in size, shape and texture of the organ. If cancer is suspected, follow-up tests will be needed, such as the transrectal ultrasound (TRUS) and prostate biopsy. A stage of the cancer is then determined based on the comprehensive evaluation of all the results from these diagnostic tests, which helps the cancer care team to choose treatment options and to predict a patient's outlook for survival. At early stage, the cancerous epithelial cells are confined to the organ with an intact basement membrane and do not invade the stroma. Active surveillance or watchful waiting is usually recommended for the elderly or those with other serious health problems. If the tumor appears as a large mass, treatment options might include radical prostatectomy (often with removal of the pelvic lymph nodes) and radiation therapy (external beam radiation or brachytherapy or both). As the disease progresses, the tumor extends beyond the prostate capsule and advances to local invasion of surrounding tissues such as seminal vesicle. At this stage, besides the remedies mentioned above, hormone therapy, also called androgen deprivation therapy or androgen suppression therapy, is commonly prescribed, which includes surgical castration (i.e., orchiectomy, a surgery to permanently and irreversibly remove one or both testicles) and chemical castration (i.e., luteinizing hormone-releasing hormone agonists or antagonists, CYP17 inhibitor and anti-androgens, all of which either lower the androgen level or stop the hormone from working). Finally, cancers spread to nearby areas like the bladder, rectum, lymph nodes or even distant organs such as the bones. Unfortunately, no cure is attainable for tumors in this aggressive form, and current treatment merely helps to keep the cancer under control and to improve a man's quality of life. Initially, prostate cancer cells depend on the androgen for their growth and survival, thereby hormone therapy is the most effective way to make prostate tumors shrink or grow slowly when cancer has metastasized beyond the prostate or better effectiveness of radiation therapy is wanted. However, despite the fact that 80–90% of tumors initially respond to the hormone therapy, nearly all patients progress to a more aggressive and lethal form of the disease termed castration resistant prostate cancer (CRPC) with median time to progression of approximately 18–24 months [13]. This means that cancer cells continue to divide perpetually and grow uncontrollable in the presence of castrate levels of testosterone (≤50 ng/dL). Patients with metastatic CRPC retain a guarded prognosis. Without treatment, median survival time ranges from 9.1 to 21.7 months, and most of these patients, if not all, eventually succumb to their disease [14–16]. Over the last two decades, huge advances have been made pertaining to the biology and pathophysiology of CRPC. There have been several models proposed on the causes of CRPC. For instance, AR gene mutations and amplification, which results in altered ligand specificity and increased sensitivity of AR signaling; expression of AR splice variants that lack ligand-binding domain and are constitutively active; aberrant AR reactivation by unbalanced interaction with its co-activators or co-repressors; induction of bypass pathway, which circumvents the AR axis and utilizes other mechanisms to stimulate the proliferation of prostate cancer cell [17]. Better understanding of the disease has

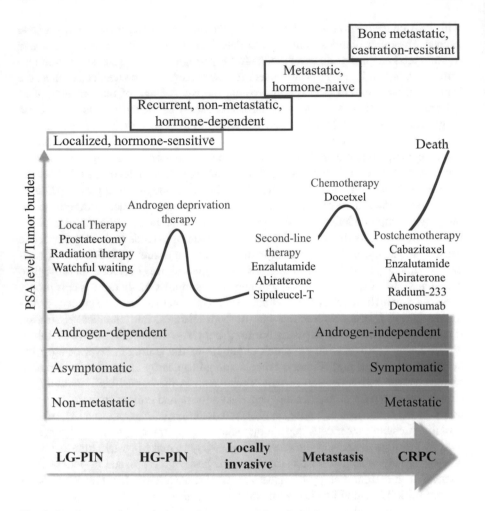

Fig. 1 Prostate cancer progression and treatment options for each stage

enabled the development of new therapeutic modalities including chemotherapy, immunotherapy, novel hormonal and palliative agents, which have gained US FDA approval and significantly improved life expectancy in men with metastatic CRPC (Fig. 1). These innovative treatment options for CRPC include:

(i) Sipuleucel-T. It is a therapeutic vaccine, and generated by first incubating the patient's antigen-presenting cells with a fusion protein consisting of antigen prostatic acid phosphatase and granulocyte-macrophage colony stimulating factor. The activated blood product is then re-infused into the patients and reprograms his immune system to attack the cancer.

(ii) Abiraterone acetate. This is an inhibitor of CYP17A1, the enzyme that catalyzes the synthesis of androgens, and thus decreases circulating levels of the hormone.

(iii) Enzalutamide. The pure anti-androgen is actually a blocker of AR signaling, which inhibits multiple steps along the axis: binding of androgens to AR, AR nuclear translocation, and recruitment of AR to target DNA.

(iv) Cabazitaxel and docetaxel. Both taxane compounds are microtubule inhibitors and thus block the mitotic cellular function, which leads to apoptosis. Cabazitaxel is a dimethyloxy derivative of docetaxel, and is superior to its predecessor because of lower substrate affinity for the drug efflux pump and ability to cross the blood-brain barrier. Therefore, cabazitaxel is the drug of choice in patients with docetaxel-refractory metastatic prostate cancer.

(v) Denosumab. As one of the bone-targeting agents in the management of CRPC, denosumab acts to prevent the maturation of osteoclast cells that break down bone tissues. Receptor activator of nuclear factor-κB (RANK) plays a critical role in osteoclast formation, and it is activated by its specific ligand RANKL. Denosumab is the human monoclonal antibody of RANKL, so it binds to RANKL and blocks the RANK signaling pathway.

(vi) Radium-223. This is another FDA-approved drug that is prescribed to prevent pain and fractures in CRPC patients with bone metastases. It is a "calcium mimetic" radioactive isotope, which means that it accumulates preferentially in areas where bone metastases are forming and emits low levels of α-particle radiation there to cause double-strand DNA breaks and kill cells.

All these new therapies have shown significant clinical improvement in men with metastatic CRPC, however prostate cancer remains the second leading cause of cancer death in American men. Further advances in prostate cancer research require definite mechanistic and molecular analyses, and the most overarching challenges in terms of clinical management include: (1) identification of prognostic markers that distinguish fatal from indolent prostate cancer; (2) exploration of mechanisms that lead to castration resistance; (3) development of strategies to enhance the well-being of men with prostate cancer; (4) recognition of new markers more sensitive and specific than PSA for prostate cancer detection. These studies will facilitate better diagnosis of primary tumors, lead to the development of novel cancer therapies, and improve quality of life for prostate cancer survivors.

2 Genetics and Epigenetics in Prostate Cancer

Like most cancers, prostate cancer is driven by genetic and non-genetic causes. Modern genetic and genome-based technologies have enabled the discoveries of somatic alterations and germline variations, which drive malignant transformation and progression of prostate cancer. Common genetic changes with well-defined roles in the disease include loss of heterozygosity (LOH) of *TP53* (in 10–20% of primary and up to 42% of advanced prostate cancer) [18] and *PTEN* (in approximately 27% of localized and 60% of metastatic tumors) genes [19], fusion of ETS transcription factor genes with androgen-responsive *TMPRSS2* promoter (in about half of prostate cancer) [20], mutations of *AR* gene (in less than 2% of untreated localized prostate cancer and up to 50% of metastatic hormone-refractory tumors) [21], and mutations of *SPOP* gene encoding the substrate-binding component of a cullin-RING-based ubiquitin ligase complex (in 6–15% of prostate cancer) [22, 23], etc. However, even with all these mutation hotspots in prostate cancer, some cases of prostate tumorigenesis still cannot be explained by definitive driving genomic events. As a consequence of divergent clonal evolution of the disease, the constellation of genetic mutations in prostate cancer can be quite heterogeneous, and many identified mutation types have low levels of recurrence. So genetic change is not the sole contributory factor to the origins of prostate cancer, and it is quite likely that other biological events precede and enforce the malignant transformation of the cells. Epigenetic alteration is one of the candidates for such early events.

Epigenetics refers to any biological process that acts upon the chromatin but does not affect the actual DNA sequences in order to modulate gene expression and subsequently control cell fate [24]. The topics that are covered in the epigenetic study have expanded rapidly, and now include DNA methylation, histone modifications, chromatin remodeling and non-coding RNA processing. A specific epigenetic pattern is highly susceptible to environmental stimuli such as dietary components and life style, hence it undergoes a real-time change upon the stimulation of the external factors and induces biological signaling cascade as an early response. It has been shown that numerous epigenetic alterations appear to be highly recurrent, and sometimes nearly universal, in prostate cancer. These alterations can affect thousands of loci across the cancer genome, reinforcing the establishment of a new transcriptional profile that favors self-renewal, survival, and invasion of prostate cancer cells. It has been demonstrated that accumulation of epigenetic aberrations eventually creates genetic or genomic instability. On the other hand, several genes encoding the enzymes for shaping the epigenetic landscape are found mutated in prostate cancer. Therefore, acquired/inherited genetic mutations and epigenetic aberrations contribute individually and cooperatively to the pathogenesis and progression of prostate cancer. In this chapter, we will mainly focus on two of the most broadly studied epigenetic modifications, DNA methylation and histone methylation. We will not only give a review of the most updated functions of these two epigenetic programs in prostate cancer, but also discuss the prospects for targeting either one of these two marks to better diagnose and treat the disease.

3   Prostate Cancer and DNA Methylation

3.1   DNA Methylation and Demethylation

DNA methylation is one of the critical epigenetic regulatory mechanisms to control gene expression. The reaction results in the addition of a methyl (−CH3) group to the 5′-carbon position of the cytosine ring (5mC). In mammals, DNA methylation predominantly occurs in the context of CpG dinucleotide (5′-Cytosine-phosphate-Guanine-3′), and approximately 60–90% of all CpGs are methylated. However, this dinucleotide is found in only 1% of human genome, less than one-quarter of the expected frequency due to the spontaneous deamination of the methylcytosines to thymines. It has been extensively documented that DNA methylation is used as an epigenetic mark for gene silencing, and several models have been proposed to explain the molecular mechanisms [25]. The modification directly retrains the binding of transcription factors to the methylated recognition elements, or it specifically attracts proteins containing a methylated-DNA binding domain (MBD) so that the preoccupied chromatin region is no longer accessible to factors required for genc induction. Besides, methylated DNA establishes a repressive and closed chromatin structure, as suggested by the evidence that methylated chromatin is insensitive to nuclease digestion and histone proteins assembled on it are significantly less acetylated. Finally, a *cis*-acting theory showed evidence that transcriptional repression does not require methylation of promoter sequences but is dependent on the position, length, or density of methylated cytosine residues. All these mechanisms of action indicate how critical and complex DNA methylation can be in terms of gene expression regulation, thus this epigenetic program must be precisely controlled. This covalent chemical modification is catalyzed by DNA methyltransferases (DNMTs), of which 3 active members (DNMT1, DNMT3A and DNMT3B) have been identified [26]. DNMT1 is the first DNA methyltransferase to be discovered and also the most abundant one in all adult human tissues. It is mainly responsible for maintaining DNA methylation patterns after DNA replication, when the parent DNA strand remains methylated while the daughter strand is not. So DNMT1 binds to CpG sites on DNA with only one strand modified, so-called hemi-methylated DNA, and methylates the cytosine on the newly synthesized strand. In contrast, both DNMT3A and B are de novo DNA methyltransferases, which means that they bind with equal affinity to hemi-methylated and non-methylated DNA and that they catalyze DNA methylation from the beginning after embryo implantation. Of course, the maintenance versus de novo function of these enzymes is not absolute, and DNMTs can fulfill the role as one or the other when their levels are modulated. Removal of methyl group from DNA is a more complicated process compared with its methylation, as there are no single enzymes directly catalyzing the reaction [27]. DNA demethylation can be achieved as a passive process simply due to the loss of methylation on daughter strand after several rounds of DNA replication, or it takes place actively by replication-independent processes. Unlike in plants where firm evidence has been identified that direct excision of the methyl group is accomplished by a subfamily of DNA glycosylases specific to 5mC, the active demethylation pathways in animal cells are hotly contested and proposed to involve various mechanisms, none of which have been conclusively proven. So far, accumulating data has suggested an affirmative role for base excision repair (BER) in active demethylation in mammals, which is initiated by either direct excision of 5mC in a locus specific manner or deamination of 5mC to thymine resulting in T-G mismatch. In another hypothetical theory, entire DNA patch containing the methylated CpG sites is removed, and the bulky lesions are then filled with unmodified nucleotides by nucleotide excision repair (NER). Recently, the discovery of Ten-eleven translocation (TET) family proteins opened up a new mechanistic route for DNA demethylation. Three members, TET1–3, have been currently identified, and all are oxygenases that catalyze the oxidation of 5mC to 5-hydroxymethyl cytosine (5hmC), then 5-formylcytosine (5fC) and finally 5-carboxylcytosine (5caC). TET-mediated removal of DNA methylation could be achieved by several ways: first, DNMT1 does not recognize 5hmC, thus the newly synthesized DNA would not be methylated so that the patterns of methylation will be diluted after several rounds of replication passively; second, BER DNA repair pathway may be activated to process the lesions that are introduced by either a 5hmC-specific or, after deamination of 5hmC to 5hmU, a 5hmU-specific glycosylase; third, the oxidative derivatives of 5hmC (5fC and 5caC) can be ultimately replaced with unmodified cytosine by a decarboxylation reaction similar to the thymidine salvage pathway. Altogether, the whole system for DNA methylation and demethylation cycling is sophisticated, which implies far-reaching effects of these epigenetic programs on the modulation of local and global chromatin structure (Fig. 2). Therefore, any step in these processes going awry may lead to deranged biological conditions, such as genomic imprinting-related diseases, psychiatric disorders and cancers.

3.2   DNA Hypermethylation in Prostate Cancer

Many human diseases, cancers in particular, are found to be associated with aberrant DNA methylation patterns, either globally or locus specifically. One of the common hallmarks in all human malignant neoplasias is the CpG island hypermethylation. By the most updated definition, CpGs are short stretches of DNA that are longer than 500 base pairs in length and have a GC content greater than 55% with an observe-to-expected CpG ratio of at least 65% [28]. In human genome, there are about 29,000 such regions, which occur at or near up to 70% of annotated gene promoters. In normal cells, most promoter CpG islands are unmethylated. However, when cells become transformed or malignant, hypermethylation of certain CpG islands occurs resulting in inappropriate transcriptional repression. This observation has been described in almost every tumor type, including prostate cancer. Although most of the target genes that are inactivated by CpG hypermethylation are supposed to act as tumor suppressors, unique sets of genes with dynamic biological functions are affected when comparing different cancer types. In prostate carcinoma, over 40 genes have been reported to be silenced by hypermethylation, and this number is still increasing probably due to the development of more

---

Fig. 2 (continued) homocysteine (SAH) and methylated cytosine (5mC). The transferred methyl group is circled. (**B**) DNA demethyation can be achieved by passive demethylation mechanism (*upper panel*) or active demethylation mechanism (*lower panel*). Passive demethylation happens during DNA replication, and the modified cytosines are either missed (5mC) or not recoganized (5hmC) by DNMTs. Active demethylation takes place through nucleotide excision repair (NER) pathway or TETs-involved base excision (BER) pathway

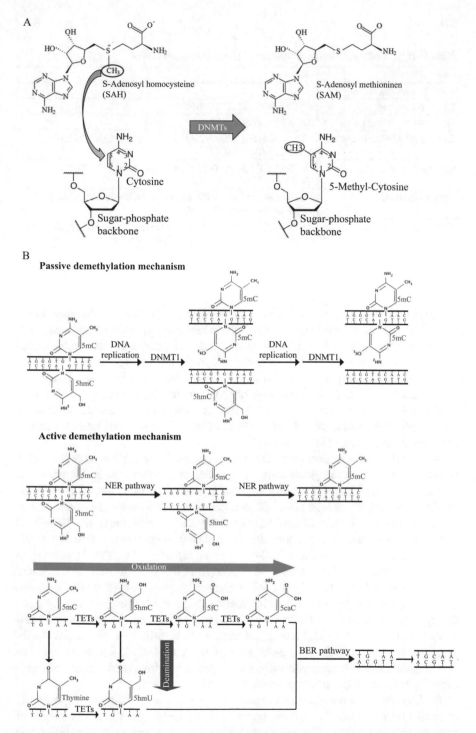

Fig. 2 DNA methylation and demethylation reactions. (**A**) DNA methylation is catalyzed by DNA methyltransferases (DNMTs), which transfers the methyl (−CH3) group from S-Adenosyl-methioninen (SAM) to the 5′-carbon position of the cytosine ring. The final products are S-Adenosyl

Table 1 Hypermethylated and hypomethylated genes in prostate cancer

Categories	Genes
DNA hypermethylation	
DNA repair genes	*GSTP1, MGMT, GPX3, hMLH1*
Hormone signaling genes	*AR, ESRα, ESRβ, RARβ, PR-α, PR-β*
Cell invasion/adhesion genes	*CDH1, CDH13, CD44, LAMA3, LAMB3, LAMC2, TIMP3, S100A2, TIG1, THBS1*
Cell-cycle genes	*CCND2, CDKN1B, RASSF1, CDKN2α, RB1, CDKN1A, CDKN1B*
Apoptotic genes	*GADD45α, PYCARD, RPRM, GLIPR1, DAPK, TNRFSF6, TNRFSR10C, CRBP1, FHIT*
Cell signaling genes	*14-3-3σ, CAV1, APC, PTEN, PTGS1, PTGS2, MDR1, EDNRB, DAB2IP, VEGFR1, HIC1, RUNX3*
DNA hypomethylation	
Gene-locus-specific	*CAGE, HPSE, PLAU, CYP1B1*

sensitive detection technologies. Some representative genes will be discussed in the following section, because their methylation is relatively prevalent in prostate cancer and they involve in a number of pivotal cellular pathways such as hormonal response, tumor cell invasion/metastasis, cell cycle control, apoptosis, and DNA damage repair. A comprehensive list of the methylated genes in prostate cancer is summarized in Table 1. Interestingly, classical tumor suppressor genes, such as *PTEN*, *RB1* and *TP53*, are rarely methylated at their promoter regions in prostate cancer, although genetic alterations like loss of heterozygosity and point mutations are detected in advanced stage cases [29].

As described above, hormones and their corresponding nuclear receptors play significant roles in carcinogenesis and progression of prostate cancer. AR activity is particularly critical for nearly every stage of the cancer growth, from the initiation to the androgen-dependent state till the metastatic, castration resistant status. However, loss of AR protein expression has been seen in as many as 20–30% of androgen-independent tumors, and this is attributed to epigenetic silencing partly by promoter hypermethylation [30–32]. It is reported that the incidence of methylation-mediated AR inactivation ranged from 0%–20% in untreated primary cancer to 13–28% in CRPC tissues. Although the frequency of AR promoter methylation in general appears to be low in prostate cancer and varies from case to case, this type of epigenetic regulation seems to be more prevalent in CRPC than in primary tumor tissues. It is highly clinical relevant to identify this AR-negative subgroup of prostate cancer, and implication of DNA methylation in mediating the downregulation of AR expression will have a profound effect on the treatment regimens for the metastatic, hormone-refractory prostate cancer.

Besides *AR*, other members of the steroid/thyroid hormone receptor superfamily have also been identified as having promoter hypermethylation in some studies of prostate cancer samples. For instance, both estrogen receptors genes, *ESR1* and *ESR2*, which encode two different forms of the receptor ERα and ERβ respectively, are frequently methylated in prostate cancer. Frequencies of *ESR1* methylation are diverse from 19% to 95% and ESR2 from 65% to 83% in prostate cancer [33–35]. However, the findings on the expression of ERα and ERβ in prostate cancer have been very conflicting [36], especially for ERα levels, although downregulation of both ERs in prostate tumor tissues has been documented in some studies and promoter hypermethylation is the primary mechanism responsible for this transcriptional inactivation [35]. Some evidence showed that higher methylation levels of the ER genes, particularly at some CpG sites, were detected in high-grade and CRPC cancer samples than in low-grade and BPH tissues [34, 35], but it also appears unlikely that alterations in the expression of either ER are associated with the progression of prostate cancer [37, 38]. Therefore, it is still very controversial and remains to be established as for the biological significance of DNA hypermethylation of both ER genes in prostate cancer. One thing we can have certainty about, however, is that DNA methylation is the main reason for gene silencing in any clinical cases when lost or decreased ER expression was noticed. Retinoic acid receptor β (RARβ) is another nuclear receptor that shows abnormal CpG island methylation patterns in prostate cancer, especially in the second promoter region of the gene (*RARβ2*). *RARβ2* methylation varies greatly across studies, for example 0–23% of normal and BPH tissues, 20–94.7% of PIN and 40–97.5% of primary prostate cancer [39–41], and it appears to happen in early stage of prostate cancer, suggesting a role in cancer initiation. There is no clear association between *RARβ2* methylation and pathological stage or Gleason score of prostate cancer [42–44].

DNA damage response (DDR) is an exquisite proofreading mechanism that repairs DNA lesions and prevents the duplication of these errors into daughter cells. Misregulation of DDR pathways leads to the deleterious genomic instability, which is a universal characteristic of cancer cells, and therefore is a major driver for carcinogenesis. So far, two genes that are involved in DNA damage repair have been reported to be hypermethylated in prostate cancer, one is the detoxifier gene glutathione S-transferase Pi (*GSTP1*) and the other is the DNA alkyl-repair gene O^6-methylguanine DNA methyltransferase (*MGMT*). GSTs are a family of metabolic enzymes that catalyze the conjugation of hydrophobic and electrophilic compounds with reduced glutathione for the purpose of detoxification. Thus, inactivation of GST proteins may lead to cell vulnerability to genotoxic foreign compounds and accumulation of DNA base adducts. Indeed, some evidence suggests that mutations or polymorphisms of GST genes can influence BER capacity and subsequent DNA stability, suggesting a potential role for these proteins in DNA damage processing. CpG island hypermethylation of *GSTP1* gene is one of the most common molecular alterations detected in prostate adenocarcinoma. This epigenetic aberrancy is absent or at very low level in nonmalignant prostate tissues, but present in 50–70% of PIN and in nearly all prostate cancers at different stages [45]. Recently, emerging evidence suggests that the extent of *GSTP1* promoter methylation is also positively correlated with the risk of recurrence in prostate cancer patients with early disease [46]. MGMT is one of the few proteins functioning in direct reversal (DR) DNA repair pathway. It transfers the methyl group from O^6-methylguanine to a nucleophilic cysteine residue in its active site. O^6-methylguanine base pairs with thymine instead of cytosine and thus is the major carcinogenic lesion in DNA. The reaction is irreversible, so the modified cysteine cannot be regenerated and the alkylated MGMT protein is degraded after the direct DNA repair. Results about the association between the status of MGMT methylation and prostate cancer have been inconsistent. Some studies reported low frequency of MGMT promoter methylation in 0–2% of prostate cancer tissues, while others observed moderate to high prevalence of this event in 19–76% of tumor samples [40, 47–49]. This discrepancy may come from technical issues, e.g., various assays used for quantifying methylation levels and different tissue processing methods, so further work or meta-analysis will be needed to resolve the inconsistent results.

Cell proliferation and programmed cell death are two coupling processes that determine the destiny of a cell to either live or die, so deregulation of the balance between cell cycle progression and apoptosis leads to pathological conditions including cancer. *CDKN2A* (p16^{INK4a}) is one of the cyclin-dependent kinase inhibitors (CDKIs) and a well-characterized tumor suppressor. Besides genetic changes such as deletion and point mutation, *CDKN2A* is inactivated by DNA hypermethylation in many tumor tissues including prostate [50]. This feature makes the gene unique because other CDKIs, such as *CDKN2B*, *CDKN1A* and *CDKN1B*, are rarely methylated in prostate tumors. However, the frequency of *CDKN2A* promoter methylation varies in prostate tumors across studies, ranging from 0% to 16%, and it appears to be indiscriminate between benign and malignant cases [51]. Interestingly, several reports indicate methylation at exon 2 of *CDKN2A*, which is present in more tumors (73%) relative to normal tissues [52]. Although there was no apparent association between the expression level of *CDKN2A* gene and the extent of its exon 2 methylation, it is plausible that this epigenetic modification may serve as a biomarker for early detection of prostate carcinoma. Another well-known tumor suppressor gene that is frequently silenced by promoter hypermethylation in prostate cancer is RAS association domain family protein 1 isoform A (*RASSF1A*). RASSF1A exerts its tumor suppressive functions by modulating microtubule stability, inducing cell cycle arrest and apoptosis. CpG islands within promoter region of *RASSF1A* gene are highly methylated in a wide range of cancers, and up to 99% of prostate tumors show this epigenetic alteration [53, 54]. In normal epithelial cells and benign prostate tissues, *RASSF1A* promoter methylation is detected in 0–40% of samples, and it also occurs in 64% of PIN [55]. In addition, the relative frequency of methylation is higher in more aggressive tumors with higher Gleason scores compared with less malignant tumors. All these findings suggest that *RASSF1A* promoter methylation may be a common event during prostate carcinogenesis and progression, and hence it can be utilized for the early detection and prognosis prediction of prostate cancer. Many other cell cycle regulators, for example *CCND2* and *SFN*, and apoptosis genes such as *DAPK* and *TNFRSF10C*, have also been found to be aberrantly hypermethylated at their promoter regions in prostate cancer [56].

Most prostate cancer-related deaths are caused by the metastasis of the original tumor cells. The process of tumor invasion and metastasis entails a series of sequential events, including the penetration of original cancer cells into surrounding tissues, spreading to distant organs through the circulatory system, and finally seeding secondary tumors in distinct target locations. During this metastatic cascade, cell adhesion molecules (CAMs) play important roles in cell-cell and cell-matrix interaction. Therefore, misregulation of CAMs expression is often observed in many human cancers, including prostate. E-cadherin, encoded by *CDH1* gene, is a CAM that distributes at the epithelial cell junctions and mediates cell-cell adhesion. In E-cadherin-negative prostate cancer cell lines, the CpG islands in the promoter of *CDH1* gene are densely methylated, which suggests that epigenetic alteration in DNA methylation contributes to the decreased or loss of E-cadherin expression [57]. Hypermethylation of *CDH1* gene has been detected in 0–77% of prostate tumors, and the overall methylation frequencies are higher in advanced prostate tumors compared with early stage samples [58]. However, several studies reported contradictory results regarding the methylation status of *CDH1* gene in prostate cancer. In two such studies, promoter region of *CDH1* was found no methylation signals in either primary or metastatic prostate tumor samples [47, 59]. In the other, unmethylated *CDH1* gene was detected in metastatic prostate cancer cells in bone, which was significantly associated with the concurrent expression of E-cadherin protein [60]. It is currently unclear why discrepancies were observed in different cases, but epigenetic alteration in promoter methylation appears to be the main explanation for E-cadherin transcriptional inactivation in prostate cancer, rather than *CDH1* gene mutations which lead to loss of E-cadherin function in other cancer types like gastric and breast [61, 62]. Adenomatous polyposis coli (*APC*) gene is also an important molecule that helps control the movement of a cell within or away from a tissue. It associates with the WNT/β-catenin signaling pathway and negatively regulates β-catenin protein stability and interaction with E-cadherin, which is a critical step in cell-cell adhesion. Mutations in *CTNNB1*, the gene encoding β-catenin protein, or truncation in *APC* have been detected in colon cancer and melanoma, which increases the stability of β-catenin. However, these genetic alterations are relatively rare in prostate cancer. In contrast, *APC* gene is commonly methylated at its promoter region, with a prevalence of 27–100% in prostate cancer samples but only 5–6% in noncancerous tissues [63, 64]. Multiple analyses also demonstrated that hypermethylation in *APC* gene is significantly associated with progression of prostate cancer [65, 66], and more frequent in patients who experienced biochemical recurrence, metastasis or death [64, 67]. Many additional genes with critical functions in tumor invasion and metastasis have been reported to undergo methylation-mediated inactivation in prostate cancer, including the cell-surface glycoprotein (*CD44*), H-cadherin (*CDH13*), the scaffolding protein on the caveolae plasma membrane caveolin-1 (*CAV1*), tissue inhibitors of matrix metalloproteinases (*TIMP-2* and *-3*), etc. [68].

3.3 DNA Hypomethylation in Prostate Cancer

Although DNA hypermethylaion has been focused as an important mechanism for inactivation of tumor suppressor genes in prostate cancer, demethylation of normally methylated genomic regions, also known as DNA hypomethylation, is shown to associate with prostate cancer development and progression as well. In contrast to DNA hypermethylation that usually occurs at specific regulatory sites of specific individual genes, loss of DNA methylation modification seems to be a genome-wide phenomenon. It predominantly occurs in the intergenic and intronic genomic areas, particularly at repeated sequences including the heterochromatic satellite DNA and interspersed transposable elements. It is postulated that DNA hypomethylation induces genomic instability and mutation events, thus contributing to oncogenesis and cancer progression. For example, aberrations on chromosome 8 were strongly correlated with the presence of hypomethylation in prostate cancer, and such genetic and epigenetic alterations tended to be more frequent in higher-stage tumors [69]. In prostate adenocarcinoma, methylation signals at repetitive DNA elements were dramatically decreased from normal prostate to PIN to cancer [70]. In another study, primary prostate cancer cells from up to 96.7% of patients exhibited dramatic decrease in overall 5mC levels compared with the paired benign and normal sections from the same patient. Interestingly, partial gain of methylation was observed in men with recurrent disease [71]. These results, together with many others, suggest that overall reduction of genomic methylcytosine content appears to occur early in prostate carcinogenesis. Global hypomethylation is thus hypothesized to precede temporally the promoter CpG island hypermethylation that later leads to aberrant silencing of specific tumor suppressor genes critical for cancer progression. However, there is emerging evidence that diffuse genomic hypomethylation in prostate cancer may not adhere to this generalized model. An early report showed that the overall DNA methylation levels were particularly lower in metastatic, androgen-refractory prostate tumors, while the 5mC content in non-metastatic prostate tumors was essentially comparable to that in normal tissues [72]. Similar conclusion was obtained when methylation of repetitive sequences like *LINE-1* retrotransposons was found diminished in 49% of prostate cancer and this hypomethylation was more pronounced in high stage and lymph-node positive tumors [73]. In the same study, hypermethylation at specific genes such as *GSTP1*, *RARB2* and *APC*, however, was neither related to tumor stage nor Gleason score. In an independent report, decreased *LINE-1* methylation was again detected in the primary prostate cancer compared with normal tissues, but the degree of reduction was more dramatic in metastatic prostate cancer. In addition, the overall genomic 5mC content was reduced only in metastatic but not primary cancer or tumors adjacent PIN/normal tissues [74]. All these findings suggest that global DNA hypomethylation may actually occur later than hypermethylation changes and play an important role in prostate cancer progression rather than initiation.

Compared with the focal hypermethylation of CpG islands containing promoters, demethylation of individual genes is much less documented in terms of its role in the initiation and progression of cancers. This type of epigenetic alteration was often ignored because localized DNA hypomethylation seems to be much less frequent in cancer and some theory suggests that specific regional demethylation may occur as a consequence of being swept by the large genomic hypomethylation [75]. Even so, a number of single copy genes have been reported to be derepressed in prostate cancer by the epigenetic mechanism of DNA hypomethylation. For instance, the *PLAU* gene, which promotes extracellular matrix tissue degradation and cell migration, is highly expressed in most prostate cancer tissues, particularly in the invasive ones [76]. Overexpression of *PLAU* is partly attributed to the unmethylated status of the CpG islands proximal to its transcription start site, which was noticeable in nearly all prostate cancer samples but rare in non-neoplastic tissues or BPH samples. Most interestingly, disruption of the demethylation condition at *PLAU* gene promoter induced higher invasive capacity of prostate cancer cells and larger xenograft prostate tumor volumes in vivo [77, 78]. One unique group of genes with regard to their methylation status in cancers is the cancer/testis antigen (*CTA*), since many of the gene members are hypomethylated in several types of cancers including prostate. As their name indicates, *CTA* genes are typically expressed in germ cells of the testis and most cancers but absent in any other normal tissues. It is well known that this exclusive expression pattern of CTAs is highly correlated with the extent of DNA methylation at their promoters [75]. In prostate carcinoma, a large fraction of *CTA* genes, especially those in the X chromosome-associated subfamily, showed CpG islands hypomethylation. More than that, some report claimed that significant DNA hypomethylation of these genes occurred only in metastatic prostate cancer [74]. Other work showed similar results that some representative *CTA* genes were highly methylated in more than 90% of primary cancer specimens, but severely unmethylated in castration resistant samples [79]. Recently, partial hypomethylation was observed in prostate cancer tissues at the promoter of *XIST* gene, which is transcribed into a non-coding RNA acting as a major effector of the X-chromosome inactivation in females [80]. Although the association between the degree of methylation and transcription of *XIST* gene was not clearly established, it is a perfect example to demonstrate the universal presence of DNA hypomethylation, affecting repeat and unique sequences at specific loci that encode proteins or not. Other hypomethylated genes in prostate cancer include *WNT5A*, *CRIP1*, *S100P*, *CYB1B1* and *HPSE*, etc., overexpression of which have all been implicated in prostate cancer progression [81–83]. Taken together, DNA methylation, both hypo- and hypermethylation, is a critical mechanism that cancer cells adapt to regulate gene expression so as to drive prostate cancer development and progression.

4 Prostate Cancer and Histone Methylation

4.1 Proteins in Regulation of Histone Methylation

Histones are the chief protein components of nucleosome, the basic structural unit of chromatin. They are highly alkaline and positively charged, so they closely associate with DNA, which is negatively charged instead, through a series of electrostatic interactions including hydrogen bonds and salt bridges. Five major families of histone proteins exist: H1/5, H2A, H2B, H3 and H4. Histone H2A, H2B, H3 and H4 are known as the core histones, so two copies of each core protein assemble in an octamerous complex, with which 146–147 base pairs of DNA wrap around in a superhelical manner. This core particle is bound by the linker histones, H1 (or H5 in avian species), at the entry and exit sites of the DNA, thus locking the DNA into place and organizing nucleosome chains into higher order structures. Interaction between histones and DNA governs the chromatin structure and thus exerts a tremendous amount of influence on gene expression. There are several regulatory mechanisms controlling the dynamic changes in this histone-DNA interaction, one of which is the post-translational modifications (PTMs) on the histone protein tails. Histone proteins feature two structurally and functionally distinct domains: the central globular domain that allows heterodimeric interactions between core histones or mediates the protection of linker DNA, and unstructured terminal tails of various length, on which specific amino acids are subject to various covalent modifications, including acetylation, phosphorylation, ADP-ribosylation, ubiquitination and methylation, etc. These enzyme-assisted modifications primarily occur at N-terminal tails of the histones. They can affect the charge properties of the histone, and thus loosen or tighten the condensed DNA that is wrapped around histones. Such modifications can also recruit other proteins specifically recognizing the modified residues, which act to alter the chromatin structure so that it becomes more closed or more accessible.

Histone methylation is a biochemical reaction by which methyl groups are transferred to specific residues on histone proteins. It can happen on all three basic amino acids: arginine (R), lysine (K) and histidine (H), although lysines on tails of histone H3 and H4 are most commonly targeted, whereas only monomethylation of histidine has been described and it is rarely observed [84, 85]. Because the addition of the methyl group leaves the charge of lysine or arginine intact, methylation of histones can be associated with either transcriptional repression or activation, depending on the specific modified residues in the histones and also the numbers of methyl groups attached. Arginine is able to be either mono- or dimethylated. When it is dimethylated, these two methyls can be added asymmetrically on the same free NH2 group or symmetrically with one on NH2 and one on NH2+ group. Even though the similar reactions end up with molecules in the same chemical formulas, these two types of dimethylation are catalyzed by two different subfamilies of enzymes. Lysine can accept up to three methyl moieties replacing each hydrogen of its NH3+ group. Site-specific methylation is catalyzed by histone modifying enzymes called the histone methyltransferases (HMTs).

Two major types of HMTs exist, lysine-specific and arginine-specific. Both types of HMTs transfer the methyl groups from S-adenosyl-L-methionine (AdoMet or SAM), which serves as the cofactor and methyl group donor, to either ε-amino group (NH_3^+) on lysine or the guanidine functional group on arginine, forming the methylated products and S-adenosyl-L-homocysteine (AdoHcy). The class of lysine-specific HTMs is subdivided into SET (Su(var)3-9, Enhancer of zeste, Trithorax) domain-containing ones and non-SET domain-containing ones. The SET domain is an evolutionary well-conserved sequence motif of 130–140 amino acid long. It contains a catalytic pocket, where cofactor SAM and the to-be-modified lysine are bound as well as properly oriented. Next, the ε-amine of the lysine substrate is deprotonated, makes a nucleophilic attack on the collinear methyl group on the sulfur of SAM, and finally completes the attachment of the methyl group to the lysine side chain. The adjacent cysteine-rich regions flanking the SET domain on either side play a crucial role in substrate recognition and maximizing enzymatic activity. Dot1 (Distruptor of telomeric silencing) is the only HMT known to date that does not contain the SET domain. Dot1 and its mammalian homolog, DOT1L (DOT1-Like, also called KMT4), are very special enzymes in terms of its substrate specificity. First, Dot1/DOT1L appears to be solely responsible for methylation of K79 on histone H3; second, unlike SET-domain-containing HMTs that target at the histone tail regions, Dot1/DOT1L is the only enzyme known to methylate a lysine residue in the globular core of the histone; finally, Dot1/DOT1L only methylates histone substrates that are actively engaged in the nucleosome but not the free ones. Despite lacking a SET domain, Dot1/DOT1L share a similar structure with other classical methyltransferases, which surprisingly more resemble histone arginine methyltransferases. However, extensive efforts have failed to demonstrate that Dot1/DOT1L can directly methylate arginine [86]. Amino acids 1–416 at the N terminus of Dot1/DOT1L contain the active histone methyltransferase catalytic sites, where several critical residues (T139, Q168, D161, E186, and D222 of human DOT1L/KMT4) align the methionyl moiety of SAM molecule and the lysine substrate for a methyl transfer reaction. The long, flexible C-terminal tail is important for substrate specificity and nucleosome binding [87]. There are at least nine members of protein arginine methyltransferase (PRMTs) in mammals, which are separated into three main types. Type I PRMTs (e.g., PRMT1, 2, 3, 4, 6, and 8) can all catalyze mono-methylation and continue to form asymmetric dimethylarginine. Type II PRMTs (e.g., PRMT5 and 9) produce monomethylarginie and symmetric dimethylarginine. PRMT7 is the single Type III enzyme described to date that generates monomethyl-ation of arginine only [88]. PRMT2 was identified by sequence homology, but demonstrated substantially low enzymatic activity in vitro [89]. Structural comparison suggests that all PRMTs contain a conserved catalytic core where the cofactor SAM binds, and a barrel-like domain where the substrate binds [90]. The sequences at both N- and C-termini are variable among different PRMTs, containing protein-protein interaction modules that may participate in determining substrate specificity or recruiting other proteins critical for enzymatic activity. Like in the methylation reaction mediated by a SET-containing HMT, the nitrogen group on target arginine residue is also first deprotonated and then acts as a nucleophile to attack the methyl group of SAM. It is suggested that a methionine in the active site of Type I PRMTs grants their abilities to catalyze asymmetric methylation, whereas in Type II PRMTs, like PRMT5, the corresponding residue is switched to a serine, so the less bulky side chain of this amino acid now allows for symmetric methylation formation [91].

For many years, histone methylation, unlike acetylation or phosphorylation, was thought to be irreversible, because of the fact that the N-CH3 bond is very stable with a half-life approximately equal to that of histones themselves. The identifica-tion of histone demethylases, enzymes that remove methyl groups from histones, completely overturned the dogma (Fig. 3). Two main classes of histone demethyl-ases have thus far been identified, which predominantly target at the lysine residues: the flavin adenine dinucleotide (FAD)-dependent amine oxidase, which includes the Lysine (K) Demethylase 1 (KDM1) family proteins, and the Fe(II) and 2-oxoglutarate

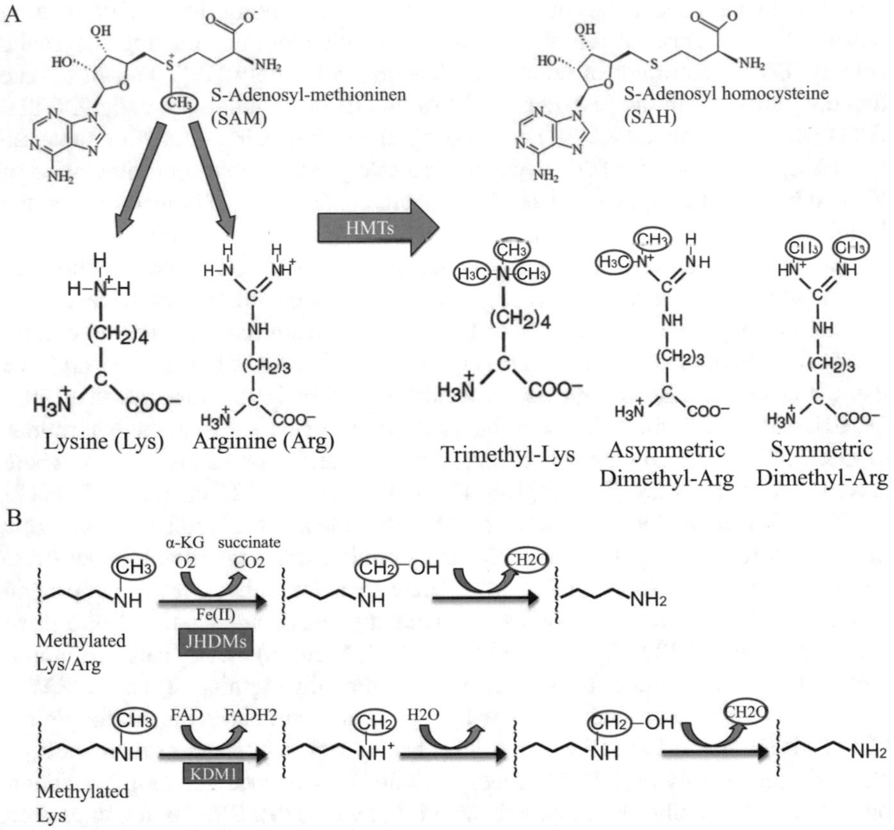

Fig. 3 Histone methylation and demethylation reactions. (**a**) Lysine or arginine can be methylated by histone methyltransferases (HMTs). The transferred methyl (−CH3) group is circled. (**b**) Histone demethylation can be catalyzed by either JmjC-domain-containing histone demethylases (JHDMs) (*upper panel*) or lysine demethylase 1 (KDM1) family proteins (*lower panel*). The removed methyl group is *circled*

(2OG)-dependent dioxygenase, which features a signature motif of JmjC domain. Both families of demethylases operate via an oxidative mechanism that releases formaldehyde as a co-product. KDM1A/LSD1 and KDM1B/LSD2 are the only two members that have been identified so far in the KDM1 family, and KDM1A/LSD1 is actually the first protein demonstrated to possess bona fide histone demethylase activity. Interestingly, both KDM1A and B can demethylate only mono- and demethylated lysines. The JmjC domain-containing histone demethylases form a larger and more versatile family, which act on multiple histone lysine residues and can accept all three methylation states. Of note, although no arginine-specific demethylases have ever been reported, some of the JmjC KDMs have demonstrated arginine demethylation activity in vitro [92, 93]. There are some other mechanisms of demethylation, much less common though, such as the nucleophilic demethylation by methylesterases [94]. The dynamic and reversible nature of histone methylation supports the hypothesis that modifications on histone tails, called the histone code, serve as marks for the recruitment of proteins or protein complexes to dictate the information of the genetic code [95, 96]. So, besides the enzymes that add or eliminate the histone modifications, there is another group of proteins that play pivotal roles in deciphering the language of the histone code: the binding partners of specific chemical moieties on histones. A large family of proteins has been identified that can recognize methylated lysine residues, and they are divided into several subfamilies based on the distinct recognition domains they contain, including PHD (plant homeodomain) domain that binds histone H3 in various methylation states, PWWP (named after a conserved Pro-Trp-Trp-Pro motif) domain that is concurrent with other motifs such as PHD, Chromo domain that is known to bind methylated H3K4/9/27, and MBT (Malignant Brain Tumor) domain that mostly binds mono- and dimethylated lysines, etc. In spite of the presence of divergent recognition motifs, their pairs with the corresponding lysine methylation do not simply fit into the "one domain-one mark" model: one single methylated lysine can be recognized by several readers and one reading module can bind multiple separate methylated substrates. Sometimes even different methylation states (mono-, di- or trimethylation) of the same residue can recruit different sets of binders [97], and the more methyl groups attached, the stronger the binding strength will be [98]. Considering all these uncertainties, here comes the question: how are the strength and specificity of one particular lysine methylation reader determined? Firstly, structural evidence suggests that the binding surfaces of distinct domains that recognize the same mark remarkably resemble each other. Secondly, flanking sequences of the methylated lysine are heavily involved in the selective recruitment process and make multiple direct contacts with the reader. Finally, according to the "histone end effects", modified lysine that locates near the end of a histone peptide, like H3K4 methylation, is easy to be read and therefore attracts more diverse binding partners. As for the readers of the methylated arginines, it is still highly ambiguous whether such specific motifs do exist. So far, only two proteins were claimed to recognize methylated arginine, one is the PHD motif within the ADD domain of DNMT3A, which may [99], or may not [100], directly bind symmetrically methylated H4R3; and the other is the Tudor domain of TDRD3 protein, which was spotted using a protein domain microarray approach as a reading module of asymmetrically methylated H3R4 and R17 [101].

All currently known methyltransferases, demethylases and recognition modules of methylated histones are summarized in Table 2, together with the corresponding methylation marks. For years, the diverse array of methylation events on histone proteins is believed to provide exceptional regulatory power of gene regulation in a context-specific manner, and considered to be essential steps in many processes that determine cell fate. Therefore it is not surprising that abnormal expression or activities of the enzymes that write, erase or read methylated histones are implicated in a variety of human disease states including cancers.

Table 2 Proteins in regulation of histone methylation

Histone-modifying enzymes	Epigenetic marks	Proposed functions
Histone Methyltransferases (HMTs)		
Lysine-specific methylation		
EZH2	H1K26me1/2/3	Transcriptional silencing
Unknown	H2BK5me1	Transcriptional activation
MLL	H3K4me1/2/3	Transcriptional activation, permissive euchromatin
G9A/EHMT2, SETDB1	H3K9me1/2/3	Transcriptional silencing, genomic imprinting
EZH1, EZH2, G9A/EHMT2	H3K27me1/2/3	Transcriptional repression, X inactivation
SET2D (tri-Me), ASH1L (mono−/di-Me)	H3K36me1/3	Transcriptional activation/ elongation
DOT1L	H3K79me1/2/3	Transcriptional activation/ elongation, euchromatin
SETDB1, SUV420H, NSD1	H4K20me1/3	Transcriptional silencing (mono-Me)/activation, heterochromatin
Unkonwn	H4K59me1/2/3	Transcriptional silencing
Arginine-specific methylation		
PRMT1/5/6/7	H2AR3me2	Transcriptional activation/ repression
PRMT5/6	H3R2me1/2	Transcriptional repression
PRMT2/5/6	H3R8me2	Transcriptional activation/ repression
CARM1	H3R17me1/2	Transcriptional activation
CARM1	H3R26me1/2	Transcriptional activation
CARM1	H3R42me1/2	Transcriptional activation
PRMT1/5/6/7	H4R3me1/2	Transcriptional activation/ repression
Histone Demethylases		
Lysine-specific demethylation		
KDM2A/JHDM1A	H3K36me2	Transcriptional repression, associated with heterochromatin
KDM2B/JHDM1B	H3K4me3, H3K36me2	Transcriptional repression
KDM3A/JMJD1A	H3K9me1/2	Transcriptional activation
KDM3B/JMJD1B	H3K9me1/2	Transcriptional activation
KDM4A/JMJD2A	H3K9me3, H3K36me3	Transcriptional repression
KDM4B/JMJD2B	H3K9me3	Unknown
KDM4C/JMJD2C	H3K9me2/3	Transcriptional activation, inhibition of heterochromatin
KDM4D/JMJD2D	H3K9me2/3, H1K25me1	Unknown
KDM5B/JARID1B	H3K4me3	Transcriptional activation
KDM5C/JARID1C	H3K4me3	Transcriptional repression

(continued)

Table 2 (continued)

Histone-modifying enzymes	Epigenetic marks	Proposed functions
KDM5D/JARID1D	H3K4me2/3	Transcriptional repression, DNA condensation
KDM6A/UTX	H3K27me3	Transcripional activation/repression
KDM6B/JMJD3	H3K27me2/3	Transcriptional silencing
JHDM1D/KDM7A	H3K9me2, H3K27me2	Transcriptional activation
JMJD5/KDM8	H3K36me2	Unknown
KDM1A	H3K4me1/2, H3K9me1/2	Transcriptional activation/ repression
KDM1B	H3K9me2	Transcriptional activation
PHF8/JHDM1F	H3K9me2, H3K4me2, H4K20me, H3K27me2	Transcriptional activation
Arginine-specific demethylation		
JMJD6	H3R2me2, H4R3me1/2	RNA splicing
KDM4E/JMJD2E	H3R2me1/2, H3R8me1/2, H3R26me1/1, H4R3me2	Unknown
KDM5C/JARID1C	H3R2me1/2, H3R8me2, H4R3me2	Unknown
Readers		
Tudor domain (e.g., SHH1)	H3K9me3	
Chromodomain (e.g., HP1, Pc proteins, MRG1/2)	H3K9me3, H3K27me3, H3K4me3, H3K36me3	
PWWP (Pro-Trp-Trp-Pro) (e.g., ZCWPW1)	H3K4me0/1/2/3	
MBT domain (e.g., L3MBTL1/2)	H4K20me1/2	
PHD domain (e.G., BPTF, ING1/2, MMD1)	H3K4me3	
WD40 repeat (e.g., WDR5, CYP71)	H3K4me3, H3K27me3	

4.2   Histone Methylation in Prostate Cancer

Increasing evidence suggests that histone methylation, together with other types of histone modifications, contributes to the onset and progression of prostate cancer. A panel of methylation marks, including mono-, di- and trimethylation of H3K4 (H3K4me, H3K4me2 and H3K4me3) and H3K9 (H3K9me, H3K9me2 and H3K9me3) as well as pan-acetylation of H3 and H4, was stained in a tissue micro-array containing 23 nonmalignant prostate tissues and 113 prostate adenocarcinoma samples in various pathological states [102]. H3K9 di- and trimethylation and acetylation of H3 and H4 were all significantly reduced in cancer samples compared to BPH and normal tissues, whereas all three methylation states of H3K4 were upregulated in androgen-independent tumors and correlated with clinical-pathological parameters. The other histone methylation mark that has been extensively investigated in prostate cancer is H3K27 methylation. Different methylation status (mono-, di- or trimethylation) of H3K27 (H3K27me, H3K27me2 or H3K27me3) showed distinct patterns in normal prostate tissue, clinically localized tumors, hormone-dependent and hormone-refractory prostate cancer [103]. Levels of H3K27 mono- and trimethylation have been reported to positively correlate with aggressive tumor features [103, 104]. Intriguingly, the global concentrations of H3K27me3 in cell-free circulating nucleosome from peripheral blood of prostate cancer patients, detected by an ELISA-based assay, were significantly lower in men with metastatic disease than in those with localized or local advanced tumors [105]. Although it is still deliberative as for how the overall levels of specific histone methylation marks change in prostate cancer, cumulative evidence implies that global patterns of histone methylation may distinguish cancer cells from their normal counterparts or even metastatic disease from organ confined tumors, and it is highly possible that they can be prognostically relevant. Indeed, multiple studies showed that certain methylation marks, either alone or in combination with other types of histone modifications, could serve as independent prognostic markers associated with clinical outcome in prostate cancer patients. In one study, five individual histone modifications, the acetylation of H3K9 (H3K9ac), H3K18 (H3K18ac) and H4K12 (H4K12ac) as well as the dimethylation of H3K4 (H3K4me2) and H4R3 (H4R3me2), were evaluated by immunohistochemical staining in 183 primary prostate cancer tissues [106]. Except H3K9ac, higher level of each one of the rest four histone modifications is correlated with higher grade of cancer samples. Interestingly, combination of the patterns of all these five modifications clearly predicted the clinical outcome of patients with lower grade (Gleason score 2–6) prostate tumors. The prognostic power of specific histone modifications was further confirmed in another prostate cancer cohort [107]. The levels of both H3K18ac and H3K4me2 were quantified immunohistochemically in 279 prostate cancer cases, and stronger intensities of both histone marks were significantly associated with increased risk of tumor relapse. In another study, H3K4 di- and trimethylation (H3K4me2 and H3K4me3), H3K36 trimethylation (H3K36me3), H4K20 trimethylation (H4K20me3) and H3K9 acetylation (H3K9ac) were assessed using immunohistochemistry in 169 primary prostatectomy tissue samples [108]. H3K4me3 alone can serve as an accurate predictor of the biochemical recurrence following radical prostatectomy for low grade (Gleason score ≤ 6) prostate cancer. Taken together, all these studies convincingly demonstrate that changes in overall levels of certain histone methylation events are associated with increased risks of prostate cancer recurrence and poor survival. Therefore, global epigenetic patterns of histone methylation may function as promising biomarkers for prostate cancer prognosis.

Not only the dissimilarity in overall levels, dynamic changes of histone methylation at individual chromatin loci also contribute to prostate cancer initiation and progression by coordinated regulation of cancer-specific gene expression. Because histone methylation has been implicated in both transcriptional activation and repression, a number of oncogenes and tumor suppressor genes were found to be epigenetically switched on or off, respectively, driving the malignant transformation of prostate epithelial cells. For instance, H3K27 trimethylation (H3K27me3), the methylation mark that is associated with gene silencing, was found to be significantly enriched at the promoter regions of a large number of tumor suppressor genes, such as *ADRB2*, *DAB2IP*, *RARβ2*, etc., in metastatic prostate cancer compared with localized tumors or normal prostates. Presence of this epigenetic mark is correlated with decreased expression of these genes and results in prostate cancer cell growth, survival and metastasis [104, 109–111]. Histone methylation is also intimately involved in controlling the transcriptional activity of AR. Methylation of H3K4 dictates the functionally active chromatin region, and its presence at AR binding sites contributes to the maintenance of the open chromatin architecture and initial recruitment of the pioneer factor FOXA1, which facilitates the transactivation of AR target genes, such as the proto-oncogene *UBE2C*, in CRPC cells [112]. In contrast, methylation of H3K9, another histone mark strongly linked to transcriptional repression, is detected at the regulatory regions of AR target genes, such as *KLK3* that encodes PSA, and constrains the transactivation of these genes. Androgen stimulation leads to transcriptional activation of *KLK3* gene, which is accompanied by a robust decrease in H3K9 methylation levels at its promoter [113]. Silencing of H3K9 demethylases LSD1, JHDM2A or JMJD2C, increased the signals of this repressive mark and subsequently decreased the expression of AR target genes [114, 115]. Recently, AR is found to act as a global transcriptional repressor, and genes being silenced by functional AR are mostly developmental regulators that play important roles in cell differentiation. Surprisingly, AR-repressed genes demonstrated strong enrichment of bivalent H3K4me3 and H3K27me3 modifications at their promoter regions, suggesting that the repressive function of AR is dictated by the status of histone methylation and that this particular epigenetic pattern contributes to prostate cancer progression through cell dedifferentiation and destabilization [116, 117]. All the above evidence offers important insights into the roles of histone methylation in prostate cancer development and progression. No matter if it is at individual genomic locations or at the overall levels, alteration in methylation pattern may directly reflect the aberrant activities or expressions of the enzymes that regulate this epigenetic program. Approximately 50% of the HMTs encoded by the human genome, for example, are now linked to diseases and in particular cancers [118]. In the following parts, only those enzymes that regulate histone methylation marks with clear links to cancer formation and progression will be discussed.

One of the best-characterized histone-modifying proteins in prostate cancer is the enhancer of zeste 2 (EZH2) that specifically methylates histone H3 at lysine 27. It is also reported to have methyltransferase activity towards the linker histone H1.4 at lysine 26. EZH2 is the catalytic subunit of the polycomb repressive complex 2 (PRC2), which also contains other core components such as EED, SUZ12 and RbAp46/48, for maximum enzymatic efficiency. EZH2 is found to be significantly increased in metastatic, hormone-refractory prostate cancer compared with clinically localized prostate tumors and normal samples. Overexpression of EZH2 is strongly associated with poor clinical outcome and prognosis in prostate cancer patients. Loss of EZH2 expression blocked the aggressive behaviors, like proliferation, metastasis and invasion, of prostate cancer cells, while overexpression of

EZH2 caused the neoplastic transformation of normal prostate epithelial cells [119]. All these observations clearly establish the oncogenic function of EZH2 in prostate cancer. Although there is still much debate about the mechanisms by which EZH2 drives prostate tumorigenesis, it is believed that H3K27me3 at regulatory chromatin regions leading to the downregulation of targeted tumor suppressor genes may in part explain the cancer-driving effects of EZH2. Indeed, a "polycomb repression signature" was identified in metastatic human prostate cancer tissues, which consists of 14 direct targets of EZH2 as they were upregulated upon EZH2 knockdown and contained high H3K27me3 signals in their promoter regions. Interestingly, the signature genes are largely downregulated in prostate cancer and can predict clinical outcome of multiple solid tumors including prostate [109]. In addition, EZH2 is reported to also involve in biological signaling other than epigenetic regulation. For example, EZH2 was recently found to serve as an AR co-activator and facilitate the recruitment of AR to target genes that are critical for the development of androgen-independent prostate cancer [120]. Although this co-activator function of EZH2 is still dependent on its methyltransferase activity, H3K27 methylation is not involved as the specific chromatin loci co-bound by EZH2 and AR was devoid of this epigenetic mark. In addition, cytosolic EZH2 was shown to regulate actin polymerization in prostate cancer cells in a methyltransferase-dependent fashion [121]. EZH2-mediated maintenance of a dynamic actin cytoskeleton controls the shape and motive force of cancer cells, subsequently promoting a metastatic phenotype. All the evidence suggests the possibilities of proteins other than histones being methylated by EZH2, which is also critical for the roles of EZH2 in oncogenic transformation. Several non-histone proteins of EZH2 have been identified albeit not in prostate cancer, such as GATA4 [122], STAT3 [123] and RORα [124]. EZH2-catalyzed methylation modulates either activities or protein stabilities of these transcription factors, which may be broadly relevant to EZH2-dependent normal development and malignancies. All these findings show diverse mechanisms by which EZH2 promotes the aggressive characteristics of cancer cells through methylation of histone or non-histone proteins, and thus pharmacological inhibition of the methyltransferase activity of EZH2 may hold great promise for the treatment of prostate cancer.

As a functionally important epigenetic mark, methylation of H3K27 is dynamically and precisely controlled. The JmjC domain-containing proteins, UTX (ubiquitously transcribed tetratricopeptide repeat, X chromosome) and JMJD3, specifically remove only the di- and tri-methyl groups though, from H3K27, counteracting the action of EZH2. Therefore, it is conceivable that UTX or JMJD3 exerts a tumor-suppressive role in prostate cancer. In support of this supposition, inactivating somatic mutations of UTX have been discovered in many types of human cancers including prostate [125]. Lack of functional UTX may result in increased levels of H3K27 methylation and subsequently have an analogous effect to the phenotypes caused by EZH2 overexpression. Genome-wide study revealed that UTX-occupied promoters were significantly underrepresented for H3K27me3 signals and that majority of the downstream target genes were functionally enriched in RB-centered cell cycle regulation. This suggests a role for UTX-catalyzed demethylation of

H3K27me3 in controlling cancer cell fate through the RB network [126]. This conclusion was further confirmed in another study, which demonstrated that UTX restricted Notch and RB signaling to suppress eye tumor formation in Drosophila, which was dependent on its demethylase activity [127]. More than that, UTX was shown to be localized at the promoters of apoptosis and autophagy genes, upregulated their expressions by removing the repressive methylation marks from H3K27, hence induced cell death of larval salivary glands [128]. In keeping with these findings, it was shown that the other only H3K27 demethylase, JMDJ3, induced the transcriptional activation of several tumor suppressor genes, such as $p16^{INK4A}$ and $p14^{ARF}$ [129, 130]. All the above indications support the idea that demethylation of H3K27 catalyzed by either UTX or JMJD3 impedes tumorigenesis. However, the exact function of UTX or JMJD3 in prostate cancer is insufficiently investigated. Recently, an oncogenic role of UTX was discovered that it cooperates with H3K4 methyltransferase MLL4 in activating transcriptional programs that are required for proliferation and invasiveness of breast cancer cells [131]. This implies that the biological effects of UTX in cancers, either tumor-promoting or tumor-suppressive, are highly tissue-specific. Considering the relatively high rate of loss-of-function mutations of UTX in prostate carcinoma, the demethylase may function as a tumor suppressor in this type of cancer. Adding to the complexity of the situation, JMJD3 was upregulated in prostate cancer with higher expression levels in metastatic samples [132]. Therefore, it is likely that UTX and JMJD3, albeit their same activities against H3K27 demethylation, may produce opposite biological outcomes in prostate cancer. Further investigation is clearly warranted to explore the dynamic and divergent functions of H3K27 demethylation in prostate carcinogenesis and tumor progression.

Unlike H3K27 methylation, which is catalyzed by only two methyltransferases EZH2 or its close homolog EZH1, H3K4 can be methylated by at least ten known or predicted methyltransferases. The major class of such enzymes is the Mixed Lineage Leukemia (MLL) family, which contains six members MLL1–4, SET1A and B. Like EZH2 and most histone-modifying enzymes, MLL-family methyltransferases exist in multiprotein complexes, and the most common components that are shared by all MLL family complexes include WDR5, RBBP5 and ASH2L [133]. Misregulation of *MLL* genes is implicated in prostate cancer development and progression. The recurrent mutations in *MLL2* gene have been identified in 8.6% of prostate cancers [125], and somatic *MLL3* mutations found in African American patients were associated with the aggressiveness of prostate cancer [23, 134]. In addition, translocation of *MLL* gene was found in two metastatic CRPC cases [135]. Besides the genetic alterations, MLL proteins together with the assisting subunits involve intimately in AR signaling through direct epigenetic regulation of AR target genes. It was demonstrated that MLL-containing complex acts as a co-activator of AR signaling, and that pharmacological blockage of MLL-AR axis reduces xenograft tumor growth in CRPC mouse models [136]. WD repeat-containing protein 5 (WDR5), an indispensible subunit of all MLL complexes, is upregulated in human prostate cancer. It directly interacts with the T11-phosphorylated histone H3 at AR-bound chromatin locations, then recruits MLL1 complex that leads to H3K4 methylation at these sites, and subsequent transactivates AR target genes [137]. Using similar mechanism of action, BPTF associated protein of 18 KDa (BAP18), which was also shown to associate with MLL complexes, facilitates the recruitment of MLL1 complex to the androgen-response elements, increases the levels of active epigenetic marks such as H3K4me3 and H4K16ac, and therefore enhances AR-induced transactivation [138]. In addition to AR signaling, MLL complex was shown to activate the transcription of *HOXA9* gene by upregulating H3K4me3 intensity at its promoter region, which induces metastatic phenotype in prostate cancer cells [139]. Another integral subunit of MLL1/2 complexes, menin encoded by the *MEN1* gene, has also been indicated in prostate carcinogenesis. Male mice carrying the loss-of heterozygosity of *MEN1* gene developed prostate cancer, suggesting a possible role of *MEN1* in suppressing tumorigenesis of the prostate gland [140]. However, increased expression of *MEN1* was also detected in metastatic prostate cancer [141–143], and gain at the gene locus was shown to independently predict disease recurrence after radical prostatectomy [144].

Similar to adding the functional methyl onto H3K4, which is catalyzed by multiple methyltransferases, eradiation of this epigenetic mark is tightly controlled by groups of demethylases, such as the JARID1 subfamily proteins (e.g., JARID1A-D) and KDM1 family members (e.g., KDM1A and B). Among them, KDM1A, also known as LSD1, is the most extensively studied demethylase in prostate cancer. Overexpression of LSD1 was detected in prostate cancer compared with benign prostatic hyperplasia, which is positively correlated with high Gleason score, distant metastases and poor prognosis [145, 146]. As the demethylase for the active histone mark H3K4me1/2, LSD1 is expected to mediate transcriptional repression, and indeed, it is found to associate tightly with several corepressors such as NuRD complex, histone deacetylases, and CoREST, etc. [147–149]. How the role of LSD1 as a transcriptional repressor leads to prostate cancer was best explicated by the discovery that LSD1 mediates AR-dependent silencing of target genes such as those involved in androgen synthesis, DNA synthesis and cell proliferation, including *AR* itself [150]. This was concomitant with a decrease of H3K4 methylation intensity at the regulatory chromatin elements of these AR-repressed genes in an androgen-dependent manner. Interestingly, LSD1 has also been repeatedly demonstrated to function as a transcriptional co-activator for AR [113, 115]. Pharmacological inhibition or genetic silencing of LSD1 abrogates androgen-induced gene activation and prostate cancer cell proliferation. In these scenarios, LSD1 stimulates AR-dependent transcription by relieving the repressive histone mark H3K9 methylation. It colocalizes with JMJD2C, the demethylase possessing an enzymatic activity towards H3K9 trimethylation, at AR-binding sites, where JMJD2C initiates the demethylation reaction followed by LSD1-catalyzed removal of remaining mono- and dimethylation marks on H3K9 [115]. Thereby, these two demethylases cooperatively stimulate AR-dependent gene expression. It is postulated that switch in the substrate specificity of LSD1 from H3K4 on AR-repressed genes to H3K9 on AR-activated genes may be determined by phosphorylation status of histone H3. Phosphorylation of H3 on threonine 11 (H3T11ph), which is catalyzed by protein kinase C-related kinase 1 (PRK1), increases the activities of LSD1 (mono- and dimethylation) and

JMJD2C (trimethylation) for H3K9 demethylation [151], while PKCβ1-induced phosphorylation of H3 on threonine 6 (H3T6ph) prevents LSD1 from demethylating H3K4me1/2 [152]. This is an excellent example of the close and dynamic crosstalk among distinct epigenetic patterns in establishing specific chromatin structure for transcriptional regulation. Apart from engaging in AR signaling, LSD1 also controls aggressive features of prostate cancer cells, such as angiogenesis, invasion and metastasis. This attributes to the fact that the demethylase epigenetically activates or represses expression of critical genes in these processes, including lysophosphatidic acid receptor 6 (*LPAR6*) and vascular endothelial growth factor (*VEGF-A*), etc. [153, 154]. Although implied, further mechanisms, such as demethylation of non-histone substrates, need to be explored, which likely contribute to the biological function of LSD1 in prostate cancer [155, 156].

Not only the above mentioned histone-modifying enzymes, many additional proteins that are involved in regulation of histone methylation have been implicated pivotal roles in prostate cancer development and progression. For example, the levels of arginine methyltransferases, such as CARM1, PRMT1 and PRMT2, are elevated in metastatic, hormone-refractory prostate cancer [157–159], and they regulate the transcriptional activity of AR, which is dependent on the arginine methylation states of histone H3 [158–160]. Equally interesting, SET7/9, which can write monomethylation on H3K4, was reported to directly methylate AR at K630 and K632, potentiating transcriptional activity of the nuclear receptor and stimulating prostate cancer cell proliferation [161, 162]. This list of histone-methylation-regulating proteins can keep growing, but their precise functions in prostate cancer development and progression need to be deliberately evaluated. It is intriguing to find that a lot of these enzymes as well as the corresponding histone methylation marks are involved in control of AR activity, further supporting an indispensible role of epigenetics in regulation of central signaling axis that drives prostate carcinogenesis and tumor progression.

5 DNA/Histone Methylation in Prostate Cancer Diagnosis, Prognosis and Treatment

Although in the preliminary stage, epigenetic regulatory mechanisms are gaining strength and proving their potential in terms of risk assessment, diagnosis, and therapy monitoring in prostate cancer. Even though the widespread application of PSA test has a paradigm-shifting impact on the clinical management of prostate cancer, this marker cannot effectively differentiate between cancer and non-cancerous conditions such as prostatitis and BPH. On the other hand, there are frequent occasions when PSA level is detected low but prostate cancer is actually present. Both false-positive and false-negative results of PSA test warrant the discoveries of approaches with high sensitivity and specificity for early detection of prostate cancer. Epigenetic marks hold great promise as useful diagnostic indexes, and DNA hypermethylation seems to especially fulfill this mission as several features of this epigenetic modification render it promising for risk assessment of prostate carcinogenesis. First, genome-wide and locus specific DNA methylation alterations of certain genes have been recurrently detected in prostate cancer. For instance, *GSTP1* hypermethylation is replicated in tons of independent studies that involve more than thousands of prostate cancer samples [48, 163, 164]. When considered together with methylation status of other genes such as *APC*, the specific epigenetic mark at *GSTP1* gene promoter can distinguish primary prostate cancer from benign tissues with sensitivity approaching 97.3 100% [47]. Second, somatic changes of DNA methylation pattern are usually found to occur early in prostate carcinogenesis. Acquisition of CpG island hypermethylation can already be detected in PIN lesion but is not or rarely present in BPH [49, 165]. Promoter methylation of certain genes helps discriminate between cancerous and non-cancerous prostate cells during the early development of the disease [65, 166]. This highlights the prospective character of DNA hypermethylation as an early event in prostate cancer evolution, and hence suggests that this epigenetic signature may accurately and sensitively diagnose initial stage of the disease. Third, methylated DNA can be detected in cancer tissues and body fluids of prostate malignancy. Moderate or high frequencies of methylation at several gene promoters, such as *RARβ2*, *APC*, *RASSF1A*, and *GSTP1*, were observed in the plasma, serum and urine of patients [167, 168]. One of the biggest advantages of measuring DNA methylation in body fluids is that fluctuation in the levels of this epigenetic modification can be easily and reproducibly quantified using well-developed techniques like methylation-specific PCR and bisulphite sequencing. This enables the feasibility of a non-invasive molecular approach for quick detection of epigenetic changes associated with prostate cancer. Finally, DNA hypermethylation appears to be relatively stable in a defined area of the gene. Somatic alterations of methylation can be repeatedly spotted using specific primers for the particular chromatin regions of particular genes. This is in contrast to genetic mutations, which can take place at a wide range of sites along a gene and therefore be easily missed unless the whole gene is completely sequenced. Besides, DNA is much less susceptible to degradation than protein or RNA, and thus can be maintained at steady levels throughout the sampling process. Due to its relative simplicity, safety and sensitivity, DNA methylation analysis has become a promising tool in molecular diagnostics of prostate cancer, which will substantially reduce mortality and unwanted tension of patients.

In addition to an impact on early detection, epigenetic marks have also been implicated in rapid determination of prognosis and monitor of treatment efficacy in advanced prostate cancer. DNA hypermethylation of several genes is found to correlate with clinicopathological features of poor prognosis like late stage and high Gleason scores, and accurately predict patients who are likely to experience biochemical recurrence [169–171]. While DNA hypermathylation can be an earlier event in prostate tumorigenesis, global hypomethylation and histone methylation seem to happen relatively late in prostate cancer and are more common in metastatic cases. For example, the methylation status of H4R3 positively correlates with increasing tumor grade and can be used to predict the risk of prostate cancer recurrence [106]. Loss of *LINE-1* transposable elements was observed in 67% of prostate tumors with lymph node metastases but in only 8% of tumors with no metastatic lesions [172]. More interestingly, the prognostic roles of epigenetic marks can be assessed in cell-free circulating tumor DNA (ctDNA) or nucleosome (ctNUC). Methylated ctDNA of *GSTP1* gene was found to be associated with chemotherapy response and overall survival of CRPC patients [173]. H3K27 trimethylation level in intact ctNUC discriminated metastatic prostate cancer from organ confined, locally controlled disease [105]. Taken together, specific epigenetic signatures, such as DNA methylation and histone modifications, represent a new generation of prognostic biomarkers for monitoring of cancer recurrence and therapy response. Although still in its infancy, innovative methodology has been developed so as to detect and validate these epigenetic biomarkers in an efficient and sensitive way using materials originating from body fluids of cancer patients.

Interests in targeting epigenetic modulators for anticancer therapy have never been stopped. So far, six epigenetic drugs, two DNA methyltransferase (DNMT) inhibitors and four histone deacetylase (HDAC) inhibitors, have been approved by FDA for treatment of myelodysplastic syndrome, multiple myeloma and T cell lymphoma [174–178]. In the case of prostate cancer, pharmacological inhibition of DNA methylation and histone modifications show encouraging yet limited antitumor activities. Several nucleoside analogues including those two FDA-approved DNMT inhibitors, 5-Aza-2′-deoxycytidine and 5-Azacytidine, were reported to suppress CRPC cell proliferation, reactivate AR signaling and induce cancer cell differentiation [179, 180]. Compounds that are designed to directly inhibit the enzymatic activity of human DNMTs like RG108 also exhibited some inhibitory efficacy against CRPC in vitro and in vivo [181–183]. Both types of DNMT inhibitors are thought to have the tumor-suppressive effects by specifically demethylating and reactivating tumor suppressor genes. It is indeed the case that exposure of prostate cancer cells to DNMT inhibitors significantly decreased promoter methylation signals of several genes, such as *GSTP1*, *APC*, *RASSF1A* and *RARβ2*, which, in general, is concomitant with the expression restoration of these prostate cancer specific methylated genes [183–185]. Unfortunately, in spite of all these promising results in pre-clinical settings, there are only a few clinical trials testing DNMT inhibitors in prostate cancer patients with either modest activities or severe side effects [186, 187]. A panel of small molecule inhibitors of the enzymes that regulate histone methylation is currently under intensive evaluation to assess their anticancer effectiveness. Compounds that selectively disrupt the catalytic sites of EZH2 are thought to hold great promise for treatment of prostate cancer. The very original prototype of EZH2 inhibitors is 3-dezaneplanocin-A (DZNeP), which later turned out to be a pan-HMT inhibitor [188]. DZNeP downregulates EZH2 protein, decreases the overall levels of H3K27me3, and therefore de-represses several tumor suppressor genes that are epigenetically silenced by PRC2 complex [104, 189, 190]. Exposure of prostate cancer cells to DZNeP resulted in cell cycle arrest, blocked prostatosphere formation, and diminished invasion capacity of the cancer cells [189]. More interestingly, this compound significantly reduced the expression of cancer stem cell markers and therefore abrogated self-renewal ability [189]. More specific inhibitors of EZH2 methyltransferase activity were recently developed, like GSK126,

EPZ-6438, etc. [191–193]. These drugs all demonstrated dose dependent inhibition of H3K27me3 without triggering EZH2 protein degradation. Intriguingly, both H3K27me3-dependent and -independent functions of EZH2 were indicated in mediating the antitumor effects of EZH2 inhibitors, hence the mechanism of drug action in prostate cancer cells needs further investigation [194]. Currently, there are no clinical studies involving EZH2 inhibitors in prostate cancer. Another group of epigenetic drug precursors that have been extensively studied thus far is the inhibitors of histone demethylase LSD1. Because LSD1 catalyzes lysine demethylation via an FAD-dependent monoamine oxidase (MAO) mechanism, majority of currently available compounds targeting LSD1 are actually non-selective MAO inhibitors, which include pargyline, tranylcypromine and phenelzine, etc. Pargyline blocked LSD1-catalyzed demethylation of H3K9 in prostate cancer cells, and subsequently inhibited AR-dependent transcription [113]. Furthermore, this LSD1 inhibitor reduced migration and invasion ability of prostate cancer cells and retarded the epithelial-mesenchymal transition (EMT) process in vitro and in vivo [195]. Inhibition of LSD1 by pargyline and tranylcypromine suppressed proliferation of both androgen-responsive and androgen-independent prostate cancer cells in a dose- and time-dependent manner [154]. However, in another independent study, pargyline treatment induced cell cycle arrest, whereas tranylcypromine had no effect or even promoted proliferation of prostate cancer cells [196]. The conflicting findings prompted comprehensive research on LSD1 function in prostate cancer and urged the generation of more specific inhibitors of the histone demethylase activity. Indeed, several highly selective LSD1 inhibitors have been identified recently, such as NCL-1, HCI-2509 and namoline [197–199]. All of these potent, reversible and selective LSD1 inhibitors suppressed the androgen-independent growth of CRPC cells in vitro and in vivo, with no apparent adverse effects [198–200]. Pandemethylase inhibitors have also been designed and synthesized, which can simultaneously inhibit both families of KDMs, KDM1 and JmjC-containing demethylases. Several of these compounds caused growth arrest and substantial apoptosis in cancer cells including prostate, but had little effects on nonmalignant cells [201]. Finally, two clinical trials are currently being conducted with the non-specific LSD1 inhibitor phenelzine sulfate, either alone in treating patients with relapsed prostate cancer that has not metastasized (NCT02217709) or in combination with docetaxel to treat patients with progressive prostate cancer after first-line therapy with docetaxel (NCT01253642). Tremendous efforts are ongoing to screen for compounds that target other epigenetic enzymes involving in regulation of histone methylation. For example, selective (e.g., BIX01294, UNC0638 and A-366, etc.) and non-selective (e.g., chaetocin) inhibitors of euchromatic histone methyltransferase 2 (EHMT2, also known as G9a), the HMT that is primarily responsible for H3K9 dimethylation, have been identified [202–205]. Unfortunately, although they efficiently reduce H3K9me2 in prostate cancer cells, their effects on the development and progression of the disease are quite obscure. CARM1 (PRMT4), the protein arginine methyltransferase that methylates H3 on arginines 2, 17, and 26, has been implicated as a transcriptional coactivator of AR signaling [158, 159], and therefore several pharmacological inhibitors of CARM1, such as the 1-benzyl-3,5-bis(3-

bromo-4-hydroxybenzylidene)piperidin-4-one and its analogues, dramatically reduced AR transcriptional activity in a dose-dependent fashion [206]. Additionally, a small molecule inhibitor that dissociates the menin-MLL HMT complex blocked AR signaling and prevented the growth of castration resistant tumors in vivo [136].

Overwhelming evidence supports the idea that solid tumors, such as prostate cancer, may well respond to epigenetic drugs targeting DNA methylation or histone modifications. However, the lack of success in clinical trials testing these drugs in prostate cancer raises the concerns about their potencies, specificities, and side effects. Further work is warranted in order to gain deeper understanding of the global patterns of these epigenetic modifications, such as DNA methylation and histone methylation, during prostate carcinogenesis and tumor progression. Increased insights into these epigenetic regulatory mechanisms will definitely foster successful clinical applications of these epigenetic modifications as biomarkers of cancer diagnosis and risk stratification, in predicting a patient's response to therapy or providing alternative treatment options for prostate cancer.

References

1. Griffiths J (1889) Observations on the function of the prostate gland in man and the lower animals: part II. J Anat Physiol 24:27–41
2. Schirmer HK, Walton KN, Scott WW (1964) Prostatic epithelial cells: their preparation and catalase activity. Investig Urol 1:301–306
3. Greene LF, Farrow GM, Ravits JM, Tomera FM (1979) Prostatic adenocarcinoma of ductal origin. J Urol 121:303–305
4. Merchant DJ (1976) Prostatic tissue cell growth and assessment. Semin Oncol 3:131–140
5. Hudson DL (2003) Prostate epithelial stem cell culture. Cytotechnology 41:189–196
6. Chung LW (1995) The role of stromal-epithelial interaction in normal and malignant growth. Cancer Surv 23:33–42
7. Mostofi FK, Sesterhenn IA, Davis CJ (1987) Progress in pathology of carcinoma of prostate. Prog Clin Biol Res 243A:445–475
8. Bashir MN (2015) Epidemiology of prostate cancer. Asian Pac J Cancer Prev 16:5137–5141
9. American Cancer Society (2016) Cancer facts & figures 2016. American Cancer Society, Atlanta
10. Walker AR (1986) Prostate cancer--some aspects of epidemiology, risk factors, treatment and survival. S Afr Med J 69:44–47
11. Kerr L et al (2016) A cohort analysis of men with a family history of BRCA1/2 and Lynch mutations for prostate cancer. BMC Cancer 16:529
12. Simental JA, Sar M, Wilson EM (1992) Domain functions of the androgen receptor. J Steroid Biochem Mol Biol 43:37–41
13. Denis LJ et al (1998) Maximal androgen blockade: final analysis of EORTC phase III trial 30853. EORTC Genito-Urinary Tract Cancer Cooperative Group and the EORTC Data Center. Eur Urol 33:144–151
14. Kantoff PW et al (2010) Overall survival analysis of a phase II randomized controlled trial of a Poxviral-based PSA-targeted immunotherapy in metastatic castration-resistant prostate cancer. J Clin Oncol 28:1099–1105
15. Lassi K, Dawson NA (2009) Emerging therapies in castrate-resistant prostate cancer. Curr Opin Oncol 21:260–265

16. Berry W, Dakhil S, Modiano M, Gregurich M, Asmar L (2002) Phase III study of mitoxan-trone plus low dose prednisone versus low dose prednisone alone in patients with asymptomatic hormone refractory prostate cancer. J Urol 168:2439–2443
17. Wadosky KM, Koochekpour S (2016) Molecular mechanisms underlying resistance to androgen deprivation therapy in prostate cancer. Oncotarget 7(39):64447–64470
18. Massenkeil G et al (1994) P53 mutations and loss of heterozygosity on chromosomes 8p, 16q, 17p, and 18q are confined to advanced prostate cancer. Anticancer Res 14:2785–2790
19. Phin S, Moore MW, Cotter PD (2013) Genomic rearrangements of PTEN in prostate cancer. Front Oncol 3:240
20. Tomlins SA et al (2005) Recurrent fusion of TMPRSS2 and ETS transcription factor genes in prostate cancer. Science 310:644–648
21. Linja MJ, Visakorpi T (2004) Alterations of androgen receptor in prostate cancer. J Steroid Biochem Mol Biol 92:255–264
22. Boysen G et al (2015) SPOP mutation leads to genomic instability in prostate cancer. elife 4:e09207
23. Barbieri CE et al (2012) Exome sequencing identifies recurrent SPOP, FOXA1 and MED12 mutations in prostate cancer. Nat Genet 44:685–689
24. Holliday R (1994) Epigenetics: an overview. Dev Genet 15:453–457
25. Chomet PS (1991) Cytosine methylation in gene-silencing mechanisms. Curr Opin Cell Biol 3:438–443
26. Pradhan S, Esteve PO (2003) Mammalian DNA (cytosine-5) methyltransferases and their expression. Clin Immunol 109:6–16
27. Ikeda Y, Kinoshita T (2009) DNA demethylation: a lesson from the garden. Chromosoma 118:37–41
28. Takai D, Jones PA (2002) Comprehensive analysis of CpG islands in human chromosomes 21 and 22. Proc Natl Acad Sci U S A 99:3740–3745
29. Schulz WA, Hatina J (2006) Epigenetics of prostate cancer: beyond DNA methylation. J Cell Mol Med 10:100–125
30. Kinoshita H et al (2000) Methylation of the androgen receptor minimal promoter silences transcription in human prostate cancer. Cancer Res 60:3623–3630
31. Nakayama T et al (2000) Epigenetic regulation of androgen receptor gene expression in human prostate cancers. Lab Investig 80:1789–1796
32. Jarrard DF et al (1998) Methylation of the androgen receptor promoter CpG island is associated with loss of androgen receptor expression in prostate cancer cells. Cancer Res 58:5310–5314
33. Li LC, Yeh CC, Nojima D, Dahiya R (2000) Cloning and characterization of human estrogen receptor beta promoter. Biochem Biophys Res Commun 275:682–689
34. Nojima D et al (2001) CpG hypermethylation of the promoter region inactivates the estrogen receptor-beta gene in patients with prostate carcinoma. Cancer 92:2076–2083
35. Li LC et al (2000) Frequent methylation of estrogen receptor in prostate cancer: correlation with tumor progression. Cancer Res 60:702–706
36. Royuela M et al (2001) Estrogen receptors alpha and beta in the normal, hyperplastic and carcinomatous human prostate. J Endocrinol 168:447–454
37. Nelson AW, Tilley WD, Neal DE, Carroll JS (2014) Estrogen receptor beta in prostate cancer: friend or foe? Endocr Relat Cancer 21:T219–T234
38. Yeh CR, Da J, Song W, Fazili A, Yeh S (2014) Estrogen receptors in prostate development and cancer. Am J Clin Exp Urol 2:161–168
39. Jeronimo C et al (2004) Quantitative RARbeta2 hypermethylation: a promising prostate cancer marker. Clin Cancer Res 10:4010–4014
40. Yamanaka M et al (2003) Altered methylation of multiple genes in carcinogenesis of the prostate. Int J Cancer 106:382–387
41. Nakayama T et al (2001) The role of epigenetic modifications in retinoic acid receptor beta2 gene expression in human prostate cancers. Lab Investig 81:1049–1057

42. Dumache R et al (2012) Retinoic acid receptor beta2 (RARbeta2): nonivasive biomarker for distinguishing malignant versus benign prostate lesions from bodily fluids. Chirurgia (Bucur) 107:780–784
43. Woodson K, Hanson J, Tangrea J (2004) A survey of gene-specific methylation in human prostate cancer among black and white men. Cancer Lett 205:181–188
44. Gao T et al (2013) The association of retinoic acid receptor beta2(RARbeta2) methylation status and prostate cancer risk: a systematic review and meta-analysis. PLoS One 8:e62950
45. Martignano F et al (2016) GSTP1 methylation and protein expression in prostate cancer: diagnostic implications. Dis Markers 2016:4358292
46. Maldonado L et al (2014) GSTP1 promoter methylation is associated with recurrence in early stage prostate cancer. J Urol 192:1542–1548
47. Yegnasubramanian S et al (2004) Hypermethylation of CpG islands in primary and metastatic human prostate cancer. Cancer Res 64:1975–1986
48. Konishi N et al (2002) DNA hypermethylation status of multiple genes in prostate adenocarcinomas. Jpn J Cancer Res 93:767–773
49. Kang GH, Lee S, Lee HJ, Hwang KS (2004) Aberrant CpG island hypermethylation of multiple genes in prostate cancer and prostatic intraepithelial neoplasia. J Pathol 202:233–240
50. Jarrard DF et al (1997) Deletional, mutational, and methylation analyses of CDKN2 (p16/MTS1) in primary and metastatic prostate cancer. Genes Chromosomes Cancer 19:90–96
51. Gu K, Mes-Masson AM, Gauthier J, Saad F (1998) Analysis of the p16 tumor suppressor gene in early-stage prostate cancer. Mol Carcinog 21:164–170
52. Nguyen TT et al (2000) Analysis of cyclin-dependent kinase inhibitor expression and methylation patterns in human prostate cancers. Prostate 43:233–242
53. Liu L, Yoon JH, Dammann R, Pfeifer GP (2002) Frequent hypermethylation of the RASSF1A gene in prostate cancer. Oncogene 21:6835–6840
54. Kawamoto K et al (2007) Epigenetic modifications of RASSF1A gene through chromatin remodeling in prostate cancer. Clin Cancer Res 13:2541–2548
55. Singal R, Ferdinand L, Reis IM, Schlesselman JJ (2004) Methylation of multiple genes in prostate cancer and the relationship with clinicopathological features of disease. Oncol Rep 12:631–637
56. Park JY (2010) Promoter hypermethylation in prostate cancer. Cancer Control 17:245–255
57. Graff JR et al (1995) E-cadherin expression is silenced by DNA hypermethylation in human breast and prostate carcinomas. Cancer Res 55:5195–5199
58. Li LC et al (2001) Methylation of the E-cadherin gene promoter correlates with progression of prostate cancer. J Urol 166:705–709
59. Woodson K, Hayes R, Wideroff L, Villaruz L, Tangrea J (2003) Hypermethylation of GSTP1, CD44, and E-cadherin genes in prostate cancer among US Blacks and Whites. Prostate 55:199–205
60. Saha B et al (2008) Unmethylated E-cadherin gene expression is significantly associated with metastatic human prostate cancer cells in bone. Prostate 68:1681–1688
61. Guilford P et al (1998) E-cadherin germline mutations in familial gastric cancer. Nature 392:402–405
62. Dossus L, Benusiglio PR (2015) Lobular breast cancer: incidence and genetic and non-genetic risk factors. Breast Cancer Res 17:37
63. Richiardi L et al (2009) Promoter methylation in APC, RUNX3, and GSTP1 and mortality in prostate cancer patients. J Clin Oncol 27:3161–3168
64. Henrique R et al (2007) High promoter methylation levels of APC predict poor prognosis in sextant biopsies from prostate cancer patients. Clin Cancer Res 13:6122–6129
65. Chen Y et al (2013) APC gene hypermethylation and prostate cancer: a systematic review and meta-analysis. Eur J Hum Genet 21:929–935
66. Yaqinuddin A et al (2013) Frequent DNA hypermethylation at the RASSF1A and APC Gene loci in prostate cancer patients of Pakistani origin. ISRN Urol 2013:627249
67. Rosenbaum E et al (2005) Promoter hypermethylation as an independent prognostic factor for relapse in patients with prostate cancer following radical prostatectomy. Clin Cancer Res 11:8321–8325

68. Majumdar S, Buckles E, Estrada J, Koochekpour S (2011) Aberrant DNA methylation and prostate cancer. Curr Genomics 12:486–505
69. Schulz WA et al (2002) Genomewide DNA hypomethylation is associated with alterations on chromosome 8 in prostate carcinoma. Genes Chromosomes Cancer 35:58–65
70. Cho NY, Kim JH, Moon KC, Kang GH (2009) Genomic hypomethylation and CpG island hypermethylation in prostatic intraepithelial neoplasm. Virchows Arch 454:17–23
71. Brothman AR et al (2005) Global hypomethylation is common in prostate cancer cells: a quantitative predictor for clinical outcome? Cancer Genet Cytogenet 156:31–36
72. Bedford MT, van Helden PD (1987) Hypomethylation of DNA in pathological conditions of the human prostate. Cancer Res 47:5274–5276
73. Florl AR et al (2004) Coordinate hypermethylation at specific genes in prostate carcinoma precedes LINE-1 hypomethylation. Br J Cancer 91:985–994
74. Yegnasubramanian S et al (2008) DNA hypomethylation arises later in prostate cancer progression than CpG island hypermethylation and contributes to metastatic tumor heterogeneity. Cancer Res 68:8954–8967
75. Kim R, Kulkarni P, Hannenhalli S (2013) Derepression of cancer/testis antigens in cancer is associated with distinct patterns of DNA hypomethylation. BMC Cancer 13:144
76. Van Veldhuizen PJ, Sadasivan R, Cherian R, Wyatt A (1996) Urokinase-type plasminogen activator expression in human prostate carcinomas. Am J Med Sci 312:8–11
77. Pulukuri SM, Estes N, Patel J, Rao JS (2007) Demethylation-linked activation of urokinase plasminogen activator is involved in progression of prostate cancer. Cancer Res 67:930–939
78. Pakneshan P, Xing RH, Rabbani SA (2003) Methylation status of uPA promoter as a molecular mechanism regulating prostate cancer invasion and growth in vitro and in vivo. FASEB J 17:1081–1088
79. Suyama T et al (2010) Expression of cancer/testis antigens in prostate cancer is associated with disease progression. Prostate 70:1778–1787
80. Laner T, Schulz WA, Engers R, Muller M, Florl AR (2005) Hypomethylation of the XIST gene promoter in prostate cancer. Oncol Res 15:257–264
81. Wang Q et al (2007) Hypomethylation of WNT5A, CRIP1 and S100P in prostate cancer. Oncogene 26:6560–6565
82. Tokizane T et al (2005) Cytochrome P450 1B1 is overexpressed and regulated by hypomethylation in prostate cancer. Clin Cancer Res 11:5793–5801
83. Li LC, Carroll PR, Dahiya R (2005) Epigenetic changes in prostate cancer: implication for diagnosis and treatment. J Natl Cancer Inst 97:103–115
84. Gershey EL, Haslett GW, Vidali G, Allfrey VG (1969) Chemical studies of histone methylation. Evidence for the occurrence of 3-methylhistidine in avian erythrocyte histone fractions. J Biol Chem 244:4871–4877
85. Borun TW, Pearson D, Paik WK (1972) Studies of histone methylation during the HeLa S-3 cell cycle. J Biol Chem 247:4288–4298
86. van Leeuwen F, Gafken PR, Gottschling DE (2002) Dot1p modulates silencing in yeast by methylation of the nucleosome core. Cell 109:745–756
87. Min J, Feng Q, Li Z, Zhang Y, Xu RM (2003) Structure of the catalytic domain of human DOT1L, a non-SET domain nucleosomal histone methyltransferase. Cell 112:711–723
88. Feng Y et al (2013) Mammalian protein arginine methyltransferase 7 (PRMT7) specifically targets RXR sites in lysine- and arginine-rich regions. J Biol Chem 288:37010–37025
89. Lakowski TM, Frankel A (2009) Kinetic analysis of human protein arginine N-methyltransferase 2: formation of monomethyl- and asymmetric dimethyl-arginine residues on histone H4. Biochem J 421:253–261
90. Schapira M, Ferreira de Freitas R (2014) Structural biology and chemistry of protein arginine methyltransferases. Medchemcomm 5:1779–1788
91. Branscombe TL et al (2001) PRMT5 (Janus kinase-binding protein 1) catalyzes the formation of symmetric dimethylarginine residues in proteins. J Biol Chem 276:32971–32976
92. Walport LJ et al (2016) Arginine demethylation is catalysed by a subset of JmjC histone lysine demethylases. Nat Commun 7:11974

93. Chang B, Chen Y, Zhao Y, Bruick RK (2007) JMJD6 is a histone arginine demethylase. Science 318:444–447
94. Walport LJ, Hopkinson RJ, Schofield CJ (2012) Mechanisms of human histone and nucleic acid demethylases. Curr Opin Chem Biol 16:525–534
95. Jenuwein T, Allis CD (2001) Translating the histone code. Science 293:1074–1080
96. Strahl BD, Allis CD (2000) The language of covalent histone modifications. Nature 403:41–45
97. Wang Y, Jia S (2009) Degrees make all the difference: the multifunctionality of histone H4 lysine 20 methylation. Epigenetics 4:273–276
98. Li B et al (2009) Histone H3 lysine 36 dimethylation (H3K36me2) is sufficient to recruit the Rpd3s histone deacetylase complex and to repress spurious transcription. J Biol Chem 284:7970–7976
99. Zhao Q et al (2009) PRMT5-mediated methylation of histone H4R3 recruits DNMT3A, coupling histone and DNA methylation in gene silencing. Nat Struct Mol Biol 16:304–311
100. Otani J et al (2009) Structural basis for recognition of H3K4 methylation status by the DNA methyltransferase 3A ATRX-DNMT3-DNMT3L domain. EMBO Rep 10:1235–1241
101. Yang Y et al (2010) TDRD3 is an effector molecule for arginine-methylated histone marks. Mol Cell 40:1016–1023
102. Ellinger J et al (2010) Global levels of histone modifications predict prostate cancer recurrence. Prostate 70:61–69
103. Ellinger J et al (2012) Global histone H3K27 methylation levels are different in localized and metastatic prostate cancer. Cancer Investig 30:92–97
104. Ngollo M et al (2014) The association between histone 3 lysine 27 trimethylation (H3K27me3) and prostate cancer: relationship with clinicopathological parameters. BMC Cancer 14:994
105. Deligezer U et al (2010) Post-treatment circulating plasma BMP6 mRNA and H3K27 methylation levels discriminate metastatic prostate cancer from localized disease. Clin Chim Acta 411:1452–1456
106. Seligson DB et al (2005) Global histone modification patterns predict risk of prostate cancer recurrence. Nature 435:1262–1266
107. Bianco-Miotto T et al (2010) Global levels of specific histone modifications and an epigenetic gene signature predict prostate cancer progression and development. Cancer Epidemiol Biomark Prev 19:2611–2622
108. Zhou LX et al (2010) Application of histone modification in the risk prediction of the biochemical recurrence after radical prostatectomy. Asian J Androl 12:171–179
109. Yu J et al (2007) A polycomb repression signature in metastatic prostate cancer predicts cancer outcome. Cancer Res 67:10657–10663
110. Yu J et al (2007) Integrative genomics analysis reveals silencing of beta-adrenergic signaling by polycomb in prostate cancer. Cancer Cell 12:419–431
111. Chen H, Tu SW, Hsieh JT (2005) Down-regulation of human DAB2IP gene expression mediated by polycomb Ezh2 complex and histone deacetylase in prostate cancer. J Biol Chem 280:22437–22444
112. Wang Q et al (2009) Androgen receptor regulates a distinct transcription program in androgen-independent prostate cancer. Cell 138:245–256
113. Metzger E et al (2005) LSD1 demethylates repressive histone marks to promote androgen-receptor-dependent transcription. Nature 437:436–439
114. Yamane K et al (2006) JHDM2A, a JmjC-containing H3K9 demethylase, facilitates transcription activation by androgen receptor. Cell 125:483–495
115. Wissmann M et al (2007) Cooperative demethylation by JMJD2C and LSD1 promotes androgen receptor-dependent gene expression. Nat Cell Biol 9:347–353
116. Zhao JC et al (2012) Cooperation between Polycomb and androgen receptor during oncogenic transformation. Genome Res 22:322–331
117. Chng KR et al (2012) A transcriptional repressor co-regulatory network governing androgen response in prostate cancers. EMBO J 31:2810–2823
118. Cohen I, Poreba E, Kamieniarz K, Schneider R (2011) Histone modifiers in cancer: friends or foes? Genes Cancer 2:631–647

119. Karanikolas BD, Figueiredo ML, Wu L (2009) Polycomb group protein enhancer of zeste 2 is an oncogene that promotes the neoplastic transformation of a benign prostatic epithelial cell line. Mol Cancer Res 7:1456–1465

120. Xu K et al (2012) EZH2 oncogenic activity in castration-resistant prostate cancer cells is Polycomb-independent. Science 338:1465–1469

121. Bryant RJ, Winder SJ, Cross SS, Hamdy FC, Cunliffe VT (2008) The Polycomb Group protein EZH2 regulates actin polymerization in human prostate cancer cells. Prostate 68:255–263

122. He A et al (2012) PRC2 directly methylates GATA4 and represses its transcriptional activity. Genes Dev 26:37–42

123. Kim E et al (2013) Phosphorylation of EZH2 activates STAT3 signaling via STAT3 methylation and promotes tumorigenicity of glioblastoma stem-like cells. Cancer Cell 23:839–852

124. Lee JM et al (2012) EZH2 generates a methyl degron that is recognized by the DCAF1/DDB1/CUL4 E3 ubiquitin ligase complex. Mol Cell 48:572–586

125. Gonzalez-Perez A, Jene-Sanz A, Lopez-Bigas N (2013) The mutational landscape of chromatin regulatory factors across 4,623 tumor samples. Genome Biol 14:r106

126. Wang JK et al (2010) The histone demethylase UTX enables RB-dependent cell fate control. Genes Dev 24:327–332

127. Herz HM et al (2010) The H3K27me3 demethylase dUTX is a suppressor of Notch- and Rb-dependent tumors in Drosophila. Mol Cell Biol 30:2485–2497

128. Denton D et al (2013) UTX coordinates steroid hormone-mediated autophagy and cell death. Nat Commun 4:2916

129. Agger K et al (2009) The H3K27me3 demethylase JMJD3 contributes to the activation of the INK4A-ARF locus in response to oncogene- and stress-induced senescence. Genes Dev 23:1171–1176

130. Barradas M et al (2009) Histone demethylase JMJD3 contributes to epigenetic control of INK4a/ARF by oncogenic RAS. Genes Dev 23:1177–1182

131. Kim JH et al (2014) UTX and MLL4 coordinately regulate transcriptional programs for cell proliferation and invasiveness in breast cancer cells. Cancer Res 74:1705–1717

132. Xiang Y et al (2007) JMJD3 is a histone H3K27 demethylase. Cell Res 17:850–857

133. Li Y et al (2016) Structural basis for activity regulation of MLL family methyltransferases. Nature 530:447–452

134. Kumar A et al (2011) Exome sequencing identifies a spectrum of mutation frequencies in advanced and lethal prostate cancers. Proc Natl Acad Sci U S A 108:17087–17092

135. Brenner JC, Chinnaiyan AM (2009) Translocations in epithelial cancers. Biochim Biophys Acta 1796:201–215

136. Malik R et al (2015) Targeting the MLL complex in castration-resistant prostate cancer. Nat Med 21:344–352

137. Kim JY et al (2014) A role for WDR5 in integrating threonine 11 phosphorylation to lysine 4 methylation on histone H3 during androgen signaling and in prostate cancer. Mol Cell 54:613–625

138. Sun S et al (2016) BAP18 coactivates androgen receptor action and promotes prostate cancer progression. Nucleic Acids Res 44(17):8112

139. Gajula RP et al (2013) The twist box domain is required for Twist1-induced prostate cancer metastasis. Mol Cancer Res 11:1387–1400

140. Seigne C et al (2010) Characterisation of prostate cancer lesions in heterozygous Men1 mutant mice. BMC Cancer 10:395

141. Tomlins SA et al (2007) Integrative molecular concept modeling of prostate cancer progression. Nat Genet 39:41–51

142. Varambally S et al (2005) Integrative genomic and proteomic analysis of prostate cancer reveals signatures of metastatic progression. Cancer Cell 8:393–406

143. Dhanasekaran SM et al (2001) Delineation of prognostic biomarkers in prostate cancer. Nature 412:822–826

144. Paris PL et al (2009) An oncogenic role for the multiple endocrine neoplasia type 1 gene in prostate cancer. Prostate Cancer Prostatic Dis 12:184–191

145. Kahl P et al (2006) Androgen receptor coactivators lysine-specific histone demethylase 1 and four and a half LIM domain protein 2 predict risk of prostate cancer recurrence. Cancer Res 66:11341–11347
146. Wang M et al (2015) Relationship between LSD1 expression and E-cadherin expression in prostate cancer. Int Urol Nephrol 47:485–490
147. Shi YJ et al (2005) Regulation of LSD1 histone demethylase activity by its associated factors. Mol Cell 19:857–864
148. Hakimi MA et al (2002) A core-BRAF35 complex containing histone deacetylase mediates repression of neuronal-specific genes. Proc Natl Acad Sci U S A 99:7420–7425
149. Wang Y et al (2009) LSD1 is a subunit of the NuRD complex and targets the metastasis programs in breast cancer. Cell 138:660–672
150. Cai C et al (2011) Androgen receptor gene expression in prostate cancer is directly suppressed by the androgen receptor through recruitment of lysine-specific demethylase 1. Cancer Cell 20:457–471
151. Metzger E et al (2008) Phosphorylation of histone H3 at threonine 11 establishes a novel chromatin mark for transcriptional regulation. Nat Cell Biol 10:53–60
152. Metzger E et al (2010) Phosphorylation of histone H3T6 by PKCbeta(I) controls demethylation at histone H3K4. Nature 464:792–796
153. Ketscher A et al (2014) LSD1 controls metastasis of androgen-independent prostate cancer cells through PXN and LPAR6. Oncogene 3:e120
154. Kashyap V et al (2013) The lysine specific demethylase-1 (LSD1/KDM1A) regulates VEGF-A expression in prostate cancer. Mol Oncol 7:555–566
155. Huang J et al (2007) p53 is regulated by the lysine demethylase LSD1. Nature 449:105–108
156. Cho HS et al (2011) Demethylation of RB regulator MYPT1 by histone demethylase LSD1 promotes cell cycle progression in cancer cells. Cancer Res 71:655–660
157. Yang Y, Bedford MT (2013) Protein arginine methyltransferases and cancer. Nat Rev Cancer 13:37–50
158. Hong H et al (2004) Aberrant expression of CARM1, a transcriptional coactivator of androgen receptor, in the development of prostate carcinoma and androgen-independent status. Cancer 101:83–89
159. Majumder S, Liu Y, Ford OH 3rd, Mohler JL, Whang YE (2006) Involvement of arginine methyltransferase CARM1 in androgen receptor function and prostate cancer cell viability. Prostate 66:1292–1301
160. Meyer R, Wolf SS, Obendorf M (2007) PRMT2, a member of the protein arginine methyltransferase family, is a coactivator of the androgen receptor. J Steroid Biochem Mol Biol 107:1–14
161. Gaughan L et al (2011) Regulation of the androgen receptor by SET9-mediated methylation. Nucleic Acids Res 39:1266–1279
162. Ko S et al (2011) Lysine methylation and functional modulation of androgen receptor by Set9 methyltransferase. Mol Endocrinol 25:433–444
163. Lee WH, Isaacs WB, Bova GS, Nelson WG (1997) CG island methylation changes near the GSTP1 gene in prostatic carcinoma cells detected using the polymerase chain reaction: a new prostate cancer biomarker. Cancer Epidemiol Biomark Prev 6:443–450
164. Bastian PJ et al (2004) Molecular biomarker in prostate cancer: the role of CpG island hypermethylation. Eur Urol 46:698–708
165. Brooks JD et al (1998) CG island methylation changes near the GSTP1 gene in prostatic intraepithelial neoplasia. Cancer Epidemiol Biomark Prev 7:531–536
166. Jeronimo C et al (2011) Epigenetics in prostate cancer: biologic and clinical relevance. Eur Urol 60:753–766
167. Gonzalgo ML, Pavlovich CP, Lee SM, Nelson WG (2003) Prostate cancer detection by GSTP1 methylation analysis of postbiopsy urine specimens. Clin Cancer Res 9:2673–2677
168. Roupret M et al (2007) Molecular detection of localized prostate cancer using quantitative methylation-specific PCR on urinary cells obtained following prostate massage. Clin Cancer Res 13:1720–1725

169. Suzuki M et al (2006) Methylation of apoptosis related genes in the pathogenesis and prognosis of prostate cancer. Cancer Lett 242:222–230
170. Maruyama R et al (2002) Aberrant promoter methylation profile of prostate cancers and its relationship to clinicopathological features. Clin Cancer Res 8:514–519
171. Stott-Miller M et al (2014) Validation study of genes with hypermethylated promoter regions associated with prostate cancer recurrence. Cancer Epidemiol Biomark Prev 23:1331–1339
172. Santourlidis S, Florl A, Ackermann R, Wirtz HC, Schulz WA (1999) High frequency of alterations in DNA methylation in adenocarcinoma of the prostate. Prostate 39:166–174
173. Mahon KL et al (2014) Methylated Glutathione S-transferase 1 (mGSTP1) is a potential plasma free DNA epigenetic marker of prognosis and response to chemotherapy in castrate-resistant prostate cancer. Br J Cancer 111:1802–1809
174. Kaminskas E et al (2005) Approval summary: azacitidine for treatment of myelodysplastic syndrome subtypes. Clin Cancer Res 11:3604–3608
175. Kantarjian H et al (2006) Decitabine improves patient outcomes in myelodysplastic syndromes: results of a phase III randomized study. Cancer 106:1794–1803
176. Mann BS, Johnson JR, Cohen MH, Justice R, Pazdur R (2007) FDA approval summary: vorinostat for treatment of advanced primary cutaneous T-cell lymphoma. Oncologist 12:1247–1252
177. VanderMolen KM, McCulloch W, Pearce CJ, Oberlies NH (2011) Romidepsin (Istodax, NSC 630176, FR901228, FK228, depsipeptide): a natural product recently approved for cutaneous T-cell lymphoma. J Antibiot (Tokyo) 64:525–531
178. Poole RM (2014) Belinostat: first global approval. Drugs 74:1543–1554
179. Tian J et al (2012) Targeting the unique methylation pattern of androgen receptor (AR) promoter in prostate stem/progenitor cells with 5-aza-2′-deoxycytidine (5-AZA) leads to suppressed prostate tumorigenesis. J Biol Chem 287:39954–39966
180. Gravina GL et al (2008) Chronic azacitidine treatment results in differentiating effects, sensitizes against bicalutamide in androgen-independent prostate cancer cells. Prostate 68:793–801
181. Valente S et al (2014) Selective non-nucleoside inhibitors of human DNA methyltransferases active in cancer including in cancer stem cells. J Med Chem 57:701–713
182. Chuang JC et al (2005) Comparison of biological effects of non-nucleoside DNA methylation inhibitors versus 5-aza-2′-deoxycytidine. Mol Cancer Ther 4:1515–1520
183. Graca I et al (2014) Anti-tumoral effect of the non-nucleoside DNMT inhibitor RG108 in human prostate cancer cells. Curr Pharm Des 20:1803–1811
184. Vardi A et al (2010) Soy phytoestrogens modify DNA methylation of GSTP1, RASSF1A, EPH2 and BRCA1 promoter in prostate cancer cells. In Vivo 24:393–400
185. Jagadeesh S, Sinha S, Pal BC, Bhattacharya S, Banerjee PP (2007) Mahanine reverses an epigenetically silenced tumor suppressor gene RASSF1A in human prostate cancer cells. Biochem Biophys Res Commun 362:212–217
186. Singal R et al (2015) Phase I/II study of azacitidine, docetaxel, and prednisone in patients with metastatic castration-resistant prostate cancer previously treated with docetaxel-based therapy. Clin Genitourin Cancer 13:22–31
187. Thibault A et al (1998) A phase II study of 5-aza-2′deoxycytidine (decitabine) in hormone independent metastatic (D2) prostate cancer. Tumori 84:87–89
188. Miranda TB et al (2009) DZNep is a global histone methylation inhibitor that reactivates developmental genes not silenced by DNA methylation. Mol Cancer Ther 8:1579–1588
189. Crea F et al (2011) Pharmacologic disruption of Polycomb Repressive Complex 2 inhibits tumorigenicity and tumor progression in prostate cancer. Mol Cancer 10:40
190. Hibino S et al (2014) Inhibitors of enhancer of zeste homolog 2 (EZH2) activate tumor-suppressor microRNAs in human cancer cells. Oncogene 3:e104
191. Knutson SK et al (2012) A selective inhibitor of EZH2 blocks H3K27 methylation and kills mutant lymphoma cells. Nat Chem Biol 8:890–896
192. McCabe MT et al (2012) EZH2 inhibition as a therapeutic strategy for lymphoma with EZH2-activating mutations. Nature 492:108–112

193. Qi W et al (2012) Selective inhibition of Ezh2 by a small molecule inhibitor blocks tumor cells proliferation. Proc Natl Acad Sci U S A 109:21360–21365
194. Wu C et al (2016) Inhibition of EZH2 by chemo- and radiotherapy agents and small molecule inhibitors induces cell death in castration-resistant prostate cancer. Oncotarget 7:3440–3452
195. Wang M et al (2015) Inhibition of LSD1 by Pargyline inhibited process of EMT and delayed progression of prostate cancer in vivo. Biochem Biophys Res Commun 467:310–315
196. Lee HT, Choi MR, Doh MS, Jung KH, Chai YG (2013) Effects of the monoamine oxidase inhibitors pargyline and tranylcypromine on cellular proliferation in human prostate cancer cells. Oncol Rep 30:1587–1592
197. Ueda R et al (2009) Identification of cell-active lysine specific demethylase 1-selective inhibitors. J Am Chem Soc 131:17536–17537
198. Sorna V et al (2013) High-throughput virtual screening identifies novel N'-(1-phenylethylidene)-benzohydrazides as potent, specific, and reversible LSD1 inhibitors. J Med Chem 56:9496–9508
199. Willmann D et al (2012) Impairment of prostate cancer cell growth by a selective and reversible lysine-specific demethylase 1 inhibitor. Int J Cancer 131:2704–2709
200. Etani T et al (2015) NCL1, a highly selective lysine-specific demethylase 1 inhibitor, suppresses prostate cancer without adverse effect. Oncotarget 6:2865 2878
201. Rotili D et al (2014) Pan-histone demethylase inhibitors simultaneously targeting Jumonji C and lysine-specific demethylases display high anticancer activities. J Med Chem 57:42–55
202. Greiner D, Bonaldi T, Eskeland R, Roemer E, Imhof A (2005) Identification of a specific inhibitor of the histone methyltransferase SU(VAR)3-9. Nat Chem Biol 1:143–145
203. Kubicek S et al (2007) Reversal of H3K9me2 by a small-molecule inhibitor for the G9a histone methyltransferase. Mol Cell 25:473–481
204. Liu F et al (2010) Protein lysine methyltransferase G9a inhibitors: design, synthesis, and structure activity relationships of 2,4-diamino-7-aminoalkoxy-quinazolines. J Med Chem 53:5844–5857
205. Sweis RF et al (2014) Discovery and development of potent and selective inhibitors of histone methyltransferase g9a. ACS Med Chem Lett 5:205–209
206. Lee E et al (2013) Inhibition of androgen receptor and beta-catenin activity in prostate cancer. Proc Natl Acad Sci U S A 110:15710–15715

Part V
DNA and Histone Modifications in Diagnosis and Therapy of Cancer

DNA and Histone Modifications in Cancer Diagnosis

Masaki Kinehara, Yuki Yamamoto, Yoshitomo Shiroma, Mariko Ikuo, Akira Shimamoto, and Hidetoshi Tahara

Abstract A number of epigenetic alterations occur during carcinogenesis, and inactivation of tumor suppressor genes is a major determinant of cancer development. Hypermethylation of tumor suppressor genes, histone modification, DNA methylation are major epigenetic alteration in cancers. These alterations may cause a change in gene expression in cells as well as in secretory factors, which include proteins and nucleic acid. Aberrant miRNA expression associated with promoter methylation has been found in body fluids such as plasma and serum, and liquid biopsy can therefore be used to identify significant biomarkers in the early detection of cancer. In addition, telomeres are a key regulator of chromosome stability in cancer. Epigenetic modification by histone methylation is associated with the maintenance of telomere length. This maintenance is essential for cancer to maintain an immortal phenotype. Telomeric repeat-containing RNA (TERRA) is also a regulator of epigenetic modification. In this review, we describe recent advances in our understanding of epigenetic regulation in cancers, including DNA and histone modifications, as well as regulation by non-coding RNAs.

Keywords Senescence • MicroRNA • Telomere • Stem cell • Liquid biopsy • Cancer diagnosis • Histone modification

1 Epigenetic Changes as Biomarkers for Cancer Diagnosis

1.1 Altered and Hypermethylation of Tumor-Suppressor Genes

DNA methylation occurs in cytosines that precede a guanine nucleotide (CpG) in DNA. CpG-rich regions, known as CpG islands, are distributed in the regulatory region of many genes [1]. Abnormal DNA hypermethylation at CpG islands of gene promoters contributes to tight transcriptional silencing of many genes in cancer [1].

M. Kinehara • Y. Yamamoto • Y. Shiroma • M. Ikuo • A. Shimamoto • H. Tahara (✉)
Department of Cellular and Molecular Biology, Basic Life Sciences, Institute of Biomedical and Health Sciences, Hiroshima University, Hiroshima 734-8553, Japan
e-mail: kinehara@hiroshima-u.ac.jp; yyamamoto@hiroshima-u.ac.jp; shiroma1023@hiroshima-u.ac.jp; ikuo@hiroshima-u.ac.jp; shim@hiroshima-u.ac.jp; toshi@hiroshima-u.ac.jp

© Springer International Publishing AG 2017
A. Kaneda, Y.-i. Tsukada (eds.), *DNA and Histone Methylation as Cancer Targets*, Cancer Drug Discovery and Development, DOI 10.1007/978-3-319-59786-7_19

In 1989, epigenetic silencing was first reported to be associated with retinoblastoma protein (RB) [2, 3], known as a tumor suppressor gene [4–6]. RB plays an important role in negative control of the cell cycle and in cancer progression [7]. These findings suggest that epigenetic pathways play an important role in tumor-suppressor gene silencing. In addition to RB, several groups have reported that hypermethylation of other tumor-suppressor genes is associated with epigenetic gene inactivation in cancer [8, 9]. For example, *CDKN2A*, which encodes two proteins [10] – p16^{INK4a}, a cyclin-dependent kinase inhibitor, and the alternative reading frame (ARF) – is associated with dense CpG methylation of its promoter regions in cancer [8, 9]. Hypermethylation in the CpG island occurs early in tumorigenesis and leads to transcriptional silencing of *CDKN2A*. On the other hand, Serrano et al., reported that p16^{INK4a} and ARF function to suppress tumor development [11], and that both p16^{INK4a} and ARF were induced by constitutive activation of the oncogenic Ras signaling pathway, and lead to premature cell senescence associated with activation of p53 and RB [12]. In addition, the relationship between tumor-suppressor activity and DNA methylation was demonstrated by the potency of demethylating drugs or by gene silencing of DNA methyltransferases (DNMTs) [13–15]. These early studies reveal that CpG-island methylation as well as cancer-specific mutation play an important role in tumor-suppressor gene silencing in tumorigenesis. Hence, it has been recognized that tumor-suppressor genes protect tumor development. In fact, tumor-suppressor genes such as p16^{INK4a}, ARF, p53, and RB have been found to be disable in many tumor types [10].

1.2 Histone Modification Connected to DNA Methylation in Tumor Suppressor Genes

DNA methylation changes have been associated with other epigenetic changes, such as histone modification, to maintain the silent epigenetic state. The development of genomic technologies has revealed a link between DNA and histone methylation events over the last few years. These technologies, particularly next-generation sequencing (NGS) and chromatin immunoprecipitation (ChIP), have generated comprehensive maps of DNA and histone methylation, and uncovered the recruitment of protein complexes to methylated DNA and modified histones [16]. In human cancer, DNA methylation profiles with ChIP-Seq data for histone methylation have indicated a correlation between cancer-associated DNA methylation and genes marked with histone methylation [17, 18]. These genes are marked by bivalent histone modifications, namely trimethylation of histone H3 lysine 4 (H3K4me3), which is strongly associated with transcriptional activation, and trimethylation of histone H3 lysine 27 (H3K27me3), which is frequently associated with gene silencing. For example, H3K27me3 occurs with gene silencing of the *CDKN2A* tumor suppressor in cancer cells [19–23]. In addition, de novo DNA hypermethylation is mediated by the presence of H3K27me3 [24]. This evidence suggests the presence of crosstalk between histone modification and DNA methylation. While it is possible to detect tumor-associated alterations in histone modifications for cancer diagnosis, assessment of histone modifications in cancer diagnosis remains technically challenging compared with the diagnostic potential of DNA methylation [25]. Because histone modifications have been shown to be more dynamic and unstable, their assessment using antibodies is more difficult to apply in cancer diagnosis.

1.3 Advantage of Aberrant DNA Methylation in Cancer Diagnosis

Aberrant DNA methylation and genetic mutation in tumor-suppressor genes is recognized as an important cause of tumor formation and progression [26]. DNA methylation changes have been associated with the alteration of gene expression in some tumor-suppressor genes, suggesting that aberrant DNA methylation can be exploited in cancer diagnosis. DNA methylation-based diagnostic techniques present advantages over genetic mutational analysis in cancer diagnosis. In many types of cancers, DNA hypermethylation occurs more frequently at CpG islands, facilitating detection compared with genetic mutations and allowing higher sensitivity in the assessment of cancer risk and cancer diagnosis [25, 27, 28]. Moreover, the diagnostic use of genetic mutation is limited by the low frequency of point mutations, making them technically complicated to detect. In marked contrast, changes in methylation of circulating tumor DNA (ctDNA) in blood can be reliably identified by commonly used techniques, such as the methylation-specific PCR (MSP) method. This method converts unmethylated cytosines to uracil by sodium bisulphite treatment of DNA, and analyses the modified DNA using either specific PCR with primers for methylated and unmethylated DNA, or DNA sequencing. As an example, the diagnostic potential of DNA methylation in the vimentin gene in plasma or stool has been well studied in human colorectal cancer [29, 30]. In addition, cancer-specific DNA hypermethylation has been detected in fluids, including blood, stool, saliva and urine (Table 1) [91, 92]. Detection of methylated ctDNA in fluids might serve as a liquid biopsy, which would be useful in assessing cancer risk and cancer diagnosis.

1.4 Liquid Biopsy and Epigenetics

Although epigenetic alterations are events in the nucleus, there are evolving approaches to diagnosing such abnormalities with minimally invasive methods, such as liquid biopsy.

Liquid biopsy requires body fluid samples such as blood, plasma, serum, urine, saliva, and cerebrospinal fluid, and does not use affected tissue area or cell samples

Table 1 Detectable circulating tumor DNA methylation in fluid

	DNA source	Genes	References
Bladder	Plasma	*CDKN2A (ARF and INK4A)*	[31]
	Serum	*CDKN2A (INK4A)*	[32]
	Urine	*RARB(RAR-β), DAPK1, CDH1(E-cadherin), and CDKN2A (INK4A)*	[33]
Breast	Plasma	*CDKN2A (INK4A)*	[34, 35]
	Serum	*RASSF1A*	[36]
	Plasma	*RASSF1A und IIIC-1*	[37]
	Serum	*MDR1*	[38]
	Serum	*BRCA1, MGMT, and GSTP1*	[39]
	Plasma	*RASSF1A, RARB (RAR-β), and HIC-1*	[40]
	Ductal lavage fluid	*RARB (RAR-β), CCND2 (cyclin D2), and TWIST*	[41]
Cervical	Plasma	*FHIT and CDH1(E-cadherin)*	[42]
	Serum	*CALCA, hTERT, MYOD1, PGR, and TIMP3*	[43]
Colorectal	Plasma	*SEPT9*	[44, 45]
	Plasma/serum	*CDKN2A (INK4A)*	[46–48]
	Plasma	*ALX4, SEPT9, and TMEFF2*	[49]
	Serum	*MLH1*	[50]
Liver	Serum	*RASSF1A*	[51]
	Plasma/serum	*CDKN2A (INK4A) and CDKN2B (INK4B)*	[52]
	Serum	*GSTP1*	[53]
	Plasma/serum	*CDKN2A (INK4A)*	[54]
Lung	Plasma	*CDKN2A (INK4A)*	[55–58]
	Sputum/plasma	*CDKN2A (INK4A)*	[59]
	Plasma	*SFN(14-3-3σ)*	[60]
	Serum	*CDKN2A (INK4A), GSTP1, MGMT, and DAPK1*	[61]
	Plasma/serum	*APC*	[62]
	Sputum	*CDKN2A (INK4A)*	[63, 64]
	Bronchoalveolar lavage fluid	*CDKN2A (INK4A)*	[64, 65]
	Sputum	*CDKN2A (INK4A) and MGMT,*	[66]
	Sputum	*CDKN2A (INK4A), MGMT, DAPK1, and RASSF1A*	[67]
Lymphoma	Plasma	*CDKN2A (INK4A)*	[68]
Melanoma	Serum	*RASSF1A and RARB2(RAR-β2)*	[69]
	Serum	*RASSF1A, MGMT, and RARB2(RAR-β2)*	[70]
Ovarian	Plasma	*BRCA1, PGR, HIC1, PAX5, and THBS1*	[71]
	Peritoneal fluid	*TIMP3, CDH1, CDH13, APC, PPP1R13B, HSPA2, HSD17B4, ESR1, GSTP1, CYP1B1, BRCA1, MYOD1, SOCS1, TITF1, and GSTM3*	[72]

(continued)

Table 1 (continued)

	DNA source	Genes	References
Pancreatic	Plasma	*CCND2, DAPK1, ESR1, HMLH1, MGMT, MUC2, MYOD1, CDKN2B, CDKN1C, PGK1, PGR, RARB(RAR-β), RB1, and SYK*	[73]
	Plasma	*CCND2, SOCS1, THBS1, PLAU, and VHL*	[74]
Prostate	Plasma and urine	*GSTP1*	[75, 76]
	Plasma/serum, urine, and ejaculate	*GSTP1*	[77, 78]
	Serum	*GSTP1*	[79]
	Serum	*RASSF1, RARB2(RAR-β2), and GSTP1*	[80]
	Blood	*GSTP1, RASSF1A, APC, and RARB(RARβ)*	[81]
	Ejaculate	*GSTP1*	[82]
	Urine	*GSTP1*	[83, 84]
	Biopsy lavage fluid	*GSTP1*	[85]
Esophageal	Plasma	*APC*	[86]
	Serum	*CDKN2A (INK4A)*	[87]
Head and neck	Serum	*DAPK1, MGMT, and CDKN2A (INK4A)*	[88]
	Plasma	*DAPK1*	[89]
	Saliva	*DAPK1, MGMT, and CDKN2A (INK4A)*	[90]

directly. The noninvasive character of most of these enables the use of liquid biopsy in healthy persons to predict cancer risk; in pre- or less-symptomatic patients to detect early-stage cancer; pre-treatment patients to predict therapeutic efficacy; patients under treatments to test therapeutic effects; and post-treatment patients to detect cancer recurrence. Cancer cells and their microenvironment secrete cancer-specific small molecules, peptides, proteins, lipids, and nucleic acids into body fluids. DNA and histone modification-related molecules are no exception.

1.5 Nucleic Acids for Liquid Biopsy

Nucleic acids circulating in body fluids, including free, protein-bound and vesicle-contained nucleic acids (exosomes, microvesicles and apoptotic bodies *etc.*), are also potent biomarkers for cancer diagnosis. Circulating nucleic acids in plasma/serum were first reported in 1948 [93]. Circulating DNAs with oncogenic mutation, mutated *K-ras* gene and mutated *N-ras* gene, were found in 1994 and are the first convincing evidences of the existence of cancer-derived nucleic acids in body fluid [94, 95]. Cancer-related circulating RNAs were not discovered for another 5 years. Kopreski *et al.* detected tyrosinase mRNAs in the cell-free serum of a patients with malignant melanoma [96], while Lo *et al.* detected Epstein-Barr virus (EBV) coding RNAs from the plasma of patients with nasopharyngeal carcinoma [97].

Serum DNA reflects the DNA methylation status of cancer cells. Methylation of the *transmembrane protein containing epidermal growth factor and follistatin domains* (*TPEF*) gene locus was detected in peripheral blood from colorectal tumor patients [98]. Fujiwara *et al.* detected methylation of serum DNA derived from the promoter region of tumor suppressive genes such as *MGMT, p16^{INK4a}, RASSF1A, DAPK* and *RAR-β* from lung cancer patients [99]. Since promoter methylation leads to low promoter activity, serum DNA is expected to be a novel cancer diagnostic tool. DNA hypomethylation is not limited to specific tumor suppressive genes. Shotgun massively parallel bisulfite sequencing in 2013 revealed the cancer-type independent genome-wide hypomethylation of plasma DNA [100]. Genome-wide hypomethylation was observed in plasma DNA from hepatocellular carcinoma (HCC), breast cancer, lung cancer, nasopharyngeal cancer, smooth muscle sarcoma and neuroendocrine cancer patients. Analysis in 26 HCC patients versus 32 healthy subjects gave 81% sensitivity and 94% specificity for HCC detection.

Plasma RNA expression levels are also linked with the epigenetic status of cancer cells. Plasma EBV coding RNA is associated with epigenetic changes in host nasopharyngeal carcinoma cells [97]. EBV is a double stranded DNA (dsDNA) virus which causes mononucleosis and is also associated with wide range of cancers. EBV keeps its virus genome in the host cell as episomal circular dsDNA and silences its lytic genes by promoter CpG methylation [101]. EBV also modifies DNA methylation of host genome DNA and alters gene expression pattern of the host cell [102]. In EBV latency, promoter regions of host genomic DNA are also highly methylated. The tumor-suppressor gene promoters *CDH1, p14* and *p16* are densely methylated in EBV-associated gastric carcinoma [103–105].

Circulating noncoding RNA (ncRNA) such as microRNA (miRNA) and long ncRNA (lncRNA) is another potent epigenetic RNA biomarker for cancer diagnosis. miR-155 expression is regulated by miR-155 promoter methylation in cancers, including chronic lymphocyte leukemia (CLL) [106–110]. High expression of plasma miR-155 is a potent prognostic marker which predicts the response to chemotherapy and overall survival of CLL patients [111]. Plasma miR-155 is secreted within microvesicles derived from leukemia cells or platelets. Cellular miR-155 levels are elevated in early-stage CLL cells and involved in the transition of monoclonal B lymphocytosis (MBL) to CLL. The expression of cellular and plasma miR-155 levels may be regulated in the early stage of cancer progression and their DNA and histone methylation status are associated with miR-155 expression. The next section describes the aberrant expression of miRNA in cancer in detail.

Circulating lncRNAs are also detected in body fluids. In 2004, a lncRNA, *differential display code 3* ^{prostate cancer associated 3} (DD3^{PCA3}), was detected in the urine of patients with prostate cancer [112]. This discovery has lead to the challenge to find lncRNA biomarkers for cancer diagnosis. Numerous lncRNAs are associated with DNA and histone modifications. Conversely, lncRNA expression is often regulated by these epigenetic changes. Liquid biopsy lncRNA markers that reflect epigenetic changes are waiting to be discovered.

The mechanisms by which circulating nucleic acids are protected from degradation are still under investigation. Initially, the source of these nucleic acids was considered to be dead cancer cells and cancer-surrounding cells. It is natural to consider apoptotic bodies as stable sources of circulating nucleic acids [113]. In 2007, Valadi *et al.* reported that the transfer of circulating RNAs was mediated by exosomes, termed endosome-originated secreted vesicles [114]. This finding shed light on the nature of circulating nucleic acids as not only fragments of dead cells but also as intercellular communication tools. Circulating nucleic acids are potential biomarkers of the epigenetic status of the originating cells and might also reflect the condition of the recipient cells.

1.6 Other Epigenetic Markers for Liquid Biopsy

A number of examples of epigenetic-related protein markers for liquid biopsy in the diagnosis of cancer are available. Histone modifications within circulating nucleosomes are proposed as possible biomarkers [115, 116]. Histones make a complex with DNA to form a nucleosome. Histones within nucleosomes have N-terminal amino acid tails which are post-translationally methylated, acetylated and phosphorylated. These histone modifications change nucleosome folding into heterochromatin or euchromatin to control gene expressions coded in the chromatin region. Histone modifications such as H3K9me3 and H4K20me3 ratio changes are observed in many types of cancer cell. Nucleosomes with modified histones are secreted into and circulate in plasma/serum collected from colorectal cancer or breast cancer patients [115, 116].

Liquid biopsy test using plasma nucleic acids is already in clinical use. In June 2016, the US Food and Drug Administration (FDA) approved the first blood-based genetic liquid biopsy test for non-small cell lung cancer (NSCLC). The presence of a specific mutation in the *epidermal growth factor receptor* (*EGFR*) gene in plasma DNA indicates eligibility for erlotinib treatment. Although liquid biopsy techniques based on epigenetic changes are still in the developmental stage, the numerous studies to date, a few of which are introduced above, will enable their practical applications.

2 Aberrant Expression of microRNA in Cancer: Diagnosis of Liquid Biopsy

2.1 Biogenesis and Function of miRNA

MicroRNAs (miRNAs) are endogenous small non-coding RNAs which regulate target genes by degrading mRNA or repressing translation of mRNA. In 1993, the first functional small non-coding RNA, *lin-4*, was reported to regulate the development of *C. elegans* by repressing its target, *LIN-14* [117]. Since this discovery, many miRNAs have been identified. 35,828 mature miRNAs in 223 species, including *C. elegans*, mouse and human, are currently stored in miRNA database miRBase (Release 21; June 2014, http://www.mirbase.org), including 2585 mature human miRNAs. The sequences of miRNAs are well-conserved among various species in eukaryotes [118]. Moreover, several miRNAs are expressed in a tissue-specific manner: examples include miR-1 and miR-133, which are expressed in skeletal and cardiac muscle, and miR-122 and miR-124, which are expressed in liver and brain, respectively [119]. miRNAs have accordingly received attention as key effectors of biological processes.

MiRNAs are transcribed by RNA polymerase II as primary miRNAs (pri-miR-NAs), which are long form of transcripts. These are then cleaved by a microprocessor complex consisting of the RNase III enzyme Drosha and the double-strand RNA binding protein DGCR8 in the nucleus. This leads to the generation of precursor miRNAs (pre-miRNAs) of 60–70 nt in length. Pre-miRNAs are exported from the nucleus to the cytoplasm by Ran-GTP-dependent RNA binding protein Exportin-5, wherein the RNase III enzyme Dicer processes pre-miRNAs to approximately 22 nt double-strand mature miRNAs. The guide strand of mature miRNA is distinguished from the passenger strand, and selectively incorporated into the RNA-induced silencing complex (RISC) [120]. RISC specifically bind the 3′ untranslated region (3′ UTR) of target mRNA, resulting in the suppression of translation with or without the cleavage of target mRNA [121]. As many miRNAs bind partially complementary sequences on the target mRNAs, one miRNA could target multiple genes, and one mRNA could be targeted by several miRNAs [122]. Accordingly, miRNAs are thought to regulate various genes through concomitant translational suppression of multiple target genes; indeed, a study using an algorithm to predict miRNA targets reported the targeting of one-third of genes in the human genome [123, 124]. In addition, a recent study showed that miRNAs bind not only 3′ UTR but also 5′ UTR and CDS of target mRNAs [125, 126]. Thus, miRNA has more target genes than predicted. Thus, miRNAs appear to be involved in various biological processes, including development, differentiation and apoptosis [122], and the changes in miRNAs expression are thought to be associated with various diseases, such as cancer, diabetes, and neurological disorders.

2.2 Alteration of miRNA Expression in Cancers

In fact, aberrant miRNA expression has been revealed in human cancer. Calin demonstrated that miR-15 and miR-16, located at human chromosome 13q14, were deleted or down-regulated in B cell chronic lymphocytic leukemia. Moreover, both miRNAs exert tumor suppressor function by targeting genes associated with apoptosis and cell cycle [127]. Following this finding, abnormal expression profiles of miRNAs were shown in various cancer cell lines, in which one cluster of miRNAs, the miR-17-92 polycistron, was amplified and involved in tumorigenesis [128]. It was revealed that the expression level of miR-21 was elevated in glioblastoma tissues, and that knockdown of miR-21 triggered activation of caspases, leading to apoptosis [129]. In contrast, it was also reported that some miRNAs were decreased in cancer; for example, expression of let-7 was decreased in lung cancer, and over-expression of let-7 in lung cancer cells inhibited cancer cell proliferation [130]. In addition, several lines of evidence revealed that miR-34a was reduced in various cancers and that it had the ability to suppress cancer cell growth by inducing apoptosis or senescence [131–133]. Intriguingly, expression of miR-34a is activated directly by p53 tumor suppressor protein [134]. In this way, some miRNAs function as oncogenic genes and are up-regulated in cancer cells – these are called "OncomiRs" – whereas conversely, other miRNAs function as tumor suppressors and are down-regulated in cancer cells. These latter miRNAs are called "Tumor Suppressor miRNAs". These studies suggest that the aberrant expression of miRNA is associated with diseases, included cancer.

2.3 Epigenetic Regulation of miRNAs

As described above, abnormal expression of miRNAs is associated with cancer progression. What then is involved in the abnormal expression of miRNAs in cancer? As summarized in Table 2, aberrant expression of miRNAs is partly caused by a single nucleotide polymorphism (SNP) in miRNA sequence, copy number variation (CNV) and epigenetic change. Examples of the major causes are shown below.

2.3.1 Single Nucleotide Polymorphisms

A SNP is a variation in a single nucleotide, occurring at a specific position in the genome sequence among human beings, and generally associated with differences among individuals. Since they approximately occur once in every 300 nucleotides, they are also found in genomic regions which include miRNA genes, resulting in the aberrant expression of miRNAs. Polymorphisms in genomic sequences encoding pri-miRNAs might affect their secondary stem-loop structures and alter pri-miRNA stability, leading to changes in the efficiency of miRNA processing. SNP rs531564, a C/G polymorphism in the genomic sequence encoding pri-miR-124, affects its secondary structure and processing efficiency, and the expression level of the mature form of miR-124 is consequently upregulated [183]. In addition, SNPs in the promoter region of miRNA genes affect the transcriptional regulation of pri-miRNAs. Dysregulated miR-107 in gastric adenocarcinomas is caused by an SNP in the promoter region of miR-107 [155]. Moreover, SNPs in miRNA processing genes are associated with the efficiency of miRNA biogenesis [184]. These findings indicate that the SNPs occurring in miRNA genes affect not only their biogenesis but also their function.

Table 2 Epigenetic alteration of miRNA in cancers

Cancer types	miRNA	Epigenetic regulation	References
Glioblastoma	miR-214, miR-328 and miR-1224-3p	Promoter methylation	[135]
	miR-181c	Promoter methylation	[136]
	miR-200a/b and miR-429	Promoter methylation and H3K27 tri-methylation	[137]
	miR-142-3p	Promoter methylation	[138]
Head and neck	miR-10b	H3K79 mono-methylation	[139]
	miR-137 and miR-196a	Promoter methylation	[140, 141]
Breast	miR-181a/b, miR-200a/b/c and miR-203	H3K9 and H3K27 tri-methylation	[142]
	miR-200a/b/c	Promoter demethylation	[143]
	miR-205	SNP	[144]
	miR-125b-1	H3K9 and H3K27 tri-methylation	[145]
	miR-29c	Promoter methylation	[146]
	miR-146b	Promoter methylation	[147]
	miR-31	Promoter methylation	[148]
	miR-335a/b	CNV	[149]
Lung	miR-139	Histone methylation	[150]
	miR-205	SNP	[144]
	miR-373	Histone deacetylation	[151]
	miR-200b	Histone deacetylation	[152]
	let-7a-3	Promoter demethylation	[153]
Gastric	miR-30b-5p	Promoter methylation	[154]
	miR-107	SNP	[155]
	miR-23a, miR-27a, miR-24-2 and miR-181c/d	CNV	[156]
	miR-196b	Promoter demethylation	[157]
	miR-181c	Promoter methylation	[158]
Liver	miR-101	Histone methylation	[159]
	miR-148a	Promoter methylation	[160]
	miR-191	Promoter demethylation	[161]
Pancreatic	miR-132	Promoter methylation	[162]
	miR-124	Promoter methylation	[163]
	miR-615	Promoter methylation	[164]
	miR-506	Promoter methylation	[165]
Colorectal	miR-9, miR-129 and miR-137	Histone deacetylation	[166]
	miR-34b/c	Promoter methylation	[167]
	miR-612	SNP	[168]

(continued)

Table 2 (continued)

Cancer types	miRNA	Epigenetic regulation	References
Prostate	miR-181a/b, miR-200a/b/c and miR-203	Histone methylation	[142]
	miR-29a and miR-1256	Promoter methylation	[169]
	miR-612	SNP	[168]
	miR-205	Promoter methylation	[170]
	miR-31	H3K27 tri-methylation	[171]
Ovarian	let-7a-3	Promoter methylation	[172]
	miR-182, miR-103, miR-140, miR-184 and miR-15	CNV	[173]
	miR-337, miR-432, miR-495, miR-368, miR-376a/b, miR-337 and miR-419	Promoter methylation	[173]
	miR-29	Promoter methylation	[174]
Cervical	miR-432, miR-1286, miR-641, miR-1290, miR-1287 and miR-95	Promoter methylation	[175]
	miR-155	SNP	[176]
	miR-23b	Promoter methylation	[177]
Leukemia	miR-15 and miR-16	CNV	[127]
	miR-31	H3K9 and H3K27 tri-methylation	[178]
	miR-9-2, miR-124-2, miR-129-2, miR-551b and miR-708	Promoter methylation	[179]
	miR-21, miR-29a/b-1, miR-34a, miR-155, miR-574 and miR-1204	Promoter demethylation	[179]
	miR-203	Promoter methylation	[180]
Lymphoma	miR-17-92 cluster	CNV	[128]
	miR-29	Histone deacetylation and tri-methylation	[181]
	miR-155	Promoter demethylation	[182]

2.3.2 Copy Number Variation

CNV is an alteration in the copy number of a genomic region, wherein some regions are duplicated and others deleted. Alterations in the copy number of genomic regions which include miRNA genes is reported to affect expression levels of miR-NAs. When the genomic loci corresponding to 186 miRNAs were mapped on the human genome and compared with nonrandom genomic alterations, 52.5% of miRNA gene loci were associated with genomic regions altered in cancer, many of which were found to be located in the deleted regions in cancer cells and reduced in their expression levels in cancer samples [185]. For example, miR-15 and miR-16 are located at human chromosome 13q14, which is frequently deleted in B-CLL and associated with tumorigenesis, so that expression levels of miR-15 and miR-16 are down-regulated. In contrast, amplification of human chromosome 19p13.13, which includes loci of five miRNAs (miR-23a, miR-27a, miR-24-2, miR-181c and miR-181d), was observed in gastric cancer, and up-regulation of these miRNAs promoted their proliferation [156]. These findings suggest that aberrant expression of miRNA resulting from CNVs is closely associated with cancer progression.

2.3.3 Epigenetic Change

Aberrant expression of miRNAs is associated with alteration of epigenetic regulation, which also affect miRNAs. The best-known factors in epigenetic regulation are DNA and histone modifications. For example, the DNA methylation involved in gene silencing is associated with downregulation of miRNA expression in cancer cells. Hyper-methylation of CpG islands in the promoter region of let-7a-3 was identified in epithelial ovarian cancer, resulting in down-regulation of let-7a-3 [172]. Similarly, miR-137 and miR-193a located around these CpG islands were silenced by DNA hyper-methylation in oral cancer, and these miRNAs were identified as tumor suppressors [140]. On the other hand, expression levels of miRNAs were upregulated by hypomethylation of CpG islands in their promoter regions. Expression levels of miR-196a and miR-196b are relatively low in normal lung and stomach tissues, but highly expressed in non-small cell lung carcinoma and gastric cancer cell lines due to the lack of methylation in the promoter region. Moreover, hypomethylation in the promoter region of miR-196 was observed in gastric cancer [157].

DNA methylation is regulated by DNA methyltransferases (DNMTs) and Ten-eleven translocation methylcytosine dioxygenases (TETs). The MiR-29 family (miR-29a, 29b and 29c) is known to directly target both DNMT3A and DNMT3B. In lung cancer, down-regulation of miR-29s were observed, and DNMT3A/3B mRNA expression was accordingly upregulated [186]. Moreover, DNMT3A/3B was recently shown to suppress miR-29b expression through methylation of the CpG island in the promoter region. As a consequence, miR-29 and DNMT3A/3B reciprocally affect their expression levels [174]. In addition, miR-22 suppresses expression of the TET family, which is associated with DNA demethylation, resulting in downregulation of mir-200 through lack of demethylation of the promoter region of the mir-200 gene [143].

Histone modifications are another example of epigenetic regulation. These occur via acetylation, methylation, phosphorylation, etc. For instance, histone deacetylation promoted by HDAC downregulated expression levels of miR-9, miR-129 and miR-137. HDAC1 is suppressed by miR-449a, resulting in cell cycle arrest [166, 187]. In addition, histone deacetylation of the promoter region in the miR-29 gene was enhanced though binding of c-myc through a corepressor complex with HDAC3 and EZH2, resulting in silencing of miR-29 expression. Moreover, HDAC3 and EZH2 are regulated by miR-494 and miR-26a, respectively [181]. Together, these findings indicate that aberrant expression of miRNAs could alter DNA and histone modifications, leading to repression of miRNA expression, and that epigenetic regulation is deeply involved in the regulation of miRNA expression.

2.4 Detection of Aberrant miRNA Expression for Cancer Diagnosis

Expression profiles of miRNA are unique in each tissue, enabling the detection of a cancer's tissue of origin [188]. Moreover, expression profiles of miRNA reflect the developmental lineage and differentiation state in various cancer types, and expression levels of various miRNAs are globally down-regulated in tumors compared with normal tissues [189]. These findings indicate that aberrant expression profiles of miRNA are a biomarker for cancer detection. Furthermore, it was revealed that miRNAs exist not only inside but also outside cells in almost all body fluids containing serum, plasma or urine [190–192]. In the first study of the miRNA profile in serum, miR-21 level was higher in serum from patients with B-cell lymphoma than from healthy controls, and a high level of miR-21 was associated with relapse-free survival [190]. By contrast, miR-21 level is up-regulated in the activated B cell-like subtype of B-cell lymphoma [193]. These studies indicate that the miRNA profile in serum does not necessarily reflect the cellular profile of miRNA expression. Aberrant miRNA profiles in body fluids might therefore be biomarkers for the diagnosis, progression, prognosis, and prediction of therapeutics effects in several diseases, including cancer. As reviewed by Kosaka et al., various miRNAs, including miR-21, have been revealed as biomarkers for the early diagnosis for cancer [194]. Recent reports of miRNA profiles in body fluids are summarized in Table 3. Additionally, it has been noted that the combination of miRNA levels in serum would represent a more sensitive, specific and accurate biomarker for cancer diagnosis than the single miRNA level [237]. Non-invasive diagnosis using miRNA profiles in body fluids is therefore expected to find practical applications.

3 Association of Epigenetic Alterations in Telomeres with Expression of TERRA and Telomerase

3.1 Relationship Between Telomere Length and Epigenetic Modification

In eukaryotes, chromosome ends are composed of tandem repeat DNA sequences known as telomeres, which protect them from inappropriate DNA transactions. Telomeres have epigenetic marks of constitutive heterochromatin, and play a key role in chromosome stability (Fig. 1). In mammals, telomeric and subtelomeric chromatin abounds in trimethylated histone H3 lysine 9 (H3K9), trimethylated histone H4 lysine 20 (H4K20) and HP1 [238]. These histone modifications are known to require deacetylase and methyltransferases. SIRT 6 deacetylates H3K9, and SUV39-H1 and SUV39-H2 mediates trimethylation of H3K9 [239–241]. Consequently, trimethylated H3K9 interacts with HP1, contributing to chromatin

Table 3 Aberrant miRNA levels in body fluids of cancer patients

Cancer types	Body fluid	miRNA	References
Glioblastoma	Serum	miR-137	[195]
	Plasma	miR-211, miR-212	[196]
	Serum	miR-320, miR-574-3p	[197]
	Cerebrospinal fluid	miR-21	[198]
Head and neck	Saliva	miR-139-5p	[199]
	Saliva	miR-9, miR-134, miR-191	[200]
	Saliva	miR-31	[201]
Esophageal	Serum	miR-1246	[202]
	Plasma	miR-21, miR-375	[203]
Breast	Serum	miR-1246, miR-1307-3p, miR-4634, miR-6861-5p, miR-6875-5p	[204]
	Plasma	miR-145, miR-451	[205]
	Serum	miR-181a	[206]
Lung	Serum	miR-29c, miR-93, miR-429	[207]
	Serum	miR-15b, miR-27b	[208]
	Serum	miR-1254, miR-574-5p	[209]
Gastric	Plasma	miR-16, miR-25, miR-92a, miR-451, miR-486-5p	[210]
	Plasma	miR-199a-3p	[211]
	Serum	miR-378	[212]
	Plasma	miR-17-5p, miR-20a	[213]
Liver	Plasma	miR-483-5p	[214]
	Serum	miR-15b, miR-130b	[215]
	Serum	miR-885-5p	[216]
Pancreatic	Serum	miR-17-5p, miR-21	[217]
	Serum	miR-1290	[218]
	Serum	miR-20a, miR-21, miR-24, miR-25, miR-99a, miR-185, miR-191	[219]
Renal	Serum	miR-193a-3p, miR-362, miR-572, miR-28-5p, miR-378	[220]
	Serum	miR-378, miR-451	[221]
Colorectal	Serum	miR-19a	[222]
	Serum	let-7a, miR-1224-5p, miR-1229, miR-1246, miR-150, miR-21, miR-223, miR-23a	[223]
	Serum	miR-200c	[224]
	Plasma	miR-378	[225]
Bladder	Urine	miR-96	[226]
	Urinary sediment	miR-200a/b/c, miR-192, miR-155	[227]
Prostate	Serum	miR-375	[228]
	Plasma	let-7c/e, miR-30c, miR-622, miR-1285	[229]
Ovarian	Serum	miR-92	[230]

(continued)

Table 3 (continued)

Cancer types	Body fluid	miRNA	References
Cervical	Serum	miR-16-2, miR-195, miR-2861, miR-497	[231]
	Serum	miR-20a, miR-203	[232]
Leukemia	Serum	miR-150, miR-155, miR-1246	[233]
	Plasma	miR-150, miR-342	[234]
Lymphoma	Cerebrospinal fluid	miR-21, miR-19, miR-92a	[235]
	Plasma	miR-92a	[236]

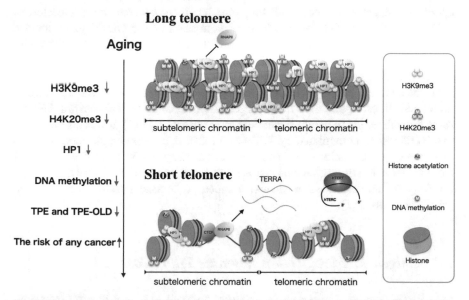

Fig. 1 Epigenetic alterations of telomeres with aging. In mammals, telomere regions are rich in heterochromatic marks, such as subtelomeric DNA hypermethylation, modified histones including H3K9me3 and H4K20me3, and HP1, which suppress TERRA expression, while telomeres regulate the expression of hTERT though the TPE-OLD mechanism. Not only do these heterochromatic marks decrease in telomeric and subtelomeric regions, but also the influence of TPE-OLD is attenuated, as the length of the telomere shortens with age. Consequently, telomeric and subtelomeric chromatin became "open" chromatin, and transcription of TERRA is increased. Therefore, the risk of any cancer, such as head and neck cancer and gastrointestinal tumors, increases as the telomeres get shorter

compaction [242]. In addition, the Rb family facilitates methylation of H4K20 by SUV4-20H1 and SUV4-20H2 [243]. Downregulation of SUV39H1 and SUV39H2, as well as Rb deficiency, are reported to cause abnormal telomere elongation [241, 243, 244]. Meanwhile, telomere shortening induces hypomethylation of subtelomeric DNA, leading to decreased binding of H3K9me3 and HP1 in the region [245]. These findings suggest that telomere length is epigenetically regulated by telomeric and subtelomeric histone and subtelomeric DNA modifications.

3.2   Telomere Length and Chromatin Modification Regulate Transcription of Genes Near and Far from Telomere

Telomeres have the ability to reversibly silence genes located near them. This phenomenon is called the telomere position effect (TPE) [246]. TPE depends on telomere length, distance from the telomere, and histone acetylation. A specific HDAC inhibitor, Tricostatin A, impaired TPE, while overexpression of human telomerase catalytic subunit gene hTERT enhanced TPE in HeLa cells [247]. Moreover, SIRT6-deficient cells induced hyper-acetylation of telomeric and subtelomeric H3K9 and resulted in gain of TPE [240]. These findings suggest the possibility that epigenetic status associated with telomere length modulates the expression of genes located near the telomere. In fact, expression of the DUX4 gene, located 25–60 kb from the telomere, increased in cells derived from patients with facio-scapulo-humeral-dystrophy (FSHD) with shortened telomeres; and in general, the range of TPE is possibly within 100 kb from the telomere [248]. Recently, however, the telomere position effect over long distance (TPE-OLD) was reported to affect gene transcription over much larger distances of up to 10 Mb from the telomere through telomere length-dependent loop formation [249]. It was also reported that hTERT gene is regulated by TPE-OLD [250]. Thus, epigenetic modifications of subtelomeric and telomeric regions affect gene expression located near and far from the telomere through mechanisms involved in TPE and TPE-OLD. Although not fully understood, these mechanisms appear to be associated with human diseases [248, 250, 251].

3.3   Epigenetic Modification Regulate Telomerase

Mammalian telomeres are composed of repetitive DNA sequence $5'$-(TTAGGG)-$3'_n$ and bound to a complex of six proteins, known as shelterin [252, 254]. The protein complex regulates telomere length homeostasis and protects telomeres from DNA damage repair processing at chromosome ends [253, 254]. Critically shortened telomeres or lack of shelterin complex induce DNA damage responses including activation of checkpoint kinases, accumulation of gamma H2AX and repair factors, resulting in growth arrest or apoptosis [255]. Telomeres of most normal somatic cells in humans are gradually shortened as cells divide, referred to as the end replication problem [256]. By contrast, the telomere lengths of human germinal stem cells as well as most cancer cells are maintained by telomerase, an enzyme responsible for extension of the ends of the chromosomes by *de novo* synthesis. Telomerase consists of protein subunits including human telomerase associated protein (hTEP1), human telomerase RNA (hTERC), hTERT, and other RNA-binding proteins. Since telomerase components excepting hTERT are constitutively expressed, and expression of hTERT is strictly limited in tissue stem cells in adults, dysregulation of hTERT expression is associated with cell immortalization and tumorigenesis.

Transcription of the hTERT gene is regulated by epigenetic modification, such as DNA and histone modifications [257, 258]. hTERT promoter in certain somatic cell species is unmethylated or hypomethylated [259, 260], but by contrast is methylated in many telomerase-positive cancer cells [261]. These paradoxical observations between the methylation status of the hTERT promoter and expression levels of hTERT are partially explained by CTCF, a transcriptional repressor which binds the unmethylated TERT promoter in normal cells but not in hTERT-positive cells, resulting in higher expression of hTERT in cancer cells than in normal cells, even though the hTERT promoter is methylated in cancer cells [262].

In addition, histone modifications were also reported to affect expression of hTERT. Treatment of normal cells with HDAC inhibitors induces expression of hTERT and telomerase activity [263, 264]. Conversely, in cancer cells, HDAC inhibitors inhibit hTERT expression and telomerase activity [265]. Moreover, a decrease in trimethylation levels of H3K9 and H4K20 in telomeric regions was observed in cancer cells [266], whereas telomeric regions in telomerase-positive cells were associated with methylated H3K4 and hyperacetylated H3 and H4 [267]. Accordingly, alterations in DNA and histone modifications are common in telomerase-positive cancers.

3.4 Alternative Lengthening of Telomeres

While most cancer cells, around 90%, are telomerase-positive, the remaining 10% are telomerase-negative. These have a unique telomere elongation mechanism which is independent of telomerase [268, 269]. These cells, called Alternative lengthening of telomeres (ALT) cells, maintain telomere length by homologous recombination between telomeric regions of sister chromosomes [270]. ALT cells are often found in cancer cells with a mesenchymal origin, such as neuroendocrine tumors, neuroblastomas, and pediatric glioblastomas [271–274]. In these cells, the ATRX gene, which is associated with chromatin remodeling, has a high probability of being mutated [275, 276]. In addition, hypomethylation of subtelomeric DNA has been observed in cells from ATRX patients [276]. Mutation in histone H3.3 chaperone DAXX gene has also been found in ALT cells [277, 278], and other factors activating the ALT pathway have been identified [271, 273, 274]. Furthermore, ATRX depletion did not activate the ALT pathway in epithelial or telomerase-positive cells, while suppression of ATRX expression induced activation of ALT pathway in fibroblasts. Moreover, overexpression ATRX was reported to suppress ALT phenotype in ALT cells [279]. These results suggest that mutation of ATRX plays a key although inadequate role in acquiring the ALT mechanism, and that cells with the ALT mechanism express ATRX [280]. However, it is unclear how these cells acquire the traits of the ALT mechanism, and further studies to the elucidate ALT mechanism are required.

3.5   Telomeric Repeat Containing RNA

ALT cells are known to exhibit higher expression of telomeric repeat-containing RNA (TERRA) than other normal and telomerase-positive cells [281, 282]. TERRA is long non-coding RNA (lncRNA) transcribed from sub-telomeric CpG islands toward chromosomal telomeric ends by RNAPII [283]. Deng and colleagues found that siRNA-mediated knockdown of CTCF decreased RNAPII binding to subtelomeric DNA, resulting in reduction of TERRA expression, and suggested that TERRA transcription required CTCF [284]. The 5' ends of TERRAs contain a 7-methylguanosine cap structure. Meanwhile, in only about 7% of TERRA, the 3' ends contain a poly (A) tail, which is unable to bind chromatin. Non-polyadenylated TERRA was found to have the ability to bind chromatin and contribute to HR [285]. Additionally, overexpression of hTERT in HeLa and HT1080 cells caused elongation of telomeres, from which longer TERRA was transcribed [286], suggesting that TERRA length depends on telomere length. In fact, TERRA length varies from 100 bases to 9 kb in mammals [285]. Since telomeres and subtelomeres in normal cells form heterochromatin with enriched heterochromatin markers such as H3K9me3 and H3K27me3, expression of genes located near telomeres was suppressed [247, 287]. Telomere shortening induces a decrease in methylated H3K9 and H3K27 and DNA methylation in CpG islands, leading to 'open' chromatin and upregulation of TERRA transcription [288].

In addition to epigenetic modification, TERRA expression is regulated through the cell cycle. Expression of TERRA increases during M/G1 phase and decreases during S/G2 phase [286, 288]. siRNA-mediated depletion of ATRX sustained the expression level of TERRA in G2 phase, implicating a role for ATRX in regulation of TERRA expression through the cell cycle [289]. Expression level of TERRA also changes in gametogenesis and is reported to increase during meiosis. Further, TERRA is colocalized with telomerase catalytic subunit and TRF2, a member of the shelterin complex, in prophase [290].

It is also known that TERRA binds and interacts with many factors. TERRA is associated with origin recognition complex (ORC) and is recruited at telomeres via the GAR domain of TRF2 [291]. TERRA directly binds LSD1, which catalyzes the removal of mono and dimethyl groups from H3K4 and H3K9, and mediates the interaction of LSD1 with MRE 11, which is required for telomere 3'overhang processing [292]. In addition, introduction of recombinant TERRA into telomerase-positive cells reduces the accessibility of telomerase to chromosomal ends [293]. On the other hand, hnRNPA1 binds TERRA and inhibits its function by suppressing telomerase accessibility [294]. Thus, it has become clear that TERRA plays key roles in telomere biology, and further studies will provide important new findings.

3.6 TERRA Associates with Epigenetic Modification

TERRA transcription is regulated by epigenetic modification. It has been reported that a correlation was found between the expression of TERRA and histone code preferentially modified with H3K4me3 and H3K27ac in the TERRA promoter [295]. Subtelomeric hypomethylation in human cells by depletion of the DNA methyltransferases DNMT1 and DNMT3b resulted in the elevated expression of TERRA and elongated telomere [296]. In addition to DNA modification, methylation of H3K4 mediated by the methyltransferase MLL was associated with TERRA transcription activity [297], and moreover, HDAC inhibitor induced upregulation of TERRA [285]. These results suggest that TERRA expression is regulated by epigenetic modification. On the other hand, it was shown that trimethylation of H3K9 bound by TERRA was reduced at telomeric chromatin when TERRA was knocked down [291]. Therefore, TERRA affects DNA and histone modification, although it is unknown how TERRA influences epigenetic status.

ALT cells commonly show high expression of TERRA, as do some normal mammalian cells [298]. Novakovic and colleagues reported that the promoter region of TERRA in human placenta is hypomethylated compared to other somatic cells and ALT cancer cells, and that telomere length in human placenta is longer than that in other somatic cells [299]. Furthermore, they suggested that the ALT mechanism is involved in maturation of the placenta [299]. In summary, because TERRA is closely associated with epigenetic status of telomeres, further accumulation of evidence will help us to understand the biology of TERRA and ALT.

3.7 Diagnosis for Prevention and Early Detection of Cancer

In general, since cancer therapy becomes more difficult as cancer progresses, early detection is extremely important for radical cure of cancer. Exosomes are known to be secreted into the blood from various cell species including cancer cells [300]. Recently, Wang and colleagues reported that a cell-free form of TERRA (cfTERRA) was secreted from cells through exosomes, and that cfTERRA levels were increased with telomere dysfunction induced by the expression of the dominant negative TRF2. Furthermore, cfTERRA-containing exosomes stimulated the expression of genes encoding inflammatory cytokines in peripheral blood mononuclear cells [301, 302]. These results suggest that cfTERRA-containing exosomes might be a promising biomarker for the early detection of cancers with telomere dysfunction.

In addition, because telomere shortening induces chromosomal instability as well as expression of hTERT and TERRA, shortened telomeres have been recognized as a risk factor of oncogenesis [303–305]. Recently, a meta-analysis of 51 papers with 23,379 cancer cases and 68,792 controls showed an association between telomere shortening and the increased risk of head and neck cancer and gastrointestinal tumor [306]. These reports suggest that monitoring of telomere length might be important for the prevention of cancer.

As described above, cancer cells are roughly classified as telomerase-positive cells and ALT cells [268, 269]. Anticancer drugs targeting telomerase are considered to be effective against telomerase-positive cells, and telomerase inhibitors is under development [307, 308]. On the other hand, it was recently reported that inhibitors of ATR checkpoint kinase, which plays a critical role in genomic integrity, selectively induced cell death in ALT cells [289].

The accumulating evidence and understanding of telomere biology associated with cancer diagnosis and therapy described above, including epigenetic alterations, liquid biopsies, and anticancer drugs, is expected to contribute to clinical application in the near future.

4 Disseminated Tumor Cells with Stem Cell Properties and Epigenetic Plasticity for Early Diagnosis of Cancer Metastasis and Recurrence

Cancer stem cells are profoundly implicated in resistance to chemotherapy and molecular target treatment, and cancer stem cell dormancy is a major cause of therapy resistance, metastasis, and recurrence. Although cancer metastasis is widely considered as a late event in cancer progression, recent findings suggest that cancer cells are disseminated throughout the body from epithelial precancerous lesions early in carcinogenesis [309]. Disseminated tumor cells (DTCs) dispersed throughout the body exhibit the plasticity required for metastasis, dormancy and recurrence, suggesting that DTCs have properties of cancer stem cells, which is mainly regulated by epigenetic mechanisms.

Epigenetic regulation of gene expression through information not encoded in DNA sequences themselves, such as DNA methylation, histone modification, and nucleosome positioning play pivotal roles as a program of developmental progression and generation of tissue-specific cell species. Epigenetic properties are inherited through mitosis, and are predisposed to be affected by environmental alteration and external stimuli. Thus, epigenetic plasticity allows adaptation to environmental change and epigenetic aberration, termed "Epimutation", and plays an important part in tumorigenesis [310]. The existence of DTCs not only predicts cancer metastasis and recurrence, but might also indicate a target for the development of new DTC-focused therapeutic strategies aimed at preventing metastasis or keeping DTCs in dormancy through revealing epigenetic alteration in DTCs.

4.1 Significance of Cancer Dormancy and Recurrence in Metastatic Disease

Patients with breast, colorectal, and prostate cancer can experience recurrence years after complete resection of a primary tumor [311–315]. Dormancy is deeply involved in cancer recurrence. In the case of breast cancer, patients have a disease latency of 10–15 years from primary diagnosis to recurrence in a distant organ, and despite complete resection of a primary tumor and tumor-free regional lymph nodes, 20–25% of patients potentially experience cancer recurrence in distant organ [315]. The border between dormancy and recurrence is the first 20–25 years after surgery, and recurrence hardly occurs after that [312]. Moreover, metastasis of melanoma cells in the dormant state mediated by organ transplantation from a donor to a recipient has been reported: the recipient of a lung transplant from a donor who had not experienced recurrence in the 32 years since resection of the primary melanoma lesion developed metastatic melanoma, suggesting that melanoma cells were in a dormant state via immune system activity in the donor for a significant period of time [316]. As cancer recurrence results in death in most cases, elucidation of the mechanism of relapse after prolonged dormancy is a most important task for the identification of new therapy targets and development of diagnostic methods.

4.2 Significance of Disseminated Tumor Cells in Cancer Dormancy and Recurrence

DTCs dispersed throughout the body from the primary lesion and occult in tissues, including bone marrow, are implicated in cancer dormancy and recurrence. Death in patients who had successful complete resection of a primary tumor seems to be caused by early metastasis which cannot be detected at primary diagnosis. DTCs are thought to be already dispersed throughout the body at primary surgery, most of which might be nonproliferated and in a dormant state [317]. According to an epidemiological study of 12,423 breast cancer patients, it is predicted that metastatic disease had already occurred in more than 80% of patients at primary diagnosis, and that metastasis was initiated more than 5 years before diagnosis [318]. These findings might enable us to identify patients before overt metastasis, who are predicted to die due to metastatic disease. Therapeutic strategies determined by tumor size and lymph node status only will result in misjudgment about whether to perform adjuvant therapy to prevent recurrence. Therefore, detection of occult metastasis in patients with early-stage cancer is important for prognosis after surgical resection and appropriate therapy selection. Furthermore, as DTCs exhibit resistance to known adjuvant therapy [319], in addition to developing detection methods for dormant cancer cells, revealing the molecular mechanisms of dormancy and recurrence would enable the development of adjuvant therapy targeting DTCs in the dormant state.

4.3   Characteristics of Disseminated Tumor Cells

Solid tumors have three possible routes for metastasis: invasion to adjacent organs from the primary lesion and subsequent proliferation, and the lymphatic and hematogenic pathways. Although metastasis through the two former pathways would be detectable by imaging and histopathological analyses, it is difficult to detect dissemination via the hematogenic pathway. Detection of DTCs or circulating tumor cells (CTCs) provides a clue to linking the primary lesion with distant metastasis. Highly sensitive immunocytochemical methods were developed to detect DTCs/ CTCs in the 1980s, and a study using bone aspirate revealed that DTCs were enriched in bone marrow, and that bone marrow played an important role as an organ sustaining DTCs [320]. Antibodies against intermediate filament protein cytokeratin or epithelial specific antigen EpCAM expressed on the cell surface are mainly used for detection of DTCs/CTCs derived from epithelial cancer tissue such as breast cancer [321], and studies using these antibodies indicated the profound association of epithelial cells in bone marrow with recurrence after surgical resection and poor prognosis [322]. Moreover, since postoperative adjuvant therapy with drugs targeting proliferating cells had little effect on cytokeratin-positive cells [319], cytokeratin-positive cells are thought to be DTCs which are disseminated early through the body from the primary lesion, and have the ability to sustain a dormant state by adapting to niches in tissues such as bone marrow. Additionally, as the early stage of hematogenic metastasis followed by transition to the dormant state through dissemination throughout the body is extremely efficient, the colonization ability of DTCs in distant organs is considered to determine the prognosis of metastatic disease.

As described below, DTCs might include cancer stem cells with phenotypic plasticity, which might contribute to cancer recurrence through adaptation and proliferation in microenvironmental niches in distant organs. Thus, detection and analysis of DTCs in a dormant state is a valuable strategy to preventing cancer recurrence by appropriate choice of adjuvant therapy. The presence of DTCs in bone marrow predicts recurrence and poor prognosis in pancreatic and prostate cancer, as well as in breast cancer [323, 324], and is also a critical factor in the selection of adjuvant therapy in these cancers. However, as invasive bone aspiration is not only burdensome on patients but needs skills in aseptic procedure and anesthesia, it is difficult to standardize bone aspirate testing in clinical practice. On the other hand, CTC testing by blood collection is simpler, repeatable, and imposes a lesser burden on the patient. In addition, since the detection of CTCs correlates with the presence of DTCs, and the proliferative ability of CTC is reported to be weak, as is that of DTCs [325], CTC testing is expected to be an alternative to DTC testing in the future [326].

4.4   Cancer Stem Cell Properties in Disseminated Tumor Cells

It is reported that CD44+ CD24/low cancer stem cells were enriched in cytokeratin-positive DTCs derived from patients with breast cancer [327]. An increase in the positive rate for cancer stem cell markers in CTCs correlated with stage of cancer progression, and expression of EMT (epithelial-mesenchymal transition) markers was induced in CTCs enriched with antibody against EpCAM [328, 329]. Given that chemotherapy resistance and sustained dormancy of DTCs/CTCs are common properties of cancer stem cells [330], DTCs/CTCs appear relevant to cancer stem cells.

Mutations in genes such as Ras, p53, and Idh which are observed in various cancers and are known to serve as drivers which not only promote cancer cell growth but also affect the epigenetic states of cancer cells, involving changes in expression of epigenetic modifier genes. Activated Ras oncogene is known to epigenetically suppress genes related to apoptosis induction and growth inhibition via chromatin modifiers such as polycomb and DNA methyltransferase [331]. By contrast, gain-of-function mutation in tumor suppressor p53 increased histone methylation and acetylation in a genome-wide manner through increased expression of epigenetic modifier genes required for stem cell self-renewal, including acetyltransferase [332]. Moreover, mutation in the metabolic enzyme gene Idh induced repressive histone methylation and contributed to differentiation resistance of gliomas [333]. These findings suggest the possibility that the well-known mechanism of tumorigenesis provokes aberration in epigenetic regulation, and play a crucial role in the acquisition of stem cell properties during tumorigenesis.

For example, alteration of epigenetic regulation due to driver mutations in oncogenes or tumor suppressor genes would provide cancer cells with cancer stem cell properties by epigenetically inducing pluripotency genes, such as Oct3/4, Sox2, and Nanog. Whereas these pluripotency genes are known to form a transcriptional network to sustain their undifferentiated state [334], and have an ability to provide somatic cells with stem cell properties by reprogramming them into an undifferentiated state [335], transient induced expression of reprogramming factors in vivo generated tumors in various tissues [336]. In this regard, highly attractive findings were more recently reported by Mu *et al.*, who showed that suppression of p53 and the function of Rb tumor suppressors in androgen-dependent prostate cancer cells lead to phenotypic conversion into androgen-independent prostate cancer cells though increased expression of Sox2 [337].

These pluripotency genes were also reported to be expressed in tumor tissues, including breast cancer, and to be associated with cancer progression, such as EMT [338–341]. Expression of Sox2 and Nanog in gliomas and germ cell tumors, respectively, undergo epigenetic regulation [342, 343]. Furthermore, these pluripotency genes induce epigenetic alterations in cancer cells and are involved in phenotypic plasticity [344–346]. Therefore, they likely play a pivotal role in the phenotypic plasticity possibly involved in the dormancy and recurrence in cancer stem cells. Moreover, epigenetic traits are inherited through cell division, but unlike genetic information, they exhibit flexibility in response to environmental change. Epigenetic alterations might therefore arise early in tumor development and be crucially involved in the extravasation of cancer cells from the primary lesion to blood vessels, and metastasis to and dormancy in distant organs, including bone marrow [347]. Thus, establishing a relationship of these cells with cancer stem cells would facilitate effective strategies in appropriate diagnosis and the choice of adjuvant therapy. A possible mechanism underlying how epigenetic alterations are involved in the acquisition of cancer stem cell properties is shown in Fig. 2.

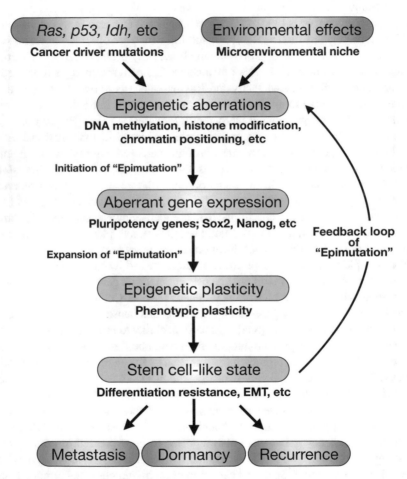

Fig. 2 Possible mechanism underlying how epigenetic alterations are involved in the acquisition of cancer stem cell properties. Cells harboring driver mutations in genes such as Ras, p53, and Idh are predisposed to alterations in epigenetic regulation mechanisms, including DNA methylation, histone modification, and chromatin positioning. Microenvironmental insults in the niche can also result in epigenetic aberrations. Initial "Epimutations" are initiated from this point, possibly leading to aberrant expression of pluripotency genes such as Sox2 and Nanog. Expression of pluripotency genes results in expansion of "Epimutations", providing the epigenetic and phenotypic plasticity involved in the stem cell-like state, including differentiation resistance and epithelial-to-mesenchymal transition (EMT). Cells acquiring epigenetic plasticity and a stem cell-like state probably form a feedback loop enhancing "Epimutations" toward the cancer stem cells implicated in metastasis, dormancy, and recurrence

4.5   Enrichment of Disseminated Tumor Cells

As DTCs in bone marrow and CTCs in the blood are distributed among millions of blood cells, an enrichment process in the detection and isolation of these cells is indispensable. Density gradient centrifugation is used as the first choice for simple enrichment of DTCs/CTCs from nucleated cells in the blood [325]. In addition, filtration by size differences between DTCs/CTCs and blood cells is used for higher enrichment [348–350]. The most widely used enrichment procedure is actually immunomagnetic separation, which effectively concentrates DTCs/CTCs using antibodies against cytokeratin or EpCAM [351, 352]. FACS [353], laser capture microdissection [354], and microfluidics [355, 356] are also used to isolate cells as single cells, and isolation of single DTCs/CTCs has been done by a method which first separates fluorescence-labeled cells by dielectrophoresis using cartridges developed by a combination of microfluidic and silicon-based biochip technologies, and then selects and isolates single cells with a fluorescence microscope and CMOS camera [357, 358].

4.6   Procedures for Epigenetic Analysis of DTCs/CTCs

Epigenetic properties inheritable though cell division are not encoded in DNA sequences themselves and are predisposed to modification by environmental changes and external stimuli. Thus, epigenetic plasticity enables cells to adapt to alterations in the environment, and aberration of epigenetic regulation, so-called "epimutation," has important roles in tumorigenesis [310]. The best-known inheritable substances in epigenetic regulation are DNA and histone modifications, and mechanisms based on accessible chromatin are also important epigenetic information. Accurate detection and measurement of epigenetic marks not only identify the epigenetic alterations associated with cancer, but will also help understanding of the mechanisms by which epimutations regulate processes in tumorigenesis, dormancy and metastasis as drivers. Evaluation methods are described below for DNA methylation, histone modification, and accessible chromatin in single cells. A flow diagram of single-cell epigenetic analysis, including the enrichment and isolation of DTCs/CTCs and epigenetic analysis procedure, is shown in Fig. 3.

4.6.1   DNA Methylation

The methylation status of cytosine residues in gene promoter regions, showing inverse correlation with activation state of the genes is major targets of epigenetic aberrations. When genomic DNA is treated with sodium bisulfite, non-methylated cytosine residues are deaminated into uracil, and 5-methylated

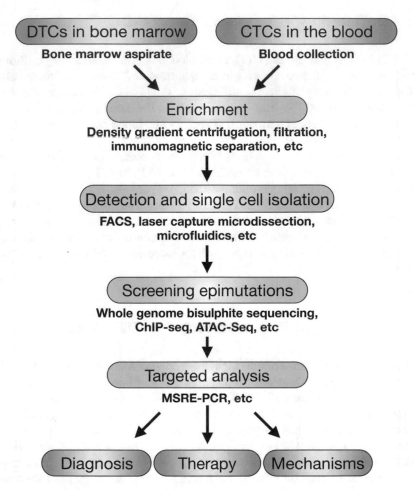

Fig. 3 Flow diagram of single-cell epigenetic analysis. Enrichment of DTCs/CTCs is an indispensable process for the detection and isolation of these cells. Density gradient centrifugation, filtration, and immunomagnetic separation are used in the enrichment process, followed by detection and single cell isolation using FACS, laser capture microdissection, and microfluidics. Isolated DTCs/CTCs are subjected to whole genome epigenetic analyses including whole genome bisulphite sequencing, ChIP-seq, and ATAC-Seq to identify "Epimutations" distinguishing cancer stem cells from other malignant cancer cells. These "Epimutations" are used as targets for DTC/CTC testing to determine diagnosis and therapeutic measures, and elucidate epigenetic mechanisms in cancer stem cell properties

cytosine residues remain intact [359]. The methylation status of each cytosine can be evaluated by whether or not it is converted to uracil with treatment. This method is the gold standard in DNA methylation analysis, and can be analyze in single nucleotide resolution across the whole genome. Although several whole-genome bisulfite sequencing methods of single cells have been recently reported

[360, 361], DNA degradation during bisulfite conversion is a hurdle in diagnosis requiring highly reliable data and a constant and stable analysis range. Comprehensive single cell bisulfite sequencing is therefore used for genome-wide screening of methylated sites as targets for diagnosis. In contrast, a method which combines methylation-sensitive restriction enzyme (MSRE) digestion and PCR is valuable for reliable analysis of DNA methylation status in the target sites of single cells [362, 363], and will be applicable to analysis of DNA methylation status in single DTCs/CTCs.

4.6.2 Histone Modification

Variation in cell species in multicellular organisms depends on the whole genome chromatin structure, which regulates the accessibility of transcriptional regulators to gene promoters and other regulatory elements, and consequently the gene expression profile [364]. Histone modification and nucleosome positioning play critical roles in chromatin organization, and mutations and aberrant expression of histone modifiers and chromatin remodeling factors are involved in cancer etiology [365]. ChIP-Seq, with a combination of chromatin immunoprecipitation and DNA sequencing, is widely used for genome-wide mapping of binding sites of modified histones, transcription factors, and other DNA-binding proteins [366], and is therefore an important tool for genome-wide elucidation of cell species-specific and transcriptionally active or silent epigenetic status through the mapping of overlapped sites among modified histone, transcription factors, and DNA-binding proteins [367]. Because epigenetic aberrations in chromatin organization are associated with phenotypic plasticity and heterogeneity of cancer cells, genome-wide mapping of these binding sites in single cells would provide important clues to understanding the epigenetic status of individual cancer cells. However, as a large amount of DNA is required as input material, the ChIP-Seq method has the disadvantage that data is obtained as an average value of the cell population, and is thus unsuitable for heterogeneity in individual single cells. Recently, the epigenetic heterogeneity of embryonic stem cells was successfully demonstrated by genome-wide mapping of methylated histones and transcription factor binding sites using single cell ChIP-Seq with combination of a cell sorting method based on microfluidics and indexing of chromatin fragments using barcode sequences [356]. Although the number of captured promoters and enhancers was about one thousand, if transcription factors defining cancer stem cells, such as Sox2 and/or Nanog, were employed by the targets, the existence of cancer stem cells would be identified in DTC/CTC populations.

4.6.3 Accessible Chromatin

Transcriptionally active regions on the genome are DNase I-sensitive, and DNase-Seq is a technique for identifying these accessible chromatin regions. In particular, analysis of genome-wide accessible chromatin regions in a variety of cell species or tissues has made it possible to efficiently identify regulatory sequences across a variety of cell species [368]. However, the standard DNase-Seq method involves in the order of 10^6–10^7 cells, and is therefore unsuitable for single cell analysis. Assay of transposase-accessible chromatin sequencing (ATAC-Seq) allows the detection of active chromatin regions sensitively and comprehensively by next-generation sequencing analysis of genomic libraries constructed by introducing adaptor sequences into open chromatin regions using Tn5 transposase in vitro [369]. More recently, diversity in accessible chromatin among different cell species was reported by analysis of individual single cells captured by applying microfluidics and using single-cell ATAC-Seq with barcode sequences [370]. Matching of data obtained from single-cell ATAC-Seq with a database of ChIP-seq and binding motifs for transcription factors allows us to speculate on what transcription factors bind to accessible chromatin. Although promoter elements accounted for fewer than 10% of accessible chromatin regions by ATAC-Seq [370], the existence of cancer stem cells would be identified as single DTCs/CTCs by matching with ChIP-seq data of transcription factors defining cancer stem cells.

In single cell analysis, separation and isolation of individual cells is indispensable before the epigenetic analysis procedure. Although not described here, the advantages of microfluidics are its automation of high-throughput experiments and reduction in the amount of samples and reagents required for single cell analysis [371]. Moreover, as microfluidics integrate the processes of cell separation and isolation with experiments such as enzymatic reaction and quantitative detection into one device, this technology will increasingly develop in the epigenetics and single cell analysis fields [372].

References

1. Jones PA (2012) Functions of DNA methylation: islands, start sites, gene bodies and beyond. Nat Rev Genet 13(7):484–492. doi:10.1038/nrg3230
2. Greger V, Passarge E, Hopping W, Messmer E, Horsthemke B (1989) Epigenetic changes may contribute to the formation and spontaneous regression of retinoblastoma. Hum Genet 83(2):155–158
3. Sakai T, Toguchida J, Ohtani N, Yandell DW, Rapaport JM, Dryja TP (1991) Allele-specific hypermethylation of the retinoblastoma tumor-suppressor gene. Am J Hum Genet 48(5):880–888
4. Friend SH, Bernards R, Rogelj S, Weinberg RA, Rapaport JM, Albert DM, Dryja TP (1986) A human DNA segment with properties of the gene that predisposes to retinoblastoma and osteosarcoma. Nature 323(6089):643–646. doi:10.1038/323643a0
5. Knudson AG Jr (1971) Mutation and cancer: statistical study of retinoblastoma. Proc Natl Acad Sci U S A 68(4):820–823

6. Benedict WF, Murphree AL, Banerjee A, Spina CA, Sparkes MC, Sparkes RS (1983) Patient with 13 chromosome deletion: evidence that the retinoblastoma gene is a recessive cancer gene. Science 219(4587):973–975

7. Ohtani-Fujita N, Fujita T, Aoike A, Osifchin NE, Robbins PD, Sakai T (1993) CpG methylation inactivates the promoter activity of the human retinoblastoma tumor-suppressor gene. Oncogene 8(4):1063–1067

8. Gonzalez-Zulueta M, Bender CM, Yang AS, Nguyen T, Beart RW, Van Tornout JM, Jones PA (1995) Methylation of the 5′ CpG island of the p16/CDKN2 tumor suppressor gene in normal and transformed human tissues correlates with gene silencing. Cancer Res 55(20):4531–4535

9. Merlo A, Herman JG, Mao L, Lee DJ, Gabrielson E, Burger PC, Baylin SB, Sidransky D (1995) 5′ CpG island methylation is associated with transcriptional silencing of the tumour suppressor p16/CDKN2/MTS1 in human cancers. Nat Med 1(7):686–692

10. Ruas M, Peters G (1998) The p16INK4a/CDKN2A tumor suppressor and its relatives. Biochim Biophys Acta 1378(2):F115–F177

11. Serrano M, Lee H, Chin L, Cordon-Cardo C, Beach D, DePinho RA (1996) Role of the INK4a locus in tumor suppression and cell mortality. Cell 85(1):27–37

12. Serrano M, Lin AW, McCurrach ME, Beach D, Lowe SW (1997) Oncogenic ras provokes premature cell senescence associated with accumulation of p53 and p16INK4a. Cell 88(5):593–602

13. West RW, Barrett JC (1993) Inactivation of a tumor suppressor function in immortal Syrian hamster cells by N-methyl-N′-nitro-N-nitrosoguanidine and by 5-aza-2′-deoxycytidine. Carcinogenesis 14(2):285–289

14. Rhee I, Bachman KE, Park BH, Jair KW, Yen RW, Schuebel KE, Cui H, Feinberg AP, Lengauer C, Kinzler KW, Baylin SB, Vogelstein B (2002) DNMT1 and DNMT3b cooperate to silence genes in human cancer cells. Nature 416(6880):552–556. doi:10.1038/416552a

15. Robert MF, Morin S, Beaulieu N, Gauthier F, Chute IC, Barsalou A, MacLeod AR (2003) DNMT1 is required to maintain CpG methylation and aberrant gene silencing in human cancer cells. Nat Genet 33(1):61–65. doi:10.1038/ng1068

16. Dawson MA, Kouzarides T (2012) Cancer epigenetics: from mechanism to therapy. Cell 150(1):12–27. doi:10.1016/j.cell.2012.06.013

17. Ohm JE, McGarvey KM, Yu X, Cheng L, Schuebel KE, Cope L, Mohammad HP, Chen W, Daniel VC, Yu W, Berman DM, Jenuwein T, Pruitt K, Sharkis SJ, Watkins DN, Herman JG, Baylin SB (2007) A stem cell-like chromatin pattern may predispose tumor suppressor genes to DNA hypermethylation and heritable silencing. Nat Genet 39(2):237–242. doi:10.1038/ng1972

18. Easwaran H, Johnstone SE, Van Neste L, Ohm J, Mosbruger T, Wang Q, Aryee MJ, Joyce P, Ahuja N, Weisenberger D, Collisson E, Zhu J, Yegnasubramanian S, Matsui W, Baylin SB (2012) A DNA hypermethylation module for the stem/progenitor cell signature of cancer. Genome Res 22(5):837–849. doi:10.1101/gr.131169.111

19. Nguyen CT, Weisenberger DJ, Velicescu M, Gonzales FA, Lin JC, Liang G, Jones PA (2002) Histone H3-lysine 9 methylation is associated with aberrant gene silencing in cancer cells and is rapidly reversed by 5-aza-2′-deoxycytidine. Cancer Res 62(22):6456–6461

20. Bachman KE, Park BH, Rhee I, Rajagopalan H, Herman JG, Baylin SB, Kinzler KW, Vogelstein B (2003) Histone modifications and silencing prior to DNA methylation of a tumor suppressor gene. Cancer Cell 3(1):89–95

21. Bracken AP, Kleine-Kohlbrecher D, Dietrich N, Pasini D, Gargiulo G, Beekman C, Theilgaard-Monch K, Minucci S, Porse BT, Marine JC, Hansen KH, Helin K (2007) The Polycomb group proteins bind throughout the INK4A-ARF locus and are disassociated in senescent cells. Genes Dev 21(5):525–530. doi:10.1101/gad.415507

22. Agger K, Cloos PA, Rudkjaer L, Williams K, Andersen G, Christensen J, Helin K (2009) The H3K27me3 demethylase JMJD3 contributes to the activation of the INK4A-ARF locus in response to oncogene- and stress-induced senescence. Genes Dev 23(10):1171–1176. doi:10.1101/gad.510809

23. Barradas M, Anderton E, Acosta JC, Li S, Banito A, Rodriguez-Niedenfuhr M, Maertens G, Banck M, Zhou MM, Walsh MJ, Peters G, Gil J (2009) Histone demethylase JMJD3 contributes to epigenetic control of INK4a/ARF by oncogenic RAS. Genes Dev 23(10):1177–1182. doi:10.1101/gad.511109

24. Schlesinger Y, Straussman R, Keshet I, Farkash S, Hecht M, Zimmerman J, Eden E, Yakhini Z, Ben-Shushan E, Reubinoff BE, Bergman Y, Simon I, Cedar H (2007) Polycomb-mediated methylation on Lys27 of histone H3 pre-marks genes for de novo methylation in cancer. Nat Genet 39(2):232–236. doi:10.1038/ng1950

25. Heyn H, Esteller M (2012) DNA methylation profiling in the clinic: applications and challenges. Nat Rev Genet 13(10).679–692. doi:10.1038/nrg3270

26. Esteller M (2008) Epigenetics in cancer. N Engl J Med 358(11):1148–1159. doi:10.1056/NEJMra072067

27. Esteller M, Corn PG, Baylin SB, Herman JG (2001) A gene hypermethylation profile of human cancer. Cancer Res 61(8):3225–3229

28. Ushijima T, Asada K (2010) Aberrant DNA methylation in contrast with mutations. Cancer Sci 101(2):300–305. doi:10.1111/j.1349-7006.2009.01434.x

29. Li M, Chen WD, Papadopoulos N, Goodman SN, Bjerregaard NC, Laurberg S, Levin B, Juhl H, Arber N, Moinova H, Durkee K, Schmidt K, He Y, Diehl F, Velculescu VE, Zhou S, Diaz LA Jr, Kinzler KW, Markowitz SD, Vogelstein B (2009) Sensitive digital quantification of DNA methylation in clinical samples. Nat Biotechnol 27(9):858–863. doi:10.1038/nbt.1559

30. Ned RM, Melillo S, Marrone M (2011) Fecal DNA testing for colorectal cancer screening: the ColoSure test. PLoS Curr 3:RRN1220. doi:10.1371/currents.RRN1220

31. Dominguez G, Carballido J, Silva J, Silva JM, Garcia JM, Menendez J, Provencio M, Espana P, Bonilla F (2002) p14ARF promoter hypermethylation in plasma DNA as an indicator of disease recurrence in bladder cancer patients. Clin Cancer Res 8(4):980–985

32. Valenzuela MT, Galisteo R, Zuluaga A, Villalobos M, Nunez MI, Oliver FJ, Ruiz de Almodovar JM (2002) Assessing the use of p16(INK4a) promoter gene methylation in serum for detection of bladder cancer. Eur Urol 42 (6):622–628; discussion 628-630

33. Chan MW, Chan LW, Tang NL, Tong JH, Lo KW, Lee TL, Cheung HY, Wong WS, Chan PS, Lai FM, To KF (2002) Hypermethylation of multiple genes in tumor tissues and voided urine in urinary bladder cancer patients. Clin Cancer Res 8(2):464–470

34. Silva JM, Dominguez G, Garcia JM, Gonzalez R, Villanueva MJ, Navarro F, Provencio M, San Martin S, Espana P, Bonilla F (1999) Presence of tumor DNA in plasma of breast cancer patients: clinicopathological correlations. Cancer Res 59(13):3251–3256

35. Silva JM, Dominguez G, Villanueva MJ, Gonzalez R, Garcia JM, Corbacho C, Provencio M, Espana P, Bonilla F (1999) Aberrant DNA methylation of the p16INK4a gene in plasma DNA of breast cancer patients. Br J Cancer 80(8):1262–1264. doi:10.1038/sj.bjc.6690495

36. Fiegl H, Millinger S, Mueller-Holzner E, Marth C, Ensinger C, Berger A, Klocker H, Goebel G, Widschwendter M (2005) Circulating tumor-specific DNA: a marker for monitoring efficacy of adjuvant therapy in cancer patients. Cancer Res 65(4):1141–1145. doi:10.1158/0008-5472.CAN-04-2438

37. Rykova EY, Laktionov PP, Skvortsova TE, Starikov AV, Kuznetsova NP, Vlassov VV (2004) Extracellular DNA in breast cancer: cell-surface-bound, tumor-derived extracellular DNA in blood of patients with breast cancer and nonmalignant tumors. Ann N Y Acad Sci 1022:217–220. doi:10.1196/annals.1318.033

38. Sharma G, Mirza S, Parshad R, Srivastava A, Datta Gupta S, Pandya P, Ralhan R (2010) CpG hypomethylation of MDR1 gene in tumor and serum of invasive ductal breast carcinoma patients. Clin Biochem 43(4–5):373–379. doi:10.1016/j.clinbiochem.2009.10.009

39. Sharma G, Mirza S, Parshad R, Srivastava A, Gupta SD, Pandya P, Ralhan R (2010) Clinical significance of promoter hypermethylation of DNA repair genes in tumor and serum DNA in invasive ductal breast carcinoma patients. Life Sci 87(3–4):83–91. doi:10.1016/j.lfs.2010.05.001

40. Skvortsova TE, Rykova EY, Tamkovich SN, Bryzgunova OE, Starikov AV, Kuznetsova NP, Vlassov VV, Laktionov PP (2006) Cell-free and cell-bound circulating DNA in breast tumours: DNA quantification and analysis of tumour-related gene methylation. Br J Cancer 94(10):1492–1495. doi:10.1038/sj.bjc.6603117

41. Evron E, Dooley WC, Umbricht CB, Rosenthal D, Sacchi N, Gabrielson E, Soito AB, Hung DT, Ljung B, Davidson NE, Sukumar S (2001) Detection of breast cancer cells in ductal lavage fluid by methylation-specific PCR. Lancet 357(9265):1335–1336

42. Ren CC, Miao XH, Yang B, Zhao L, Sun R, Song WQ (2006) Methylation status of the fragile histidine triad and E-cadherin genes in plasma of cervical cancer patients. Int J Gynecol Cancer 16(5):1862–1867. doi:10.1111/j.1525-1438.2006.00669.x

43. Widschwendter A, Muller HM, Fiegl H, Ivarsson L, Wiedemair A, Muller-Holzner E, Goebel G, Marth C, Widschwendter M (2004) DNA methylation in serum and tumors of cervical cancer patients. Clin Cancer Res 10(2):565–571

44. deVos T, Tetzner R, Model F, Weiss G, Schuster M, Distler J, Steiger KV, Grutzmann R, Pilarsky C, Habermann JK, Fleshner PR, Oubre BM, Day R, Sledziewski AZ, Lofton-Day C (2009) Circulating methylated SEPT9 DNA in plasma is a biomarker for colorectal cancer. Clin Chem 55(7):1337–1346. doi:10.1373/clinchem.2008.115808

45. Grutzmann R, Molnar B, Pilarsky C, Habermann JK, Schlag PM, Saeger HD, Miehlke S, Stolz T, Model F, Roblick UJ, Bruch HP, Koch R, Liebenberg V, Devos T, Song X, Day RH, Sledziewski AZ, Lofton-Day C (2008) Sensitive detection of colorectal cancer in peripheral blood by septin 9 DNA methylation assay. PLoS One 3(11):e3759. doi:10.1371/journal.pone.0003759

46. Lecomte T, Berger A, Zinzindohoue F, Micard S, Landi B, Blons H, Beaune P, Cugnenc PH, Laurent-Puig P (2002) Detection of free-circulating tumor-associated DNA in plasma of colorectal cancer patients and its association with prognosis. Int J Cancer 100(5):542–548. doi:10.1002/ijc.10526

47. Zou HZ, Yu BM, Wang ZW, Sun JY, Cang H, Gao F, Li DH, Zhao R, Feng GG, Yi J (2002) Detection of aberrant p16 methylation in the serum of colorectal cancer patients. Clin Cancer Res 8(1):188–191

48. Nakayama H, Hibi K, Taguchi M, Takase T, Yamazaki T, Kasai Y, Ito K, Akiyama S, Nakao A (2002) Molecular detection of p16 promoter methylation in the serum of colorectal cancer patients. Cancer Lett 188(1–2):115–119

49. He Q, Chen HY, Bai EQ, Luo YX, Fu RJ, He YS, Jiang J, Wang HQ (2010) Development of a multiplex MethyLight assay for the detection of multigene methylation in human colorectal cancer. Cancer Genet Cytogenet 202(1):1–10. doi:10.1016/j.cancergencyto.2010.05.018

50. Grady WM, Rajput A, Lutterbaugh JD, Markowitz SD (2001) Detection of aberrantly methylated hMLH1 promoter DNA in the serum of patients with microsatellite unstable colon cancer. Cancer Res 61(3):900–902

51. Chan KC, Lai PB, Mok TS, Chan HL, Ding C, Yeung SW, Lo YM (2008) Quantitative analysis of circulating methylated DNA as a biomarker for hepatocellular carcinoma. Clin Chem 54(9):1528–1536. doi:10.1373/clinchem.2008.104653

52. Wong IH, Lo YM, Yeo W, Lau WY, Johnson PJ (2000) Frequent p15 promoter methylation in tumor and peripheral blood from hepatocellular carcinoma patients. Clin Cancer Res 6(9):3516–3521

53. Wang J, Qin Y, Li B, Sun Z, Yang B (2006) Detection of aberrant promoter methylation of GSTP1 in the tumor and serum of Chinese human primary hepatocellular carcinoma patients. Clin Biochem 39(4):344–348. doi:10.1016/j.clinbiochem.2006.01.008

54. Wong IH, Lo YM, Zhang J, Liew CT, Ng MH, Wong N, Lai PB, Lau WY, Hjelm NM, Johnson PJ (1999) Detection of aberrant p16 methylation in the plasma and serum of liver cancer patients. Cancer Res 59(1):71–73

55. An Q, Liu Y, Gao Y, Huang J, Fong X, Li L, Zhang D, Cheng S (2002) Detection of p16 hypermethylation in circulating plasma DNA of non-small cell lung cancer patients. Cancer Lett 188(1–2):109–114

56. Bearzatto A, Conte D, Frattini M, Zaffaroni N, Andriani F, Balestra D, Tavecchio L, Daidone MG, Sozzi G (2002) p16(INK4A) Hypermethylation detected by fluorescent methylation-specific PCR in plasmas from non-small cell lung cancer. Clin Cancer Res 8(12):3782–3787

57. Ng CS, Zhang J, Wan S, Lee TW, Arifi AA, Mok T, Lo DY, Yim AP (2002) Tumor p16M is a possible marker of advanced stage in non-small cell lung cancer. J Surg Oncol 79(2):101–106

58. Kurakawa E, Shimamoto T, Utsumi K, Hirano T, Kato H, Ohyashiki K (2001) Hypermethylation of p16(INK4a) and p15(INK4b) genes in non-small cell lung cancer. Int J Oncol 19(2):277–281

59. Liu Y, An Q, Li L, Zhang D, Huang J, Feng X, Cheng S, Gao Y (2003) Hypermethylation of p16INK4a in Chinese lung cancer patients: biological and clinical implications. Carcinogenesis 24(12):1897–1901. doi:10.1093/carcin/bgg169

60. Ramirez JL, Rosell R, Taron M, Sanchez-Ronco M, Alberola V, de Las PR, Sanchez JM, Moran T, Camps C, Massuti B, Sanchez JJ, Salazar F, Catot S, Spanish Lung Cancer G (2005) 14-3-3sigma methylation in pretreatment serum circulating DNA of cisplatin-plus-gem-citabine-treated advanced non-small-cell lung cancer patients predicts survival: the Spanish Lung Cancer Group. J Clin Oncol 23(36):9105–9112. doi:10.1200/JCO.2005.02.2905

61. Esteller M, Sanchez-Cespedes M, Rosell R, Sidransky D, Baylin SB, Herman JG (1999) Detection of aberrant promoter hypermethylation of tumor suppressor genes in serum DNA from non-small cell lung cancer patients. Cancer Res 59(1):67–70

62. Usadel H, Brabender J, Danenberg KD, Jeronimo C, Harden S, Engles J, Danenberg PV, Yang S, Sidransky D (2002) Quantitative adenomatous polyposis coli promoter methylation analysis in tumor tissue, serum, and plasma DNA of patients with lung cancer. Cancer Res 62(2):371–375

63. Belinsky SA, Nikula KJ, Palmisano WA, Michels R, Saccomanno G, Gabrielson E, Baylin SB, Herman JG (1998) Aberrant methylation of p16(INK4a) is an early event in lung cancer and a potential biomarker for early diagnosis. Proc Natl Acad Sci U S A 95(20):11891–11896

64. Kersting M, Friedl C, Kraus A, Behn M, Pankow W, Schuermann M (2000) Differential frequencies of p16(INK4a) promoter hypermethylation, p53 mutation, and K-ras mutation in exfoliative material mark the development of lung cancer in symptomatic chronic smokers. J Clin Oncol 18(18):3221–3229. doi:10.1200/JCO.2000.18.18.3221

65. Ahrendt SA, Chow JT, Xu LH, Yang SC, Eisenberger CF, Esteller M, Herman JG, Wu L, Decker PA, Jen J, Sidransky D (1999) Molecular detection of tumor cells in bronchoalveolar lavage fluid from patients with early stage lung cancer. J Natl Cancer Inst 91(4):332–339

66. Palmisano WA, Divine KK, Saccomanno G, Gilliland FD, Baylin SB, Herman JG, Belinsky SA (2000) Predicting lung cancer by detecting aberrant promoter methylation in sputum. Cancer Res 60(21):5954–5958

67. Belinsky SA, Palmisano WA, Gilliland FD, Crooks LA, Divine KK, Winters SA, Grimes MJ, Harms HJ, Tellez CS, Smith TM, Moots PP, Lechner JF, Stidley CA, Crowell RE (2002) Aberrant promoter methylation in bronchial epithelium and sputum from current and former smokers. Cancer Res 62(8):2370–2377

68. Deligezer U, Yaman F, Erten N, Dalay N (2003) Frequent copresence of methylated DNA and fragmented nucleosomal DNA in plasma of lymphoma patients. Clin Chim Acta 335(1–2):89–94

69. Koyanagi K, Mori T, O'Day SJ, Martinez SR, Wang HJ, Hoon DS (2006) Association of circulating tumor cells with serum tumor-related methylated DNA in peripheral blood of melanoma patients. Cancer Res 66(12):6111–6117. doi:10.1158/0008-5472.CAN-05-4198

70. Mori T, O'Day SJ, Umetani N, Martinez SR, Kitago M, Koyanagi K, Kuo C, Takeshima TL, Milford R, Wang HJ, Vu VD, Nguyen SL, Hoon DS (2005) Predictive utility of circulating methylated DNA in serum of melanoma patients receiving biochemotherapy. J Clin Oncol 23(36):9351–9358. doi:10.1200/JCO.2005.02.9876

71. Melnikov A, Scholtens D, Godwin A, Levenson V (2009) Differential methylation profile of ovarian cancer in tissues and plasma. J Mol Diagn 11(1):60–65. doi:10.2353/jmoldx.2009.080072

72. Muller HM, Millinger S, Fiegl H, Goebel G, Ivarsson L, Widschwendter A, Muller-Holzner E, Marth C, Widschwendter M (2004) Analysis of methylated genes in peritoneal fluids of ovarian cancer patients: a new prognostic tool. Clin Chem 50(11):2171–2173. doi:10.1373/clinchem.2004.034090

73. Liggett T, Melnikov A, Yi QL, Replogle C, Brand R, Kaul K, Talamonti M, Abrams RA, Levenson V (2010) Differential methylation of cell-free circulating DNA among patients with pancreatic cancer versus chronic pancreatitis. Cancer 116(7):1674–1680. doi:10.1002/cncr.24893

74. Melnikov AA, Scholtens D, Talamonti MS, Bentrem DJ, Levenson VV (2009) Methylation profile of circulating plasma DNA in patients with pancreatic cancer. J Surg Oncol 99(2):119–122. doi:10.1002/jso.21208

75. Bryzgunova OE, Morozkin ES, Yarmoschuk SV, Vlassov VV, Laktionov PP (2008) Methylation-specific sequencing of GSTP1 gene promoter in circulating/extracellular DNA from blood and urine of healthy donors and prostate cancer patients. Ann N Y Acad Sci 1137:222–225. doi:10.1196/annals.1448.039

76. Jeronimo C, Usadel H, Henrique R, Silva C, Oliveira J, Lopes C, Sidransky D (2002) Quantitative GSTP1 hypermethylation in bodily fluids of patients with prostate cancer. Urology 60(6):1131–1135

77. Goessl C, Muller M, Heicappell R, Krause H, Miller K (2001) DNA-based detection of prostate cancer in blood, urine, and ejaculates. Ann N Y Acad Sci 945:51–58

78. Goessl C, Krause H, Muller M, Heicappell R, Schrader M, Sachsinger J, Miller K (2000) Fluorescent methylation-specific polymerase chain reaction for DNA-based detection of prostate cancer in bodily fluids. Cancer Res 60(21):5941–5945

79. Bastian PJ, Palapattu GS, Lin X, Yegnasubramanian S, Mangold LA, Trock B, Eisenberger MA, Partin AW, Nelson WG (2005) Preoperative serum DNA GSTP1 CpG island hypermethylation and the risk of early prostate-specific antigen recurrence following radical prostatectomy. Clin Cancer Res 11(11):4037–4043. doi:10.1158/1078-0432.CCR-04-2446

80. Sunami E, Shinozaki M, Higano CS, Wollman R, Dorff TB, Tucker SJ, Martinez SR, Mizuno R, Singer FR, Hoon DS (2009) Multimarker circulating DNA assay for assessing blood of prostate cancer patients. Clin Chem 55(3):559–567. doi:10.1373/clinchem.2008.108498

81. Roupret M, Hupertan V, Catto JW, Yates DR, Rehman I, Proctor LM, Phillips J, Meuth M, Cussenot O, Hamdy FC (2008) Promoter hypermethylation in circulating blood cells identifies prostate cancer progression. Int J Cancer 122(4):952–956. doi:10.1002/ijc.23196

82. Suh CI, Shanafelt T, May DJ, Shroyer KR, Bobak JB, Crawford ED, Miller GJ, Markham N, Glode LM (2000) Comparison of telomerase activity and GSTP1 promoter methylation in ejaculate as potential screening tests for prostate cancer. Mol Cell Probes 14(4):211–217. doi:10.1006/mcpr.2000.0307

83. Cairns P, Esteller M, Herman JG, Schoenberg M, Jeronimo C, Sanchez-Cespedes M, Chow NH, Grasso M, Wu L, Westra WB, Sidransky D (2001) Molecular detection of prostate cancer in urine by GSTP1 hypermethylation. Clin Cancer Res 7(9):2727–2730

84. Goessl C, Muller M, Heicappell R, Krause H, Straub B, Schrader M, Miller K (2001) DNA-based detection of prostate cancer in urine after prostatic massage. Urology 58(3):335–338

85. Goessl C, Muller M, Heicappell R, Krause H, Schostak M, Straub B, Miller K (2002) Methylation-specific PCR for detection of neoplastic DNA in biopsy washings. J Pathol 196(3):331–334. doi:10.1002/path.1063

86. Kawakami K, Brabender J, Lord RV, Groshen S, Greenwald BD, Krasna MJ, Yin J, Fleisher AS, Abraham JM, Beer DG, Sidransky D, Huss HT, Demeester TR, Eads C, Laird PW, Ilson DH, Kelsen DP, Harpole D, Moore MB, Danenberg KD, Danenberg PV, Meltzer SJ (2000) Hypermethylated APC DNA in plasma and prognosis of patients with esophageal adenocarcinoma. J Natl Cancer Inst 92(22):1805–1811

87. Hibi K, Taguchi M, Nakayama H, Takase T, Kasai Y, Ito K, Akiyama S, Nakao A (2001) Molecular detection of p16 promoter methylation in the serum of patients with esophageal squamous cell carcinoma. Clin Cancer Res 7(10):3135–3138

88. Sanchez-Cespedes M, Esteller M, Wu L, Nawroz-Danish H, Yoo GH, Koch WM, Jen J, Herman JG, Sidransky D (2000) Gene promoter hypermethylation in tumors and serum of head and neck cancer patients. Cancer Res 60(4):892–895
89. Wong TS, Chang HW, Tang KC, Wei WI, Kwong DL, Sham JS, Yuen AP, Kwong YL (2002) High frequency of promoter hypermethylation of the death-associated protein-kinase gene in nasopharyngeal carcinoma and its detection in the peripheral blood of patients. Clin Cancer Res 8(2):433–437
90. Rosas SL, Koch W, da Costa Carvalho MG, Wu L, Califano J, Westra W, Jen J, Sidransky D (2001) Promoter hypermethylation patterns of p16, O6-methylguanine-DNA-methyltransferase, and death-associated protein kinase in tumors and saliva of head and neck cancer patients. Cancer Res 61(3):939–942
91. Schwarzenbach H, Hoon DS, Pantel K (2011) Cell-free nucleic acids as biomarkers in cancer patients. Nat Rev Cancer 11(6):426–437. doi:10.1038/nrc3066
92. Crowley E, Di Nicolantonio F, Loupakis F, Bardelli A (2013) Liquid biopsy: monitoring cancer-genetics in the blood. Nat Rev Clin Oncol 10(8):472–484. doi:10.1038/nrclinonc.2013.110
93. Mandel P, Metais P (1948) Les acides nucléiques du plasma sanguin chez l'homme. Comptes rendus des seances de la Societe de biologie et de ses filiales 142(3–4):241–243
94. Sorenson GD, Pribish DM, Valone FH, Memoli VA, Bzik DJ, Yao SL (1994) Soluble normal and mutated DNA sequences from single-copy genes in human blood. Cancer Epidemiol Biomarkers Prev Publ Am Assoc Cancer Res Cospo Am Soc Prev Onco 3(1):67–71
95. Vasioukhin V, Anker P, Maurice P, Lyautey J, Lederrey C, Stroun M (1994) Point mutations of the N-ras gene in the blood plasma DNA of patients with myelodysplastic syndrome or acute myelogenous leukaemia. Br J Haematol 86(4):774–779
96. Kopreski MS, Benko FA, Kwak LW, Gocke CD (1999) Detection of tumor messenger RNA in the serum of patients with malignant melanoma. Clin Cancer Res 5(8):1961–1965
97. Lo KW, Lo YM, Leung SF, Tsang YS, Chan LY, Johnson PJ, Hjelm NM, Lee JC, Huang DP (1999) Analysis of cell-free Epstein-Barr virus associated RNA in the plasma of patients with nasopharyngeal carcinoma. Clin Chem 45(8 Pt 1):1292–1294
98. Sabbioni S, Miotto E, Veronese A, Sattin E, Gramantieri L, Bolondi L, Calin GA, Gafa R, Lanza G, Carli G, Ferrazzi E, Feo C, Liboni A, Gullini S, Negrini M (2003) Multigene methylation analysis of gastrointestinal tumors: TPEF emerges as a frequent tumor-specific aberrantly methylated marker that can be detected in peripheral blood. Mol Diagn J Devo Underst Hum Dis Clin Appl Mol Biol 7(3–4):201–207
99. Fujiwara K, Fujimoto N, Tabata M, Nishii K, Matsuo K, Hotta K, Kozuki T, Aoe M, Kiura K, Ueoka H, Tanimoto M (2005) Identification of epigenetic aberrant promoter methylation in serum DNA is useful for early detection of lung cancer. Clin Cancer Res 11(3):1219–1225
100. Chan KC, Jiang P, Chan CW, Sun K, Wong J, Hui EP, Chan SL, Chan WC, Hui DS, Ng SS, Chan HL, Wong CS, Ma BB, Chan AT, Lai PB, Sun H, Chiu RW, Lo YM (2013) Noninvasive detection of cancer-associated genome-wide hypomethylation and copy number aberrations by plasma DNA bisulfite sequencing. Proc Natl Acad Sci U S A 110(47):18761–18768. doi:10.1073/pnas.1313995110
101. Fernandez AF, Rosales C, Lopez-Nieva P, Grana O, Ballestar E, Ropero S, Espada J, Melo SA, Lujambio A, Fraga MF, Pino I, Javierre B, Carmona FJ, Acquadro F, Steenbergen RD, Snijders PJ, Meijer CJ, Pineau P, Dejean A, Lloveras B, Capella G, Quer J, Buti M, Esteban JI, Allende H, Rodriguez-Frias F, Castellsague X, Minarovits J, Ponce J, Capello D, Gaidano G, Cigudosa JC, Gomez-Lopez G, Pisano DG, Valencia A, Piris MA, Bosch FX, Cahir-McFarland E, Kieff E, Esteller M (2009) The dynamic DNA methylomes of double-stranded DNA viruses associated with human cancer. Genome Res 19(3):438–451. doi:10.1101/gr.083550.108
102. Szyf M, Eliasson L, Mann V, Klein G, Razin A (1985) Cellular and viral DNA hypomethylation associated with induction of Epstein-Barr virus lytic cycle. Proc Natl Acad Sci U S A 82(23):8090–8094

103. Sudo M, Chong JM, Sakuma K, Ushiku T, Uozaki H, Nagai H, Funata N, Matsumoto Y, Fukayama M (2004) Promoter hypermethylation of E-cadherin and its abnormal expression in Epstein-Barr virus-associated gastric carcinoma. Int J Cancer 109(2):194–199. doi:10.1002/ijc.11701

104. Sakuma K, Chong JM, Sudo M, Ushiku T, Inoue Y, Shibahara J, Uozaki H, Nagai H, Fukayama M (2004) High-density methylation of p14ARF and p16INK4A in Epstein-Barr virus-associated gastric carcinoma. Int J Cancer 112(2):273–278. doi:10.1002/ijc.20420

105. Osawa T, Chong JM, Sudo M, Sakuma K, Uozaki H, Shibahara J, Nagai H, Funata N, Fukayama M (2002) Reduced expression and promoter methylation of p16 gene in Epstein-Barr virus-associated gastric carcinoma. Jpn J Cancer Res Gann 93(11):1195–1200

106. Doxaki C, Kampranis SC, Tsatsanis C (2015) Coordinated regulation of miR-155 and miR-146a genes during induction of endotoxin tolerance in macrophages. J Immunol 195(12):5750–5761. doi:10.4049/jimmunol.1500615

107. Li CL, Nie H, Wang M, Su LP, Li JF, Yu YY, Yan M, Qu QL, Zhu ZG, Liu BY (2012) microRNA-155 is downregulated in gastric cancer cells and involved in cell metastasis. Oncol Rep 27(6):1960–1966. doi:10.3892/or.2012.1719

108. Sohlberger MG, Claus R, Hielscher T, Grimm C, Weichenhan D, Blaes J, Wiestler B, Hau P, Schramm J, Sahm F, Weiss EK, Weiler M, Baer C, Schmidt-Graf F, Schackert G, Westphal M, Hertenstein A, Roth P, Galldiks N, Hartmann C, Pietsch T, Felsberg J, Reifenberger G, Sabel MC, Winkler F, von Deimling A, Meisner C, Vajkoczy P, Platten M, Weller M, Plass C, Wick W (2016) Prognostic relevance of miRNA-155 methylation in anaplastic glioma. Oncotarget 7(50):82028–82045. doi:10.18632/oncotarget.13452

109. Yin Q, Wang X, Roberts C, Flemington EK, Lasky JA (2016) Methylation status and AP1 elements are involved in EBV-mediated miR-155 expression in EBV positive lymphoma cells. Virology 494:158–167. doi:10.1016/j.virol.2016.04.005

110. Zhang G, Esteve PO, Chin HG, Terragni J, Dai N, Correa IR Jr, Pradhan S (2015) Small RNA-mediated DNA (cytosine-5) methyltransferase 1 inhibition leads to aberrant DNA methylation. Nucleic Acids Res 43(12):6112–6124. doi:10.1093/nar/gkv518

111. Ferrajoli A, Shanafelt TD, Ivan C, Shimizu M, Rabe KG, Nouraee N, Ikuo M, Ghosh AK, Lerner S, Rassenti LZ, Xiao L, Hu J, Reuben JM, Calin S, You MJ, Manning JT, Wierda WG, Estrov Z, O'Brien S, Kipps TJ, Keating MJ, Kay NE, Calin GA (2013) Prognostic value of miR-155 in individuals with monoclonal B-cell lymphocytosis and patients with B chronic lymphocytic leukemia. Blood 122(11):1891–1899. doi:10.1182/blood-2013-01-478222

112. Tinzl M, Marberger M, Horvath S, Chypre C (2004) DD3PCA3 RNA analysis in urine--a new perspective for detecting prostate cancer. Eur Urol 46(2):182–186. doi:10.1016/j.eururo.2004.06.004. discussion 187

113. Hasselmann DO, Rappl G, Tilgen W, Reinhold U (2001) Extracellular tyrosinase mRNA within apoptotic bodies is protected from degradation in human serum. Clin Chem 47(8):1488–1489

114. Valadi H, Ekstrom K, Bossios A, Sjostrand M, Lee JJ, Lotvall JO (2007) Exosome-mediated transfer of mRNAs and microRNAs is a novel mechanism of genetic exchange between cells. Nat Cell Biol 9(6):654–659. doi:10.1038/ncb1596

115. Deligezer U, Akisik EZ, Akisik EE, Kovancilar M, Bugra D, Erten N, Holdenrieder S, Dalay N (2011) H3K9me3/H4K20me3 ratio in circulating nucleosomes as potential biomarker for colorectal cancer. In: Gahan P (ed) Circulating nucleic acids in plasma and serum, 1st edn. Springer, Heidelberg, pp 97–103. doi:10.1007/978-90-481-9382-0_14

116. Leszinski G, Gezer U, Siegele B, Stoetzer O, Holdenrieder S (2012) Relevance of histone marks H3K9me3 and H4K20me3 in cancer. Anticancer Res 32(5):2199–2205

117. Lee RC, Feinbaum RL, Ambros V (1993) The C. elegans heterochronic gene lin-4 encodes small RNAs with antisense complementarity to lin-14. Cell 75(5):843–854

118. Pasquinelli AE, Reinhart BJ, Slack F, Martindale MQ, Kuroda MI, Maller B, Hayward DC, Ball EE, Degnan B, Muller P, Spring J, Srinivasan A, Fishman M, Finnerty J, Corbo J, Levine

M, Leahy P, Davidson E, Ruvkun G (2000) Conservation of the sequence and temporal expression of let-7 heterochronic regulatory RNA. Nature 408(6808):86–89. doi:10.1038/35040556

119. Sempere LF, Freemantle S, Pitha-Rowe I, Moss E, Dmitrovsky E, Ambros V (2004) Expression profiling of mammalian microRNAs uncovers a subset of brain-expressed microRNAs with possible roles in murine and human neuronal differentiation. Genome Biol 5(3):R13. doi:10.1186/gb-2004-5-3-r13

120. Ha M, Kim VN (2014) Regulation of microRNA biogenesis. Nat Rev Mol Cell Biol 15(8):509–524. doi:10.1038/nrm3838

121. Ameres SL, Zamore PD (2013) Diversifying microRNA sequence and function. Nat Rev Mol Cell Biol 14(8):475–488. doi:10.1038/nrm3611

122. Small EM, Olson EN (2011) Pervasive roles of microRNAs in cardiovascular biology. Nature 469(7330):336–342. doi:10.1038/nature09783

123. Lewis BP, Shih IH, Jones-Rhoades MW, Bartel DP, Burge CB (2003) Prediction of mammalian microRNA targets. Cell 115(7):787–798

124. Agarwal V, Bell GW, Nam JW, Bartel DP (2015) Predicting effective microRNA target sites in mammalian mRNAs. eLife 4. doi:10.7554/eLife.05005

125. Tay Y, Zhang J, Thomson AM, Lim B, Rigoutsos I (2008) MicroRNAs to Nanog, Oct4 and Sox2 coding regions modulate embryonic stem cell differentiation. Nature 455(7216):1124–1128. doi:10.1038/nature07299

126. Lytle JR, Yario TA, Steitz JA (2007) Target mRNAs are repressed as efficiently by microRNA-binding sites in the 5′ UTR as in the 3′ UTR. Proc Natl Acad Sci U S A 104(23):9667–9672. doi:10.1073/pnas.0703820104

127. Calin GA, Dumitru CD, Shimizu M, Bichi R, Zupo S, Noch E, Aldler H, Rattan S, Keating M, Rai K, Rassenti L, Kipps T, Negrini M, Bullrich F, Croce CM (2002) Frequent deletions and down-regulation of micro- RNA genes miR15 and miR16 at 13q14 in chronic lymphocytic leukemia. Proc Natl Acad Sci U S A 99(24):15524–15529. doi:10.1073/pnas.242606799

128. He L, Thomson JM, Hemann MT, Hernando-Monge E, Mu D, Goodson S, Powers S, Cordon-Cardo C, Lowe SW, Hannon GJ, Hammond SM (2005) A microRNA polycistron as a potential human oncogene. Nature 435(7043):828–833. doi:10.1038/nature03552

129. Chan JA, Krichevsky AM, Kosik KS (2005) MicroRNA-21 is an antiapoptotic factor in human glioblastoma cells. Cancer Res 65(14):6029–6033. doi:10.1158/0008-5472.CAN-05-0137

130. Takamizawa J, Konishi H, Yanagisawa K, Tomida S, Osada H, Endoh H, Harano T, Yatabe Y, Nagino M, Nimura Y, Mitsudomi T, Takahashi T (2004) Reduced expression of the let-7 microRNAs in human lung cancers in association with shortened postoperative survival. Cancer Res 64(11):3753–3756. doi:10.1158/0008-5472.CAN-04-0637

131. Liu C, Kelnar K, Liu B, Chen X, Calhoun-Davis T, Li H, Patrawala L, Yan H, Jeter C, Honorio S, Wiggins JF, Bader AG, Fagin R, Brown D, Tang DG (2011) The microRNA miR-34a inhibits prostate cancer stem cells and metastasis by directly repressing CD44. Nat Med 17(2):211–215. doi:10.1038/nm.2284

132. Li N, Fu H, Tie Y, Hu Z, Kong W, Wu Y, Zheng X (2009) miR-34a inhibits migration and invasion by down-regulation of c-Met expression in human hepatocellular carcinoma cells. Cancer Lett 275(1):44–53. doi:10.1016/j.canlet.2008.09.035

133. Tazawa H, Tsuchiya N, Izumiya M, Nakagama H (2007) Tumor-suppressive miR-34a induces senescence-like growth arrest through modulation of the E2F pathway in human colon cancer cells. Proc Natl Acad Sci U S A 104(39):15472–15477. doi:10.1073/pnas.0707351104

134. Chang TC, Wentzel EA, Kent OA, Ramachandran K, Mullendore M, Lee KH, Feldmann G, Yamakuchi M, Ferlito M, Lowenstein CJ, Arking DE, Beer MA, Maitra A, Mendell JT (2007) Transactivation of miR-34a by p53 broadly influences gene expression and promotes apoptosis. Mol Cell 26(5):745–752. doi:10.1016/j.molcel.2007.05.010

135. Wang Y, Wang M, Wei W, Han D, Chen X, Hu Q, Yu T, Liu N, You Y, Zhang J (2016) Disruption of the EZH2/miRNA/beta-catenin signaling suppresses aerobic glycolysis in glioma. Oncotarget 7(31):49450–49458. doi:10.18632/oncotarget.10370

136. Ayala-Ortega E, Arzate-Mejia R, Perez-Molina R, Gonzalez-Buendia E, Meier K, Guerrero G, Recillas-Targa F (2016) Epigenetic silencing of miR-181c by DNA methylation in glioblastoma cell lines. BMC Cancer 16:226. doi:10.1186/s12885-016-2273-6
137. Ning X, Shi Z, Liu X, Zhang A, Han L, Jiang K, Kang C, Zhang Q (2015) DNMT1 and EZH2 mediated methylation silences the microRNA-200b/a/429 gene and promotes tumor progression. Cancer Lett 359(2):198–205. doi:10.1016/j.canlet.2015.01.005
138. Chiou GY, Chien CS, Wang ML, Chen MT, Yang YP, Yu YL, Chien Y, Chang YC, Shen CC, Chio CC, Lu KH, Ma HI, Chen KH, Liu DM, Miller SA, Chen YW, Huang PI, Shih YH, Hung MC, Chiou SH (2013) Epigenetic regulation of the miR142-3p/interleukin-6 circuit in glioblastoma. Mol Cell 52(5):693–706. doi:10.1016/j.molcel.2013.11.009
139. Bourguignon LY, Wong G, Shiina M (2016) Up-regulation of histone methyltransferase, DOT1L, by matrix hyaluronan promotes MicroRNA-10 expression leading to tumor cell invasion and chemoresistance in cancer stem cells from head and neck squamous cell carcinoma. J Biol Chem 291(20):10571–10585. doi:10.1074/jbc.M115.700021
140. Kozaki K, Imoto I, Mogi S, Omura K, Inazawa J (2008) Exploration of tumor-suppressive microRNAs silenced by DNA hypermethylation in oral cancer. Cancer Res 68(7):2094–2105. doi:10.1158/0008-5472.CAN-07-5194
141. Langevin SM, Stone RA, Bunker CH, Lyons-Weiler MA, LaFramboise WA, Kelly L, Seethala RR, Grandis JR, Sobol RW, Taioli E (2011) MicroRNA-137 promoter methylation is associated with poorer overall survival in patients with squamous cell carcinoma of the head and neck. Cancer 117(7):1454–1462. doi:10.1002/cncr.25689
142. Cao Q, Mani RS, Ateeq B, Dhanasekaran SM, Asangani IA, Prensner JR, Kim JH, Brenner JC, Jing X, Cao X, Wang R, Li Y, Dahiya A, Wang L, Pandhi M, Lonigro RJ, Wu YM, Tomlins SA, Palanisamy N, Qin Z, Yu J, Maher CA, Varambally S, Chinnaiyan AM (2011) Coordinated regulation of polycomb group complexes through microRNAs in cancer. Cancer Cell 20(2):187–199. doi:10.1016/j.ccr.2011.06.016
143. Song SJ, Poliseno L, Song MS, Ala U, Webster K, Ng C, Beringer G, Brikbak NJ, Yuan X, Cantley LC, Richardson AL, Pandolfi PP (2013) MicroRNA-antagonism regulates breast cancer stemness and metastasis via TET-family-dependent chromatin remodeling. Cell 154(2):311–324. doi:10.1016/j.cell.2013.06.026
144. Zou F, Li J, Jie X, Peng X, Fan R, Wang M, Wang J, Liu Z, Li H, Deng H, Yang X, Luo D (2016) Rs3842530 polymorphism in MicroRNA-205 host gene in lung and breast cancer patients. Med Sci Monit 22:4555–5464. doi:10.12659/MSM.901042
145. Cisneros-Soberanis F, Andonegui MA, Herrera LA (2016) miR-125b-1 is repressed by histone modifications in breast cancer cell lines. Spring 5(1):959. doi:10.1186/s40064-016-2475-z
146. Poli E, Zhang J, Nwachukwu C, Zheng Y, Adedokun B, Olopade OI, Han YJ (2015) Molecular subtype-specific expression of MicroRNA-29c in breast cancer is associated with CpG dinucleotide methylation of the promoter. PLoS One 10(11):e0142224. doi:10.1371/journal.pone.0142224
147. Xiang M, Birkbak NJ, Vafaizadeh V, Walker SR, Yeh JE, Liu S, Kroll Y, Boldin M, Taganov K, Groner B, Richardson AL, Frank DA (2014) STAT3 induction of miR-146b forms a feedback loop to inhibit the NF-kappaB to IL-6 signaling axis and STAT3-driven cancer phenotypes. Sci Signal 7(310):ra11. doi:10.1126/scisignal.2004497
148. Augoff K, McCue B, Plow EF, Sossey-Alaoui K (2012) miR-31 and its host gene lncRNA LOC554202 are regulated by promoter hypermethylation in triple-negative breast cancer. Mol Cancer 11(5). doi:10.1186/1476-4598-11-5
149. Png KJ, Yoshida M, Zhang XH, Shu W, Lee H, Rimner A, Chan TA, Comen E, Andrade VP, Kim SW, King TA, Hudis CA, Norton L, Hicks J, Massague J, Tavazoie SF (2011) MicroRNA-335 inhibits tumor reinitiation and is silenced through genetic and epigenetic mechanisms in human breast cancer. Genes Dev 25(3):226–231. doi:10.1101/gad.1974211
150. Watanabe K, Amano Y, Ishikawa R, Sunohara M, Kage H, Ichinose J, Sano A, Nakajima J, Fukayama M, Yatomi Y, Nagase T, Ohishi N, Takai D (2015) Histone methylation-medi-

ated silencing of miR-139 enhances invasion of non-small-cell lung cancer. Cancer Med 4(10):1573–1582. doi:10.1002/cam4.505

151. Seol HS, Akiyama Y, Shimada S, Lee HJ, Kim TI, Chun SM, Singh SR, Jang SJ (2014) Epigenetic silencing of microRNA-373 to epithelial-mesenchymal transition in non-small cell lung cancer through IRAK2 and LAMP1 axes. Cancer Lett 353(2):232–241. doi:10.1016/j.canlet.2014.07.019

152. Chen DQ, Pan BZ, Huang JY, Zhang K, Cui SY, De W, Wang R, Chen LB (2014) HDAC 1/4-mediated silencing of microRNA-200b promotes chemoresistance in human lung adeno-carcinoma cells. Oncotarget 5(10):3333–3349. doi:10.18632/oncotarget.1948

153. Brueckner B, Stresemann C, Kuner R, Mund C, Musch T, Meister M, Sultmann H, Lyko F (2007) The human let-7a-3 locus contains an epigenetically regulated microRNA gene with oncogenic function. Cancer Res 67(4):1419–1423. doi:10.1158/0008-5472.CAN-06-4074

154. Qiao F, Zhang K, Gong P, Wang L, Hu J, Lu S, Fan H (2014) Decreased miR-30b-5p expres-sion by DNMT1 methylation regulation involved in gastric cancer metastasis. Mol Biol Rep 41(9):5693–5700. doi:10.1007/s11033-014-3439-4

155. Wang S, Lv C, Jin H, Xu M, Kang M, Chu H, Tong N, Wu D, Zhu H, Gong W, Zhao Q, Tao G, Zhou J, Zhang Z, Wang M (2014) A common genetic variation in the promoter of miR-107 is associated with gastric adenocarcinoma susceptibility and survival. Mutat Res 769:35–41. doi:10.1016/j.mrfmmm.2014.07.002

156. An J, Pan Y, Yan Z, Li W, Cui J, Yuan J, Tian L, Xing R, Lu Y (2013) MiR-23a in amplified 19p13.13 loci targets metallothionein 2A and promotes growth in gastric cancer cells. J Cell Biochem 114(9):2160–2169. doi:10.1002/jcb.24565

157. Tsai KW, Hu LY, Wu CW, Li SC, Lai CH, Kao HW, Fang WL, Lin WC (2010) Epigenetic reg-ulation of miR-196b expression in gastric cancer. Genes Chromosomes Cancer 49(11):969–980. doi:10.1002/gcc.20804

158. Hashimoto Y, Akiyama Y, Otsubo T, Shimada S, Yuasa Y (2010) Involvement of epigeneti-cally silenced microRNA-181c in gastric carcinogenesis. Carcinogenesis 31(5):777–784. doi:10.1093/carcin/bgq013

159. Huang D, Wang XB, Zhuang CB, Shi WH, Liu M, Tu QM, Zhang DT, Hu LH (2016) Reciprocal negative feedback loop between EZH2 and miR-101-1 contributes to miR-101 deregulation in hepatocellular carcinoma. Oncol Rep 35(2):1083–1090. doi:10.3892/or.2015.4467

160. Long XR, He Y, Huang C, Li J (2014) MicroRNA-148a is silenced by hypermethylation and interacts with DNA methyltransferase 1 in hepatocellular carcinogenesis. Int J Oncol 44(6):1915–1922. doi:10.3892/ijo.2014.2373

161. He Y, Cui Y, Wang W, Gu J, Guo S, Ma K, Luo X (2011) Hypomethylation of the hsa-miR-191 locus causes high expression of hsa-mir-191 and promotes the epithelial-to-mesen-chymal transition in hepatocellular carcinoma. Neoplasia 13(9):841–853

162. Zhang SY, Hao J, Xie F, Hu XG, Liu C, Tong J, Zhou JD, Wu JC, Shao CH (2011) Downregulation of miR-132 by promoter methylation contributes to pancreatic cancer devel-opment. Carcinogenesis 32(8):1183–1189. doi:10.1093/carcin/bgr105

163. Wang P, Chen L, Zhang J, Chen H, Fan J, Wang K, Luo J, Chen Z, Meng Z, Liu L (2014) Methylation-mediated silencing of the miR-124 genes facilitates pancreatic cancer progres-sion and metastasis by targeting Rac1. Oncogene 33(4):514–524. doi:10.1038/onc.2012.598

164. Gao W, Gu Y, Li Z, Cai H, Peng Q, Tu M, Kondo Y, Shinjo K, Zhu Y, Zhang J, Sekido Y, Han B, Qian Z, Miao Y (2015) miR-615-5p is epigenetically inactivated and functions as a tumor suppressor in pancreatic ductal adenocarcinoma. Oncogene 34(13):1629–1640. doi:10.1038/onc.2014.101

165. Li J, Wu H, Li W, Yin L, Guo S, Xu X, Ouyang Y, Zhao Z, Liu S, Tian Y, Tian Z, Ju J, Ni B, Wang H (2016) Downregulated miR-506 expression facilitates pancreatic cancer progression and chemoresistance via SPHK1/Akt/NF-kappa B signaling. Oncogene 35(42):5501–5514. doi:10.1038/onc.2016.90

166. Bandres E, Agirre X, Bitarte N, Ramirez N, Zarate R, Roman-Gomez J, Prosper F, Garcia-Foncillas J (2009) Epigenetic regulation of microRNA expression in colorectal cancer. Int J Cancer 125(11):2737–2743. doi:10.1002/ijc.24638

167. Toyota M, Suzuki H, Sasaki Y, Maruyama R, Imai K, Shinomura Y, Tokino T (2008) Epigenetic silencing of microRNA-34b/c and B-cell translocation gene 4 is associated with CpG island methylation in colorectal cancer. Cancer Res 68(11):4123–4132. doi:10.1158/0008-5472. Can-08-0325

168. Kim HK, Prokunina-Olsson L, Chanock SJ (2012) Common genetic variants in miR-1206 (8q24.2) and miR-612 (11q13.3) affect biogenesis of mature miRNA forms. PLoS One 7(10):ARTN e47454. doi:10.1371/journal.pone.0047454

169. Li YW, Kong DJ, Ahmad A, Bao B, Dyson G, Sarkar FH (2012) Epigenetic deregulation of miR-29a and miR-1256 by isoflavone contributes to the inhibition of prostate cancer cell growth and invasion. Epigenetics-Us 7(8):940–949. doi:10.4161/epi.21236

170. Hulf T, Sibbritt T, Wiklund ED, Patterson K, Song JZ, Stirzaker C, Qu W, Nair S, Horvath LG, Armstrong NJ, Kench JG, Sutherland RL, Clark SJ (2013) Epigenetic-induced repression of microRNA-205 is associated with MED1 activation and a poorer prognosis in localized prostate cancer. Oncogene 32(23):2891–2899. doi:10.1038/onc.2012.300

171. Zhang Q, Padi SKR, Tindall DJ, Guo B (2014) Polycomb protein EZH2 suppresses apoptosis by silencing the proapoptotic miR-31. Cell Death Dis 5:ARTN e1486. doi:10.1038/cddis.2014.454

172. Lu L, Katsaros D, de la Longrais IA, Sochirca O, Yu H (2007) Hypermethylation of let-7a-3 in epithelial ovarian cancer is associated with low insulin-like growth factor-II expression and favorable prognosis. Cancer Res 67(21):10117–10122. doi:10.1158/0008-5472. CAN-07-2544

173. Zhang L, Volinia S, Bonome T, Calin GA, Greshock J, Yang N, Liu CG, Giannakakis A, Alexiou P, Hasegawa K, Johnstone CN, Megraw MS, Adams S, Lassus H, Huang J, Kaur S, Liang S, Sethupathy P, Leminen A, Simossis VA, Sandaltzopoulos R, Naomoto Y, Katsaros D, Gimotty PA, DeMichele A, Huang Q, Butzow R, Rustgi AK, Weber BL, Birrer MJ, Hatzigeorgiou AG, Croce CM, Coukos G (2008) Genomic and epigenetic alterations deregulate microRNA expression in human epithelial ovarian cancer. P Natl Acad Sci USA 105(19):7004–7009. doi:10.1073/pnas.0801615105

174. Teng Y, Zuo X, Hou M, Zhang Y, Li C, Luo W, Li X (2016) A double-negative feedback interaction between MicroRNA-29b and DNMT3A/3B contributes to ovarian cancer progression. Cell Physiol Biochem 39(6):2341–2352. doi:10.1159/000447926

175. Yao TT, Rao QX, Liu LY, Zheng CY, Xie QS, Liang JX, Lin ZQ (2013) Exploration of tumor-suppressive microRNAs silenced by DNA hypermethylation in cervical cancer. Virol J 10:Artn 175. doi:10.1186/1743-422x-10-175

176. Wang SZ, Cao XL, Ding B, Chen JF, Cui MJ, Xu YL, Lu XY, Zhang ZD, He AQ, Jin H (2016) The rs767649 polymorphism in the promoter of miR-155 contributes to the decreased risk for cervical cancer in a Chinese population. Gene 595(1):109–114. doi:10.1016/j.gene.2016.10.002

177. Campos-Viguri GE, Jimenez-Wences H, Peralta-Zaragoza O, Torres-Altamirano G, Soto-Flores DG, Hernandez-Sotelo D, Alarcon-Romero LD, Jimenez-Lopez MA, Illades-Aguiar B, Fernandez-Tilapa G (2015) miR-23b as a potential tumor suppressor and its regulation by DNA methylation in cervical cancer. Infect Agents Cancer 10:ARTN 42. doi:10.1186/s13027-015-0037-6

178. Yamagishi M, Nakano K, Miyake A, Yamochi T, Kagami Y, Tsutsumi A, Matsuda Y, Sato-Otsubo A, Muto S, Utsunomiya A, Yamaguchi K, Uchimaru K, Ogawa S, Watanabe T (2012) Polycomb-mediated loss of miR-31 activates NIK-dependent NF-kappa B pathway in adult T cell leukemia and other cancers. Cancer Cell 21(1):121–135. doi:10.1016/j.ccr.2011.12.015

179. Baer C, Claus R, Frenzel LP, Zucknick M, Park YJ, Gu L, Weichenhan D, Fischer M, Pallasch CP, Herpel E, Rehli M, Byrd JC, Wendtner CM, Plass C (2012) Extensive promoter DNA hypermethylation and hypomethylation is associated with aberrant MicroRNA expression

in chronic lymphocytic leukemia. Cancer Res 72(15):3775–3785. doi:10.1158/0008-5472. Can-12-0803

180. Chim CS, Wong KY, Leung CY, Chung LP, Hui PK, Chan SY, Yu L (2011) Epigenetic inactivation of the hsa-miR-203 in haematological malignancies. J Cell Mol Med 15(12):2760–2767. doi:10.1111/j.1582-4934.2011.01274.x

181. Zhang X, Zhao X, Fiskus W, Lin J, Lwin T, Rao R, Zhang Y, Chan JC, Fu K, Marquez VE, Chen-Kiang S, Moscinski LC, Seto E, Dalton WS, Wright KL, Sotomayor E, Bhalla K, Tao J (2012) Coordinated silencing of MYC-mediated miR-29 by HDAC3 and EZH2 as a therapeutic target of histone modification in aggressive B-cell lymphomas. Cancer Cell 22(4):506–523. doi:10.1016/j.ccr.2012.09.003

182. Merkel O, Hamacher F, Griessl R, Grabner L, Schiefer AI, Prutsch N, Baer C, Egger G, Schlederer M, Krenn PW, Hartmann TN, Simonitsch-Klupp I, Plass C, Staber PB, Moriggl R, Turner SD, Greil R, Kenner L (2015) Oncogenic role of miR-155 in anaplastic large cell lymphoma lacking the t(2;5) translocation. J Pathol 236(4):445–456. doi:10.1002/path.4539

183. Qi L, Hu Y, Zhan Y, Wang J, Wang BB, Xia HF, Ma X (2012) A SNP site in pri-miR-124 changes mature miR-124 expression but no contribution to Alzheimer's disease in a Mongolian population. Neurosci Lett 515(1):1–6. doi:10.1016/j.neulet.2012.02.061

184. Zhao Y, Du Y, Zhao S, Guo Z (2015) Single-nucleotide polymorphisms of microRNA processing machinery genes and risk of colorectal cancer. Onco Targets Ther 8:421–425. doi:10.2147/OTT.S78647

185. Calin GA, Sevignani C, Dumitru CD, Hyslop T, Noch E, Yendamuri S, Shimizu M, Rattan S, Bullrich F, Negrini M, Croce CM (2004) Human microRNA genes are frequently located at fragile sites and genomic regions involved in cancers. Proc Natl Acad Sci U S A 101(9):2999–3004. doi:10.1073/pnas.0307323101

186. Fabbri M, Garzon R, Cimmino A, Liu Z, Zanesi N, Callegari E, Liu S, Alder H, Costinean S, Fernandez-Cymering C, Volinia S, Guler G, Morrison CD, Chan KK, Marcucci G, Calin GA, Huebner K, Croce CM (2007) MicroRNA-29 family reverts aberrant methylation in lung cancer by targeting DNA methyltransferases 3A and 3B. Proc Natl Acad Sci U S A 104(40):15805–15810. doi:10.1073/pnas.0707628104

187. Noonan EJ, Place RF, Pookot D, Basak S, Whitson JM, Hirata H, Giardina C, Dahiya R (2009) miR-449a targets HDAC-1 and induces growth arrest in prostate cancer. Oncogene 28(14):1714–1724. doi:10.1038/onc.2009.19

188. Rosenfeld N, Aharonov R, Meiri E, Rosenwald S, Spector Y, Zepeniuk M, Benjamin H, Shabes N, Tabak S, Levy A, Lebanony D, Goren Y, Silberschein E, Targan N, Ben-Ari A, Gilad S, Sion-Vardy N, Tobar A, Feinmesser M, Kharenko O, Nativ O, Nass D, Perelman M, Yosepovich A, Shalmon B, Polak-Charcon S, Fridman E, Avniel A, Bentwich I, Bentwich Z, Cohen D, Chajut A, Barshack I (2008) MicroRNAs accurately identify cancer tissue origin. Nat Biotechnol 26(4):462–469. doi:10.1038/nbt1392

189. Lu J, Getz G, Miska EA, Alvarez-Saavedra E, Lamb J, Peck D, Sweet-Cordero A, Ebert BL, Mak RH, Ferrando AA, Downing JR, Jacks T, Horvitz HR, Golub TR (2005) MicroRNA expression profiles classify human cancers. Nature 435(7043):834–838. doi:10.1038/nature03702

190. Lawrie CH, Gal S, Dunlop HM, Pushkaran B, Liggins AP, Pulford K, Banham AH, Pezzella F, Boultwood J, Wainscoat JS, Hatton CS, Harris AL (2008) Detection of elevated levels of tumour-associated microRNAs in serum of patients with diffuse large B-cell lymphoma. Br J Haematol 141(5):672–675. doi:10.1111/j.1365-2141.2008.07077.x

191. Mitchell PS, Parkin RK, Kroh EM, Fritz BR, Wyman SK, Pogosova-Agadjanyan EL, Peterson A, Noteboom J, O'Briant KC, Allen A, Lin DW, Urban N, Drescher CW, Knudsen BS, Stirewalt DL, Gentleman R, Vessella RL, Nelson PS, Martin DB, Tewari M (2008) Circulating microRNAs as stable blood-based markers for cancer detection. Proc Natl Acad Sci U S A 105(30):10513–10518. doi:10.1073/pnas.0804549105

192. Weber JA, Baxter DH, Zhang S, Huang DY, Huang KH, Lee MJ, Galas DJ, Wang K (2010) The microRNA spectrum in 12 body fluids. Clin Chem 56(11):1733–1741. doi:10.1373/clinchem.2010.147405

193. Lawrie CH, Soneji S, Marafioti T, Cooper CD, Palazzo S, Paterson JC, Cattan H, Enver T, Mager R, Boultwood J, Wainscoat JS, Hatton CS (2007) MicroRNA expression distinguishes between germinal center B cell-like and activated B cell-like subtypes of diffuse large B cell lymphoma. Int J Cancer 121(5):1156–1161. doi:10.1002/ijc.22800

194. Kosaka N, Iguchi H, Ochiya T (2010) Circulating microRNA in body fluid: a new potential biomarker for cancer diagnosis and prognosis. Cancer Sci 101(10):2087–2092. doi:10.1111/j.1349-7006.2010.01650.x

195. Li HY, Li YM, Li Y, Shi XW, Chen H (2016) Circulating microRNA-137 is a potential biomarker for human glioblastoma. Eur Rev Med Pharmacol Sci 20(17):3599–3604

196. Zhang R, Pang B, Xin T, Guo H, Xing Y, Xu SC, Feng B, Liu B, Pang Q (2016) Plasma miR-221/222 family as novel descriptive and prognostic biomarkers for Glioma. Mol Neurobiol 53(3):1452–1460. doi:10.1007/s12035-014-9079-9

197. Manterola L, Guruceaga E, Perez-Larraya JG, Gonzalez-Huarriz M, Jauregui P, Tejada S, Diez-Valle R, Segura V, Sampron N, Barrena C, Ruiz I, Agirre A, Ayuso A, Rodriguez J, Gonzalez A, Xipell E, Matheu A, de Munain AL, Tunon T, Zazpe I, Garcia-Foncillas J, Paris S, Delattre JY, Alonso MM (2014) A small noncoding RNA signature found in exosomes of GBM patient serum as a diagnostic tool. Neuro-Oncology 16(4):520–527. doi:10.1093/neuonc/not218

198. Akers JC, Ramakrishnan V, Kim R, Skog J, Nakano I, Pingle S, Kalinina J, Hua W, Kesari S, Mao Y, Breakefield XO, Hochberg FH, Van Meir EG, Carter BS, Chen CC (2013) miR-21 in the extracellular vesicles (EVs) of cerebrospinal fluid (CSF): a platform for glioblastoma biomarker development. PLoS One 8(10):ARTN e78115. doi:10.1371/journal.pone.0078115

199. Duz MB, Karatas OF, Guzel E, Turgut NF, Yilmaz M, Creighton CJ, Ozen M (2016) Identification of miR-139-5p as a saliva biomarker for tongue squamous cell carcinoma: a pilot study. Cell Oncol 39(2):187–193. doi:10.1007/s13402-015-0259-z

200. Salazar C, Nagadia R, Pandit P, Cooper-White J, Banerjee N, Dimitrova N, Coman WB, Punyadeera C (2014) A novel saliva-based microRNA biomarker panel to detect head and neck cancers. Cell Oncol 37(5):331–338. doi:10.1007/s13402-014-0188-2

201. Liu CJ, Lin SC, Yang CC, Cheng HW, Chang KW (2012) Exploiting salivary miR-31 as a clinical biomarker of oral squamous cell carcinoma. Head Neck-J Sci Spec 34(2):219–224. doi:10.1002/hed.21713

202. Takeshita N, Hoshino I, Mori M, Akutsu Y, Hanari N, Yoneyama Y, Ikeda N, Isozaki Y, Maruyama T, Akanuma N, Komatsu A, Jitsukawa M, Matsubara H (2013) Serum microRNA expression profile: miR-1246 as a novel diagnostic and prognostic biomarker for oesophageal squamous cell carcinoma. Brit J Cancer 108(3):644–652. doi:10.1038/bjc.2013.8

203. Komatsu S, Ichikawa D, Takeshita H, Tsujiura M, Morimura R, Nagata H, Kosuga T, Iitaka D, Konishi H, Shiozaki A, Fujiwara H, Okamoto K, Otsuji E (2011) Circulating microRNAs in plasma of patients with oesophageal squamous cell carcinoma. Brit J Cancer 105(1):104–111. doi:10.1038/bjc.2011.198

204. Shimomura A, Shiino S, Kawauchi J, Takizawa S, Sakamoto H, Matsuzaki J, Ono M, Takeshita F, Niida S, Shimizu C, Fujiwara Y, Kinoshita T, Tamura K, Ochiya T (2016) Novel combination of serum microRNA for detecting breast cancer in the early stage. Cancer Sci 107(3):326–334. doi:10.1111/cas.12880

205. Ng EKO, Li RFN, Shin VY, Jin HC, Leung CPH, Ma ESK, Pang R, Chua D, Chu KM, Law WL, Law SYK, Poon RTP, Kwong A (2013) Circulating microRNAs as specific biomarkers for breast cancer detection. PLoS One 8(1):ARTN e53141. doi:10.1371/journal.pone.0053141

206. Guo LJ, Zhang QY (2012) Decreased serum miR-181a is a potential new tool for breast cancer screening. Int J Mol Med 30(3):680–686. doi:10.3892/ijmm.2012.1021

207. Zhu WY, He JY, Chen DD, Zhang BJ, Xu LY, Ma HJ, Liu XG, Zhang YK, Le HB (2014) Expression of miR-29c, miR-93, and miR-429 as potential biomarkers for detection of early stage non-small lung cancer. PLoS One 9(s):ARTN e87780. doi:10.1371/journal.pone.0087780

208. Hennessey PT, Sanford T, Choudhary A, Mydlarz WW, Brown D, Adai AT, Ochs MF, Ahrendt SA, Mambo E, Califano JA (2012) Serum microRNA biomarkers for detection of non-small cell lung cancer. PLoS One 7(2):ARTN e32307. doi:10.1371/journal.pone.0032307

209. Foss KM, Sima C, Ugolini D, Neri M, Allen KE, Weiss GJ (2011) miR-1254 and miR-574-5p serum-based microRNA biomarkers for early-stage non-small cell lung cancer. J Thorac Oncol 6(3):482–488. doi:10.1097/JTO.0b013e318208c785

210. Zhu C, Ren C, Han J, Ding Y, Du J, Dai N, Dai J, Ma H, Hu Z, Shen H, Xu Y, Jin G (2014) A five-microRNA panel in plasma was identified as potential biomarker for early detection of gastric cancer. Brit J Cancer 110(9):2291–2299. doi:10.1038/bjc.2014.119

211. Li C, Li JF, Cai Q, Qiu QQ, Yan M, Liu BY, Zhu ZG (2013) MiRNA-199a 3p: a potential circulating diagnostic biomarker for early gastric cancer. J Surg Oncol 108(2):89–92. doi:10.1002/jso.23358

212. Liu HS, Zhu L, Liu BY, Yang L, Meng XX, Zhang W, Ma YY, Xiao HS (2012) Genome-wide microRNA profiles identify miR-378 as a serum biomarker for early detection of gastric cancer. Cancer Lett 316(2):196–203. doi:10.1016/j.canlet.2011.10.034

213. Wang M, Gu HB, Wang S, Qian H, Zhu W, Zhang L, Zhao CH, Tao Y, Xu WR (2012) Circulating miR-17-5p and miR-20a: molecular markers for gastric cancer. Mol Med Rep 5(6):1514–1520. doi:10.3892/mmr.2012.828

214. Shen J, Wang AT, Wang Q, Gurvich I, Siegel AB, Remotti H, Santella RM (2013) Exploration of genome-wide circulating MicroRNA in hepatocellular carcinoma: MiR-483-5p as a potential biomarker. Cancer Epidemiol Biomarkers Prev 22(12):2364–2373. doi:10.1158/1055-9965.Epi-13-0237

215. Liu AM, Yao TJ, Wang W, Wong KF, Lee NP, Fan ST, Poon RTP, Gao CF, Luk JM (2012) Circulating miR-15b and miR-130b in serum as potential markers for detecting hepatocellular carcinoma: a retrospective cohort study. BMJ Open 2(2):ARTN e000825. doi:10.1136/bmjopen-2012-000825

216. Gui JH, Tian YP, Wen XY, Zhang WH, Zhang PJ, Gao J, Run W, Tian LY, Jia XW, Gao YH (2011) Serum microRNA characterization identifies miR-885-5p as a potential marker for detecting liver pathologies. Clin Sci 120(5–6):183–193. doi:10.1042/Cs20100297

217. Que RS, Ding GP, Chen JH, Cao LP (2013) Analysis of serum exosomal microRNAs and clinicopathologic features of patients with pancreatic adenocarcinoma. World J Surg Oncol 11:Artn 219. doi:10.1186/1477-7819-11-219

218. Chabre O, Libé R, Assie G, Barreau O, Bertherat J, Bertagna X, Feige JJ, Cherradi N (2013) Serum miR-483-5p and miR-195 are predictive of recurrence risk in adrenocortical cancer patients. Endocr Relat Cancer 20(4):579–594. doi:10.1530/ERC-13-0051

219. Liu R, Chen X, Du YQ, Yao WY, Shen L, Wang C, Hu ZB, Zhuang R, Ning G, Zhang CN, Yuan YZ, Li ZS, Zen K, Ba Y, Zhang CY (2012) Serum MicroRNA expression profile as a biomarker in the diagnosis and prognosis of pancreatic cancer. Clin Chem 58(3):610–618. doi:10.1373/clinchem.2011.172767

220. Wang C, Hu JC, Lu ML, Gu HW, Zhou XJ, Chen X, Zen K, Zhang CY, Zhang TH, Ge JP, Wang JJ, Zhang CN (2015) A panel of five serum miRNAs as a potential diagnostic tool for early-stage renal cell carcinoma. Sci Rep-Uk 5:UNSP 7610. doi:10.1038/srep07610

221. Redova M, Poprach A, Nekvindova J, Iliev R, Radova L, Lakomy R, Svoboda M, Vyzula R, Slaby O (2012) Circulating miR-378 and miR-451 in serum are potential biomarkers for renal cell carcinoma. J Transl Med 10:Artn 55. doi:10.1186/1479-5876-10-55

222. Matsumura T, Sugimachi K, Iinuma H, Takahashi Y, Kurashige J, Sawada G, Ueda M, Uchi R, Ueo H, Takano Y, Shinden Y, Eguchi H, Yamamoto H, Doki Y, Mori M, Ochiya T, Mimori K (2015) Exosomal microRNA in serum is a novel biomarker of recurrence in human colorectal cancer. Brit J Cancer 113(2):275–281. doi:10.1038/bjc.2015.201

223. Ogata-Kawata H, Izumiya M, Kurioka D, Honma Y, Yamada Y, Furuta K, Gunji T, Ohta H, Okamoto H, Sonoda H, Watanabe M, Nakagama H, Yokota J, Kohno T, Tsuchiya N (2014) Circulating Exosomal microRNAs as biomarkers of Colon cancer. PLoS One 9(4):ARTN e92921. doi:10.1371/journal.pone.0092921

224. Toiyama Y, Hur K, Tanaka K, Inoue Y, Kusunoki M, Boland CR, Goel A (2014) Serum miR-200c is a novel prognostic and metastasis-predictive biomarker in patients with colorectal cancer. Ann Surg 259(4):735–743. doi:10.1097/SLA.0b013e3182a6909d

225. Zanutto S, Pizzamiglio S, Ghilotti M, Bertan C, Ravagnani F, Perrone F, Leo E, Pilotti S, Verderio P, Gariboldi M, Pierotti MA (2014) Circulating miR-378 in plasma: a reliable, haemolysis-independent biomarker for colorectal cancer. Brit J Cancer 110(4):1001–1007. doi:10.1038/bjc.2013.819

226. Eissa S, Habib H, Ali E, Kotb Y (2015) Evaluation of urinary miRNA-96 as a potential biomarker for bladder cancer diagnosis. Med Oncol 32(1):ARTN 413. doi:10.1007/s12032-014-0413-x

227. Wang G, Chan ESY, Kwan BCH, Li PKT, Yip SKH, Szeto CC, Ng CF (2012) Expression of microRNAs in the urine of patients with bladder cancer. Clin Genitourin Cancer 10(2):106–113. doi:10.1016/j.clgc.2012.01.001

228. Wach S, Al-Janabi O, Weigelt K, Fischer K, Greither T, Marcou M, Theil G, Nolte E, Holzhausen HJ, Stohr R, Huppert V, Hartmann A, Fornara P, Wullich B, Taubert H (2015) The combined serum levels of miR-375 and urokinase plasminogen activator receptor are suggested as diagnostic and prognostic biomarkers in prostate cancer. Int J Cancer 137(6):1406–1416. doi:10.1002/ijc.29505

229. Chen ZH, Zhang GL, Li HR, Luo JD, Li ZX, Chen GM, Yang J (2012) A panel of five circulating microRNAs as potential biomarkers for prostate cancer. Prostate 72(13):1443–1452. doi:10.1002/pros.22495

230. Guo FJ, Tian JY, Lin Y, Jin YM, Wang L, Cui MH (2013) Serum microRNA-92 expression in patients with ovarian epithelial carcinoma. J Int Med Res 41(5):1456–1461. doi:10.1177/0300060513487652

231. Zhang YJ, Zhang DH, Wang F, Xu DF, Guo Y, Cui W (2015) Serum miRNAs panel (miR-16-2*, miR-195, miR-2861, miR-497) as novel non-invasive biomarkers for detection of cervical cancer. Sci Rep-Uk 5:17942

232. Zhao S, Yao DS, Chen JY, Ding N (2013) Circulating miRNA-20a and miRNA-203 for screening lymph node metastasis in early stage cervical cancer. Genet Test Mol Biomarkers 17(8):631–636. doi:10.1089/gtmb.2013.0085

233. Hornick NI, Huan J, Doron B, Goloviznina NA, Lapidus J, Chang BH, Kurre P (2015) Serum Exosome MicroRNA as a minimally-invasive early biomarker of AML. Sci Rep-Uk 5:ARTN 11295. doi:10.1038/srep11295

234. Fayyad-Kazan H, Bitar N, Najar M, Lewalle P, Fayyad-Kazan M, Badran R, Hamade E, Daher A, Hussein N, ElDirani R, Berri F, Vanhamme L, Burny A, Martiat P, Rouas R, Badran B (2013) Circulating miR-150 and miR-342 in plasma are novel potential biomarkers for acute myeloid leukemia. J Transl Med 11:Artn 31. doi:10.1186/1479-5876-11-31

235. Baraniskin A, Kuhnhenn J, Schlegel U, Chan A, Deckert M, Gold R, Maghnouj A, Zollner H, Reinacher-Schick A, Schmiegel W, Hahn SA, Schroers R (2011) Identification of microRNAs in the cerebrospinal fluid as marker for primary diffuse large B-cell lymphoma of the central nervous system. Blood 117(11):3140–3146. doi:10.1182/blood-2010-09-308684

236. Ohyashiki K, Umezu T, Yoshizawa S, Ito Y, Ohyashiki M, Kawashima H, Tanaka M, Kuroda M, Ohyashiki JH (2011) Clinical impact of down-regulated plasma miR-92a levels in non-Hodgkin's lymphoma. PLoS One 6(2):ARTN e16408. doi:10.1371/journal.pone.0016408

237. Chen X, Ba Y, Ma L, Cai X, Yin Y, Wang K, Guo J, Zhang Y, Chen J, Guo X, Li Q, Li X, Wang W, Zhang Y, Wang J, Jiang X, Xiang Y, Xu C, Zheng P, Zhang J, Li R, Zhang H, Shang X, Gong T, Ning G, Wang J, Zen K, Zhang J, Zhang CY (2008) Characterization of microRNAs in serum: a novel class of biomarkers for diagnosis of cancer and other diseases. Cell Res 18(10):997–1006. doi:10.1038/cr.2008.282

238. Gonzalo S, Jaco I, Fraga MF, Chen T, Li E, Esteller M, Blasco MA (2006) DNA methyltransferases control telomere length and telomere recombination in mammalian cells. Nat Cell Biol 8(4):416–424. doi:10.1038/ncb1386

239. Peters AH, O'Carroll D, Scherthan H, Mechtler K, Sauer S, Schofer C, Weipoltshammer K, Pagani M, Lachner M, Kohlmaier A, Opravil S, Doyle M, Sibilia M, Jenuwein T (2001) Loss of the Suv39h histone methyltransferases impairs mammalian heterochromatin and genome stability. Cell 107(3):323–337

240. Tennen RI, Bua DJ, Wright WE, Chua KF (2011) SIRT6 is required for maintenance of telomere position effect in human cells. Nat Commun 2:433. doi:10.1038/ncomms1443

241. Garcia-Cao M, O'Sullivan R, Peters AH, Jenuwein T, Blasco MA (2004) Epigenetic regulation of telomere length in mammalian cells by the Suv39h1 and Suv39h2 histone methyltransferases. Nat Genet 36(1):94–99. doi:10.1038/ng1278

242. Lachner M, O'Carroll D, Rea S, Mechtler K, Jenuwein T (2001) Methylation of histone H3 lysine 9 creates a binding site for HP1 proteins. Nature 410(6824):116–120. doi:10.1038/35065132

243. Gonzalo S, Garcia-Cao M, Fraga MF, Schotta G, Peters AH, Cotter SE, Eguia R, Dean DC, Esteller M, Jenuwein T, Blasco MA (2005) Role of the RB1 family in stabilizing histone methylation at constitutive heterochromatin. Nat Cell Biol 7(4):420–428. doi:10.1038/ncb1235

244. Dang-Nguyen TQ, Haraguchi S, Furusawa T, Somfai T, Kaneda M, Watanabe S, Akagi S, Kikuchi K, Tajima A, Nagai T (2013) Downregulation of histone methyltransferase genes SUV39H1 and SUV39H2 increases telomere length in embryonic stem-like cells and embryonic fibroblasts in pigs. J Reprod Dev 59(1):27–32

245. Rodriguez-Rodero S, Fernandez-Morera JL, Fernandez AF, Menendez-Torre E, Fraga MF (2010) Epigenetic regulation of aging. Discov Med 10(52):225–233

246. Gottschling DE, Aparicio OM, Billington BL, Zakian VA (1990) Position effect at S. cerevisiae telomeres: reversible repression of pol II transcription. Cell 63(4):751–762

247. Baur JA, Zou Y, Shay JW, Wright WE (2001) Telomere position effect in human cells. Science 292(5524):2075–2077. doi:10.1126/science.1062329

248. Stadler G, Rahimov F, King OD, Chen JC, Robin JD, Wagner KR, Shay JW, Emerson CP Jr, Wright WE (2013) Telomere position effect regulates DUX4 in human facioscapulohumeral muscular dystrophy. Nat Struct Mol Biol 20(6):671–678. doi:10.1038/nsmb.2571

249. Robin JD, Ludlow AT, Batten K, Magdinier F, Stadler G, Wagner KR, Shay JW, Wright WE (2014) Telomere position effect: regulation of gene expression with progressive telomere shortening over long distances. Genes Dev 28(22):2464–2476. doi:10.1101/gad.251041.114

250. Kim W, Ludlow AT, Min J, Robin JD, Stadler G, Mender I, Lai TP, Zhang N, Wright WE, Shay JW (2016) Regulation of the human telomerase Gene TERT by telomere position effect-over long distances (TPE-OLD): implications for aging and cancer. PLoS Biol 14(12):e2000016. doi:10.1371/journal.pbio.2000016

251. Surace C, Berardinelli F, Masotti A, Roberti MC, Da Sacco L, D'Elia G, Sirleto P, Digilio MC, Cusmai R, Grotta S, Petrocchi S, El Hachem M, Pisaneschi E, Ciocca L, Russo S, Lepri FR, Sgura A, Angioni A (2014) Telomere shortening and telomere position effect in mild ring 17 syndrome. Epigenetics Chromatin 7(1):1. doi:10.1186/1756-8935-7-1

252. Moyzis RK, Buckingham JM, Cram LS, Dani M, Deaven LL, Jones MD, Meyne J, Ratliff RL, Wu JR (1988) A highly conserved repetitive DNA sequence, (TTAGGG)n, present at the telomeres of human chromosomes. Proc Natl Acad Sci U S A 85(18):6622–6626

253. O'Sullivan RJ, Karlseder J (2010) Telomeres: protecting chromosomes against genome instability. Nat Rev Mol Cell Biol 11(3):171–181. doi:10.1038/nrm2848

254. de Lange T (2005) Shelterin: the protein complex that shapes and safeguards human telomeres. Genes Dev 19(18):2100–2110. doi:10.1101/gad.1346005

255. Sfeir A, de Lange T (2012) Removal of shelterin reveals the telomere end-protection problem. Science 336(6081):593–597. doi:10.1126/science.1218498

256. Levy MZ, Allsopp RC, Futcher AB, Greider CW, Harley CB (1992) Telomere end-replication problem and cell aging. J Mol Biol 225(4):951–960

257. Lopatina NG, Poole JC, Saldanha SN, Hansen NJ, Key JS, Pita MA, Andrews LG, Tollefsbol TO (2003) Control mechanisms in the regulation of telomerase reverse transcriptase expression in differentiating human teratocarcinoma cells. Biochem Biophys Res Commun 306(3):650–659

258. Shin KH, Kang MK, Dicterow E, Park NH (2003) Hypermethylation of the hTERT promoter inhibits the expression of telomerase activity in normal oral fibroblasts and senescent normal oral keratinocytes. Br J Cancer 89(8):1473–1478. doi:10.1038/sj.bjc.6601291

259. Devereux TR, Horikawa I, Anna CH, Annab LA, Afshari CA, Barrett JC (1999) DNA methylation analysis of the promoter region of the human telomerase reverse transcriptase (hTERT) gene. Cancer Res 59(24):6087–6090

260. Dessain SK, Yu H, Reddel RR, Beijersbergen RL, Weinberg RA (2000) Methylation of the human telomerase gene CpG island. Cancer Res 60(3):537–541

261. Barthel FP, Wei W, Tang M, Martinez-Ledesma E, Hu X, Amin SB, Akdemir KC, Seth S, Song X, Wang Q, Lichtenberg T, Hu J, Zhang J, Zheng S, Verhaak RG (2017) Systematic analysis of telomere length and somatic alterations in 31 cancer types. Nat Genet 49(3). doi:10.1038/ng.3781

262. Renaud S, Loukinov D, Abdullaev Z, Guilleret I, Bosman FT, Lobanenkov V, Benhattar J (2007) Dual role of DNA methylation inside and outside of CTCF-binding regions in the transcriptional regulation of the telomerase hTERT gene. Nucleic Acids Res 35(4):1245–1256. doi:10.1093/nar/gkl1125

263. Takakura M, Kyo S, Sowa Y, Wang Z, Yatabe N, Maida Y, Tanaka M, Inoue M (2001) Telomerase activation by histone deacetylase inhibitor in normal cells. Nucleic Acids Res 29(14):3006–3011

264. Hou M, Wang X, Popov N, Zhang A, Zhao X, Zhou R, Zetterberg A, Bjorkholm M, Henriksson M, Gruber A, Xu D (2002) The histone deacetylase inhibitor trichostatin a derepresses the telomerase reverse transcriptase (hTERT) gene in human cells. Exp Cell Res 274(1):25–34. doi:10.1006/excr.2001.5462

265. Khaw AK, Silasudjana M, Banerjee B, Suzuki M, Baskar R, Hande MP (2007) Inhibition of telomerase activity and human telomerase reverse transcriptase gene expression by histone deacetylase inhibitor in human brain cancer cells. Mutat Res 625(1–2):134–144. doi:10.1016/j.mrfmmm.2007.06.005

266. Blasco MA (2007) The epigenetic regulation of mammalian telomeres. Nat Rev Genet 8(4):299–309. doi:10.1038/nrg2047

267. Atkinson SP, Hoare SF, Glasspool RM, Keith WN (2005) Lack of telomerase gene expression in alternative lengthening of telomere cells is associated with chromatin remodeling of the hTR and hTERT gene promoters. Cancer Res 65(17):7585–7590. doi:10.1158/0008-5472. CAN-05-1715

268. Shay JW, Bacchetti S (1997) A survey of telomerase activity in human cancer. Eur J Cancer 33(5):787–791. doi:10.1016/S0959-8049(97)00062-2

269. Bryan TM, Englezou A, Dalla-Pozza L, Dunham MA, Reddel RR (1997) Evidence for an alternative mechanism for maintaining telomere length in human tumors and tumor-derived cell lines. Nat Med 3(11):1271–1274

270. Cesare AJ, Reddel RR (2010) Alternative lengthening of telomeres: models, mechanisms and implications. Nat Rev Genet 11(5):319–330. doi:10.1038/nrg2763

271. Sturm D, Witt H, Hovestadt V, Khuong-Quang DA, Jones DT, Konermann C, Pfaff E, Tonjes M, Sill M, Bender S, Kool M, Zapatka M, Becker N, Zucknick M, Hielscher T, Liu XY, Fontebasso AM, Ryzhova M, Albrecht S, Jacob K, Wolter M, Ebinger M, Schuhmann MU, van Meter T, Fruhwald MC, Hauch H, Pekrun A, Radlwimmer B, Niehues T, von Komorowski G, Durken M, Kulozik AE, Madden J, Donson A, Foreman NK, Drissi R, Fouladi M, Scheurlen W, von Deimling A, Monoranu C, Roggendorf W, Herold-Mende C, Unterberg A, Kramm CM, Felsberg J, Hartmann C, Wiestler B, Wick W, Milde T, Witt O, Lindroth AM, Schwartzentruber J, Faury D, Fleming A, Zakrzewska M, Liberski PP, Zakrzewski K, Hauser P, Garami M, Klekner A, Bognar L, Morrissy S, Cavalli F, Taylor MD, van Sluis P, Koster J, Versteeg R, Volckmann R, Mikkelsen T, Aldape K, Reifenberger G, Collins VP, Majewski J, Korshunov A, Lichter P, Plass C, Jabado N, Pfister SM (2012) Hotspot mutations in H3F3A and IDH1 define distinct epigenetic and biological subgroups of glioblastoma. Cancer Cell 22(4):425–437. doi:10.1016/j.ccr.2012.08.024

272. Kannan K, Inagaki A, Silber J, Gorovets D, Zhang J, Kastenhuber ER, Heguy A, Petrini JH, Chan TA, Huse JT (2012) Whole-exome sequencing identifies ATRX mutation as a key molecular determinant in lower-grade glioma. Oncotarget 3(10):1194–1203. doi:10.18632/oncotarget.689

273. Jiao Y, Shi C, Edil BH, de Wilde RF, Klimstra DS, Maitra A, Schulick RD, Tang LH, Wolfgang CL, Choti MA, Velculescu VE, Diaz LA Jr, Vogelstein B, Kinzler KW, Hruban RH, Papadopoulos N (2011) DAXX/ATRX, MEN1, and mTOR pathway genes are frequently altered in pancreatic neuroendocrine tumors. Science 331(6021):1199–1203. doi:10.1126/science.1200609

274. Durant ST (2012) Telomerase-independent paths to immortality in predictable cancer subtypes. J Cancer 3:67–82. doi:10.7150/jca.3965

275. Wong LH, McGhie JD, Sim M, Anderson MA, Ahn S, Hannan RD, George AJ, Morgan KA, Mann JR, Choo KH (2010) ATRX interacts with H3.3 in maintaining telomere structural integrity in pluripotent embryonic stem cells. Genome Res 20(3):351–360. doi:10.1101/gr.101477.109

276. Gibbons RJ, McDowell TL, Raman S, O'Rourke DM, Garrick D, Ayyub H, Higgs DR (2000) Mutations in ATRX, encoding a SWI/SNF-like protein, cause diverse changes in the pattern of DNA methylation. Nat Genet 24(4):368–371. doi:10.1038/74191

277. Drane P, Ouararhni K, Depaux A, Shuaib M, Hamiche A (2010) The death-associated protein DAXX is a novel histone chaperone involved in the replication-independent deposition of H3.3. Genes Dev 24(12):1253–1265. doi:10.1101/gad.566910

278. Lewis PW, Elsaesser SJ, Noh KM, Stadler SC, Allis CD (2010) Daxx is an H3.3-specific histone chaperone and cooperates with ATRX in replication-independent chromatin assembly at telomeres. Proc Natl Acad Sci U S A 107(32):14075–14080. doi:10.1073/pnas.1008850107

279. Napier CE, Huschtscha LI, Harvey A, Bower K, Noble JR, Hendrickson EA, Reddel RR (2015) ATRX represses alternative lengthening of telomeres. Oncotarget 6(18):16543–16558. doi:10.18632/oncotarget.3846

280. O'Sullivan RJ, Almouzni G (2014) Assembly of telomeric chromatin to create ALTernative endings. Trends Cell Biol 24(11):675–685. doi:10.1016/j.tcb.2014.07.007

281. Ng LJ, Cropley JE, Pickett HA, Reddel RR, Suter CM (2009) Telomerase activity is associated with an increase in DNA methylation at the proximal subtelomere and a reduction in telomeric transcription. Nucleic Acids Res 37(4):1152–1159. doi:10.1093/nar/gkn1030

282. Episkopou H, Draskovic I, Van Beneden A, Tilman G, Mattiussi M, Gobin M, Arnoult N, Londono-Vallejo A, Decottignies A (2014) Alternative lengthening of telomeres is characterized by reduced compaction of telomeric chromatin. Nucleic Acids Res 42(7):4391–4405. doi:10.1093/nar/gku114

283. Feuerhahn S, Iglesias N, Panza A, Porro A, Lingner J (2010) TERRA biogenesis, turnover and implications for function. FEBS Lett 584(17):3812–3818. doi:10.1016/j.febslet.2010.07.032

284. Deng Z, Wang Z, Stong N, Plasschaert R, Moczan A, Chen HS, Hu S, Wikramasinghe P, Davuluri RV, Bartolomei MS, Riethman H, Lieberman PM (2012) A role for CTCF and cohesin in subtelomere chromatin organization, TERRA transcription, and telomere end protection. EMBO J 31(21):4165–4178. doi:10.1038/emboj.2012.266

285. Azzalin CM, Reichenbach P, Khoriauli L, Giulotto E, Lingner J (2007) Telomeric repeat containing RNA and RNA surveillance factors at mammalian chromosome ends. Science 318(5851):798–801. doi:10.1126/science.1147182

286. Arnoult N, Van Beneden A, Decottignies A (2012) Telomere length regulates TERRA levels through increased trimethylation of telomeric H3K9 and HP1alpha. Nat Struct Mol Biol 19(9):948–956. doi:10.1038/nsmb.2364

287. Benetti R, Garcia-Cao M, Blasco MA (2007) Telomere length regulates the epigenetic status of mammalian telomeres and subtelomeres. Nat Genet 39(2):243–250. doi:10.1038/ng1952

288. Thijssen PE, Tobi EW, Balog J, Schouten SG, Kremer D, El Bouazzaoui F, Henneman P, Putter H, Eline Slagboom P, Heijmans BT, van der Maarel SM (2013) Chromatin remodeling of human subtelomeres and TERRA promoters upon cellular senescence: commonalities and differences between chromosomes. Epigenetics Off J DNA Meth Soc 8(5):512–521. doi:10.4161/epi.24450

289. Flynn RL, Cox KE, Jeitany M, Wakimoto H, Bryll AR, Ganem NJ, Bersani F, Pineda JR, Suva ML, Benes CH, Haber DA, Boussin FD, Zou L (2015) Alternative lengthening of telomeres renders cancer cells hypersensitive to ATR inhibitors. Science 347(6219):273–277. doi:10.1126/science.1257216

290. Reig-Viader R, Vila-Cejudo M, Vitelli V, Busca R, Sabate M, Giulotto E, Caldes MG, Ruiz-Herrera A (2014) Telomeric repeat-containing RNA (TERRA) and telomerase are components of telomeres during mammalian gametogenesis. Biol Reprod 90(5):103. doi:10.1095/biolreprod.113.116954

291. Deng Z, Norseen J, Wiedmer A, Riethman H, Lieberman PM (2009) TERRA RNA binding to TRF2 facilitates heterochromatin formation and ORC recruitment at telomeres. Mol Cell 35(4):403–413. doi:10.1016/j.molcel.2009.06.025

292. Porro A, Feuerhahn S, Lingner J (2014) TERRA-reinforced association of LSD1 with MRE11 promotes processing of uncapped telomeres. Cell Rep 6(4):765–776. doi:10.1016/j.celrep.2014.01.022

293. Redon S, Reichenbach P, Lingner J (2010) The non-coding RNA TERRA is a natural ligand and direct inhibitor of human telomerase. Nucleic Acids Res 38(17):5797–5806. doi:10.1093/nar/gkq296

294. Redon S, Zemp I, Lingner J (2013) A three-state model for the regulation of telomerase by TERRA and hnRNPA1. Nucleic Acids Res 41(19):9117–9128. doi:10.1093/nar/gkt695

295. Negishi Y, Kawaji H, Minoda A, Usui K (2015) Identification of chromatin marks at TERRA promoter and encoding region. Biochem Biophys Res Commun 467(4):1052–1057. doi:10.1016/j.bbrc.2015.09.176

296. Nergadze SG, Farnung BO, Wischnewski H, Khoriauli L, Vitelli V, Chawla R, Giulotto E, Azzalin CM (2009) CpG-island promoters drive transcription of human telomeres. RNA 15(12):2186–2194. doi:10.1261/rna.1748309

297. Caslini C, Connelly JA, Serna A, Broccoli D, Hess JL (2009) MLL associates with telomeres and regulates telomeric repeat-containing RNA transcription. Mol Cell Biol 29(16):4519–4526. doi:10.1128/MCB.00195-09

298. Neumann AA, Watson CM, Noble JR, Pickett HA, Tam PP, Reddel RR (2013) Alternative lengthening of telomeres in normal mammalian somatic cells. Genes Dev 27(1):18–23. doi:10.1101/gad.205062.112

299. Novakovic B, Napier CE, Vryer R, Dimitriadis E, Manuelpillai U, Sharkey A, Craig JM, Reddel RR, Saffery R (2016) DNA methylation mediated up-regulation of TERRA non-coding RNA is coincident with elongated telomeres in the human placenta. Mol Hum Reprod 22(11):791–799. doi:10.1093/molehr/gaw053

300. Peinado H, Aleckovic M, Lavotshkin S, Matei I, Costa-Silva B, Moreno-Bueno G, Hergueta-Redondo M, Williams C, Garcia-Santos G, Ghajar C, Nitadori-Hoshino A, Hoffman C, Badal K, Garcia BA, Callahan MK, Yuan J, Martins VR, Skog J, Kaplan RN, Brady MS, Wolchok JD, Chapman PB, Kang Y, Bromberg J, Lyden D (2012) Melanoma exosomes educate bone marrow progenitor cells toward a pro-metastatic phenotype through MET. Nat Med 18(6):883–891. doi:10.1038/nm.2753

301. Wang Z, Deng Z, Dahmane N, Tsai K, Wang P, Williams DR, Kossenkov AV, Showe LC, Zhang R, Huang Q, Conejo-Garcia JR, Lieberman PM (2015) Telomeric repeat-containing RNA (TERRA) constitutes a nucleoprotein component of extracellular inflammatory exosomes. Proc Natl Acad Sci U S A 112(46):E6293–E6300. doi:10.1073/pnas.1505962112

302. Wang Z, Lieberman PM (2016) The crosstalk of telomere dysfunction and inflammation through cell-free TERRA containing exosomes. RNA Biol 13(8):690–695. doi:10.1080/15476286.2016.1203503

303. Willeit P, Willeit J, Mayr A, Weger S, Oberhollenzer F, Brandstatter A, Kronenberg F, Kiechl S (2010) Telomere length and risk of incident cancer and cancer mortality. JAMA 304(1):69–75. doi:10.1001/jama.2010.897

304. Prescott J, Wentzensen IM, Savage SA, De Vivo I (2012) Epidemiologic evidence for a role of telomere dysfunction in cancer etiology. Mutat Res 730(1–2):75–84. doi:10.1016/j. mrfmmm.2011.06.009
305. Pellatt AJ, Wolff RK, Torres-Mejia G, John EM, Herrick JS, Lundgreen A, Baumgartner KB, Giuliano AR, Hines LM, Fejerman L, Cawthon R, Slattery ML (2013) Telomere length, telomere-related genes, and breast cancer risk: the breast cancer health disparities study. Genes Chromosomes Cancer 52(7):595–609. doi:10.1002/gcc.22056
306. Zhu X, Han W, Xue W, Zou Y, Xie C, Du J, Jin G (2016) The association between telomere length and cancer risk in population studies. Sci Rep 6:22243. doi:10.1038/srep22243
307. Doi T, Shibata K, Yoshida M, Takagi M, Tera M, Nagasawa K, Shin-ya K, Takahashi T (2011) (S)-stereoisomer of telomestatin as a potent G-quadruplex binder and telomerase inhibitor. Org Biomol Chem 9(2):387–393. doi:10.1039/c0ob00513d
308. Tefferi A, Lasho TL, Begna KH, Patnaik MM, Zblewski DL, Finke CM, Laborde RR, Wassie E, Schimek L, Hanson CA, Gangat N, Wang X, Pardanani A (2015) A pilot study of the telomerase inhibitor Imetelstat for Myelofibrosis. N Engl J Med 373(10):908–919. doi:10.1056/NEJMoa1310523
309. Husemann Y, Geigl JB, Schubert F, Musiani P, Meyer M, Burghart E, Forni G, Eils R, Fehm T, Riethmuller G, Klein CA (2008) Systemic spread is an early step in breast cancer. Cancer Cell 13(1):58–68. doi:10.1016/j.ccr.2007.12.003
310. Dobrovic A, Kristensen LS (2009) DNA methylation, epimutations and cancer predisposition. Int J Biochem Cell Biol 41(1):34–39. doi:10.1016/j.biocel.2008.09.006
311. Quiet CA, Ferguson DJ, Weichselbaum RR, Hellman S (1995) Natural history of node-negative breast cancer: a study of 826 patients with long-term follow-up. J Clin Oncol 13(5):1144–1151. doi:10.1200/jco.1995.13.5.1144
312. Karrison TG, Ferguson DJ, Meier P (1999) Dormancy of mammary carcinoma after mastectomy. J Natl Cancer Inst 91(1):80–85
313. Luna-Perez P, Rodriguez-Coria DF, Arroyo B, Gonzalez-Macouzet J (1998) The natural history of liver metastases from colorectal cancer. Arch Med Res 29(4):319–324
314. Pound CR, Partin AW, Eisenberger MA, Chan DW, Pearson JD, Walsh PC (1999) Natural history of progression after PSA elevation following radical prostatectomy. JAMA 281(17):1591–1597
315. Fisher B, Anderson S, Bryant J, Margolese RG, Deutsch M, Fisher ER, Jeong JH, Wolmark N (2002) Twenty-year follow-up of a randomized trial comparing total mastectomy, lumpectomy, and lumpectomy plus irradiation for the treatment of invasive breast cancer. N Engl J Med 347(16):1233–1241. doi:10.1056/NEJMoa022152
316. Strauss DC, Thomas JM (2010) Transmission of donor melanoma by organ transplantation. Lancet Oncol 11(8):790–796. doi:10.1016/S1470-2045(10)70024-3
317. Pantel K, Cote RJ, Fodstad O (1999) Detection and clinical importance of micrometastatic disease. J Natl Cancer Inst 91(13):1113–1124
318. Engel J, Eckel R, Kerr J, Schmidt M, Furstenberger G, Richter R, Sauer H, Senn HJ, Holzel D (2003) The process of metastasisation for breast cancer. Eur J Cancer 39(12):1794–1806
319. Braun S, Kentenich C, Janni W, Hepp F, de Waal J, Willgeroth F, Sommer H, Pantel K (2000) Lack of effect of adjuvant chemotherapy on the elimination of single dormant tumor cells in bone marrow of high-risk breast cancer patients. J Clin Oncol 18(1):80–86. doi:10.1200/jco.2000.18.1.80
320. Mansi JL, Berger U, Easton D, McDonnell T, Redding WH, Gazet JC, McKinna A, Powles TJ, Coombes RC (1987) Micrometastases in bone marrow in patients with primary breast cancer: evaluation as an early predictor of bone metastases. Br Med J (Clin Res Ed) 295(6606):1093–1096
321. Klein CA (2000) The biology and analysis of single disseminated tumour cells. Trends Cell Biol 10(11):489–493
322. Hartkopf AD, Taran FA, Wallwiener M, Hahn M, Becker S, Solomayer EF, Brucker SY, Fehm TN, Wallwiener D (2014) Prognostic relevance of disseminated tumour cells from the bone marrow of early stage breast cancer patients – results from a large single-centre analysis. Eur J Cancer 50(15):2550–2559. doi:10.1016/j.ejca.2014.06.025

323. Effenberger KE, Schroeder C, Eulenburg C, Reeh M, Tachezy M, Riethdorf S, Vashist YK, Izbicki JR, Pantel K, Bockhorn M (2012) Disseminated tumor cells in pancreatic cancer-an independent prognosticator of disease progression and survival. Int J Cancer 131(4):E475–E483. doi:10.1002/ijc.26439

324. Lilleby W, Stensvold A, Mills IG, Nesland JM (2013) Disseminated tumor cells and their prognostic significance in nonmetastatic prostate cancer patients. Int J Cancer 133(1):149–155. doi:10.1002/ijc.28002

325. Muller V, Stahmann N, Riethdorf S, Rau T, Zabel T, Goetz A, Janicke F, Pantel K (2005) Circulating tumor cells in breast cancer: correlation to bone marrow micrometastases, heterogeneous response to systemic therapy and low proliferative activity. Clin Cancer Res 11(10):3678–3685. doi:10.1158/1078-0432.CCR-04-2469

326. Schindlbeck C, Andergassen U, Hofmann S, Juckstock J, Jeschke U, Sommer H, Friese K, Janni W, Rack B (2013) Comparison of circulating tumor cells (CTC) in peripheral blood and disseminated tumor cells in the bone marrow (DTC-BM) of breast cancer patients. J Cancer Res Clin Oncol 139(6):1055–1062. doi:10.1007/s00432-013-1418-0

327. Balic M, Lin H, Young L, Hawes D, Giuliano A, McNamara G, Datar RH, Cote RJ (2006) Most early disseminated cancer cells detected in bone marrow of breast cancer patients have a putative breast cancer stem cell phenotype. Clin Cancer Res 12(19):5615 5621. doi:10.1158/1078-0432.CCR-06-0169

328. Aktas B, Tewes M, Fehm T, Hauch S, Kimmig R, Kasimir-Bauer S (2009) Stem cell and epithelial-mesenchymal transition markers are frequently overexpressed in circulating tumor cells of metastatic breast cancer patients. Breast Cancer Res 11(4):R46. doi:10.1186/bcr2333

329. Raimondi C, Gradilone A, Naso G, Vincenzi B, Petracca A, Nicolazzo C, Palazzo A, Saltarelli R, Spremberg F, Cortesi E, Gazzaniga P (2011) Epithelial-mesenchymal transition and stemness features in circulating tumor cells from breast cancer patients. Breast Cancer Res Treat 130(2):449–455. doi:10.1007/s10549-011-1373-x

330. Visvader JE, Lindeman GJ (2008) Cancer stem cells in solid tumours: accumulating evidence and unresolved questions. Nat Rev Cancer 8(10):755–768. doi:10.1038/nrc2499

331. Gazin C, Wajapeyee N, Gobeil S, Virbasius CM, Green MR (2007) An elaborate pathway required for Ras-mediated epigenetic silencing. Nature 449(7165):1073–1077. doi:10.1038/nature06251

332. Zhu J, Sammons MA, Donahue G, Dou Z, Vedadi M, Getlik M, Barsyte-Lovejoy D, Al-awar R, Katona BW, Shilatifard A, Huang J, Hua X, Arrowsmith CH, Berger SL (2015) Gain-of-function p53 mutants co-opt chromatin pathways to drive cancer growth. Nature 525(7568):206–211. doi:10.1038/nature15251

333. Lu C, Ward PS, Kapoor GS, Rohle D, Turcan S, Abdel-Wahab O, Edwards CR, Khanin R, Figueroa ME, Melnick A, Wellen KE, O'Rourke DM, Berger SL, Chan TA, Levine RL, Mellinghoff IK, Thompson CB (2012) IDH mutation impairs histone demethylation and results in a block to cell differentiation. Nature 483(7390):474–478. doi:10.1038/nature10860

334. Boyer LA, Lee TI, Cole MF, Johnstone SE, Levine SS, Zucker JP, Guenther MG, Kumar RM, Murray HL, Jenner RG, Gifford DK, Melton DA, Jaenisch R, Young RA (2005) Core transcriptional regulatory circuitry in human embryonic stem cells. Cell 122(6):947–956. doi:10.1016/j.cell.2005.08.020

335. Takahashi K, Yamanaka S (2016) A decade of transcription factor-mediated reprogramming to pluripotency. Nat Rev Mol Cell Biol 17(3):183–193. doi:10.1038/nrm.2016.8

336. Ohnishi K, Semi K, Yamamoto T, Shimizu M, Tanaka A, Mitsunaga K, Okita K, Osafune K, Arioka Y, Maeda T, Soejima H, Moriwaki H, Yamanaka S, Woltjen K, Yamada Y (2014) Premature termination of reprogramming in vivo leads to cancer development through altered epigenetic regulation. Cell 156(4):663–677. doi:10.1016/j.cell.2014.01.005

337. Mu P, Zhang Z, Benelli M, Karthaus WR, Hoover E, Chen CC, Wongvipat J, Ku SY, Gao D, Cao Z, Shah N, Adams EJ, Abida W, Watson PA, Prandi D, Huang CH, de Stanchina E, Lowe SW, Ellis L, Beltran H, Rubin MA, Goodrich DW, Demichelis F, Sawyers CL (2017) SOX2 promotes lineage plasticity and antiandrogen resistance in TP53- and RB1-deficient prostate cancer. Science 355(6320):84–88. doi:10.1126/science.aah4307

338. Wang D, Lu P, Zhang H, Luo M, Zhang X, Wei X, Gao J, Zhao Z, Liu C (2014) Oct-4 and Nanog promote the epithelial-mesenchymal transition of breast cancer stem cells and are associated with poor prognosis in breast cancer patients. Oncotarget 5(21):10803–10815. doi:10.18632/oncotarget.2506

339. Rudin CM, Durinck S, Stawiski EW, Poirier JT, Modrusan Z, Shames DS, Bergbower EA, Guan Y, Shin J, Guillory J, Rivers CS, Foo CK, Bhatt D, Stinson J, Gnad F, Haverty PM, Gentleman R, Chaudhuri S, Janakiraman V, Jaiswal BS, Parikh C, Yuan W, Zhang Z, Koeppen H, Wu TD, Stern HM, Yauch RL, Huffman KE, Paskulin DD, Illei PB, Varella-Garcia M, Gazdar AF, de Sauvage FJ, Bourgon R, Minna JD, Brock MV, Seshagiri S (2012) Comprehensive genomic analysis identifies SOX2 as a frequently amplified gene in small-cell lung cancer. Nat Genet 44(10):1111–1116. doi:10.1038/ng.2405

340. Luo W, Li S, Peng B, Ye Y, Deng X, Yao K (2013) Embryonic stem cells markers SOX2, OCT4 and Nanog expression and their correlations with epithelial-mesenchymal transition in nasopharyngeal carcinoma. PLoS One 8(2):e56324. doi:10.1371/journal.pone.0056324

341. Chiou SH, Wang ML, Chou YT, Chen CJ, Hong CF, Hsieh WJ, Chang HT, Chen YS, Lin TW, Hsu HS, Wu CW (2010) Coexpression of Oct4 and Nanog enhances malignancy in lung adenocarcinoma by inducing cancer stem cell-like properties and epithelial-mesenchymal trans-differentiation. Cancer Res 70(24):10433–10444. doi:10.1158/0008-5472.CAN-10-2638

342. Alonso MM, Diez-Valle R, Manterola L, Rubio A, Liu D, Cortes-Santiago N, Urquiza L, Jauregi P, Lopez de Munain A, Sampron N, Aramburu A, Tejada-Solis S, Vicente C, Odero MD, Bandres E, Garcia-Foncillas J, Idoate MA, Lang FF, Fueyo J, Gomez-Manzano C (2011) Genetic and epigenetic modifications of Sox2 contribute to the invasive phenotype of malignant gliomas. PLoS One 6(11):e26740. doi:10.1371/journal.pone.0026740

343. Nettersheim D, Biermann K, Gillis AJ, Steger K, Looijenga LH, Schorle H (2011) NANOG promoter methylation and expression correlation during normal and malignant human germ cell development. Epigenetics Off J DNA Meth Soc 6(1):114–122. doi:10.4161/epi.6.1.13433

344. Berezovsky AD, Poisson LM, Cherba D, Webb CP, Transou AD, Lemke NW, Hong X, Hasselbach LA, Irtenkauf SM, Mikkelsen T, de Carvalho AC (2014) Sox2 promotes malignancy in glioblastoma by regulating plasticity and astrocytic differentiation. Neoplasia 16 (3):193–206, 206 e119–125. doi:10.1016/j.neo.2014.03.006

345. Pandian V, Ramraj S, Khan FH, Azim T, Aravindan N (2015) Metastatic neuroblastoma cancer stem cells exhibit flexible plasticity and adaptive stemness signaling. Stem Cell Res Ther 6:2. doi:10.1186/s13287-015-0002-8

346. Lin SC, Chou YT, Jiang SS, Chang JL, Chung CH, Kao YR, Chang IS, Wu CW (2016) Epigenetic switch between SOX2 and SOX9 regulates cancer cell plasticity. Cancer Res 76(23):7036–7048. doi:10.1158/0008-5472.CAN-15-3178

347. Baylin SB, Ohm JE (2006) Epigenetic gene silencing in cancer – a mechanism for early oncogenic pathway addiction? Nat Rev Cancer 6(2):107–116. doi:10.1038/nrc1799

348. Kahn HJ, Presta A, Yang LY, Blondal J, Trudeau M, Lickley L, Holloway C, McCready DR, Maclean D, Marks A (2004) Enumeration of circulating tumor cells in the blood of breast cancer patients after filtration enrichment: correlation with disease stage. Breast Cancer Res Treat 86(3):237–247. doi:10.1023/B:BREA.0000036897.92513.72

349. Lin HK, Zheng S, Williams AJ, Balic M, Groshen S, Scher HI, Fleisher M, Stadler W, Datar RH, Tai YC, Cote RJ (2010) Portable filter-based microdevice for detection and characterization of circulating tumor cells. Clin Cancer Res 16(20):5011–5018. doi:10.1158/1078-0432. CCR-10-1105

350. Coumans FA, van Dalum G, Beck M, Terstappen LW (2013) Filter characteristics influencing circulating tumor cell enrichment from whole blood. PLoS One 8(4):e61770. doi:10.1371/journal.pone.0061770

351. Kruger W, Datta C, Badbaran A, Togel F, Gutensohn K, Carrero I, Kroger N, Janicke F, Zander AR (2000) Immunomagnetic tumor cell selection--implications for the detection of disseminated cancer cells. Transfusion 40(12):1489–1493

352. Weihrauch MR, Skibowski E, Draube A, Geller A, Tesch H, Diehl V, Bohlen H (2002) Immunomagnetic enrichment and detection of isolated tumor cells in bone marrow of patients with epithelial malignancies. Clin Exp Metastasis 19(7):617–621

353. Dalerba P, Kalisky T, Sahoo D, Rajendran PS, Rothenberg ME, Leyrat AA, Sim S, Okamoto J, Johnston DM, Qian D, Zabala M, Bueno J, Neff NF, Wang J, Shelton AA, Visser B, Hisamori S, Shimono Y, van de Wetering M, Clevers H, Clarke MF, Quake SR (2011) Single-cell dissection of transcriptional heterogeneity in human colon tumors. Nat Biotechnol 29(12):1120–1127. doi:10.1038/nbt.2038

354. Yachida S, Jones S, Bozic I, Antal T, Leary R, Fu B, Kamiyama M, Hruban RH, Eshleman JR, Nowak MA, Velculescu VE, Kinzler KW, Vogelstein B, Iacobuzio-Donahue CA (2010) Distant metastasis occurs late during the genetic evolution of pancreatic cancer. Nature 467(7319):1114–1117. doi:10.1038/nature09515

355. Fan HC, Wang J, Potanina A, Quake SR (2011) Whole-genome molecular haplotyping of single cells. Nat Biotechnol 29(1):51–57. doi:10.1038/nbt.1739

356. Rotem A, Ram O, Shoresh N, Sperling RA, Goren A, Weitz DA, Bernstein BE (2015) Single-cell ChIP-seq reveals cell subpopulations defined by chromatin state. Nat Biotechnol 33(11):1165–1172. doi:10.1038/nbt.3383

357. Polzer B, Medoro G, Pasch S, Fontana F, Zorzino L, Pestka A, Andergassen U, Meier-Stiegen F, Czyz ZT, Alberter B, Treitschke S, Schamberger T, Sergio M, Bregola G, Doffini A, Gianni S, Calanca A, Signorini G, Bolognesi C, Hartmann A, Fasching PA, Sandri MT, Rack B, Fehm T, Giorgini G, Manaresi N, Klein CA (2014) Molecular profiling of single circulating tumor cells with diagnostic intention. EMBO Mol Med 6(11):1371–1386. doi:10.15252/emmm.201404033

358. De Luca F, Rotunno G, Salvianti F, Galardi F, Pestrin M, Gabellini S, Simi L, Mancini I, Vannucchi AM, Pazzagli M, Di Leo A, Pinzani P (2016) Mutational analysis of single circulating tumor cells by next generation sequencing in metastatic breast cancer. Oncotarget 7(18):26107–26119. doi:10.18632/oncotarget.8431

359. Frommer M, McDonald LE, Millar DS, Collis CM, Watt F, Grigg GW, Molloy PL, Paul CL (1992) A genomic sequencing protocol that yields a positive display of 5-methylcytosine residues in individual DNA strands. Proc Natl Acad Sci U S A 89(5):1827–1831

360. Guo H, Zhu P, Yan L, Li R, Hu B, Lian Y, Yan J, Ren X, Lin S, Li J, Jin X, Shi X, Liu P, Wang X, Wang W, Wei Y, Li X, Guo F, Wu X, Fan X, Yong J, Wen L, Xie SX, Tang F, Qiao J (2014) The DNA methylation landscape of human early embryos. Nature 511(7511):606–610. doi:10.1038/nature13544

361. Smallwood SA, Lee HJ, Angermueller C, Krueger F, Saadeh H, Peat J, Andrews SR, Stegle O, Reik W, Kelsey G (2014) Single-cell genome-wide bisulfite sequencing for assessing epigenetic heterogeneity. Nat Methods 11(8):817–820. doi:10.1038/nmeth.3035

362. Kantlehner M, Kirchner R, Hartmann P, Ellwart JW, Alunni-Fabbroni M, Schumacher A (2011) A high-throughput DNA methylation analysis of a single cell. Nucleic Acids Res 39(7):e44. doi:10.1093/nar/gkq1357

363. Cheow LF, Quake SR, Burkholder WF, Messerschmidt DM (2015) Multiplexed locus-specific analysis of DNA methylation in single cells. Nat Protoc 10(4):619–631. doi:10.1038/nprot.2015.041

364. Rivera CM, Ren B (2013) Mapping human epigenomes. Cell 155(1):39–55. doi:10.1016/j.cell.2013.09.011

365. Baylin SB, Jones PA (2011) A decade of exploring the cancer epigenome – biological and translational implications. Nat Rev Cancer 11(10):726–734. doi:10.1038/nrc3130

366. Ernst J, Kheradpour P, Mikkelsen TS, Shoresh N, Ward LD, Epstein CB, Zhang X, Wang L, Issner R, Coyne M, Ku M, Durham T, Kellis M, Bernstein BE (2011) Mapping and analysis of chromatin state dynamics in nine human cell types. Nature 473(7345):43–49. doi:10.1038/nature09906

367. Consortium EP (2012) An integrated encyclopedia of DNA elements in the human genome. Nature 489(7414):57–74. doi:10.1038/nature11247

368. Thurman RE, Rynes E, Humbert R, Vierstra J, Maurano MT, Haugen E, Sheffield NC, Stergachis AB, Wang H, Vernot B, Garg K, John S, Sandstrom R, Bates D, Boatman L, Canfield TK, Diegel M, Dunn D, Ebersol AK, Frum T, Giste E, Johnson AK, Johnson EM, Kutyavin T, Lajoie B, Lee BK, Lee K, London D, Lotakis D, Neph S, Neri F, Nguyen ED, Qu H, Reynolds AP, Roach V, Safi A, Sanchez ME, Sanyal A, Shafer A, Simon JM, Song L, Vong S, Weaver M, Yan Y, Zhang Z, Zhang Z, Lenhard B, Tewari M, Dorschner MO, Hansen RS, Navas PA, Stamatoyannopoulos G, Iyer VR, Lieb JD, Sunyaev SR, Akey JM, Sabo PJ, Kaul R, Furey TS, Dekker J, Crawford GE, Stamatoyannopoulos JA (2012) The accessible chromatin landscape of the human genome. Nature 489(7414):75–82. doi:10.1038/nature11232
369. Buenrostro JD, Giresi PG, Zaba LC, Chang HY, Greenleaf WJ (2013) Transposition of native chromatin for fast and sensitive epigenomic profiling of open chromatin, DNA-binding proteins and nucleosome position. Nat Methods 10(12):1213–1218. doi:10.1038/nmeth.2688
370. Buenrostro JD, Wu B, Litzenburger UM, Ruff D, Gonzales ML, Snyder MP, Chang HY, Greenleaf WJ (2015) Single-cell chromatin accessibility reveals principles of regulatory variation. Nature 523(7561):486–490. doi:10.1038/nature14590
371. Yin H, Marshall D (2012) Microfluidics for single cell analysis. Curr Opin Biotechnol 23(1):110–119. doi:10.1016/j.copbio.2011.11.002
372. Bheda P, Schneider R (2014) Epigenetics reloaded: the single-cell revolution. Trends Cell Biol 24(11):712–723. doi:10.1016/j.tcb.2014.08.010

DNA and Histone Modifications in Cancer Therapy

Takayoshi Suzuki

Abstract Epigenetic mechanisms, including DNA methylation and posttranslational histone modifications, play a pivotal role in DNA replication/repair and gene expression regulation. These epigenetic mechanisms are responsible for controlling cellular functions, such as cell cycle progression, immunoresponse, and signal transduction. Among the epigenetic mechanisms, the methylation of DNA and histones is closely associated with the oncogenesis and proliferation of cancer cells, and alterations of DNA methylation and histone methylation have been identified in many cancer cells. Several enzymes that control the methylation of DNA or histones have been identified, including DNA methyltransferases, ten-eleven translocation proteins, lysine methyltransferases, lysine demethylases, protein arginine methyltransferases, and peptidyl arginine deiminases. As some of the enzymes are involved in cancer, their inhibitors are considered useful not only as chemical tools for probing the biology of DNA and histone methylation, but also as anticancer agents. In this chapter, hitherto reported enzyme inhibitors are presented and their potential as anticancer agents is discussed.

Keywords Epigenetics • Methylation • DNA • Histone • Lysine • Arginine • Enzyme • Inhibitor • Cancer

1 Introduction

DNA methylation and posttranslational histone modifications, including acetylation and methylation, regulate the expression of various genes independently of the changes in DNA sequence. Such epigenetic mechanisms are crucial for regulating cellular functions, including development and differentiation [1, 2]. They are also involved in various disease states, such as cancer [3]. In particular, the methylation of DNA and histones is closely associated with the oncogenesis and proliferation of cancer cells, and alterations of DNA methylation and histone methylation have been

T. Suzuki (✉)
Graduate School of Medical Science, Kyoto Prefectural University of Medicine, Kyoto, Japan
e-mail: suzukit@koto.kpu-m.ac.jp

© Springer International Publishing AG 2017   585
A. Kaneda, Y.-i. Tsukada (eds.), *DNA and Histone Methylation as Cancer Targets*,
Cancer Drug Discovery and Development, DOI 10.1007/978-3-319-59786-7_20

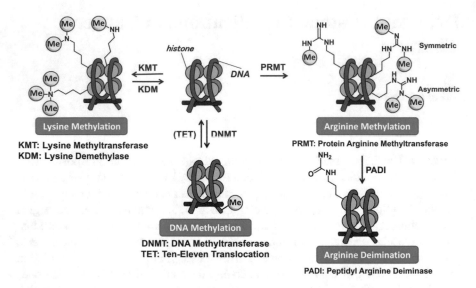

Fig. 1 Drug target enzymes involved in methylation of DNA and histones

identified in many cancer cells. Basically, the methylation of DNA and histones is controlled by enzymes (Fig. 1). DNA methyltransferases (DNMTs), lysine methyltransferases (KMTs), and protein arginine methyltransferases (PRMTs) add methyl groups to DNA, histone lysine residue, and histone arginine residue, respectively. In contrast, ten-eleven translocation proteins (TETs), lysine demethylases (KDMs), and peptidyl arginine deiminases (PADIs) are involved in erasing the methyl groups of DNA, the histone lysine residue, and the histone arginine residue, respectively. Epigenetic aberrations, such as increased levels of DNA methylation and abnormal methylation of histones, are associated with oncogenesis and proliferation of cancer cells via the repression of tumor suppressor genes, such as p53. Therefore, small-molecule modulators of epigenetic enzymes are of interest as potential anticancer agents. In this chapter, hitherto reported epigenetic enzyme inhibitors are presented and their potential as antitumor agents is discussed.

2　DNA Methylation in Cancer Therapy

2.1　DNA Methyltransferase (DNMT) Inhibitors

The methylation of deoxycytidines in DNA plays a key role in epigenetic regulation and occurs at CpG sites that are enriched in the so-called islands essentially located in gene promoters [4]. In general, hypermethylation of the gene promoters' CpG islands induces gene silencing, whereas hypomethylation induces gene expression [5]. In cancer cells, hypermethylation is observed in the promoter regions of some

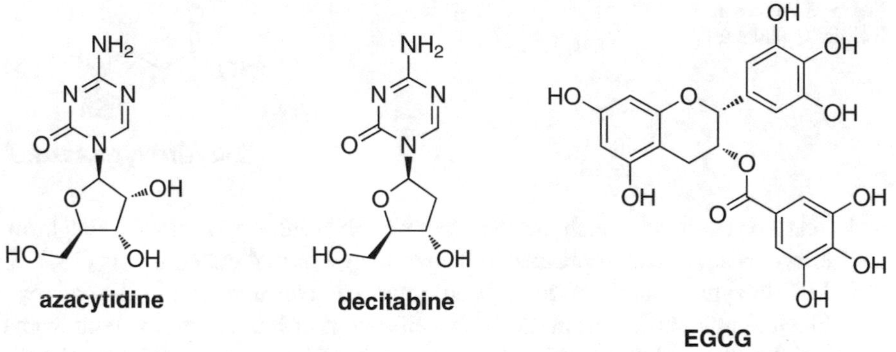

Fig. 2 Structures of DNMT inhibitors

tumor suppressor genes, such as p16 and mutL homolog 1, which are involved in mechanisms relevant to the tumorigenic process, including DNA repair, cell cycle regulation, and apoptosis [6]. DNA hypermethylation and the subsequent silencing of tumor suppressor genes occur frequently during oncogenesis.

DNA methylation is catalyzed by DNA methyltransferases (DNMTs) (Fig. 1) that transfer a methyl group from the universal methyl donor *S*-adenosyl-L-methionine (SAM) to the 5-position of cytosine [7]. Two families of catalytically active DNMTs have been identified so far: DNMT1 and DNMT3A/B. DNMT1 is responsible for DNA methylation maintenance during replication, whereas DNMT3A and 3B are responsible for *de novo* DNA methylation. The activities of DNMT1, 3A, and 3B in cancers are essential for perpetuating gene silencing in tumor suppressor genes, and elevated levels of DNMTs in cancers contribute to tumorigenesis by improper de novo methylation and silencing of tumor suppressor genes [8]. Thus, DNMT inhibitors should be useful for the treatment of cancers. Two DNMT inhibitors, azacytidine and decitabine, (Fig. 2) are the most successful epigenetic drugs for the treatment of myelodysplastic syndrome (MDS) and the most widely used as epigenetic modulators [9]. However, their clinical use is restricted by their low bioavailability, instability in physiological media, and toxicity. To resolve this issue, chemically stable non-nucleoside DNMT inhibitors have been developed [10]. For example, the green tea major polyphenol (-)-epigallocatechin-3-gallate (EGCG) (Fig. 2), which is a DNMT inhibitor that acts on human skin cancer cells, is being tested in phase II clinical trials [11].

2.2 Ten-Eleven Translocation (TET) Inhibitors

Members of the ten-eleven translocation (TET 1–3) family of Fe(II)/α-ketoglutarate-dependent dioxygenases are involved in DNA demethylation (Fig. 1) by catalyzing the conversion of 5-methylcytosine into 5-hydroxymethylcytosine [12]. TET proteins also catalyze the conversion of 5-hydroxy methylcytosine into 5-formylcytosine

2-hydroxyglutarate

and 5-carboxycytosine, which are then repaired to restore cytosine. Although the
TET enzymes have been implicated in the pathology of malignant tumors [13, 14],
few TET enzyme inhibitors have been reported. Navarro et al. showed that
5-hydroxymethylcytosine promoted the proliferation of human uterine leiomyoma
cells and 2-hydroxyglutarate (Fig. 3), a competitive TET enzyme inhibitor, significantly decreased both 5-hydroxymethylcytosine content and leiomyoma cell proliferation [15].

3 Histone Lysine Methylation in Cancer Therapy

3.1 Lysine Methyltransferase (KMT) Inhibitors

The methylation of histone (H) lysine (K) residues occurs at H1K26, H3K4, H3K9,
H3K27, H3K36, H3K79, and H4K20, and is responsible for transcriptional activation
as well as silencing [16, 17]. In addition, the ε-amino group of lysine residues can
undergo mono-, di- or trimethylation, and this differential methylation gives functional diversity to each lysine methylation site. For example, the dimethylation of
H3K4 occurs in both inactive and active genes, whereas the trimethylation is exclusive to active genes [18]. Similarly, the monomethylation of H3K9 is seen in active
genes, whereas the trimethylation of H3K9 is associated with gene repression [19].

To date, a number of histone lysine methyltransferases (KMTs) have been identified, and many of them display substrate specificity [16]. KMTs catalyze the methylation of histones (Fig. 1) using SAM as the methyl donor. In cancer cells, the
mutation and/or overexpression of KMTs, including disruptor of telomeric silencing 1-like (DOT1L), G9a, and enhancer of zeste homolog 2 (EZH2), yields abnormal methylation patterns that lead to oncogenesis. Therefore, KMTs are interesting
as targets of cancer therapy [20].

DOT1L is unique in that it does not have the evolutionarily conserved SET
domain that is necessary for KMT activities [21]. In addition, the DOT1L substrate
H3K79 is located in the ordered core structure of histone H3, whereas the substrates
of the other KMTs are situated in the unordered histone tails. Several studies have
demonstrated the critical role of DOT1L in mixed lineage leukemia (MLL) fusion-
driven leukemias [22–24]. It was shown that the genetic inactivation of DOT1L
leads to a decrease in MLL fusion target gene expression, including a rapid decrease
in HOX cluster gene expression, which is related to an anti-proliferative response.
In addition, small-molecule inhibitors targeting DOT1L exhibited potent activity

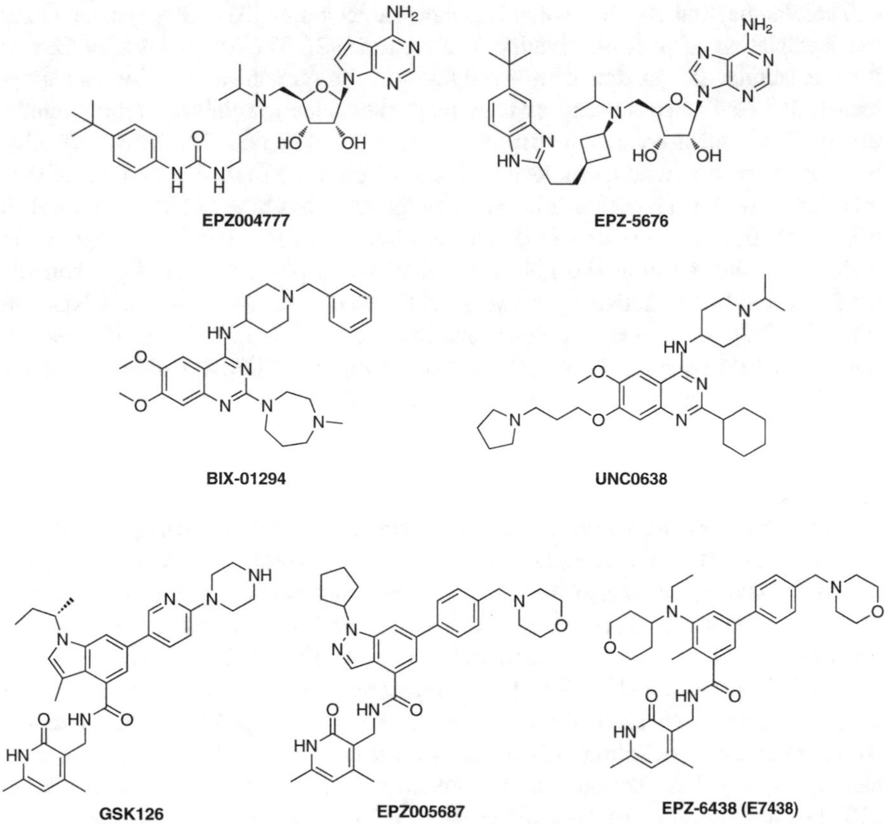

Fig. 4 Structures of KMT inhibitors

against MLL-rearranged leukemias in preclinical studies. Thus, DOT1L inhibitors could be used as a therapeutic agent for MLL. EPZ004777, which binds to the SAM binding site, is a potent and selective inhibitor of DOT1L [25–27]. EPZ004777 (Fig. 4) showed a minimum selectivity of >1000-fold for DOT1L relative to the other KMTs tested. Treatment of MLL cells with EPZ004777 selectively inhibited H3K79 methylation and repressed the expression of leukemogenic genes. In addition, EPZ004777 improved survival in a mouse MLL xenograft model. Currently, EPZ-5676 (Fig. 4), a derivative of EPZ004777, is being evaluated in clinical trials as an antileukemic agent [28].

G9a, a member of the SUV39H subgroup of SET domain-containing molecules, is a KMT that catalyzes the mono- and dimethylation of H3K9. The G9a-catalyzed H3K9 methylation induces transcriptional silencing, heterochromatin formation, and DNA methylation under physiological conditions [29, 30]. G9a expression is high in many cancers compared with normal tissues. Cancer transcriptome analysis has revealed high G9a expression in many cancers, including bladder cancer, hepatocellular cancer, colon cancer, prostate cancer, lung cancer, invasive transitional cell carcinoma, and B-cell chronic lymphocytic leukemia [31]. G9a also catalyzes the methylation of p53, inactivating its function [32]. The knockdown of G9a in lung, leukemia, and prostate cancer cell lines caused growth suppression and apoptosis [33]. G9a is also overexpressed in pancreatic adenocarcinoma and the inhibition of G9a induces cellular senescence in this type of cancer [34]. Therefore, G9a has been viewed as a target molecule for cancer therapy. To date, a number of G9a inhibitors have been reported (Fig. 4), although none has been subjected to clinical trials. BIX-01294 is the first G9a-selective inhibitor that binds to the groove in which the lysine substrate lies [35]. As BIX-01294 displays cytotoxicity despite its moderate inhibitory activity, its use in cell-based assays is limited. UNC0638 (Fig. 4), which has improved potency and lower toxicity than BIX-01294, was discovered in 2011 by Jin and co-workers [36]. Although UNC0638 still has problems regarding metabolism and pharmacokinetics, its high stability under cellular assay conditions, coupled with high potency (G9a; IC_{50} = 15 nM) and selectivity (other epigenetic targets; IC_{50} > 4500 nM), makes it an excellent chemical tool for cell-based studies.

EZH2 is a KMT that catalyzes the methylation of H3K27 [37]. Along with cofactors SUZ12, EED, and RbAp46/48, EZH2 forms the Polycomb Repressive Complex 2 (PRC2), which functions to silence target genes by trimethylating H3K27. Unlike most other genetic markers that are mediated by multiple enzymes, the trimethylation of H3K27 appears to be mediated primarily by EZH2 [38]. The increased levels of trimethylated H3K27 due to an increased expression of EZH2 contribute to cancer aggressiveness, metastasis, short patient survival, and high death rate in a variety of cancers, including melanoma, prostate cancer, breast cancer, and ovarian cancer [39–42]. Furthermore, the maintenance of cancer stem cells depends on EZH2 expression, and the knockdown of EZH2 in cancer cells blocks cancer cell growth [43–45]. In addition, somatic mutations and deletions in EZH2 were identified in hematological malignancies [46]. Approximately 30% of diffuse large B-cell lymphomas and 10% of follicular lymphomas contain a mutation at tyrosine 641 (Y641) within the SET domain, which results in a change in substrate preference from the non-methylated H3K27 to the mono- and dimethylated ones [47]. Accordingly, diffuse large B-cell lymphoma cells with EZH2Y641X display increased levels of trimethylated H3K27, which stimulate the malignant transformation of diffuse large B-cell lymphomas. Thus, there is strong evidence that the selective inhibition of EZH2 is useful for the treatment of cancer, and it is desirable to identify small-molecule EZH2-selective inhibitors. GlaxoSmithKline and Epizyme Inc. have reported potent EZH2-selective inhibitors GSK126 and EPZ005687 (Fig. 4), respectively [48, 49]. These inhibitors show high EZH2 selectivity against the other protein methyltransferases, including the closely related enzyme EZH1. In addition, they reduced H3K27 methylation in various lymphoma cells and killed lymphoma cells bearing genetic mutations in EZH2, but had minimal effects on the proliferation of wild-type cells. Epizyme Inc. developed EPZ-6438 (E7438) (Fig. 4), which shows potent antitumor activity against EZH2-mutant non-Hodgkin lymphoma and is currently being evaluated in phase I/II trials for the treatment thereof [50].

3.2 Lysine Demethylase (KDM) Inhibitors

3.2.1 LSD1 Inhibitors

In contrast to other histone modifications, such as acetylation and phosphorylation, histone lysine methylation had been regarded as an irreversible process because of the high thermodynamic stability of the N-C bond. Indeed, whereas a number of KMTs had been identified by 2003 [16], no KDMs had been identified. However, two classes of KDMs (Fig. 1) have been identified since 2004 [51]. One class includes lysine-specific demethylase 1 (LSD1, also known as KDM1A) and LSD2 (also known as KDM1B), which are flavin-dependent amine oxidase domain-containing enzymes [52, 53]. The other class comprises the recently discovered Jumonji domain-containing protein (JMJD) histone demethylases (JHDMs) [54, 55], which are Fe(II)/α-ketoglutarate-dependent enzymes.

LSD1 is the first histone demethylase to have been discovered [52]. As this enzyme induces the oxidative imination of methyl amino groups, the substrates of LSD1 are limited to mono- and dimethyllysines [56]. LSD1 removes methyl groups from mono- and dimethylated Lys4 of histone H3 (H3K4me1/2), which is a well-characterized gene activation mark, through flavin adenine dinucleotide (FAD)-dependent enzymatic oxidation [52]. In prostate cell lines, LSD1 also demethylates H3K9me1/2 and regulates androgen receptor-mediated transcription [57].

LSD1 represents an interesting target for epigenetic drugs as supported by data related to its overexpression in many types of cancers, including neuroblastoma, glioma, and breast cancer cells [58–61]. In addition, the overexpression of LSD1 is correlated to tumor recurrence in prostate cancer [62]. Moreover, LSD1 inhibition reactivates silenced tumor suppressor genes to target selectively cancer cells with pluripotent stem cell properties [63, 64]. Indeed, LSD1 maintains an undifferentiated tumor initiating or cancer stem cell phenotype in a spectrum of cancers [65, 66]. Acute myeloid leukemias (AMLs) are an example of neoplastic cells that retain some of their less differentiated stem cell like phenotype or leukemia stem cell potential. Analysis of AML cells by gene expression arrays and chromatin immuno-precipitation with next-generation sequencing (ChIP-Seq) revealed that LSD1 regulates a subset of genes involved in multiple oncogenic programs to maintain leukemia stem cells [67, 68]. These results suggest the potential therapeutic benefit of LSD1 inhibitors targeting cancers.

As mentioned above, LSD1 is an amine oxidase that catalyzes the demethylation of mono- or dimethylated histone lysine residues and shows homology with mono-amine oxidases (MAOs) A and B [69]. Indeed, trans-2-phenylcyclopropylamine (PCPA) (Fig. 5), a MAO inhibitor used as an antidepressant, was found to be also able to inhibit LSD1. It was shown that PCPA is a mechanism-based irreversible inhibitor of LSD1. Kinetics, MS, and X-ray analysis data suggested that PCPA inhibits LSD1 through the formation of a covalent adduct with the flavin ring following one-electron oxidation and cyclopropyl ring opening [69, 70]. PCPA at high concentrations induced an increase of global H3K4 methylation and growth inhibition of

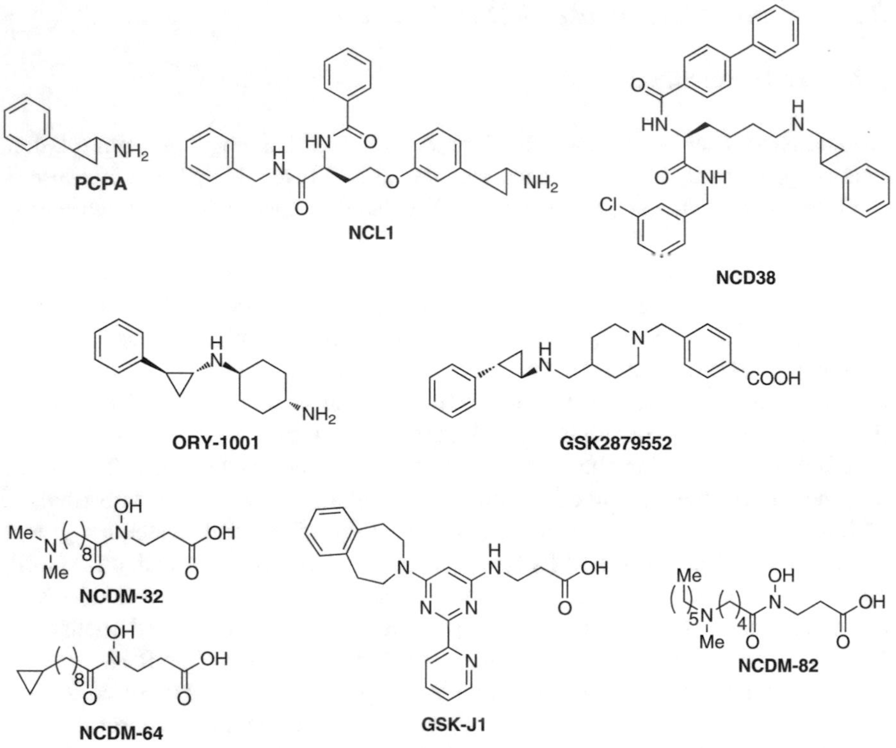

Fig. 5 Structures of KDM inhibitors

neuroblastoma cells and bladder cancer cells [58, 71]. In addition, the combination of PCPA and all-*trans* retinoic acid (ATRA) is an effective therapy for AML [68].

Many of the identified LSD1 inhibitors are PCPA analogs. NCL1 (Fig. 5), a lysine-PCPA hybrid compound designed on the basis of crystallographic data, was the first cell-active LSD1-selective inhibitor to be reported [72, 73]. NCL1 inhibited the growth of cancer cells at µM concentrations, consistent with its effect on H3K4 methylation. In addition, combination therapy with anti-estrogen and NCL1 showed potential therapeutic effects by inhibiting the growth of drug-resistant breast cancer cells [74]. NCL1 also reduced tumor volume in mice injected subcutaneously with hormone-resistant prostate cancer PCai1 cells without adverse effects, suggesting the potential of LSD1 inhibitors as therapeutic agents for hormone-resistant prostate cancer [75]. NCD38 (Fig. 5) was discovered on the basis of the concept that LSD1 could be potently and selectively inactivated by delivering PCPA directly to the enzyme's active site [76]. Biological and mechanistic studies revealed that NCD38 inhibits LSD1 potently and selectively by delivering PCPA directly to the enzyme's active site. Interestingly, NCD38 was also able to inhibit both cancer stem cell formation and the maintenance of human metastatic breast cancer cells by inducing their reversion to the epithelial form [77].

GlaxoSmithKline and Oryzon Genomics discovered potent LSD1-selective inhibitors GSK2879552 and ORY-1001, respectively (Fig. 5) [78, 79]. GSK2879552 and ORY-1001 exhibit anti-leukemia activity and are currently undergoing clinical trials for AML treatment. In addition, a screen of cancer cell lines showed that small cell lung carcinoma (SCLC) is sensitive to LSD1 inhibition by PCPA analogs, including GSK2879552 [78]. GSK2879552 exhibited DNA hypomethylation in SCLC lines, suggesting that DNA hypomethylation can be used as a predictive bio-marker of LSD1 inhibitory activity.

3.2.2 Jumonji Domain-Containing Protein (JMJD) Histone Demethylase (JHDM) Inhibitors

JHDMs catalyze the demethylation of methylated histone lysine residues through $Fe(II)/\alpha$-ketoglutarate-dependent enzymatic oxidation [54, 55, 80]. Unlike LSD1, JHDMs can demethylate all the three methylated lysine states, namely, mono-, di- and trimethylated lysines, because the demethylation by JHDMs does not require the lone-pair electrons on the nitrogen atom of lysines to initiate catalysis. To date, a number of JHDM family members have been identified, including KDM2–8, NO66, Mina53, and PHF2 [51]. The demethylation of methylated histone lysine residues by JHDMs regulates the expression of a number of genes and controls various cellular functions [51]. For example, H3K9 demethylation by KDM3A is responsible for the gene expression of HOXA1, which is upregulated in a variety of human cancer lesions [81–85]. KDM4A, KDM4C, and KDM4D, the demethylases of methylated H3K9 and H3K36, are associated with both transcriptional activation and inactivation [86–89]. KDM7B contributes to gene activation in prostate cancer cells through the demethylation of H3K9me1/2, H3K27me2, and H4K20me1 [90–93]. Furthermore, several JHDMs are involved in the growth of cancers, including leukemia, breast cancer, and prostate cancer [94–96]. Therefore, JHDM inhibitors are expected as candidates for anticancer agents.

It has been reported that KDM4C, a demethylase of H3K9me2/3, is associated with cancer. The demethylase activity of KDM4C increases the expression of Mdm2 oncogene, which leads to a decrease of p53 tumor suppressor gene product in cancer cells [97]. Moreover, KDM4C is associated with cell growth of many cancers, including esophageal squamous cancer, prostate cancer, breast cancer, and AML [87, 91, 95, 96, 98]. NCDM-32 (Fig. 5) was identified as a KDM4C inhibitor [99]. NCDM-32 inhibited KDM4C with an IC_{50} value of 1.0 μM without inhibiting prolyl hydroxylases 1 and 2, other $Fe(II)/\alpha$-ketoglutarate-dependent enzymes. Furthermore, the ester prodrug of NCDM-32 showed synergistic inhibition of cancer cells when used in combination with an inhibitor of LSD1. The ester prodrug of NCDM-32 impaired several critical pathways that drive cellular proliferation and transformation in aggressive breast cancer, suggesting the possibility of using KDM4 inhibitors as novel therapeutic agents for aggressive breast cancer [100].

KDM5A is an H3K4me2/3 demethylase [101, 102]. It is overexpressed in many cancer cells, including lung cancer and gastric cancer, and its gene is amplified in cervix carcinoma [103–107]. KDM5A has been implicated in the development of drug tolerance in cancers, including lung cancer, breast cancer, and glioblastoma [108–110]. Therefore, there is a need to develop KDM5A inhibitors for cancer therapy. Recently, NCDM-82 (Fig. 5) has been identified as a KDM5A inhibitor [111]. NCDM-82 selectively inhibits KDM5A over KDM4A, KDM4C, and KDM7B.The methyl ester prodrug of NCDM-82 induced a selective increase in the expression of H3K4me3, the substrate of KDM5A. The methyl ester prodrug of NCDM-82 also synergistically enhanced A549 human lung cancer cell growth inhibition induced by vorinostat, a histone deacetylase (HDAC) inhibitor.

KDM6B functions as an H3K27me2/3-specific demethylase [112]. It facilitates gene transcription by demethylating H3K27me2/3, which are repressive histone marks. KDM6B regulates the differentiation state of the epidermis and activates the tumor suppressor INK4-Arf in response to stress-induced signals [113, 114]. Furthermore, KDM6B is overexpressed in many cancers, such as renal cell carcinoma, MDS, colorectal cancer, and melanoma, and is involved in the growth of cancer cells [115–118]. These reports suggest the possibility of using KDM6B inhibitors as anticancer agents. Kruidenier et al. reported the first small-molecule catalytic site inhibitor GSK-J1 (Fig. 5) that showed selectivity for H3K27me3-specific KDM6A and KDM6B [119]. The ethyl ester prodrug of GSK-J1 modulated proinflammatory macrophage response that was dependent on the accumulation of H3K27me3. In addition to the anti-inflammatory activity, the ethyl ester prodrug of GSK-J1 exhibited anticancer activity in acute lymphoblastic leukemia, ovarian cancer, and pediatric brainstem glioma [120–122].

KDM7B is known to catalyze the demethylation of H3K27me2 [123]. It has been reported to activate the transcription of the E2F1 transcription factor in HeLa cells, which promotes cell cycle progression [124]. It has also been reported that KDM7B is associated with the proliferation of prostate cancer cells, osteosarcoma cells, and esophageal squamous cell carcinoma cells [93, 125, 126]. Therefore, KDM7B inhibitors are of interest as candidates for anticancer agents. NCDM-64 (Fig. 5) was found as a KDM7B inhibitor [127]. NCDM-64 enhanced the methylation level of H3K27, increased the expression of E2F1 gene, and caused growth inhibition by G0/G1 cell cycle arrest in HeLa cells and esophagus KYSE150 cells.

4 Histone Arginine Methylation in Cancer Therapy

4.1 Protein Arginine N-Methyltransferase (PRMT) Inhibitors

The methylation of histone (H) arginine (R) residues occurs at H3R2, H3R8, H3R17, H3R26, and H4R3. The methylation at H3R17, H3R26, and H4R3 is associated with gene activation [128–130], whereas that at H3R8 is correlated with gene repression [131]. Protein arginine N-methyltransferase (PRMT) 1, PRMT4, PRMT5, and PRMT7 have been identified as histone arginine methyltransferases (Fig. 1) [132, 133]. Whereas PRMT4 catalyzes the methylation of H3R2, H3R17, and H3R26, PRMT1 and PRMT5 specifically methylate H4R3 and H3R8, respectively. It has

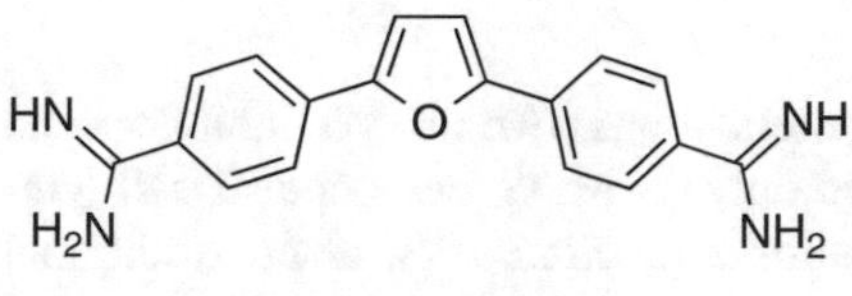

Fig. 6 Structures of PRMT inhibitors

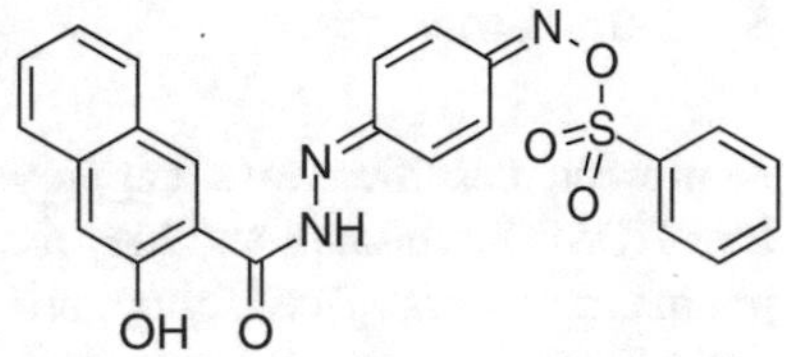

Fig. 7 Structure of
YW3-56

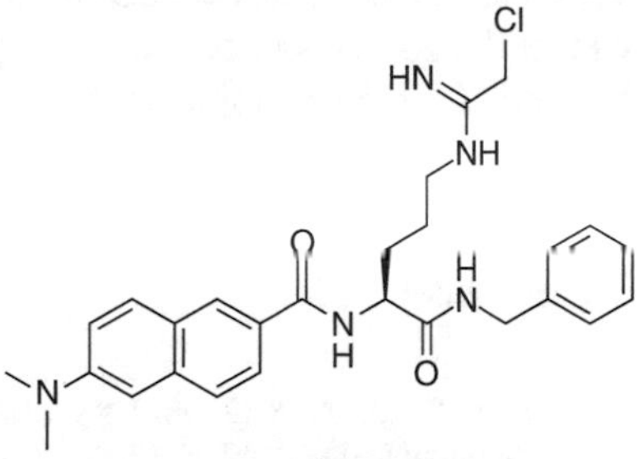

been found that PRMT1 and PRMT4 catalyze the asymmetric dimethylation of arginines, whereas PRMT5 and PRMT7 catalyze symmetric demethylation (Fig. 1).

Among the PRMTs, PRMT1 is involved in several disease states, including cancer. PRMT1 is an essential element in oncogenic MLL fusion complexes, and is involved in the transcription and transformation of the oncogenic MLL fusion complexes in leukemia cells [98, 134]. Therefore, PRMT1 inhibitors are potential anticancer agents. DB75 (Fig. 6) has been reported as a PRMT1 inhibitor [135]. DB75 inhibited PRMT1 activity in cells and showed antiproliferative activity in leukemia cell lines with different genetic lesions. A9 (Fig. 6) was also identified as a PRMT1 inhibitor [136]. A9 efficiently inhibited the growth of castration-resistant prostate cancer cells.

4.2 Peptidyl Arginine Deiminase (PADI) Inhibitors

Although it is unclear whether histone arginine methylation is reversible or irreversible, the deimination of methylated arginines has been reported. Peptidyl arginine deiminase 4 (PADI4) deiminates non-methylated or monomethylated arginine residues of R2, R8, R17, and R26 in the H3 tail (Fig. 1) [137]. The deimination by PADI4 prevents arginine methylation by PRMT4, and PADI4 represses hormone receptor-mediated gene induction. In addition, the deimination of H4R3 in HL-60 granulocytes has also been reported [138]. It is unclear whether the deimination by PADIs is related to cancer or not, but it was reported that PADI inhibitors, including YW3–56 (Fig. 7), inhibited the growth of cancer cells by regulating autophagy flux [139].

5   Summary

At present, there are only six approved epigenetic drugs (two DNMT inhibitors and four HDAC inhibitors), and they are utilized only for MDS, cutaneous T-cell lymphoma, peripheral T-cell lymphoma, or multiple myeloma treatment. Additional indications of the current epigenetic drugs are limited. In this regard, researchers need to develop an integrated understanding of cancer epigenetics in order to discover useful next-generation drugs for cancer therapy.

In this chapter, small-molecule inhibitors of DNMTs, TETs, KMTs, KDMs, PRMTs, and PADIs have been discussed from the point of view of potential use in cancer therapy. It is hoped that the epigenetic inhibitors presented here will provide the basis for the development of novel anticancer agents.

References

1. Sasaki H, Matsui Y (2008) Epigenetic events in mammalian germ-cell development: reprogramming and beyond. Nat Rev Genet 9:129–140
2. Lotem J, Sachs L (2006) Epigenetics and the plasticity of differentiation in normal and cancer stem cells. Oncogene 25:7663–7672
3. Dawson MA, Kouzarides T (2012) Cancer epigenetics: from mechanism to therapy. Cell 150:12–27
4. Berger SL, Kouzarides T, Shiekhattar R, Shilatifard A (2009) An operational definition of epigenetics. Genes Dev 23:781–783
5. Esteller N (2008) Epigenetics in cancer. N Engl J Med 358:1148–1159
6. Baylin SB, Ohm JE (2006) Epigenetic gene silencing in cancer – a mechanism for early oncogenic pathway addiction? Nat Rev Cancer 6:107–116
7. Jurkowska RZ, Jurkowski TP, Jeltsch A (2011) Structure and function of mammalian DNA methyltransferases. Chembiochem 12:206–222
8. Linhart HG, Lin H, Yamada Y, Moran E, Steine EJ, Gokhale S, Lo G, Cantu E, Ehrich M, He T, Meissner A, Jaenisch R (2007) Author information Dnmt3b promotes tumorigenesis in vivo by gene-specific de novo methylation and transcriptional silencing. Genes Dev 21:3110–2312
9. Egger G, Liang G, Aparicio A, Jones PA (2004) Epigenetics in human disease and prospects for epigenetic therapy. Nature 429:457–463
10. Erdmann A, Halby L, Fahy J, Arimondo PB (2015) Targeting DNA methylation with small molecules: what's next? J Med Chem 58:2569–2583
11. Nandakumar V, Vaid M, Katiyar SK (2011) (-)-Epigallocatechin-3-gallate reactivates silenced tumor suppressor genes, Cip1/p21 and p16INK4a, by reducing DNA methylation and increasing histones acetylation in human skin cancer cells. Carcinogenesis 32:537–544
12. Kohli RM, Zhang Y (2013) Tet enzymes, TDG and the dynamics of DNA demethylation. Nature 502:472–479
13. Takai H, Masuda K, Sato T, Sakaguchi Y, Suzuki T, Suzuki T, Koyama-Nasu R, Nasu-Nishimura Y, Katou Y, Ogawa H, Morishita Y, Kozuka-Hata H, Oyama M, Todo T, Ino Y, Mukasa A, Saito N, Toyoshima C, Shirahige K, Akiyama T (2014) 5-hydroxymethylcytosine plays a critical role in glioblastomagenesis by recruiting the chtop-methylosome complex. Cell Rep 9:48–60
14. Huang Y, Rao A (2014) Connections between tet proteins and aberrant DNA modification in cancer. Trends Genet 30:464–474

15. Navarro A, Yin P, Ono M, Monsivais D, Moravek MB, Coon JS 5th, Dyson MT, Wei JJ, Bulun SE (2014) 5-Hydroxymethylcytosine promotes proliferation of human uterine leiomyoma: a biological link to a new epigenetic modification in benign tumors. J Clin Endocrinol Metab 99:E2437–E2445

16. Kubicek S, Jenuwein T (2004) A crack in histone lysine methylation. Cell 119:903–906

17. Bannister AJ, Kouzarides T (2005) Reversing histone methylation. Nature 436:1103–1106

18. Santos-Rosa H, Schneider R, Bannister AJ, Sherriff J, Bernstein BE, Emre NC, Schreiber SL, Mellor J, Kouzarides T (2002) Active genes are tri-methylated at K4 of histone H3. Nature 419:407–411

19. Barski A, Cuddapah S, Cui K, Roh TY, Schones DE, Wang Z, Wei G, Chepelev I, Zhao K (2007) High-resolution profiling of histone methylations in the human genome. Cell 129:823–837

20. Copeland RA, Solomon ME, Richon VM (2009) Protein methyltransferases as a target class for drug discovery. Nat Rev Drug Discov 8:724–732

21. Jenuwein T (2001) Re-SET-ting heterochromatin by histone methyltransferases. Trends Cell Biol 11:266–273

22. Jo SY, Granowicz EM, Maillard I, Thomas D, Hess JL (2011) Requirement for Dot1l in murine postnatal hematopoiesis and leukemogenesis by MLL translocation. Blood 117:4759–4768

23. Nguyen AT, Taranova O, He J, Zhang Y (2011) DOT1L, the H3K79 methyltransferase, is required for MLL-AF9-mediated leukemogenesis. Blood 117:6912–6922

24. Chang MJ, Wu H, Achille NJ, Reisenauer MR, Chou CW, Zeleznik-Le NJ, Hemenway CS, Zhang W (2010) Histone H3 lysine 79 methyltransferase Dot1 is required for immortalization by MLL oncogenes. Cancer Res 70:10234–10242

25. Yao Y, Chen P, Diao J, Cheng G, Deng L, Anglin JL, Prasad BV, Song Y (2011) Selective inhibitors of histone methyltransferase DOT1L: design, synthesis, and crystallographic studies. J Am Chem Soc 133:16746–16749

26. Daigle SR, Olhava EJ, Therkelsen CA, Majer CR, Sneeringer CJ, Song J, Johnston LD, Scott MP, Smith JJ, Xiao Y, Jin L, Kuntz KW, Chesworth R, Moyer MP, Bernt KM, Tseng JC, Kung AL, Armstrong SA, Copeland RA, Richon VM, Pollock RM (2011) Selective killing of mixed lineage leukemia cells by a potent small-molecule DOT1L inhibitor. Cancer Cell 20:53–65

27. Anglin JL, Deng L, Yao Y, Cai G, Liu Z, Jiang H, Cheng G, Chen P, Dong S, Song Y (2012) Synthesis and structure-activity relationship investigation of adenosine-containing inhibitors of histone methyltransferase DOT1L. J Med Chem 55:8066–8074

28. Daigle SR, Olhava EJ, Therkelsen CA, Basavapathruni A, Jin L, Boriack-Sjodin PA, Allain CJ, Klaus CR, Raimondi A, Scott MP, Waters NJ, Chesworth R, Moyer MP, Copeland RA, Richon VM, Pollock RM (2013) Potent inhibition of DOT1L as treatment of MLL-fusion leukemia. Blood 122:1017–1025

29. Shinkai Y, Tachibana M (2011) H3K9 methyltransferase G9a and the related molecule GLP. Genes Dev 25:781–788

30. Collins RE, Tachibana M, Tamaru H, Smith KM, Jia D, Zhang X, Selker EU, Shinkai Y, Cheng X (2005) In vitro and in vivo analyses of a Phe/Tyr switch controlling product specificity of histone lysine methyltransferases. J Biol Chem 280:5563–5570

31. Shankar SR, Bahirvani AG, Rao VK, Bharathy N, Ow JR, Taneja R (2013) G9a, a multipotent regulator of gene expression. Epigenetics 8:16–22

32. Huang J, Dorsey J, Chuikov S, Pérez-Burgos L, Zhang X, Jenuwein T, Reinberg D, Berger SL (2010) G9a and Glp methylate lysine 373 in the tumor suppressor p53. J Biol Chem 285:9636–9641

33. Goyama S, Nitta E, Yoshino T, Kako S, Watanabe-Okochi N, Shimabe M, Imai Y, Takahashi K, Kurokawa M (2010) EVI-1 interacts with histone methyltransferases SUV39H1 and G9a for transcriptional repression and bone marrow immortalization. Leukemia 24:81–88

34. Yuan Y, Wang Q, Paulk J, Kubicek S, Kemp MM, Adams DJ, Shamji AF, Wagner BK, Schreiber SL (2012) A small-molecule probe of the histone methyltransferase G9a induces cellular senescence in pancreatic adenocarcinoma. ACS Chem Biol 7:1152–1157

35. Kubicek S, O'Sullivan RJ, August EM, Hickey ER, Zhang Q, Teodoro ML, Rea S, Mechtler K, Kowalski JA, Homon CA, Kelly TA, Jenuwein T (2007) Reversal of H3K9me2 by a small-molecule inhibitor for the G9a histone methyltransferase. Mol Cell 25:473–481

36. Vedadi M, Barsyte-Lovejoy D, Liu F, Rival-Gervier S, Allali-Hassani A, Labrie V, Wigle TJ, Dimaggio PA, Wasney GA, Siarheyeva A, Dong A, Tempel W, Wang SC, Chen X, Chau I, Mangano TJ, Huang XP, Simpson CD, Pattenden SG, Norris JL, Kireev DB, Tripathy A, Edwards A, Roth BL, Janzen WP, Garcia BA, Petronis A, Ellis J, Brown PJ, Frye SV, Arrowsmith CH, Jin J (2011) A chemical probe selectively inhibits G9a and GLP methyltransferase activity in cells. Nat Chem Biol 7:566–574

37. Cao R, Zhang Y (2004) The functions of E(Z)/EZH2-mediated methylation of lysine 27 in histone H3. Curr Opin Genet Dev 14:155–164

38. Hansen KH, Bracken AP, Pasini D, Dietrich N, Gehani SS, Monrad A, Rappsilber J, Lerdrup M, Helin K (2008) A model for transmission of the H3K27me3 epigenetic mark. Nat Cell Biol 10:1291–1300

39. Bachmann IM, Halvorsen OJ, Collett K, Stefansson IM, Straume O, Haukaas SA, Salvesen HB, Otte AP, Akslen LA (2006) EZH2 expression is associated with high proliferation rate and aggressive tumor subgroups in cutaneous melanoma and cancers of the endometrium, prostate, and breast. J Clin Oncol 24:268–273

40. Pietersen AM, Horlings HM, Hauptmann M, Langerød A, Ajouaou A, Cornelissen-Steijger P, Wessels LF, Jonkers J, van de Vijver MJ, van Lohuizen M (2008) EZH2 and BMI1 inversely correlate with prognosis and TP53 mutation in breast cancer. Breast Cancer Res 10:R109

41. Yu J, Yu J, Rhodes DR, Tomlins SA, Cao X, Chen G, Mehra R, Wang X, Ghosh D, Shah RB, Varambally S, Pienta KJ, Chinnaiyan AM (2007) A polycomb repression signature in metastatic prostate cancer predicts cancer outcome. Cancer Res 67:10657–10663

42. Rao ZY, Cai MY, Yang GF, He LR, Mai SJ, Hua WF, Liao YJ, Deng HX, Chen YC, Guan XY, Zeng YX, Kung HF, Xie D (2010) EZH2 supports ovarian carcinoma cell invasion and/or metastasis via regulation of TGF-β 1 and is a predictor of outcome in ovarian carcinoma patients. Carcinogenesis 31:1576–1583

43. Fussbroich B, Wagener N, Macher-Goeppinger S, Benner A, Fälth M, Sültmann H, Holzer A, Hoppe-Seyler K, Hoppe-Seyler F (2011) EZH2 depletion blocks the proliferation of colon cancer cells. PLoS One 6:e21651

44. Kamminga LM, Bystrykh LV, de Boer A, Houwer S, Douma J, Weersing E, Dontje B, de Haan G (2006) The Polycomb group gene Ezh2 prevents hematopoietic stem cell exhaustion. Blood 107:2170–2179

45. Rizzo S, Hersey JM, Mellor P, Dai W, Santos-Silva A, Liber D, Luk L, Titley I, Carden CP, Box G, Hudson DL, Kaye SB, Brown R (2011) Ovarian cancer stem cell-like side populations are enriched following chemotherapy and overexpress EZH2. Mol Cancer Ther 10:325–335

46. Morin RD, Johnson NA, Severson TM, Mungall AJ, An J, Goya R, Paul JE, Boyle M, Woolcock BW, Kuchenbauer F, Yap D, Humphries RK, Griffith OL, Shah S, Zhu H, Kimbara M, Shashkin P, Charlot JF, Tcherpakov M, Corbett R, Tam A, Varhol R, Smailus D, Moksa M, Zhao Y, Delaney A, Qian H, Birol I, Schein J, Moore R, Holt R, Horsman DE, Connors JM, Jones S, Aparicio S, Hirst M, Gascoyne RD, Marra MA (2010) Somatic mutations altering EZH2 (Tyr641) in follicular and diffuse large B-cell lymphomas of germinal-center origin. Nat Genet 42:181–185

47. Sneeringer CJ, Scott MP, Kuntz KW, Knutson SK, Pollock RM, Richon VM, Copeland RA (2010) Coordinated activities of wild-type plus mutant EZH2 drive tumor-associated hyper-trimethylation of lysine 27 on histone H3 (H3K27) in human B-cell lymphomas. Proc Natl Acad Sci U S A 107:20980–20985

48. McCabe MT, Ott HM, Ganji G, Korenchuk S, Thompson C, Van Aller GS, Liu Y, Graves AP, Della Pietra A 3rd, Diaz E, LaFrance LV, Mellinger M, Duquenne C, Tian X, Kruger RG, McHugh CF, Brandt M, Miller WH, Dhanak D, Verma SK, Tummino PJ, Creasy CL (2012) EZH2 inhibition as a therapeutic strategy for lymphoma with EZH2-activating mutations. Nature 492:108–112

49. Knutson SK, Wigle TJ, Warholic NM, Sneeringer CJ, Allain CJ, Klaus CR, Sacks JD, Raimondi A, Majer CR, Song J, Scott MP, Jin L, Smith JJ, Olhava EJ, Chesworth R, Moyer MP, Richon VM, Copeland RA, Keilhack H, Pollock RM, Kuntz KW (2012) A selective inhibitor of EZH2 blocks H3K27 methylation and kills mutant lymphoma cells. Nat Chem Biol 8:890–896

50. Knutson SK, Kawano S, Minoshima Y, Warholic NM, Huang KC, Xiao Y, Kadowaki T, Uesugi M, Kuznetsov G, Kumar N, Wigle TJ, Klaus CR, Allain CJ, Raimondi A, Waters NJ, Smith JJ, Porter-Scott M, Chesworth R, Moyer MP, Copeland RA, Richon VM, Uenaka T, Pollock RM, Kuntz KW, Yokoi A, Keilhack H (2014) Selective inhibition of EZH2 by EPZ-6438 leads to potent antitumor activity in EZH2-mutant non-Hodgkin lymphoma. Mol Cancer Ther 13:842–854

51. Suzuki T, Miyata N (2011) Lysine demethylases inhibitors. J Med Chem 54:8236–8250

52. Shi Y, Lan F, Matson C, Mulligan P, Whetstine JR, Cole PA, Casero RA, Shi Y (2004) Histone demethylation mediated by the nuclear amine oxidase homolog LSD1. Cell 119:941–953

53. Karytinos A, Forneris F, Profumo A, Ciossani G, Battaglioli E, Binda C, Mattevi A (2009) A novel mammalian flavin-dependent histone demethylase. J Biol Chem 284:17775–17782

54. Tsukada Y, Fang J, Erdjument-Bromage H, Warren ME, Borchers CH, Tempst P, Zhang Y (2006) Histone demethylation by a family of JmjC domain-containing proteins. Nature 439:811–816

55. Klose RJ, Kallin EM, Zhang Y (2006) JmjC-domain-containing proteins and histone demethylation. Nat Rev Genet 7:715–727

56. Yang M, Culhane JC, Szewczuk LM, Gocke CB, Brautigam CA, Tomchick DR, Machius M, Cole PA, Yu H (2007) Structural basis of histone demethylation by LSD1 revealed by suicide inactivation. Nat Struct Mol Biol 14:535–539

57. Metzger E, Wissmann M, Yin N, Müller JM, Schneider R, Peters AH, Günther T, Buettner R, Schüle R (2005) LSD1 demethylates repressive histone marks to promote androgen-receptor-dependent transcription. Nature 437:436–439

58. Schulte JH, Lim S, Schramm A, Friedrichs N, Koster J, Versteeg R, Ora I, Pajtler K, Klein-Hitpass L, Kuhfittig-Kulle S, Metzger E, Schüle R, Eggert A, Buettner R, Kirfel J (2009) Lysine-specific demethylase 1 is strongly expressed in poorly differentiated neuroblastoma: implications for therapy. Cancer Res 69:2065–2071

59. Singh MM, Manton CA, Bhat KP, Tsai WW, Aldape K, Barton MC, Chandra J (2011) Inhibition of LSD1 sensitizes glioblastoma cells to histone deacetylase inhibitors. Neuro-Oncology 13:894–903

60. Singh MM, Johnson B, Venkatarayan A, Flores ER, Zhang J, Su X, Barton M, Lang F, Chandra J (2015) Preclinical activity of combined HDAC and KDM1A inhibition in glioblastoma. Neuro-Oncology 17:1463–1473

61. Lim S, Janzer A, Becker A, Zimmer A, Schüle R, Buettner R, Kirfel J (2010) Lysine-specific demethylase 1 (LSD1) is highly expressed in ER-negative breast cancers and a biomarker predicting aggressive biology. Carcinogenesis 31:512–520

62. Kahl P, Gullotti L, Heukamp LC, Wolf S, Friedrichs N, Vorreuther R, Solleder G, Bastian PJ, Ellinger J, Metzger E, Schüle R, Buettner R (2006) Androgen receptor coactivators lysine-specific histone demethylase 1 and four and a half LIM domain protein 2 predict risk of prostate cancer recurrence. Cancer Res 66:11341–11347

63. Huang Y, Greene E, Murray Stewart T, Goodwin AC, Baylin SB, Woster PM, Casero RA Jr (2007) Inhibition of lysine-specific demethylase 1 by polyamine analogues results in reexpression of aberrantly silenced genes. Proc Natl Acad Sci U S A 104:8023–8028

64. Huang Y, Stewart TM, Wu Y, Baylin SB, Marton LJ, Perkins B, Jones RJ, Woster PM, Casero RA Jr (2009) Novel oligoamine analogues inhibit lysine-specific demethylase 1 and induce reexpression of epigenetically silenced genes. Clin Cancer Res 15:7217–7228

65. Zhang X, Lu F, Wang J, Yin F, Xu Z, Qi D, Wu X, Cao Y, Liang W, Liu Y, Sun H, Ye T, Zhang H (2013) Pluripotent stem cell protein Sox2 confers sensitivity to LSD1 inhibition in cancer cells. Cell Rep 5:445–457

66. Wang J, Lu F, Ren Q, Sun H, Xu Z, Lan R, Liu Y, Ward D, Quan J, Ye T, Zhang H (2011) Novel histone demethylase LSD1 inhibitors selectively target cancer cells with pluripotent stem cell properties. Cancer Res 71:7238–7249

67. Harris WJ, Huang X, Lynch JT, Spencer GJ, Hitchin JR, Li Y, Ciceri F, Blaser JG, Greystoke BF, Jordan AM, Miller CJ, Ogilvie DJ, Somervaille TC (2012) The histone demethylase KDM1A sustains the oncogenic potential of MLL-AF9 leukemia stem cells. Cancer Cell 21:473–487

68. Schenk T, Chen WC, Göllner S, Howell L, Jin L, Hebestreit K, Klein HU, Popescu AC, Burnett A, Mills K, Casero RA Jr, Marton L, Woster P, Minden MD, Dugas M, Wang JC, Dick JE, Müller-Tidow C, Petric K, Zelent A (2012) Inhibition of the LSD1 (KDM1A) demethylase reactivates the all-*trans*-retinoic acid differentiation pathway in acute myeloid leukemia. Nat Med 18:605–611

69. Schmidt DM, McCafferty DG (2007) *trans*-2-Phenylcyclopropylamine is a mechanism-based inactivator of the histone demethylase LSD1. Biochemistry 46:4408–4416

70. Yang M, Culhane JC, Szewczuk LM, Jalili P, Ball HL, Machius M, Cole PA, Yu H (2007) Structural basis for the inhibition of the LSD1 histone demethylase by the antidepressant *trans*-2-phenylcyclopropylamine. Biochemistry 46:8058–8065

71. Kauffman EC, Robinson BD, Downes MJ, Powell LG, Lee MM, Scherr DS, Gudas LJ, Mongan NP (2011) Role of androgen receptor and associated lysine-demethylase coregulators, LSD1 and JMJD2A, in localized and advanced human bladder cancer. Mol Carcinog 50:931–944

72. Ueda R, Suzuki T, Mino K, Tsumoto H, Nakagawa H, Hasegawa M, Sasaki R, Mizukami T, Miyata N (2009) Identification of cell-active lysine specific demethylase 1-selective inhibitors. J Am Chem Soc 131:17536–17537

73. Ogasawara D, Suzuki T, Mino K, Ueda R, Khan MN, Matsubara T, Koseki K, Hasegawa M, Sasaki R, Nakagawa H, Mizukami T, Miyata N (2010) Synthesis and biological activity of optically active NCL-1, a lysine-specific demethylase 1 selective inhibitor. Bioorg Med Chem 19:3702–3708

74. Cortez V, Mann M, Tekmal S, Suzuki T, Miyata N, Rodriguez-Aguayo C, Lopez-Berestein G, Sood AK, Vadlamudi RK (2012) Targeting the PELP1-KDM1 axis as a potential therapeutic strategy for breast cancer. Breast Cancer Res 14:R108

75. Etani T, Suzuki T, Naiki T, Naiki-Ito A, Ando R, Iida K, Kawai N, Tozawa K, Miyata N, Kohri K, Takahashi S (2015) NCL1, a highly selective lysine-specific demethylase 1 inhibitor, suppresses prostate cancer without adverse effect. Oncotarget 6:2865–2878

76. Ogasawara D, Itoh Y, Tsumoto H, Kakizawa T, Mino K, Fukuhara K, Nakagawa H, Hasegawa M, Sasaki R, Mizukami T, Miyata N, Suzuki T (2013) Lysine-specific demethylase 1-selective inactivators: protein-targeted drug delivery mechanism. Angew Chem Int Ed 52:8620–8624

77. Rao S, Zafar A (2014) Methods and compositions comprising lysine-specific demethylase inhibitors (LSD) for inhibiting growth of cancer stem cells. Patent Appl WO2014205511A1

78. Mohammad HP, Smitheman KN, Kamat CD, Soong D, Federowicz KE, Van Aller GS, Schneck JL, Carson JD, Liu Y, Butticello M, Bonnette WG, Gorman SA, Degenhardt Y, Bai Y, McCabe MT, Pappalardi MB, Kasparec J, Tian X, McNulty KC, Rouse M, McDevitt P, Ho T, Crouthamel M, Hart TK, Concha NO, McHugh CF, Miller WH, Dhanak D, Tummino PJ, Carpenter CL, Johnson NW, Hann CL, Kruger RG (2015) A DNA hypomethylation signature predicts antitumor activity of LSD1 inhibitors in SCLC. Cancer Cell 28:57–69

79. Maes T, Mascaró C, Ortega A, Lunardi S, Ciceri F, Somervaille TC, Buesa C (2015) KDM1 histone lysine demethylases as targets for treatments of oncological and neurodegenerative disease. Epigenomics 7:609–626

80. Shi Y (2007) Histone lysine demethylases: emerging roles in development, physiology and disease. Nat Rev Genet 8:829–833

81. Cho HS, Toyokawa G, Daigo Y, Hayami S, Masuda K, Ikawa N, Yamane Y, Maejima K, Tsunoda T, Field HI, Kelly JD, Neal DE, Ponder BA, Maehara Y, Nakamura Y, Hamamoto R (2012) The JmjC domain-containing histone demethylase KDM3A is a positive regulator of the G1/S transition in cancer cells via transcriptional regulation of the HOXA1 gene. Int J Cancer 131:E179–E189

82. Yamane K, Toumazou C, Tsukada Y, Erdjument-Bromage H, Tempst P, Wong J, Zhang Y (2006) JHDM2A, a JmjC-containing H3K9 demethylase, facilitates transcription activation by androgen receptor. Cell 125:483–495

83. Okada Y, Scott G, Ray MK, Mishina Y, Zhang Y (2007) Histone demethylase JHDM2A is critical for Tnp1 and Prm1 transcription and spermatogenesis. Nature 450:119–123

84. Tateishi K, Okada Y, Kallin EM, Zhang Y (2009) Role of Jhdm2a in regulating metabolic gene expression and obesity resistance. Nature 458:757–761

85. Uemura M, Yamamoto H, Takemasa I, Mimori K, Hemmi H, Mizushima T, Ikeda M, Sekimoto M, Matsuura N, Doki Y, Mori M (2010) Jumonji domain containing 1A is a novel prognostic marker for colorectal cancer: in vivo identification from hypoxic tumor cells. Clin Cancer Res 16:4636–4646

86. Hillringhaus L, Yue WW, Rose NR, Ng SS, Gileadi C, Loenarz C, Bello SH, Bray JE, Schofield CJ, Oppermann U (2011) Structural and evolutionary basis for the dual substrate selectivity of human KDM4 histone demethylase family. J Biol Chem 286:41616–41625

87. Cloos PA, Christensen J, Agger K, Maiolica A, Rappsilber J, Antal T, Hansen KH, Helin K (2006) The putative oncogene GASC1 demethylates tri- and dimethylated lysine 9 on histone H3. Nature 442:307–311

88. Whetstine JR, Nottke A, Lan F, Huarte M, Smolikov S, Chen Z, Spooner E, Li E, Zhang G, Colaiacovo M, Shi Y (2006) Reversal of histone lysine trimethylation by the JMJD2 family of histone demethylases. Cell 125:467–481

89. Chen Z, Zang J, Whetstine J, Hong X, Davrazou F, Kutateladze TG, Simpson M, Mao Q, Pan CH, Dai S, Hagman J, Hansen K, Shi Y, Zhang G (2006) Structural insights into histone demethylation by JMJD2 family members. Cell 125:691–702

90. Horton JR, Upadhyay AK, Qi HH, Zhang X, Shi Y, Cheng X (2010) Enzymatic and structural insights for substrate specificity of a family of jumonji histone lysine demethylases. Nat Struct Mol Biol 17:38–43

91. Crea F, Sun L, Mai A, Chiang YT, Farrar WL, Danesi R, Helgason CD (2012) The emerging role of histone lysine demethylases in prostate cancer. Mol Cancer 11:52

92. Loenarz C, Ge W, Coleman ML, Rose NR, Cooper CD, Klose RJ, Ratcliffe PJ, Schofield CJ (2010) PHF8, a gene associated with cleft lip/palate and mental retardation, encodes for an Nε-dimethyl lysine demethylase. Hum Mol Genet 19:217–222

93. Feng W, Yonezawa M, Ye J, Jenuwein T, Grummt I (2010) PHF8 activates transcription of rRNA genes through H3K4me3 binding and H3K9me1/2 demethylation. Nat Struct Mol Biol 17:445–450

94. Rui L, Emre NC, Kruhlak MJ, Chung HJ, Steidl C, Slack G, Wright GW, Lenz G, Ngo VN, Shaffer AL, Xu W, Zhao H, Yang Y, Lamy L, Davis RE, Xiao W, Powell J, Maloney D, Thomas CJ, Möller P, Rosenwald A, Ott G, Muller-Hermelink HK, Savage K, Connors JM, Rimsza LM, Campo E, Jaffe ES, Delabie J, Smeland EB, Weisenburger DD, Chan WC, Gascoyne RD, Levens D, Staudt LM (2010) Cooperative epigenetic modulation by cancer amplicon genes. Cancer Cell 18:590–605

95. Liu G, Bollig-Fischer A, Kreike B, van de Vijver MJ, Abrams J, Ethier SP, Yang ZQ (2009) Genomic amplification and oncogenic properties of the GASC1 histone demethylase gene in breast cancer. Oncogene 28:4491–4500

96. Wissmann M, Yin N, Müller JM, Greschik H, Fodor BD, Jenuwein T, Vogler C, Schneider R, Günther T, Buettner R, Metzger E, Schüle R (2007) Cooperative demethylation by JMJD2C and LSD1 promotes androgen receptor-dependent gene expression. Nat Cell Biol 9:347–353

97. Ishimura A, Terashima M, Kimura H, Akagi K, Suzuki Y, Sugano S, Suzuki T (2009) Jmjd2c histone demethylase enhances the expression of Mdm2 oncogene. Biochem Biophys Res Commun 389:366–371

98. Cheung N, Fung TK, Zeisig BB, Holmes K, Rane JK, Mowen KA, Finn MG, Lenhard B, Chan LC, So CW (2016) Targeting aberrant epigenetic networks mediated by PRMT1 and KDM4C in acute myeloid leukemia. Cancer Cell 29:32–48

99. Hamada S, Suzuki T, Mino K, Koseki K, Oehme F, Flamme I, Ozasa H, Itoh Y, Ogasawara D, Komaarashi H, Kato A, Tsumoto H, Nakagawa H, Hasegawa M, Sasaki R, Mizukami T, Miyata N (2010) Design, synthesis, enzyme-inhibitory activity, and effect on human cancer cells of a novel series of jumonji domain-containing protein 2 histone demethylase inhibitors. J Med Chem 53:5629–5638

100. Ye Q, Holowatyj A, Wu J, Liu H, Zhang L, Suzuki T, Yang ZQ (2015) Genetic alterations of KDM4 subfamily and therapeutic effect of novel demethylase inhibitor in breast cancer. Am J Cancer Res 5:1519–1530

101. Klose RJ, Yan Q, Tothova Z, Yamane K, Erdjument-Bromage H, Tempst P, Gilliland DG, Zhang Y, Kaelin WG Jr (2007) The retinoblastoma binding protein RBP2 is an H3K4 demethylase. Cell 128:889–900

102. Christensen J, Agger K, Cloos PA, Pasini D, Rose S, Sennels L, Rappsilber J, Hansen KH, Salcini AE, Helin K (2007) RBP2 belongs to a family of demethylases, specific for tri-and dimethylated lysine 4 on histone 3. Cell 128:1063–1076

103. Rasmussen PB, Staller P (2014) The KDM5 family of histone demethylases as targets in oncology drug discovery. Epigenomics 6:277–286

104. Teng YC, Lee CF, Li YS, Chen YR, Hsiao PW, Chan MY, Lin FM, Huang HD, Chen YT, Jeng YM, Hsu CH, Yan Q, Tsai MD, Juan LJ (2013) Histone demethylase RBP2 promotes lung tumorigenesis and cancer metastasis. Cancer Res 73:4711–4721

105. Liang X, Zeng J, Wang L, Fang M, Wang Q, Zhao M, Xu X, Liu Z, Li W, Liu S, Yu H, Jia J, Chen C (2013) Histone demethylase retinoblastoma binding protein 2 is overexpressed in hepatocellular carcinoma and negatively regulated by hsa-miR-212. PLoS One 8:e69784

106. Zeng J, Ge Z, Wang L, Li Q, Wang N, Björkholm M, Jia J, Xu D (2010) The histone demethylase RBP2 is overexpressed in gastric cancer and its inhibition triggers senescence of cancer cells. Gastroenterology 138:981–992

107. Hidalgo A, Baudis M, Petersen I, Arreola H, Piña P, Vázquez-Ortiz G, Hernández D, González J, Lazos M, López R, Pérez C, García J, Vázquez K, Alatorre B, Salcedo M (2005) Microarray comparative genomic hybridization detection of chromosomal imbalances in uterine cervix carcinoma. BMC Cancer 5:77

108. Sharma SV, Lee DY, Li B, Quinlan MP, Takahashi F, Maheswaran S, McDermott U, Azizian N, Zou L, Fischbach MA, Wong KK, Brandstetter K, Wittner B, Ramaswamy S, Classon M, Settleman J (2010) A chromatin-mediated reversible drug-tolerant state in cancer cell sub-populations. Cell 141:69–80

109. Hou J, Wu J, Dombkowski A, Zhang K, Holowatyj A, Boerner JL, Yang ZQ (2012) Genomic amplification and a role in drug-resistance for the KDM5A histone demethylase in breast cancer. Am J Transl Res 4:247–256

110. Banelli B, Carra E, Barbieri F, Würth R, Parodi F, Pattarozzi A, Carosio R, Forlani A, Allemanni G, Marubbi D, Florio T, Daga A, Romani M (2015) The histone demethylase KDM5A is a key factor for the resistance to temozolomide in glioblastoma. Cell Cycle 14:3418–3429

111. Itoh Y, Sawada H, Suzuki M, Tojo T, Sasaki R, Hasegawa M, Mizukami T, Suzuki T (2015) Identification of jumonji AT-rich interactive domain 1A inhibitors and their effect on cancer cells. ACS Med Chem Lett 6:665–670

112. Xiang Y, Zhu Z, Han G, Lin H, Xu L, Chen CD (2007) JMJD3 is a histone H3K27 demethylase. Cell Res 17:850–857

113. Sen GL, Webster DE, Barragan DI, Chang HY, Khavari PA (2008) Control of differentiation in a self-renewing mammalian tissue by the histone demethylase JMJD3. Genes Dev 22:1865–1870

114. Agger K, Cloos PA, Rudkjaer L, Williams K, Andersen G, Christensen J, Helin K (2009) The H3K27me3 demethylase JMJD3 contributes to the activation of the INK4A-ARF locus in response to oncogene- and stress-induced senescence. Genes Dev 23:1171–1176

115. Shen Y, Guo X, Wang Y, Qiu W, Chang Y, Zhang A, Duan X (2012) Expression and significance of histone H3K27 demethylases in renal cell carcinoma. BMC Cancer 12:470

116. Wei Y, Chen R, Dimicoli S, Bueso-Ramos C, Neuberg D, Pierce S, Wang H, Yang H, Jia Y, Zheng H, Fang Z, Nguyen M, Ganan-Gomez I, Ebert B, Levine R, Kantarjian H, Garcia-Manero G (2013) Global H3K4me3 genome mapping reveals alterations of innate immunity signaling and overexpression of JMJD3 in human myelodysplastic syndrome CD34+ cells. Leukemia 27:2177–2186

117. Tokunaga R, Sakamoto Y, Nakagawa S, Miyake K, Izumi D, Kosumi K, Taki K, Higashi T, Imamura Y, Ishimoto T, Iwatsuki M, Baba Y, Miyamoto Y, Yoshida N, Oki E, Watanabe M, Baba H (2016) The prognostic significance of histone lysine demethylase JMJD3/KDM6B in colorectal cancer. Ann Surg Oncol 23:678–685

118. Park WY, Hong BJ, Lee J, Choi C, Kim MY (2016) H3K27 demethylase JMJD3 employs the NF-κB and BMP signaling pathways to modulate the tumor microenvironment and promote melanoma progression and metastasis. Cancer Res 76:161–170

119. Kruidenier L, Chung CW, Cheng Z, Liddle J, Che K, Joberty G, Bantscheff M, Bountra C, Bridges A, Diallo H, Eberhard D, Hutchinson S, Jones E, Katso R, Leveridge M, Mander PK, Mosley J, Ramirez-Molina C, Rowland P, Schofield CJ, Sheppard RJ, Smith JE, Swales C, Tanner R, Thomas P, Tumber A, Drewes G, Oppermann U, Patel DJ, Lee K, Wilson DM (2012) A selective jumonji H3K27 demethylase inhibitor modulates the proinflammatory macrophage response. Nature 488:404–408

120. Ntziachristos P, Tsirigos A, Welstead GG, Trimarchi T, Bakogianni S, Xu L, Loizou E, Holmfeldt L, Strikoudis A, King B, Mullenders J, Becksfort J, Nedjic J, Paietta E, Tallman MS, Rowe JM, Tonon G, Satoh T, Kruidenier L, Prinjha R, Akira S, Van Vlierberghe P, Ferrando AA, Jaenisch R, Mullighan CG, Aifantis I (2014) Contrasting roles of histone 3 lysine 27 demethylases in acute lymphoblastic leukaemia. Nature 514:513–517

121. Sakaki H, Okada M, Kuramoto K, Takeda H, Watarai H, Suzuki S, Seino S, Seino M, Ohta T, Nagase S, Kurachi H, Kitanaka C (2015) GSKJ4, a selective jumonji H3K27 demethylase inhibitor, effectively targets ovarian cancer stem cells. Anticancer Res 35:6607–6614

122. Hashizume R, Andor N, Ihara Y, Lerner R, Gan H, Chen X, Fang D, Huang X, Tom MW, Ngo V, Solomon D, Mueller S, Paris PL, Zhang Z, Petritsch C, Gupta N, Waldman TA, James CD (2014) Pharmacologic inhibition of histone demethylation as a therapy for pediatric brain-stem glioma. Nat Med 20:1394–1396

123. Horton JR, Upadhyay AK, Qi HH, Zhang X, Shi Y, Cheng X (2010) Enzymatic and structural insights for substrate specificity of a family of jumonji histone lysine demethylases. Nat Struct Mol Biol 17:38–43

124. Liu W, Tanasa B, Tyurina OV, Zhou TY, Gassmann R, Liu WT, Ohgi KA, Benner C, Garcia-Bassets I, Aggarwal AK, Desai A, Dorrestein PC, Glass CK, Rosenfeld MG (2010) PHF8 mediates histone H4 lysine 20 demethylation events involved in cell cycle progression. Nature 466:508–512

125. Björkman M, Östling P, Härmä V, Virtanen J, Mpindi JP, Rantala J, Mirtti T, Vesterinen T, Lundin M, Sankila A, Rannikko A, Kaivanto E, Kohonen P, Kallioniemi O, Nees M (2012) Systematic knockdown of epigenetic enzymes identifies a novel histone demethylase PHF8 overexpressed in prostate cancer with an impact on cell proliferation, migration and invasion. Oncogene 31:3444–3456

126. Sun X, Qiu JJ, Zhu S, Cao B, Sun L, Li S, Li P, Zhang S, Dong S (2013) Oncogenic features of PHF8 histone demethylase in esophageal squamous cell carcinoma. PLoS One 8:e77353

127. Suzuki T, Ozasa H, Itoh Y, Zhan P, Sawada H, Mino K, Walport L, Ohkubo R, Kawamura A, Yonezawa M, Tsukada Y, Tumber A, Nakagawa H, Hasegawa M, Sasaki R, Mizukami T, Schofield CJ, Miyata N (2013) Identification of the KDM2/7 histone lysine demethylase subfamily inhibitor and its antiproliferative activity. J Med Chem 56:7222–7231

128. Ma H, Baumann CT, Li H, Strahl BD, Rice R, Jelinek MA, Aswad DW, Allis CD, Hager GL, Stallcup MR (2001) Hormone-dependent, CARM1-directed, arginine-specific methylation of histone H3 on a steroid-regulated promoter. Curr Biol 11:1981–1985

129. Wang H, Huang ZQ, Xia L, Feng Q, Erdjument-Bromage H, Strahl BD, Briggs SD, Allis CD, Wong J, Tempst P, Zhang Y (2001) Methylation of histone H4 at arginine 3 facilitating transcriptional activation by nuclear hormone receptor. Science 293:853–857

130. Bauer UM, Daujat S, Nielsen SJ, Nightingale K, Kouzarides T (2002) Methylation at arginine 17 of histone H3 is linked to gene activation. EMBO Rep 3:39–44
131. Pal S, Vishwanath SN, Erdjument-Bromage H, Tempst P, Sif S (2004) Human SWI/SNF-associated PRMT5 methylates histone H3 arginine 8 and negatively regulates expression of ST7 and NM23 tumor suppressor genes. Mol Cell Biol 24:9630–9645
132. Zhang Y, Reinberg D (2001) Transcription regulation by histone methylation: interplay between different covalent modifications of the core histone tails. Genes Dev 15:2343–2360
133. Lee JH, Cook JR, Yang ZH, Mirochnitchenko O, Gunderson SI, Felix AM, Herth N, Hoffmann R, Pestka S (2005) PRMT7, a new protein arginine methyltransferase that synthesizes symmetric dimethylarginine. J Biol Chem 280:3656–3664
134. Cheung N, Chan LC, Thompson A, Cleary ML, So CW (2007) Protein arginine-methyltransferase-dependent oncogenesis. Nat Cell Biol 9:1208–1215
135. Yan L, Yan C, Qian K, Su H, Kofsky-Wofford SA, Lee WC, Zhao X, Ho MC, Ivanov I, Zheng YG (2014) Diamidine compounds for selective inhibition of protein arginine methyltransferase 1. J Med Chem 57:2611–2622
136. Wang J, Chen L, Sinha SH, Liang Z, Chai H, Muniyan S, Chou YW, Yang C, Yan L, Feng Y, Li KK, Lin MF, Jiang H, Zheng YG, Luo C (2012) Pharmacophore-based virtual screening and biological evaluation of small molecule inhibitors for protein arginine methylation. J Med Chem 55:7978–7987
137. Cuthbert GL, Daujat S, Snowden AW, Erdjument-Bromage H, Hagiwara T, Yamada M, Schneider R, Gregory PD, Tempst P, Bannister AJ, Kouzarides T (2004) Histone deimination antagonizes arginine methylation. Cell 118:545–553
138. Hagiwara T, Hidaka Y, Yamada M (2005) Deimination of histone H2A and H4 at arginine 3 in HL-60 granulocytes. Biochemistry 44:5827–5834
139. Wang Y, Li P, Wang S, Hu J, Chen XA, Wu J, Fisher M, Oshaben K, Zhao N, Gu Y, Wang D, Chen G, Wang Y (2012) Anticancer peptidylarginine deiminase (PAD) inhibitors regulate the autophagy flux and the mammalian target of rapamycin complex 1 activity. J Biol Chem 287:25941–25953

Part VI
Future Directions

Future Perspective of DNA and Histone Methylation as Cancer Targets

Toward Better Epigenetic Cancer Diagnosis, Therapies, and Prevention

Hideyuki Takeshima and Toshikazu Ushijima

Abstract Epigenetic alterations are useful for cancer diagnosis and therapy, and potentially for prevention. For cancer diagnosis, epigenetic alterations in cancer cells can be utilized for cancer detection and diagnosis of cancer pathophysiology, such as drug sensitivity and patient prognosis. Measurement of epigenetic alterations in normal cells can provide cancer risk diagnosis taking account of individuals' life history. To bring these epigenetic diagnoses into clinical practice, improvement of detection technologies, strict selection of marker genes, and analysis of clinically relevant samples are important. For cancer therapy, various epigenetic inhibitors are actively being developed, and a number of clinical trials are now being conducted for solid tumors. To bring these epigenetic therapies into clinical practice, we need to pay attention to cancer cell specificity, gene specificity, the small range of the biologically effective dose, and slow response to epigenetic therapy. For cancer prevention, removal of accumulated methylation in normal tissues and repression of induction of aberrant DNA methylation can be utilized, and effectiveness has been shown in animal models. Our continual efforts based on strong basic science and mechanism-based clinical trials will bring more epigenetic diagnosis, therapy, and prevention to clinical practice.

Keywords Epigenetics • DNA methylation • Cancer diagnosis • Cancer therapy • Cancer prevention

H. Takeshima • T. Ushijima (✉)
Division of Epigenomics, National Cancer Center Research Institute,
5-1-1 Tsukiji, Chuo-ku, 104-0045 Tokyo, Japan
e-mail: tushijim@ncc.go.jp

© Springer International Publishing AG 2017
A. Kaneda, Y.-i. Tsukada (eds.), *DNA and Histone Methylation as Cancer Targets*,
Cancer Drug Discovery and Development, DOI 10.1007/978-3-319-59786-7_21

1 Introduction

Epigenetic alterations are frequently present in various types of cancers, and some of them are causally involved in cancer development and progression [1, 2]. Not only in cancer cells but also in normal cells, epigenetic alterations can be present. As described in the other chapters, these epigenetic alterations are very useful for cancer diagnosis and therapy. In addition, potential usefulness in cancer prevention has also been shown. In this final chapter, we will discuss future perspectives of how epigenetic alterations can be utilized for cancer diagnosis, therapy, and prevention.

2 Future Perspective for Cancer Diagnosis

Epigenetic alterations are present not only in cancer cells but also in normal cells due to aging or exposure to environmental factors, and the alterations both in cancer and normal cells can be utilized for cancer diagnosis. Among various epigenetic modifications, DNA methylation is considered to be especially useful as a cancer diagnostic marker for its chemical and biological stability. Cancer diagnosis can be classified into detection of cancer (cancer detection diagnosis), characterization of the cancer and cancer patients (cancer pathophysiology diagnosis), and cancer risk diagnosis.

2.1 Cancer Detection Diagnosis

Cancer cell-specific DNA methylation, such as *SEPT9* methylation in colorectal cancers [3], can be utilized for the detection of cancers. Such methylation can be detected in either (i) specimens obtained with minimal invasion but containing no or few cancer cells, such as tumor-derived cell-free DNA (cfDNA), or (ii) specimens that potentially contain cancer cells, such as urine for renal and bladder cancers, sputum for lung cancers, and stool for colorectal cancers. Tumor-derived cfDNA can be utilized for the detection of a variety of cancers, but suffers from its limited availability. The merit of detecting a variety of cancers can become a shortcoming of the lack of specificity. In contrast, specimens containing cancer cells appear to contain more tumor-derived DNA [4]. In either specimen, at this moment, the sensitivity and specificity of such methylation markers have not exceeded those of the markers currently used in clinical practice [5], and several issues should be overcome.

First, the issue of extremely small amounts of DNA in a specimen needs to be overcome. PCR is often employed to analyze such a small amount of DNA. However, the more amplification we conduct, the higher the risk of stochastic results, including contamination, we have. Potential solutions for now include digital PCR and next-generation sequencing without PCR. Also, bisulfite treatment is known to reduce the amount of DNA suitable for PCR down to approximately 10% of the initial amount. Development of technology that can detect epigenetic information on DNA without bisulfite treatment will bring a significant advancement. In addition, the use of genomic loci with high copy numbers, such as multi-copy genes and repetitive sequences, is an alternative way to overcome this issue.

Second, as described below, aberrant DNA methylation can be present even in normal cells reflecting aging or exposure to environmental factors. Therefore, to achieve sufficient specificity for detection of cancer, selection of a marker locus specifically methylated in cancer cells, not in surrounding normal cells, is necessary. Since robust techniques for genome-wide screening are readily available, strict selection of loci with specific methylation can be readily achieved.

Third, although this is applicable to any marker development, the use of clinically relevant samples is essential. It is easy by conventional blood biochemistry to distinguish liver cancer patients from entirely healthy individuals, but clinically an important issue is to distinguish liver cancer patients from patients with hepatitis or liver cirrhosis. To bring a cancer cell-specific methylation marker to clinical practice, better sensitivity and specificity in clinically relevant samples are required.

2.2 Diagnosis of Cancer Pathophysiology

Epigenetic alterations in cancer cells provide information useful for the diagnosis of cancer pathophysiology, such as drug sensitivity and patient prognosis (Fig. 1). Gliomas with aberrant DNA methylation of *MGMT* show sensitivity to an alkylating agent, temozolomide [9]. Colon cancers with the CpG island methylator phenotype (CIMP) show resistance to 5-fluorouracil (5-FU) [10]. Neuroblastoma patients with CIMP show poorer prognosis than those without, and the prognostic power of CIMP is much more informative than conventional prognostic markers and *MYCN* amplification [11].

To increase the accuracy of a methylation marker, a mechanistic basis of how methylation of a locus is associated with a phenotype is important. When the prediction power of a methylation marker is dependent upon resultant gene silencing, simultaneous analysis of mutations, which can also inactivate the gene, may be useful. It used to be cumbersome to analyze mutations of the entire coding region of a relevant gene, but recent next-generation sequencing technologies have made the analysis easy. An integration of both epigenetic and genetic information is expected to be more useful for diagnosis of cancer pathophysiology. On the other hand, as typically observed for CIMP markers, methylation of specific marker genes represents that of many additional loci in the genome. In this case, selection of a marker gene (or genes) whose methylation is closely associated with methylation of the other target genes is important.

Multiple advantages of diagnosis using aberrant DNA methylation over that using mRNA or protein expression are known. First, aberrant DNA methylation can

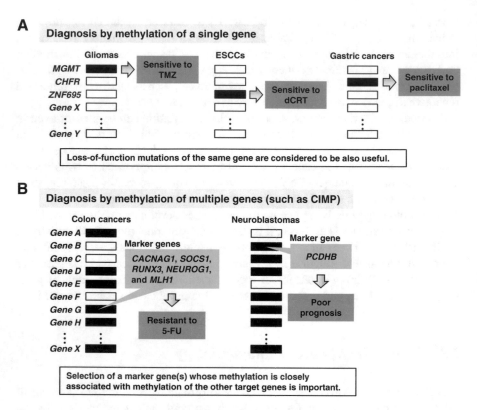

Fig. 1 Diagnosis of cancer pathophysiology, such as drug sensitivity and patient prognosis, using aberrant DNA methylation. (**a**) Diagnosis using aberrant DNA methylation of a single gene. Gliomas with aberrant DNA methylation of *MGMT* show susceptibility to an alkylating agent, temozolomide (TMZ). Esophageal squamous cell carcinomas (ESCCs) with aberrant methylation of *ZNF695* show susceptibility to definitive chemoradiotherapy (dCRT) [6]. Gastric cancers with aberrant methylation of *CHFR* show susceptibility to paclitaxel [7, 8]. Information of loss of function mutations of the same genes might improve diagnostic accuracy when loss of gene function is responsible for a pathophysiology. (**b**) Diagnosis using aberrant DNA methylation of multiple genes, exemplified by CIMP. Colon cancers with CIMP show resistance to 5-fluorouracil (5-FU). Neuroblastoma patients with CIMP show poor prognosis. Selection of a marker gene (or genes) whose methylation is closely associated with methylation of the other target genes is important

predict that a gene will not be expressed even in the future timing of drug treatment (Fig. 2). For example, *MGMT* expression can be induced by temozolomide treatment, even if it is not expressed at the time of tumor biopsy. However, if *MGMT* is methylated in a biopsy specimen, it can never be induced, even at the time of drug treatment. Second, an overall methylation level of a marker gene in a heterogeneous sample is not disturbed by a small fraction of contaminating cells. In a single cell, methylation status of an individual gene can be classified into 0 (two unmethylated alleles), 1 (one methylated and one unmethylated alleles), and 2 (two methylated alleles). In contrast, mRNA and proteins can be expressed at extremely high levels even in a single cell, and contamination of a small number of cells with extremely

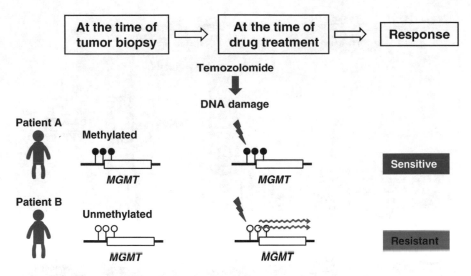

Fig. 2 Diagnosis of inability to express a gene using aberrant DNA methylation. An unexpressed gene can be induced upon transcriptional stimulation if it is not methylated in its promoter CpG island. In the case of *MGMT*, its expression can be induced by DNA damage due to temozolomide treatment even if it is not expressed at the time of tumor biopsy. However, if *MGMT* is methylated, it can never be induced. Since induction of *MGMT* leads to repair of DNA damage by temozolomide, gliomas with unmethylated *MGMT* show poorer response to temozolomide

high expression in a sample can disturb the overall expression levels in the sample. Third, DNA is chemically stable, and DNA methylation can be analyzed in a sample with partial degradation.

These confirm the potential of DNA methylation in cancer pathophysiology diagnosis and the importance of mechanistic analysis of how methylation of a marker gene is associated with cancer pathophysiology.

2.3 Cancer Risk Diagnosis by Measurement of Methylation Burden in Normal Tissues

Not only in cancer cells but also in normal cells, epigenetic alterations are accumulated [12]. Aberrant DNA methylation in normal tissues is known to be induced by aging or exposure to some environmental factors (methylation inducers), such as infectious agents [13], tobacco smoking [14], and hormones [15]. Especially, chronic inflammation, such as *Helicobacter pylori* (*H. pylori*)-induced gastritis, hepatitis virus-induced hepatitis, and ulcerative colitis, has been shown to play a critical role in aberrant DNA methylation induction [16]. Aberrant DNA methylation in normal tissues, namely methylation burden, can persist for a long time, potentially for life, even after the removal of methylation inducers, and is deeply

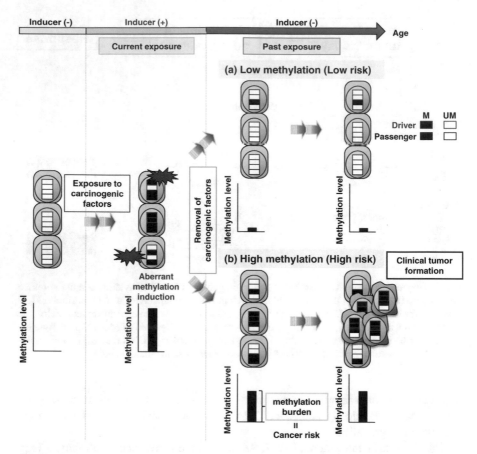

Fig. 3 Cancer risk diagnosis by measurement of methylation burden. Methylation levels after removal of methylation inducers are considered to reflect epigenomic damage of stem cells (methylation burden) in normal tissues, and their measurement has the potential to provide cancer risk diagnosis. People with low (**a**) and high (**b**) methylation levels are considered to have low and high cancer risk, respectively

involved in the formation of an epigenetic field for cancerization (an epigenetic field defect), a normal tissue predisposed to carcinogenesis [12].

Methylation burden reflects epigenomic damage in normal tissues, and its measurement has the potential to provide cancer risk diagnosis (Fig. 3). Such risk diagnosis using methylation burden is most advanced in gastric tissues. Cross-sectional studies showed that the levels of methylation burden (methylation levels after the removal of *H. pylori* infection) increased in the order of: normal gastric tissues of healthy people, those of patients with a single gastric cancer, and those of patients with multiple gastric cancers [17, 18]. Further, a multicenter prospective cohort study demonstrated that the measurement of DNA methylation levels after endoscopic submucosal dissection of a primary gastric cancer can predict the risk of developing a metachronous gastric cancer [19].

Cancer risk diagnosis using methylation burden in normal tissues is in sharp contrast with that using a single nucleotide polymorphism (SNP). SNPs define the innate cancer risk of an individual, and cannot evaluate actual exposure to environmental factors of the individual. In contrast, methylation burden reflects both the exposure and response to the exposure, which can be defined by SNPs, and thus takes account of individuals' life history. Cancer risk diagnosis using methylation burden in normal tissues potentially has a broad application since accumulation of aberrant DNA methylation is known for various organs, such as the esophagus, colon, liver, and mammary glands [20–23].

3   Future Perspective for Cancer Therapy

Various epigenetic inhibitors, which can target epigenetic writers, erasers, and readers, are actively being developed. Among such inhibitors, DNA demethylating drugs (azacytidine and decitabine) are now clinically utilized for myelodysplastic syndrome (MDS) and a part of acute myeloid leukemia (AML) [24, 25]. Histone deacetylase inhibitors (vorinostat, romidepsin, and panobinostat) are clinically utilized for cutaneous T-cell lymphoma (CTCL) and multiple myeloma [26].

3.1   Epigenetic Therapy for Solid Tumors

A large number of clinical trials are now being conducted for solid tumors, and good clinical responses have been obtained for some cancers, especially by a combination of an epigenetic drug and conventional chemotherapy [27]. A combination of azacytidine and a histone deacetylase (HDAC) inhibitor, entinostat, was effective for recurrent metastatic non-small cell lung cancers [28]. Also, a combination of decitabine and carboplatin was effective for carboplatin-resistant ovarian cancers [29], and that of decitabine and panitumumab, an anti-EGFR antibody, was effective for metastatic colorectal cancers without *KRAS* mutation [30].

To bring these promises of epigenetic therapy to clinical practice, several important issues should be addressed, including (i) cancer cell and gene specificity, (ii) the small range of the biologically effective dose, and (iii) a relatively slow response to the therapy (Fig. 4). Especially, for most epigenetic drugs, a biologically effective dose is distinct from the maximum tolerated dose (MTD). DNA demethylating agents are known to induce cell cycle arrest and thus a small degree of DNA demethylation at MTDs, while they efficiently induce DNA demethylation at doses far below the MTD, namely a biologically effective dose [31]. Usually, the maximum biological dose has a small range as expected from its definition. Also, most epigenetic drugs typically need weeks of time for their clinical responses to become visible [32].

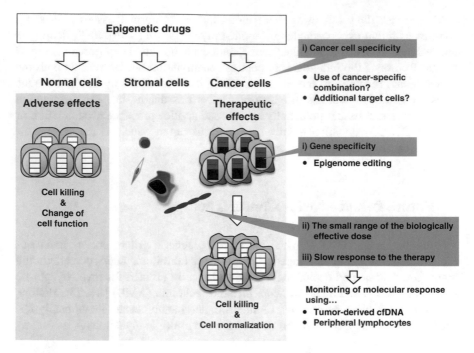

Fig. 4 Important issues to bring epigenetic therapy to solid tumors, including (i) cancer cell and gene specificity, (ii) the small range of the biologically effective dose, and (iii) slow response to the therapy. Cancer cell specificity might be achieved by targeting a cancer cell-specific combination of epigenetic modifications. At the same time, diversity of target cells for epigenetic therapy, such as stromal cells, needs attention. Gene specificity may be achieved by epigenome editing. The small range of the biologically effective dose and the slow response may be overcome by developing markers that can evaluate molecular responses before clinical responses are obtained

3.2 Monitoring of Therapeutic Efficacy

To overcome the above issues of the small range of the biologically effective dose and the slow response, we need markers that can evaluate molecular responses before clinical responses are obtained. Molecular responses can be evaluated by measuring the changes of epigenetic modifications, such as DNA demethylation, in cancer cells. Since this is for monitoring purposes, the diagnosis must be achieved using specimens obtained by minimally invasive methods, such as tumor-derived cfDNA or DNA from peripheral lymphocytes.

Regarding cfDNA, its amount is limited unless tumor necrosis (or apoptosis) is induced, tumor mass is large, or metastasis occurs. Therefore, as in the case of cancer detection, multiple pieces of invention need to be incorporated, such as (i) the use of novel technologies, such as digital-PCR and next-generation sequencing, (ii) development of a technology that can detect epigenetic information on DNA without bisulfite treatment, and iii) the use of a genomic locus with a high copy number.

In contrast, DNA from peripheral lymphocytes is available in sufficient amount, and solves the issue of small amounts of DNA. However, it has been difficult so far to develop a good monitoring marker for DNA demethylation in MDS. Recently, the potential of the long interspersed nuclear element (LINE-1) as a monitoring marker was shown [33]. In addition to the fundamental issue that therapeutic response of MDS is really due to DNA demethylation, potential reasons for the difficulty include (i) uncertainty whether DNA demethylation in peripheral leukocytes parallels that of tumor cells, and (ii) the lack of appropriate marker genes whose demethylation is in parallel with that of the genes responsible for therapeutic effects. These issues need to be solved early on for the success of epigenetic therapy in solid tumors.

3.3   Cancer Cell and Gene Specificity of Epigenetic Therapy

Not only cancer cells but also normal cells are affected by epigenetic drugs because any aberrant epigenetic modifications in a cancer cell can be physiological in other genomic regions of normal cells. To overcome this limitation, multiple attempts are being undertaken. If a combination of epigenetic modifications specifically present in cancer cells is identified, this will become a superb therapeutic target (Fig. 4). Indeed, the efficacy of a combined inhibition of DNA methylation and trimethylation of histone H3 lysine 27 (H3K27me3) has been shown in a preclinical study [34, 35]. This finding suggests that an aberrant combination of DNA methylation and H3K27me3 is specifically present in cancer cells and effectively targeted by the combination treatment. Not limited to this combination, a large-scale screening for aberrant combination of epigenetic modifications specifically present in cancer cells might lead to overcome the issue of cancer cell specificity.

Another attempt to overcome the issue of cancer cell specificity is targeting specific genes for change of an aberrant epigenetic modification in cancer cells. Such gene-specific intervention is considered to be achieved using epigenome editing technologies, and multiple reports are already available [36–38]. Third, it is noteworthy that promoter CpG islands of transcribed genes are resistant to DNA methylation induction [39–42]. This suggests that, once an aberrantly methylated promoter CpG island is partially demethylated by DNA demethylating drugs, it will become completely demethylated if it is actively transcribed. In contrast, genes without active transcription will be remethylated even after they are partially demethylated. This use of "transcription memory" may lead to a strategy of epigenetic and transcriptional restoration.

The fundamental question here is whether or not cancer cell specificity is really essential. Recent reports have shown that one of the major mechanisms of epigenetic therapy is activation of endogenous retroviruses and enhancement of antigenicity of cancer cells [43, 44]. Also, epigenetic abnormalities that are reversed by epigenetic therapy can be present not only in cancer cells but also in cells in a cancer microenvironment [45, 46]. Combining effects upon multiple genes in multiple target cells with reasonable specificity may become an effective approach.

3.4 Non-epigenetic Targets of Epigenetic Drugs

Some epigenetic drugs target not only histone proteins but also non-histone proteins. The mode of action of HDAC inhibitors is generally considered to be the reactivation of tumor-suppressor and differentiation-related genes repressed by histone deacetylation. However, a large number of proteins, such as HSP90, p53, c-Myc, and β-catenin, are also targets of HDACs, and the mode of action seems to be more complicated [47].

The mode of action of mutant IDH1/2 inhibitors is also complicated. *IDH1/2* mutations confer a novel enzymatic activity, which can catalyze the conversion of α-ketoglutarate to R(-)-2-hydroxyglutarate (2-HG) [48], and 2-HG inhibits activities of both TET enzymes [49] and histone demethylases [50], which lead to epigenetic alterations. At the same time, citric acid cycle metabolism is also affected by *IDH1* mutations [51]. Therefore, further understanding of the modes of action of individual epigenetic drugs is important, and this will lead to development of more efficient epigenetic therapy.

3.5 Novel Therapeutic Targets: Chromatin Remodelers

Recent cancer genome analysis elucidated that components of a chromatin remodeling complex, SWI/SNF, are frequently mutated in various types of cancers [52–57]. Some of these mutations are utilized to produce novel therapeutic targets. Rhabdoid tumors with *SMARCB1* mutations show up-regulation of a histone methyltransferase, EZH2 [58], and are susceptible to inhibition of EZH2 [59]. On the other hand, it is also reported that inhibition of EZH2 enzymatic activity itself is not sufficient for the growth inhibition of SWI/SNF-mutated cancer cells [60].

Synthetic lethality, due to which only cells with a specific mutation are killed by an additional mutation or lack of function of a gene, is reported for ARID1A and ARID1B [61] and also for SMARCA4 (BRG1) and SMARCA2 (BRM), ATPases of the SWI/SNF complex [62, 63]. Since ATPase is essential for survival of a cell, including a cancer cell, inhibition of the remaining ATPase subunit in cancer cells that lack one of the two ATPase subunits can induce specific cancer cell killing. Further development of therapeutic strategies against SWI/SNF-mutated cancers will be beneficial for a broad range of cancer types.

4 Future Perspective for Cancer Prevention

Methylation burden in normal tissues can persist even after the elimination of methylation inducers [64]. Therefore, in addition to suppression of methylation induction, removal of methylation burden itself is considered to be useful for cancer

Table 1 Reports about epigenetic cancer prevention using animal models

Tumor types	Inducers of cancers	Animals	Preventive treatment	Reduction of cancer incidence (or number)	Reference
Gastric cancers	*H. pylori* infection and MNU treatment	Mongolian gerbils	Decitabine	From 55% to 23%	[65]
SCCs (esophagus/ tongue)	4NQO treatment	Mouse	Hypomorphic Dnmt1	From 78% to 43% (esophagus) from 100% to 91% (tongue)	[66]
Intestinal polyps	*Apc* mutation ($Apc^{Min/+}$)	Mouse	Zebularine	From 100% to 27%	[67]
Intestinal polyps	*Apc* mutation ($Apc^{Min/+}$)	Mouse	Decitabine	From 113 polyps (n = 7) to 20 polyps (n = 12)	[68]
Intestinal tumors	*Mlh1* mutation	Mouse	Hypomorphic Dnmt1	From 83% to 0–61% (depending on Dnmt1 mutation types)	[69]
Prostate cancers	Expression of the SV40 early region, including TAg	Mouse	Decitabine	From 54% to 0%	[70]

SCC squamous cell carcinoma, *MNU* N-methyl-N-nitrosourea, *4NQO* 4-nitroquinoline 1-oxide and *TAg* large T antigen

prevention. As a proof-of-principle, administration of DNA demethylating drugs or utilization of *Dnmt1* hypomorphic alleles reduced cancer incidences in multiple animal models (Table 1). However, it is unclear whether the preventive effect was due to the repression of aberrant DNA methylation induction or due to removal of methylation burden accumulated in tissues. To address this issue, the preventive effect should be evaluated by administering a DNA demethylating agent after accumulation of methylation burden and removal of methylation inducers. Once this strategy is shown to be effective, removal of accumulated methylation burden will have immense application to cancer prevention.

To bring epigenetic cancer prevention to clinical practice, novel strategies for the removal of methylation burden need to be considered. DNA demethylating drugs currently available are not suitable for use in healthy people because of their adverse effects. A preventive intervention with currently available demethylating drugs will be potentially allowed only for a population at extremely high risk of intractable cancers, such as pancreatic cancers. At this moment, it is unclear whether DNA demethylating drugs with few adverse effects can be developed. In contrast, repression of induction of aberrant methylation can be more readily achieved, and supplementation with effective compounds for repression into food may become possible.

5 Epilogue

Epigenetic diagnosis is now coming into clinical practice. Also, a door to epigenetic therapy has now opened. At the same time, we are facing multiple challenges to bring new modes of epigenetic drugs into clinical practice. As ever, strong basic science and mechanism-based clinical trials will be required to overcome these issues. In addition to cancer, epigenetic alterations are likely to be involved in chronic disorders, such as diabetes mellitus and Alzheimer's disease. Our knowledge and technologies obtained in cancer research are valuable for research on epigenetic alterations in such disorders.

References

1. Baylin SB, Jones PA (2011) A decade of exploring the cancer epigenome – biological and translational implications. Nat Rev Cancer 11(10):726–734
2. Ushijima T (2005) Detection and interpretation of altered methylation patterns in cancer cells. Nat Rev Cancer 5(3):223–231
3. Church TR, Wandell M, Lofton-Day C, Mongin SJ, Burger M, Payne SR et al (2014) Prospective evaluation of methylated SEPT9 in plasma for detection of asymptomatic colorectal cancer. Gut 63(2):317–325
4. Sidransky D (2002) Emerging molecular markers of cancer. Nat Rev Cancer 2(3):210–219
5. Toiyama Y, Okugawa Y, Goel A (2014) DNA methylation and microRNA biomarkers for noninvasive detection of gastric and colorectal cancer. Biochem Biophys Res Commun 455(1–2):43–57
6. Takahashi T, Yamahsita S, Matsuda Y, Kishino T, Nakajima T, Kushima R et al (2015) ZNF695 methylation predicts a response of esophageal squamous cell carcinoma to definitive chemoradiotherapy. J Cancer Res Clin Oncol 141(3):453–463
7. Koga Y, Kitajima Y, Miyoshi A, Sato K, Sato S, Miyazaki K (2006) The significance of aberrant CHFR methylation for clinical response to microtubule inhibitors in gastric cancer. J Gastroenterol 41(2):133–139
8. Satoh A, Toyota M, Itoh F, Sasaki Y, Suzuki H, Ogi K et al (2003) Epigenetic inactivation of CHFR and sensitivity to microtubule inhibitors in gastric cancer. Cancer Res 63(24):8606–8613
9. Hegi ME, Diserens AC, Gorlia T, Hamou MF, de Tribolet N, Weller M et al (2005) MGMT gene silencing and benefit from temozolomide in glioblastoma. N Engl J Med 352(10):997–1003

10. Jover R, Nguyen TP, Perez-Carbonell L, Zapater P, Paya A, Alenda C et al (2011) 5-Fluorouracil adjuvant chemotherapy does not increase survival in patients with CpG island methylator phenotype colorectal cancer. Gastroenterology 140(4):1174–1181

11. Abe M, Ohira M, Kaneda A, Yagi Y, Yamamoto S, Kitano Y et al (2005) CpG island methylator phenotype is a strong determinant of poor prognosis in neuroblastomas. Cancer Res 65(3):828–834

12. Ushijima T (2007) Epigenetic field for cancerization. J Biochem Mol Biol 40(2):142–150

13. Ushijima T, Takeshima H (2011) Epigenetic epidemiology of infectious diseases. Springer.

14. Oka D, Yamashita S, Tomioka T, Nakanishi Y, Kato H, Kaminishi M et al (2009) The presence of aberrant DNA methylation in noncancerous esophageal mucosae in association with smoking history: a target for risk diagnosis and prevention of esophageal cancers. Cancer 115(15):3412–3426

15. Cheng AS, Culhane AC, Chan MW, Venkataramu CR, Ehrich M, Nasir A et al (2008) Epithelial progeny of estrogen-exposed breast progenitor cells display a cancer-like methylome. Cancer Res 68(6):1786–1796

16. Niwa T, Tsukamoto T, Toyoda T, Mori A, Tanaka H, Maekita T et al (2010) Inflammatory processes triggered by Helicobacter pylori infection cause aberrant DNA methylation in gastric epithelial cells. Cancer Res 70(4):1430–1440

17. Maekita T, Nakazawa K, Mihara M, Nakajima T, Yanaoka K, Iguchi M et al (2006) High levels of aberrant DNA methylation in Helicobacter pylori-infected gastric mucosae and its possible association with gastric cancer risk. Clin Cancer Res 12(3 Pt 1):989–995

18. Nakajima T, Maekita T, Oda I, Gotoda T, Yamamoto S, Umemura S et al (2006) Higher methylation levels in gastric mucosae significantly correlate with higher risk of gastric cancers. Cancer Epidemiol Biomark Prev 15(11):2317–2321

19. Asada K, Nakajima T, Shimazu T, Yamamichi N, Maekita T, Yokoi C et al (2015) Demonstration of the usefulness of epigenetic cancer risk prediction by a multicentre prospective cohort study. Gut 64(3):388–396

20. Eads CA, Lord RV, Kurumboor SK, Wickramasinghe K, Skinner ML, Long TI et al (2000) Fields of aberrant CpG island hypermethylation in Barrett's esophagus and associated adenocarcinoma. Cancer Res 60(18):5021–5026

21. Kondo Y, Kanai Y, Sakamoto M, Mizokami M, Ueda R, Hirohashi S (2000) Genetic instability and aberrant DNA methylation in chronic hepatitis and cirrhosis–a comprehensive study of loss of heterozygosity and microsatellite instability at 39 loci and DNA hypermethylation on 8 CpG islands in microdissected specimens from patients with hepatocellular carcinoma. Hepatology 32(5):970–979

22. Shen L, Kondo Y, Rosner GL, Xiao L, Hernandez NS, Vilaythong J et al (2005) MGMT promoter methylation and field defect in sporadic colorectal cancer. J Natl Cancer Inst 97(18):1330–1338

23. Yan PS, Venkataramu C, Ibrahim A, Liu JC, Shen RZ, Diaz NM et al (2006) Mapping geographic zones of cancer risk with epigenetic biomarkers in normal breast tissue. Clin Cancer Res 12(22):6626–6636

24. Quintas-Cardama A, Santos FP, Garcia-Manero G (2010) Therapy with azanucleosides for myelodysplastic syndromes. Nat Rev Clin Oncol 7(8):433–444

25. Wouters BJ, Delwel R (2016) Epigenetics and approaches to targeted epigenetic therapy in acute myeloid leukemia. Blood 127(1):42–52

26. West AC, Johnstone RW (2014) New and emerging HDAC inhibitors for cancer treatment. J Clin Invest 124(1):30–39

27. Nie J, Liu L, Li X, Han W (2014) Decitabine, a new star in epigenetic therapy: the clinical application and biological mechanism in solid tumors. Cancer Lett 354(1):12–20

28. Juergens RA, Wrangle J, Vendetti FP, Murphy SC, Zhao M, Coleman B et al (2011) Combination epigenetic therapy has efficacy in patients with refractory advanced non-small cell lung cancer. Cancer Discov 1(7):598–607

29. Matei D, Fang F, Shen C, Schilder J, Arnold A, Zeng Y et al (2012) Epigenetic resensitization to platinum in ovarian cancer. Cancer Res 72(9):2197–2205
30. Garrido-Laguna I, McGregor KA, Wade M, Weis J, Gilcrease W, Burr L et al (2013) A phase I/II study of decitabine in combination with panitumumab in patients with wild-type (wt) KRAS metastatic colorectal cancer. Investig New Drugs 31(5):1257–1264
31. Tsai HC, Li H, Van Neste L, Cai Y, Robert C, Rassool FV et al (2012) Transient low doses of DNA-demethylating agents exert durable antitumor effects on hematological and epithelial tumor cells. Cancer Cell 21(3):430–446
32. Issa JP, Garcia-Manero G, Giles FJ, Mannari R, Thomas D, Faderl S et al (2004) Phase 1 study of low dose prolonged exposure schedules of the hypomethylating agent 5-aza-2′-deoxycytidine (decitabine) in hematopoietic malignancies. Blood 103(5):1635–1640
33. Issa JP, Roboz G, Rizzieri D, Jabbour E, Stock W, O'Connell C et al (2015) Safety and tolerability of guadecitabine (SGI-110) in patients with myelodysplastic syndrome and acute myeloid leukaemia: a multicentre, randomised, dose-escalation phase 1 study. Lancet Oncol 16(9):1099–1110
34. Momparler RL, Idaghdour Y, Marquez VE, Momparler LF (2012) Synergistic antileukemic action of a combination of inhibitors of DNA methylation and histone methylation. Leuk Res 36(8):1049–1054
35. Takeshima H, Wakabayashi M, Hattori N, Yamashita S, Ushijima T (2015) Identification of coexistence of DNA methylation and H3K27me3 specifically in cancer cells as a promising target for epigenetic therapy. Carcinogenesis 36(2):192–201
36. Choudhury SR, Cui Y, Lubecka K, Stefanska B, Irudayaraj J (2016) CRISPR-dCas9 mediated TET1 targeting for selective DNA demethylation at BRCA1 promoter. Oncotarget 7(29):46545–46556
37. Morita S, Noguchi H, Horii T, Nakabayashi K, Kimura M, Okamura K et al (2016) Targeted DNA demethylation in vivo using dCas9-peptide repeat and scFv-TET1 catalytic domain fusions. Nat Biotechnol 34:1060–1065
38. Xu X, Tao Y, Gao X, Zhang L, Li X, Zou W et al (2016) A CRISPR-based approach for targeted DNA demethylation. Cell Discov 2:16009
39. De Smet C, Loriot A, Boon T (2004) Promoter-dependent mechanism leading to selective hypomethylation within the 5′ region of gene MAGE-A1 in tumor cells. Mol Cell Biol 24(11):4781–4790
40. Song JZ, Stirzaker C, Harrison J, Melki JR, Clark SJ (2002) Hypermethylation trigger of the glutathione-S-transferase gene (GSTP1) in prostate cancer cells. Oncogene 21(7):1048–1061
41. Takeshima H, Ushijima T (2010) Methylation destiny: Moira takes account of histones and RNA polymerase II. Epigenetics 5(2):89–95
42. Takeshima H, Yamashita S, Shimazu T, Niwa T, Ushijima T (2009) The presence of RNA polymerase II, active or stalled, predicts epigenetic fate of promoter CpG islands. Genome Res 19(11):1974–1982
43. Chiappinelli KB, Strissel PL, Desrichard A, Li H, Henke C, Akman B et al (2015) Inhibiting DNA methylation causes an interferon response in cancer via dsRNA including endogenous retroviruses. Cell 162(5):974–986
44. Roulois D, Loo Yau H, Singhania R, Wang Y, Danesh A, Shen SY et al (2015) DNA-Demethylating agents target colorectal cancer cells by inducing viral mimicry by endogenous transcripts. Cell 162(5):961–973
45. Albrengues J, Bertero T, Grasset E, Bonan S, Maiel M, Bourget I et al (2015) Epigenetic switch drives the conversion of fibroblasts into proinvasive cancer-associated fibroblasts. Nat Commun 6:10204
46. Vizoso M, Puig M, Carmona FJ, Maqueda M, Velasquez A, Gomez A et al (2015) Aberrant DNA methylation in non-small cell lung cancer-associated fibroblasts. Carcinogenesis 36(12):1453–1463
47. Xu WS, Parmigiani RB, Marks PA (2007) Histone deacetylase inhibitors: molecular mechanisms of action. Oncogene 26(37):5541–5552

48. Dang L, White DW, Gross S, Bennett BD, Bittinger MA, Driggers EM et al (2009) Cancer-associated IDH1 mutations produce 2-hydroxyglutarate. Nature 462(7274):739–744
49. Figueroa ME, Abdel-Wahab O, Lu C, Ward PS, Patel J, Shih A et al (2010) Leukemic IDH1 and IDH2 mutations result in a hypermethylation phenotype, disrupt TET2 function, and impair hematopoietic differentiation. Cancer Cell 18(6):553–567
50. Lu C, Ward PS, Kapoor GS, Rohle D, Turcan S, Abdel-Wahab O et al (2012) IDH mutation impairs histone demethylation and results in a block to cell differentiation. Nature 483(7390):474–478
51. Grassian AR, Parker SJ, Davidson SM, Divakaruni AS, Green CR, Zhang X et al (2014) IDH1 mutations alter citric acid cycle metabolism and increase dependence on oxidative mitochondrial metabolism. Cancer Res 74(12):3317–3331
52. Wiegand KC, Shah SP, Al-Agha OM, Zhao Y, Tse K, Zeng T et al (2010) ARID1A mutations in endometriosis-associated ovarian carcinomas. N Engl J Med 363(16):1532–1543
53. Fujimoto A, Totoki Y, Abe T, Boroevich KA, Hosoda F, Nguyen HH et al (2012) Whole-genome sequencing of liver cancers identifies etiological influences on mutation patterns and recurrent mutations in chromatin regulators. Nat Genet 44(7):760–764
54. Huang J, Deng Q, Wang Q, Li KY, Dai JH, Li N et al (2012) Exome sequencing of hepatitis B virus-associated hepatocellular carcinoma. Nat Genet 44(10):1117–1121
55. Takeshima H, Niwa T, Takahashi T, Wakabayashi M, Yamashita S, Ando T et al (2015) Frequent involvement of chromatin remodeler alterations in gastric field cancerization. Cancer Lett 357(1):328–338
56. Wang K, Kan J, Yuen ST, Shi ST, Chu KM, Law S et al (2011) Exome sequencing identifies frequent mutation of ARID1A in molecular subtypes of gastric cancer. Nat Genet 43(12):1219–1223
57. Zang ZJ, Cutcutache I, Poon SL, Zhang SL, McPherson JR, Tao J et al (2012) Exome sequencing of gastric adenocarcinoma identifies recurrent somatic mutations in cell adhesion and chromatin remodeling genes. Nat Genet 44(5):570–574
58. Wilson BG, Wang X, Shen X, McKenna ES, Lemieux ME, Cho YJ et al (2010) Epigenetic antagonism between polycomb and SWI/SNF complexes during oncogenic transformation. Cancer Cell 18(4):316–328
59. Knutson SK, Warholic NM, Wigle TJ, Klaus CR, Allain CJ, Raimondi A et al (2013) Durable tumor regression in genetically altered malignant rhabdoid tumors by inhibition of methyltransferase EZH2. Proc Natl Acad Sci U S A 110(19):7922–7927
60. Kim KH, Kim W, Howard TP, Vazquez F, Tsherniak A, Wu JN et al (2015) SWI/SNF-mutant cancers depend on catalytic and non-catalytic activity of EZH2. Nat Med 21(12):1491–1496
61. Helming KC, Wang X, Wilson BG, Vazquez F, Haswell JR, Manchester HE et al (2014) ARID1B is a specific vulnerability in ARID1A-mutant cancers. Nat Med 20(3):251–254
62. Hoffman GR, Rahal R, Buxton F, Xiang K, McAllister G, Frias E et al (2014) Functional epigenetics approach identifies BRM/SMARCA2 as a critical synthetic lethal target in BRG1-deficient cancers. Proc Natl Acad Sci U S A 111(8):3128–3133
63. Oike T, Ogiwara H, Tominaga Y, Ito K, Ando O, Tsuta K et al (2013) A synthetic lethality-based strategy to treat cancers harboring a genetic deficiency in the chromatin remodeling factor BRG1. Cancer Res 73(17):5508–5518
64. Nakajima T, Enomoto S, Yamashita S, Ando T, Nakanishi Y, Nakazawa K et al (2010) Persistence of a component of DNA methylation in gastric mucosae after Helicobacter pylori eradication. J Gastroenterol 45(1):37–44
65. Niwa T, Toyoda T, Tsukamoto T, Mori A, Tatematsu M, Ushijima T (2013) Prevention of Helicobacter pylori-induced gastric cancers in gerbils by a DNA demethylating agent. Cancer Prev Res (Phila) 6(4):263–270
66. Baba S, Yamada Y, Hatano Y, Miyazaki Y, Mori H, Shibata T et al (2009) Global DNA hypomethylation suppresses squamous carcinogenesis in the tongue and esophagus. Cancer Sci 100(7):1186–1191

67. Yoo CB, Chuang JC, Byun HM, Egger G, Yang AS, Dubeau L et al (2008) Long-term epigenetic therapy with oral zebularine has minimal side effects and prevents intestinal tumors in mice. Cancer Prev Res (Phila) 1(4):233–240
68. Laird PW, Jackson-Grusby L, Fazeli A, Dickinson SL, Jung WE, Li E et al (1995) Suppression of intestinal neoplasia by DNA hypomethylation. Cell 81(2):197–205
69. Trinh BN, Long TI, Nickel AE, Shibata D, Laird PW (2002) DNA methyltransferase deficiency modifies cancer susceptibility in mice lacking DNA mismatch repair. Mol Cell Biol 22(9):2906–2917
70. McCabe MT, Low JA, Daignault S, Imperiale MJ, Wojno KJ, Day ML (2006) Inhibition of DNA methyltransferase activity prevents tumorigenesis in a mouse model of prostate cancer. Cancer Res 66(1):385–392